ANESTHESIA SECRETS

JAMES DUKE, M.D.
Assistant Professor of Anesthesiology
University of Colorado Health Sciences Center
Associate Director of Anesthesiology
Denver General Hospital
Denver, Colorado

STUART G. ROSENBERG, M.D.
Assistant Professor of Anesthesiology
University of Colorado Health Sciences Center
Director of Anesthesiology
Denver General Hospital
Denver, Colorado

HANLEY & BELFUS, INC./ Philadelphia
MOSBY/ St. Louis • Baltimore • Boston • Carlsbad • Chicago • London
Madrid • Naples • New York • Philadelphia • Sydney • Tokyo • Toronto

Publisher: HANLEY & BELFUS
                    210 S. 13th Street
                    Philadelphia, PA 19107
                    (215) 546-7293
                    FAX (215) 790-9330

North American and worldwide sales and distribution:

                    MOSBY
                    11830 Westline Industrial Drive
                    St. Louis, MO 63146

In Canada: Times Mirror Professional Publishing, Ltd.
                    130 Flaska Drive
                    Markham, Ontario L6G 1B8
                    Canada

Library of Congress Cataloging-in-Publication Data

Duke James, 1957–
    Anesthesia secrets / James Duke, Stuart G. Rosenberg.
        p.   cm.
    Includes bibliographical references and index.
    ISBN 1-56053-153-3 (soft cover : alk. paper)
        1. Anesthesiology—Examinations, questions, etc.   I. Rosenberg,
    Stuart G., 1955–   .   II. Title.
        |DNLM: 1. Anesthesiology—examination questions. WO 218.2 D887a
    1995|
    RD82.3.D85   1995
    617.9'6'076—dc20
    DNLM/DLC   95-35457
    for Library of Congress   CIP

ANESTHESIA SECRETS   ISBN 1-56053-153-3

Last digit is the print number: 9   8   7   6   5   4   3   2   1

DEDICATION

To those who have inspired and challenged us,
and to all who made this book possible, including Renée, Rachelle, and Lana.

CONTENTS

CONTRIBUTORS

Richard D. Abbott, MD
Resident, Department of Anesthesiology, University of Colorado Health Sciences Center, Denver, Colorado

Olivia Vynn Adair, M.D.
Assistant Professor, Department of Medicine, University of Colorado Health Sciences Center, Denver, Colorado

David Thomas Adamson, M.D.
Chief Resident, Department of Anesthesiology, University of Colorado Health Sciences Center, Denver, Colorado

Rita Agarwal, M.D.
Assistant Professor, Department of Anesthesiology, University of Colorado Health Sciences Center, Denver, Colorado

Richard B. Allen, M.D.
Assistant Professor, Department of Anesthesiology, University of Colorado Health Sciences Center, Denver, Colorado

José M. Angel, M.D.
Assistant Professor, Department of Anesthesiology, University of Colorado Health Sciences Center, Denver, Colorado

Tanya Sue Argo, M.D.
Resident, Department of Anesthesiology, University of Colorado Health Sciences Center, Denver, Colorado

G. Samuel Baker, M.D.
Assistant Professor, Department of Anesthesiology, University of Colorado Health Sciences Center, Denver, Colorado

Barbara L. Barton, R.N., B.S.N.
Professional Research Assistant/ACLS Affiliate Faculty, Department of Anesthesiology, University of Colorado Health Sciences Center, Denver, Colorado

Robert Franklin Bossard, M.D.
Assistant Professor, Department of Anesthesiology and Pain Management, University of Texas Southwestern Medical Center, Dallas, Texas

Michael A. Duey, M.D.
Resident, Department of Anesthesiology, University of Colorado Health Sciences Center, Denver, Colorado

James Duke, M.D.
Assistant Professor, Department of Anesthesiology, University of Colorado Health Sciences Center; Associate Director, Department of Anesthesiology, Denver General Hospital, Denver, Colorado

Stephan O. Fiedler, M.D.
Resident, Department of Anesthesiology, University of Colorado Health Sciences Center, Denver, Colorado

Kevin Fitzpatrick, M.D.
Assistant Professor, Department of Anesthesiology, University of Colorado Health Sciences Center, Denver, Colorado

Matthew D. Flaherty, M.D.
Senior Instructor, Department of Anesthesiology, University of Colorado Health Sciences Center, Denver, Colorado

Timothy Griffith Fry, D.O., B.S.
Resident, Department of Anesthesiology, University of Colorado Health Sciences Center, Denver, Colorado

Frederick M. Galloway, M.D.
Associate Professor, Department of Anesthesiology, University of Colorado Health Sciences Center, Denver, Colorado

Rose Ann Gates, R.N., M.S.N., O.C.N.
Senior Instructor and Clinical Nurse Specialist, Department of Anesthesiology, University of Colorado Health Sciences Center, Denver, Colorado

David M. Glenn, M.D.
Resident, Department of Anesthesiology, University of Colorado Health Sciences Center, Denver, Colorado

Julian M. Goldman, M.D.
Assistant Professor, Department of Anesthesiology, University of Colorado Health Sciences Center, Denver, Colorado

Patricia A. Gottlob, M.D.
Staff Anesthesiologist, Colorado Permanente Medical Group, Denver, Colorado

Cindy Griffiths, M.D.
Resident, Department of Anesthesiology, University of Colorado Health Sciences Center, Denver, Colorado

Cynthia K. Hampson, M.D.
Captain, United States Air Force, Department of Anesthesiology, Fairchild Air Force Base, Spokane, Washington

James E. Hannaford, M.A., R.R.T.
Instructor, Department of Anesthesiology, University of Colorado Health Sciences Center, Denver; Technical Services Supervisor, Department of Anesthesiology, Denver General Hospital, Denver, Colorado

John Alden Hatheway, M.D.
Resident, Department of Anesthesiology, University of Colorado Health Sciences Center, Denver, Colorado

Joy L. Hawkins, M.D.
Associate Professor, and Director of Obstetric Anesthesia, Department of Anesthesiology, University of Colorado Health Sciences Center, Denver, Colorado

David Hudson, C.R.N.A,. M.S.
Staff Nurse Anesthetist, Department of Anesthesiology, St. Vincents General Hospital, Leadville, Colorado

Alma N. Juels, M.D.
Fellow, Cardiothoracic Anesthesia, University of California, Los Angeles, Los Angeles, California

Jeremy J. Katz, M.D.
Assistant Professor, Department of Anesthesiology, University of Colorado Health Sciences Center, Denver, Colorado

Theresa L. Kinnard, M.D.
Assistant Professor, Department of Anesthesiology, University of Colorado Health Sciences Center, Denver, Colorado

William V. Kinnard, M.D.
Instructor, Department of Pulmonary Sciences and Critical Care Medicine, University of Colorado Health Sciences Center, Denver, Colorado

Lyle Edward Kirson, D.D.S.
Associate Professor, Department of Anesthesiology, University of Colorado Health Sciences Center; Veterans Affairs Medical Center, Denver, Colorado

Paige Latham, M.D.
Assistant Professor, Department of Anesthesiology and Pain Management, University of Texas Southwestern Medical Center at Dallas, Dallas, Texas

Lisa A. Leonard, C.R.N.A., M.H.S.
Staff Nurse Anesthetist, Department of Anesthesiology, Denver General Hospital, Denver, Colorado

Michael Leonard, M.D.
Chief, Department of Anesthesia, Colorado Permanente Medical Group, Denver, Colorado

Ana M. Lobo, M.D., M.P.H.
Fellow, Department of Anesthesiology, University of Colorado Health Sciences Center, Denver, Colorado

John D. Lockrem, M.D.
Associate Professor, Department of Anesthesiology, University of Colorado Health Sciences Center, Denver, Colorado

Steven J. Luke, M.D.
Assistant Professor, Department of Anesthesiology and Pain Management, University of Texas Southwestern Medical Center, Dallas, Texas

Laurel L. Mahonee, M.D.
Trauma Anesthesiology Fellow, Department of Anesthesiology, Denver General Hospital, Denver, Colorado

M. Susan Mandell, M.D., Ph.D.
Assistant Professor, and Director of Anesthesia for Liver Transplantation, Department of Anesthesiology, University of Colorado Health Sciences Center, Denver, Colorado

Lora L. Manning, B.S.N., M.S.N.A., C.R.N.A.
Staff Nurse Anesthetist, Department of Anesthesiology, Denver General Hospital, Denver, Colorado

Roger A. Mattison, M.D.
Assistant Professor, Department of Anesthesiology, University of Colorado Health Sciences Center, Denver, Colorado

Stephanie Elizabeth May, M.S.A., C.R.N.A.
Staff Anesthetist, Department of Anesthesiology, Denver General Hospital, Denver, Colorado

Gladstone C. McDowell, II, M.D.
Resident, Department of Anesthesiology, University of Colorado Health Sciences Center, Denver, Colorado

Howard J. Miller, M.D.
Instructor, Department of Anesthesiology, Denver General Hospital and University of Colorado Health Sciences Center, Denver, Colorado

Christopher Alan Mills, M.D.
Assistant Professor, Department of Anesthesiology, University of Colorado Health Sciences Center, Denver, Colorado

Jefferson P. Mostellar, M.D.
Private practice, Englewood, Colorado

Jeff S. Nabonsal, M.D.
Instructor, Department of Anesthesiology, University of Colorado Health Sciences Center, Denver, Colorado

Kenneth Niejadlik, M.D.
Assistant Professor, Department of Anesthesiology, University of Colorado Health Sciences Center, Denver, Colorado

J. Todd Nilson, M.D.
Department of Anesthesiology, University of Colorado Health Sciences Center, Denver, Colorado

Michael B. Ochs, D.O.
Assistant Professor, Department of Anesthesiology, University of Colorado Health Sciences Center, Denver, Colorado

James A. Ottevaere, II, M.D.
Resident, Department of Anesthesiology, University of Colorado Health Sciences Center, Denver, Colorado

Michael T. Owens, R.R.T.
Respiratory Therapist, Department of Anesthesiology, University of Colorado Health Sciences Center, Denver, Colorado

Malcolm Packer, M.D.
Assistant Professor, Department of Anesthesiology, Denver General Hospital, Denver, Colorado

Susan K. Palmer, M.D.
Professor, Department of Anesthesiology, Faculty of Program in Ethics and Medical Humanities, University of Colorado Health Sciences Center, Denver, Colorado

Robert W. Phelps, Ph.D., M.D.
Associate Professor, Department of Anesthesiology, University of Colorado Health Sciences Center, Denver, Colorado

Philip Alan Role, M.D.
Senior Resident, Department of Anesthesiology, University of Colorado Health Sciences Center, Denver, Colorado

Stuart G. Rosenberg, M.D.
Director, Department of Anesthesiology, Denver General Hospital; Assistant Professor of Anesthesiology, University of Colorado Health Sciences Center, Denver, Colorado

James W. Rosher, M.D.
Resident, Department of Anesthesiology, University of Colorado Health Sciences Center, Denver, Colorado

Judith M. Russell, L.P.N., C.A.T.S.
Clinical Manager, Anesthesia Support Services, Department of Anesthesiology, University of Colorado Health Sciences Center, Denver, Colorado

Peter Sakas, M.D.
Department of Anesthesiology, University of Colorado Health Sciences Center, Denver, Colorado

Beth E. Schatzman, M.H.S., C.R.N.A.
Staff Anesthetist, Department of Anesthesia, Denver General Hospital, Denver, Colorado

William D. Sefton, M.D.
Chief Resident, Department of Anesthesiology, University of Colorado Health Sciences Center, Denver, Colorado

Andrew A. Shultz, M.D.
Resident, Department of Anesthesiology, University of Colorado Health Sciences Center, Denver, Colorado

Robert H. Slover, M.D.
Assistant Professor, Department of Pediatrics, University of Colorado Health Sciences Center, Denver, Colorado

Robin Baker Slover, M.D.
Assistant Professor, Department of Anesthesiology, Director, Acute Pain Service, University of Colorado Health Sciences Center, Denver, Colorado

Steven J. Stein, M.D.
Resident, Department of Anesthesiology, University of Colorado Health Sciences Center, Denver, Colorado

David E. Strick, M.D.
Resident, Department of Anesthesiology, University of Colorado Health Sciences Center, Denver, Colorado

Kenneth M. Swank, M.D.
Resident, Department of Anesthesiology, University of Colorado Health Sciences Center, Denver, Colorado

Charles A. Tinnell, R.N., M.S.P.H.
Research Assistant, Department of Anesthesiology, University of Colorado Health Sciences Center; President, Clinical Data Management, Inc., Denver, Colorado

William Clark Turner, M.D.
Resident, Department of Surgery, Washington University School of Medicine, St. Louis, Missouri

Andrew M. Veit, M.D.
Resident, Department of Anesthesiology, University of Colorado Health Sciences Center, Denver, Colorado

Douglas Paul Voorhees, R.R.T.
Ultra Imaging, Inc., Littleton, Colorado

Elizabeth F. Ward, C.R.N.A.
Staff Nurse Anesthetist, Department of Anesthesiology, Denver General Hospital, Denver, Colorado

Douglas E. Warnecke, C.R.N.A., M.S.
Chief Nurse Anesthetist, Department of Anesthesiology, Denver General Hospital, Denver, Colorado

Kelli Lambert Weiner, M.D.
Resident, Department of Anesthesiology, University of Colorado Health Sciences Center, Denver, Colorado

Lee Weiss, M.D.
Resident, Department of Anesthesiology, University of Colorado Health Sciences Center, Denver, Colorado

Charles W. Whitten, M.D.
Associate Professor, Department of Anesthesiology and Pain Management, University of Texas Southwestern Medical Center, Dallas; Director, Department of Anesthesiology and Pain Management, Parkland Memorial Hospital (Surgical Services), Dallas, Texas

Mark Wilson, C.R.T.T.
Respiratory Therapist, Instructor of Cardiopulmonary Physiology, Department of Anesthesiology, Denver General Hospital, Denver, Colorado

Gene Winkelmann, MD
Resident, Department of Anesthesiology, University of Colorado Health Sciences Center, Denver, Colorado

John H. Yang, M.D.
Resident, Department of Anesthesiology, University of Colorado Health Sciences Center, Denver, Colorado

Teresa Jo Youtz, M.D.
Resident, Department of Anesthesiology, University of Colorado Health Sciences Center, Denver, Colorado

PREFACE

An anesthesiologist is a physician first. Ensuring an insensate state within the confines of the operative theater is much too narrow an interpretation of the specialty. The practice of anesthesiology is the practice of perioperative medicine, encompassing pre-, intra-, and postoperative care. The perioperative physician understands the application of physiologic and pharmacologic principles in the care of the patient undergoing the stress of a surgical procedure. He or she must appreciate the pathophysiology involved and the human as an adaptive organism. Though the specialty is rich in technical skills mastered through continued practice, the real skill is centered about sound judgment and a substantial knowledge base. It is these attributes to which we hope this book contributes in a somewhat unique way.

This text, like all books in *The Secrets Series*®, is designed in a question and answer format. *Anesthesia Secrets* is sufficiently broad that it should be of value to the medical student recently introduced to the specialty, to house officers at all levels of training, and to all practitioners preparing for board examinations. The application of this knowledge easily extends to clinical situations outside the operating room, encompassing preoperative and postoperative evaluation, and to problems encountered in emergency and critical care settings. We challenge the reader to examine the question and formulate a response before reviewing the answer in order to participate fully in the learning experience. We trust this method will prove both fun and stimulating. We hope you find this to be true and this text to be valuable.

James Duke, M.D.
Stuart G. Rosenberg, M.D.

I. Basics of Patient Management

1. THE AUTONOMIC NERVOUS SYSTEM

William Turner, M.D., and James Duke, M.D.

1. Describe the autonomic nervous system.
The autonomic nervous system (ANS) is a network of nerves and ganglia that control involuntary physiologic parameters and maintain internal homeostasis and stress responses. The ANS innervates structures within the cardiovascular, pulmonary, endocrine, exocrine, gastrointestinal, genitourinary, and central nervous systems (CNS) and influences metabolism and thermal regulation. The ANS is divided into two parts: the sympathetic (SNS) and parasympathetic (PNS) nervous system. Activation of the sympathetic nervous system has been classically associated with the "flight or fight" response. The SNS and PNS generally have opposing effects on end-organs, with either the SNS or the PNS exhibiting a dominant resting tone.

2. Describe the functional anatomy and physiology of the sympathetic nervous system.
Preganglionic sympathetic neurons originate from the intermediolateral columns of the thoracic and lumbar region of the spinal cord (T1–L2, L3) and synapse at one of three different types of ganglia: the paired paravertebral sympathetic chain, the unpaired prevertebral ganglia, or a terminal ganglion. Preganglionic neurons may ascend or descend the sympathetic chain before synapsing. Preganglionic neurons stimulate nicotinic receptors on postganglionic sympathetic neurons by releasing acetylcholine. Postganglionic neurons synapse at targeted end-organs by releasing norepinephrine.

3. What peripheral receptors are involved in the SNS? What is the end-organ response to receptor activation?
Adrenergic receptors include the following: alpha-1 (A1), alpha-2 (A2), beta-1 (B1), and beta-2 (B2). Generally, A1, B1, and B2 receptors are postsynaptic, whereas A2 receptors are presynaptic. Alpha-1 receptor activation produces contraction of the vas deferens, trigone, ureter, splenic capsule, and prostatic capsule as well as arteriolar constriction, mydriasis, piloerection, salivation, and lacrimation. Alpha-2 receptor activation produces a negative feedback inhibition for subsequent norepinephrine release. Beta-1 receptor activation produces positive inotropic and chronotropic effects on the heart while increasing renin secretion and lipolysis. Beta-2 receptor activation produces bronchodilation, liver glycogenolysis, and skeletal muscle vascular dilation.

Quantitatively, adrenergic receptor density is inversely proportional to the amount of neurotransmitter available at the synaptic junction. This dynamic phenomenon is known as upregulation or downregulation. Clinically, it is important in desensitization to sympathomimetics (downregulation) and in abrupt withdrawal of adrenergic antagonists, such as beta blockers, producing a rebound hypersympathetic response (upregulation).

Dopamine exerts adrenergic effects but also activates a physiologically distinct class of receptors known as dopaminergic receptors. The two clinically important dopaminergic receptors are DA1 and DA2. Activation of DA1 receptors produces dilation of blood vessels in renal, coronary, and splanchnic vascular beds, whereas activation of CNS DA2 receptors produces nausea, vomiting, and psychic disturbances. Exogenous dopamine cannot cross the blood-brain barrier.

4. What are the receptor affinities for common sympathomimetics? Describe direct- and indirect-acting agents.

Direct-acting drugs are agonists at the targeted receptor, whereas indirect-acting drugs enter the presynaptic nerve terminal and release endogenous neurotransmitters into the synaptic junction. Sympathomimetics may be classified as direct-acting, indirect-acting, or mixed direct- and indirect-acting. Ephedrine and dopamine are examples of mixed direct- and indirect-acting sympathomimetics, whereas phenylephrine is an example of a direct-acting agent. Mixed and indirect-acting agents lose efficacy with repeated administration or in catecholamine-depleted states.

Receptor Activity of Adrenergic Agents and Mechanism of Action

AGENT	RECEPTOR	DIRECT/INDIRECT/MIXED
Norepinephrine	A1, A2, B1	Direct
Epinephrine	A1, A2, B1, B2	Direct
Isoproterenol	B1, B2	Direct
Dopamine	A1, B1, DA	Mixed
Clonidine	A2	Direct
Phenylephrine	A1	Direct
Ephedrine	A1, A2, B1, B2	Mixed

5. What is dose-specific receptor affinity?

Dose-specific receptor affinity describes differing adrenergic receptor affinity, which depends on the plasma concentration of the agent. Two examples are dopamine and epinephrine. Dopamine has predominantly dopaminergic effects below an infusion rate of 3 µg/kg/min, beta-adrenergic effects between 3–10 µg/kg/min, and alpha-adrenergic effects at greater than 10 µg/kg/min. Therefore, dopamine may be infused at different rates to obtain a specific pharmacologic effect. Epinephrine has predominantly B2 effects below 2 µg/min, B1 and B2 effects between 2–10 µg/min, and A1 effects at greater than 10 µg/min.

6. What is the mechanism of synthesis of norepinephrine and epinephrine?

Synthesis of norepinephrine begins with active transport of tyrosine into the adrenergic presynaptic nerve terminal cytoplasm. In the cytoplasm tyrosine is converted to dopamine by two enzymatic reactions, hydroxylation of tyrosine by tyrosine hydroxylase to dopa, and decarboxylation of dopa by aromatic l-amino acid decarboxylase to dopamine. Dopamine is then transported into storage vesicles, where it is ß-hydroxylated by dopamine ß-hydroxylase to norepinephrine. Epinephrine is synthesized in the adrenal medulla through the same sequence of enzymatic reactions as norepinephrine, except that a majority of the norephineprhine produced is converted to epinephrine via n-methylation by phenylethanolamine n-methyltransferase. Compounds from dopa to epinephrine in the synthesis process are classified as catecholamines.

7. Describe the metabolism of norepinephrine and epinephrine.

Norepinephrine is removed from the synaptic junction by two mechanisms: reuptake into the presynaptic nerve terminal and inactivation at non-neuronal tissues. Removal of norepinephrine by reuptake into the presynaptic nerve terminal produces neurotransmitters for reuse and is the most important mechanism of inactivation. Enzymatic metabolism of norepinephrine and epinephrine is by monoamine oxidase (MAO) and catecholamine O-methyl transferase (COMT); the important metabolites are 3-methoxy-4-hydroxy-mandelic acid (VMA), metanephrine, and normetanephrine.

8. Describe the pharmacology of common beta-adrenergic antagonists.

Beta-adrenergic antagonists, commonly called beta blockers, are reversible antagonists at ß1 and ß2 receptors. Beta blockers are used mainly in antihypertensive, antianginal, and antiarrhythmic therapy. Beta blockers may be cardioselective, with relatively selective B1 antagonist properties, or noncardioselective. Beta-1 blockade produces negative inotropic and chronotropic effects, decreases renin secretion, and inhibits lipolysis. Beta-2 blockade produces bronchoconstriction, peripheral vasoconstriction, and inhibition of glycogenolysis. In addition, some beta blockers have partial beta-agonist activity, and some have membrane-stabilizing, or antiarrhythmic effects.

Properties of Selective Beta Blockers

BETA BLOCKER	CARDIOSELECTIVE	PARTIAL AGONIST	MEMBRANE-STABILIZING
Propranolol	0	0	+
Timolol	0	0	0
Pindolol	0	+	+
Metoprolol	+	0	0
Atenolol	+	0	0
Acebutolol	+	+	+
Esmolol	+	0	0
Labetalol	0*	0	0

* Also an alpha-1 antagonist.
 0 = not a characteristic; + = has this characteristic.

9. Describe the pharmacology of common alpha-adrenergic antagonists.

Like beta blockers, alpha blockers may be selective or nonselective antagonists. Prazosin is the prototypical selective alpha-1 blocker, whereas phentolamine and phenoxybenzamine are examples of nonselective alpha blockers. Alpha blockers produce vasodilation and are used in the management of hypertension. When used as an antihypertensive, nonselective alpha blockers may be associated with reflex tachycardia. As a consequence, selective alpha-1 blockers are primarily used as antihypertensives. Labetalol is a nonselective beta blocker and a selective alpha-1 blocker used for treatment of angina, hypertension, glaucoma, and pheochromocytoma.

10. Describe the functional anatomy and physiology of the parasympathetic nervous system.

Preganglionic parasympathetic neurons originate from cranial nerves 3, 7, 9, and 10 and sacral segments 2–4. Preganglionic parasympathetic neurons tend to synapse with postganglionic neurons close to the targeted end-organ, creating a more discrete physiologic effect. Both pre- and postganglionic parasympathetic neurons release acetylcholine as the neurotransmitter. The receptors are subclassified as nicotinic (ganglionic and neuromuscular cholinergic receptors) or muscarinic (postganglionic cholinergic receptors). The vagus nerve is the dominant nerve of the PNS. Vagal discharge affects the heart, respiratory tree, spleen, liver, kidney, bladder, and proximal intestinal tract. The PNS tends to maintain baseline function of visceral organs. Important effects of the PNS include bronchoconstriction, activation of the gastrointestinal system, miosis, increase in secretions, and bradycardia.

11. Describe the synthesis and degradation of acetylcholine.

Acetylcholine is synthesized within the presynaptic nerve terminal mitochondria by esterification of acetylCoA and choline by the enzyme choline acetyltransferase; it is stored in synaptic vesicles until release. After release acetylcholine is principally metabolized by acetylcholinesterase, a membrane-bound enzyme located in the synaptic junction. Acetylcholinesterase is also located in other nonneuronal tissues, such as erythrocytes. Butyrylcholinesterase, also known as plasma cholinesterase, is produced in the liver and also metabolizes acetylcholine, but to a minor extent.

12. Describe the pharmacology of common muscarinic antagonists.

Muscarinic antagonists block all muscarinic receptors equally, with the exception of charged quaternary forms that do not cross the blood-brain barrier. Muscarinic antagonists produce bronchodilation, inhibition of secretions, and mydriasis, along with antispasmodic and positive chronotropic effects. Centrally acting muscarinic antagonists may produce delirium. There are four commonly used muscarinic antagonists: atropine, scopolamine, glycopyrrolate, and ipratropium bromide. Glycopyrrolate is a quaternary ammonium compound that cannot cross the blood-brain barrier and therefore lacks CNS activity. Ipratropium bromide is a poorly absorbed inhaled agent that is useful in the management of asthma by antagonizing the bronchoconstrictive effects of acetylcholine.

13. What features of the history and physical exam suggest autonomic dysfunction?
The signs and symptoms of autonomic dysfunction include orthostatic blood pressure changes as well as vasomotor, bladder, bowel, and sexual dysfunction. Patients should be asked about orthostatic symptoms, blurred vision, reduced or excessive sweating, dry or excessively moist eyes and mouth, cold or discolored extremities, incontinence or incomplete voiding, diarrhea or constipation, and impotence. A history of use of medications, illicit drugs or alcohol is also important. Evaluation of orthostatic blood pressure and heart rate changes is of key importance during the physical exam.

14. List some causes of autonomic dysfunction.

Diabetes mellitus	Rheumatoid arthritis
Hyperthyroidism	Systemic lupus erythematosus
Horner's syndrome	Paraneoplastic autonomic dysfunction
Pheochromocytoma	Shy-Drager syndrome
Human immunodeficiency virus	Fabry's disease
Amlyoidosis	Heavy metal autonomic neuropathy
Uremia	Cis-platinum and vincristine chemotherapy
Alcohol use and withdrawal	Tetanus
Guillain-Barré syndrome	Botulism
Eaton-Lambert syndrome	

15. List some commonly used drugs that have autonomic effects.
Commonly used medications with anticholinergic effects include antipsychotics, antihistamines, tricyclic antidepressants, cyclobenzaprine (Flexeril), and amantadine. Sympathomimetic medications should be avoided when a patient has recently consumed monoamine oxidase inhibitors (a class of antidepressants) or illicit stimulants, such as amphetamines and cocaine. A combination of these drugs may produce a toxic, hypersympathetic response.

16. How can renal and splanchnic blood flow be preserved when sympathomimetics are used?
Dopamine is the agent of choice to increase renal blood flow when a sympathomimetic is needed because it dilates renal and splanchnic vasculature. However, at an infusion rate greater than 10 µg/kg/min, dopamine constricts renal and splanchnic vasculature by exhibiting alpha-agonist properties.

17. How is pheochromocytoma diagnosed and treated?
Pheochromocytoma is a catecholamine-secreting tumor of chromaffin tissue. Most tumors are located in the adrenal medulla. Signs and symptoms include paroxysms of hypertension, headache, palpitations, flushing, and sweating. Pheochromocytoma is confirmed by detecting elevated levels of plasma and urinary catecholamines and urinary VMA, normetanephrines, and metanephrines. The treatment for pheochromocytoma is surgical excision. Preoperatively, the patient should be given an alpha antagonist (to control hypertension) and hydrated. If the patient becomes tachycardic, a beta blocker is instituted. Intraoperatively, invasive monitoring is needed to detect fluctuations in blood pressure and to guide therapy. Intraoperative hypertension is controlled by intravenous infusion of an alpha antagonist or nitroprusside. Once the tumor is removed, the patient should be monitored for hypoglycemia and hypotension.

18. What is the function of anesthesia in relation to the autonomic nervous system?
The purpose of anesthesia in relation to the autonomic nervous system is to maintain homeostasis, to modulate stress responses, and to control disease states with autonomic dysfunction,without producing significant side effects, throughout the perioperative period.

BIBLIOGRAPHY

1. Drug Evaluations Annual, 1994. Chicago, American Medical Association, 1994, pp 210–211, 539–549, 680–683.
2. Andreoli T, Claude-Bennet J, Carpenter C, et al (eds): Cecil's Essentials of Medicine, 3rd ed. Philadelphia, W.B. Saunders, 1993, pp 67–69, 491–492.
3. Low P: Clinical Autonomic Disorders: Evaluation and Management. Boston, Little, Brown, 1993, pp 157–197.
4. Moss J, Craigo P: The autonomic nervous system. In Miller R (ed): Anesthesia, 4th ed. New York, Churchill Livingstone, 1994, pp 523–577.
5. Smith C, Reynard A: Textbook of Pharmacology. Philadelphia, W.B. Saunders, 1992, pp 141–169.
6. Stoelting R, Miller R: Basics of Anesthesia, 2nd ed. New York, Churchill Livingstone, 1989, pp 25–41.

2. OXYGENATION AND VENTILATION

David T. Adamson, M.D., and Christopher A. Mills, M.D.

1. What are the major causes of hypoxemia?

Low inspired oxygen (O_2) concentration: Common causes of decreased oxygen concentration (FiO_2) are low O_2 mixtures, depleted O_2 supply, or breathing circuit disconnection. In the normal situation, arterial oxygenation is a function of alveolar oxygen concentration. A hypoxic gas mixture delivered to the alveoli (low PAO_2) will result in a low arterial oxygen tension (PaO_2). This relationship is described by the alveolar gas equation where Pb is the barometric pressure, $P_{vapor\ H_2O}$ is the vapor pressure of water and $PaCO_2$ is the alveolar pressure of carbon dioxide (CO_2):

$$PAO_2 = FiO_2\ (Pb - P_{vapor\ H_2O}) - (PaCO_2/0.8)$$

This equation reveals a direct relationship between FiO_2 and PAO_2. The denominator of the equation is called the respiratory quotient (RQ). The RQ is a ratio of CO_2 production to O_2 consumption, and in a healthy patient the RQ averages about 0.8. The RQ is considered to be constant but can change with the patient's metabolic state and dietary consumption.

Hypoventilation: Most patients under the effects of general anesthesia are incapable of maintaining an adequate minute ventilation to deliver sufficient O_2 to the alveoli. This may be due to muscular paralysis or the ventilatory depressant effects of virtually any of the anesthetic agents used. This effect is usually overcome by using O_2–enriched inspiratory gases and by mechanically ventilating the lungs.

Shunt: In the normal healthy patient, arteriovenous shunting accounts for about 2% of the cardiac output (CO) mainly due to blood flow through the thebesian veins of the heart and the pulmonary bronchial veins. With adequate CO, this physiologic shunt is well tolerated. Disease states such as sepsis, liver failure, arteriovenous malformations, pulmonary emboli, and right–to–left cardiac shunts can create significant shunting that will result in hypoxemia. As shunted blood is not exposed to alveoli, hypoxemia caused by shunt cannot be overcome by increasing FiO_2.

Ventilation Perfusion (V/Q) Inequality or Mismatch: Ventilation and perfusion of the alveoli in the lung ideally have a 1 to 1 relationship that allows for efficient oxygen exchange between alveoli and blood. When alveolar ventilation and perfusion to the lungs are abnormal (V/Q mismatching), hypoxemia can result. Some causes of V/Q mismatching are atelectasis, patient positioning, bronchial intubation, purposeful one–lung ventilation, bronchospasm, pneumonia, mucus plugging, acute respiratory distress syndrome (ARDS), and airway obstruction. Hypoxemia due to V/Q mismatching can usually be overcome by increasing FiO_2.

Cardiac Output (CO)/Oxygen Carrying Capacity: Oxygenation of tissues depends on the carrying capacity of oxygen in the blood and delivery of blood to the tissues. This concept is described by the oxygen delivery (DO_2) equation:

$$DO_2 = (O_2\ capacity)(CO)$$

where O_2 capacity is equal to: $(1.39 \times Hb \times \%Sat) + (0.003 \times PaO_2)$. The 1.39 is the ml of O_2 that each gram of hemoglobin can carry, Hb is the hemoglobin concentration, and %Sat is the hemoglobin saturation. Multiplying the PaO_2 by .003 gives the amount of O_2 that can be carried in the blood as a dissolved gas (a very very small amount). From this equation it is apparent that as cardiac output or O_2 capacity falls, so will the DO_2, which ultimately results in hypoxemia.

Diffusion: Efficient O_2 exchange depends on a healthy interface between the alveoli and the blood stream. In severe pulmonary diseases, such as pulmonary fibrosis, pulmonary edema, and ARDS, oxygenation can be adversely affected, as O_2 cannot diffuse from the alveoli into the blood.

2. How is pCO_2 related to alveolar ventilation?

The amount of CO_2 in the blood, or pCO_2, is inversely related to the alveolar ventilation. This is described by the equation:

$$pCO_2 = (V_{CO_2}/V_{alveolar})$$

where V_{CO_2} is the CO_2 production of the body (for our purposes considered constant), and $V_{alveolar}$ is the alveolar ventilation (defined as minute volume less the dead space of ventilation). In general, minute ventilation and pCO_2 are inversely related.

3. What are the causes of hypercarbia?

Hypoventilation: As stated, decreasing the minute ventilation will ultimately decrease alveolar ventilation, increasing pCO_2. Some common causes of hypoventilation include muscle paralysis, inadequate mechanical ventilation, inhalational anesthetics, and narcotics.

Increased CO_2 production: Although CO_2 production is assumed to be constant, there are certain situations in which metabolism and CO_2 production are increased. Malignant hyperthermia, fever, thyrotoxicosis, and other hypercatabolic states are some examples.

Iatrogenic: The anesthesiologist can administer certain drugs to increase CO_2. The most common is sodium bicarbonate, which is metabolized by the enzyme carbonic anhydrase to form CO_2. Rarely, CO_2-enriched gases can be administered. Depletion of the CO_2 absorbent in the anesthesia breathing circuit can result in rebreathing of exhaled gases and may also result in hypercarbia.

4. What physiologic effects occur in a hypoxic and hypercarbic anesthetized patient?

The most common effects of mild hypoxia and/or hypercarbia are hypertension and tachycardia due to reflex sympathetic stimulation. Effects of profound hypoxia and hypercarbia include myocardial irritability and depression, cyanosis, bradycardia, and circulatory collapse.

5. Describe the oxyhemoglobin dissociation curve.

The relationship between oxyhemoglobin saturation and arterial pO_2 is demonstrated by the oxyhemoglobin dissociation curve illustrated below.

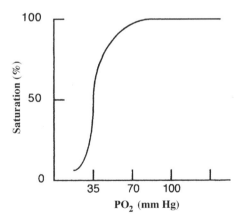

Oxyhemoglobin dissociation curve.

The saturation of normal hemoglobin at a PaO_2 of 100 is 100%, at a PaO_2 of 60 is approximately 90%, and at a PaO_2 of 40 is approximately 75% (that of normal mixed venous blood). Hemoglobin saturation is a nonlinear function of PaO_2. Within a relatively narrow range (PaO_2 ~ 35–85 mm Hg), percent saturation changes profoundly. Above a PaO_2 of 95, there is little change in the percent saturation despite increasing PaO_2.

6. How does pulse oximetry work?

Pulse oximetry is a noninvasive method by which arterial oxygenation can be approximated. Pulse oximetry is based on the Beer-Lambert law and spectrophotometric analysis. The Beer-Lambert equation is as follows:

$$I_{trans} = I_{in}\, e^{-DCa}$$

where I_{trans} is the intensity of transmitted light, I_{in} is the intensity of the incident light, D is the distance that the light is transmitted through the medium, C is the concentration of the solute (hemoglobin), and the extinction coefficient "a" is a constant for a given solute at a specified wavelength.

Using two wavelengths of light, red at 660 nanometers (nm) and infrared at 940 nm, the changes in absorption of light shone through a pulsatile vascular bed are measured. Given a constant hemoglobin concentration and light intensity, the oxygen saturation of hemoglobin becomes a logarithmic function of the absorption of light through the blood at the sight of the pulse oximeter probe (see figure below).

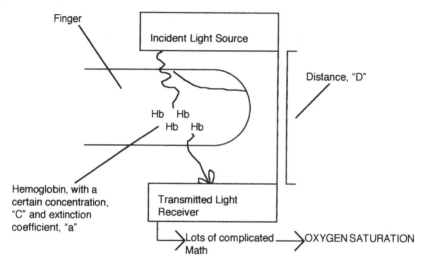

Schematic showing pulse oximetry in action. To understand the complicated math, please read Clinical Anesthesia, 2nd ed, 1992, pp 165–168.[1]

The above figure shows the use of a finger probe; however, pulse oximetry can be used on any digit or across any accessible vascular bed such as the ears, nose, and tongue. Pulse oximetry is fairly accurate between hemoglobin saturations of 80% and 100%. Accuracy is adversely affected by the presence of methemoglobin, carboxyhemoglobin, nail polish, bright background light, vasoconstriction, shivering, and motion.

7. What effects do the inhalational anesthetics have on ventilation?

In the unanesthetized patient, ventilation is usually regulated to maintain pCO_2 and pO_2 at normal values (about 40 and 80 torr, respectively). While the drive to maintain ventilation is regulated by both CO_2 and O_2, the most important regulator is CO_2. This is made possible by chemoreceptors in the medulla and receptors in the carotid bifurcations and on the aortic arch. Chemoreceptors in the medulla are primarily sensitive to changes in CO_2 and subsequent changes in cerebrospinal fluid pH, whereas the carotid and aortic bodies are sensitive to changes in pO_2. The potent inhalational anesthetics such as halothane, isoflurane, and enflurane all greatly attenuate the ventilatory response to hypercarbia and hypoxemia (see figure, next page).

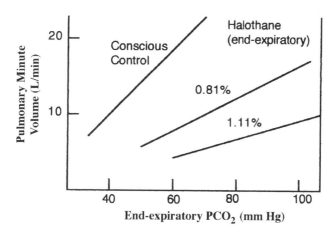

The CO_2 response curve shows the effects of inhalational anesthetics on the pulmonary minute volume with increasing pCO_2. As the inhalational agent is increased, the curve is shifted to the right, showing a decreased minute volume response to increasing hypercarbia. (Borrowed and modified with permission from Foltz B, Benumof J: Mechanisms of hypoxemia and hypercapnia in the perioperative period. Crit Care Clin 3:279, 1987.)

8. What might be done to improve oxygenation?
Increase FiO_2
Increase minute ventilation
Increase cardiac output (oxygen delivery to tissues)
Increase oxygen carrying capacity (hemoglobin)
Optimize V/Q relationships (i.e., PEEP/CPAP)
Cardiopulmonary bypass
Decrease oxygen consumption from pain, shivering, or fever

9. How does positive end–expiratory pressure (PEEP) work?
Positive end expiratory pressure (PEEP) increases oxygenation by maximizing the ventilation–perfusion relationship in the lung. By maintaining this positive pressure at the end of exhalation, alveoli that would tend to become collapsed are maintained in the open state, allowing for continued ventilation and O_2 exchange in lung units that would otherwise be perfused but not ventilated (V/Q mismatch). The lung volume at the end of exhalation is called the functional residual capacity (FRC). The FRC is the lung volume at the end of a normal expiration, and is about 2.5 liters.The volume at which alveoli begin to collapse is called the closing capacity (CC). When the CC is greater than the FRC, airway collapse occurs. PEEP maximizes the FRC, keeping lung volumes greater than closing capacity, therefore maintaining airways open and functional. Some causes of an increased CC are obesity, increased abdominal pressure, supine position, ARDS, aspiration, pregnancy, and pulmonary edema.

10. What is the purpose of pre-oxygenation before the induction of anesthesia?
Pre-oxygenation is an important part of any general anesthetic. In an unanesthetized person, inspired room air contains approximately 21% O_2, with the majority of the rest being nitrogen (N_2). Not many people can go more than a few minutes without ventilation before desaturation occurs. Should patients breath 100% oxygen for several minutes, they may not desaturate for up to 3–5 minutes, as the FRC of the lung is completely washed of N_2 and filled with O_2. The FRC is much less in patients who are obese, pregnant, or have increased abdominal pressure. Neonates also have a disproportionately small FRC and will desaturate very quickly, even with adequate pre-oxygenation.

11. What is diffusion hypoxia?

Diffusion hypoxia is a decrease in pO_2 usually observed as the patient is emerging from an inhalational anesthetic where nitrous oxide (N_2O) is a component. The rapid outpouring of insoluble N_2O can displace alveolar oxygen, resulting in hypoxia. All patients should receive supplemental O_2 at the end of an anesthetic and during the immediate recovery period.

12. You are on call (your first) and, much to your dismay, your beeper goes off. You answer the page and are informed that Mr. Smith in the ICU has acute pulmonary edema and needs to be intubated. Your senior resident and attending are both unavailable. What will you need to intubate Mr. Smith?

When intubating a patient, whether inside or outside of the operating room, there are certain bare essentials that must be present to ensure a safe intubation. They can be remembered by the mnemonic **SALT.**

   Suction. This is extremely important. Often patients will have material in the pharynx, making visualization of the vocal cords difficult. Also, suction needs to be present to avoid the aspiration of vomitus or other material. Aspiration is **bad.**

   Airway. The oral airway is a device that lifts the tongue off the posterior pharynx, often making it easier to mask ventilate a patient. The inability to ventilate a patient is **bad**. Also a source of O_2 with a delivery mechanism (ambu-bag and mask) must be available.

   Laryngoscope. This lighted tool is vital to placing an endotracheal tube. Not having a laryngoscope present at an intubation is **very bad.**

   Tube. Endotracheal tubes come in many sizes. In the average adult a size 7.0 or 8.0 oral endotracheal tube will work just fine. Not having an endotracheal tube available at an intubation is **extremely bad.**

13. You have successfully intubated Mr. Smith and now he requires a ventilator while his pulmonary edema is treated. The nurse turns to you and asks, "What settings would you like, Doctor?"

There are several easy rules to remember that will take the terror out of managing a patient who needs to be placed on a ventilator. They are **mode, tidal volume, rate,** and **FiO_2**. (First, you have listened for bilateral breath sounds.)

   Mode. Whenever a patient has just been placed on a ventilator, the easiest mode to remember (which will work just fine initially) is intermittent mandatory ventilation (IMV). In this mode a patient is given all the breaths you set and can also receive breaths that he or she initiates.

   Tidal volume. The average tidal volume for a normal patient is 10–12 ml/kg. For a 100-kg patient, a tidal volume between 1000 and 1200 ml would be adequate.

   Rate. A good place to start the rate is 10–12 breaths per minute. With an adequate tidal volume, this will usually deliver a reasonable minute ventilation and maintain an acceptable pCO_2.

   FiO_2. Always start with an FiO_2 of 1.0.

   All of these settings will have to be adjusted to maintain an acceptable pCO_2 and pO_2.

14. After returning to your call room, you receive yet another page from Mr. Smith's nurse. He informs you that he has received the blood gas analysis for Mr. Smith, which reveals: pH 7.50/pCO_2 30/pO_2 50/Sat 84%. His ventilator settings are: tidal volume, 1000 ml; respiratory rate, 12 breaths/min; FiO_2, 1.0 (100% O_2); PEEP, 0. What can you do to improve Mr. Smith's oxygenation?

It would appear from the blood gas that Mr. Smith has a respiratory alkalosis, appropriate for the low pCO_2, indicating that he is receiving an adequate minute ventilation. However, Mr. Smith is clearly hypoxic despite his inspired O_2 concentration of 100%. Pulmonary edema prohibits lung alveoli from functioning properly, which has resulted in V/Q mismatch, causing the low PaO_2. The addition of PEEP can help to improve alveolar function and improve oxygenation and is usually administered between pressures of 5 and 15 cm H_2O. The most common initial level is 5 cm H_2O.

15. What adverse effects could the addition of PEEP have on Mr. Smith?

1. Decreased cardiac output
2. Hypotension
3. Worsening hypoxia
4. Barotrauma (pneumothorax)
5. Increased intracranial pressure
6. Decreased urine output

PEEP can be a very useful tool to improve oxygenation; however, it is not without risks. Positive pressure is transmitted throughout the thorax when PEEP is applied. Any level of PEEP can decrease venous return to the heart and result in deceased CO, producing hypotension and hypoxemia. High levels of PEEP can result in trauma to lung tissue. Those most susceptible to barotrauma include patients with COPD, bullous lung disease, necrotizing infections, tuberculosis, and lung transplants. Positive pressure transmitted to the venous system limits egress of blood from the cranium, elevating intracranial pressure. Sudden decreases in urine output with the institution of PEEP have been reported and are thought to be due to release of atrial natriuretic factor.

16. During a general anesthetic for which you are using nitrous oxide (N_2O) at a flow of 2 L/min and O_2 at 2 L/min, the wall supply disconnect alarm sounds. Upon turning on your E cylinder tanks of N_2O and O_2, you note that the pressure gauge for the N_2O tank reads 750 pounds per square inch (psi) and the O_2 tank's gauge reads 1000 psi. How long will you be able to deliver these gas flows before the tanks are empty?

All contemporary anesthesia machines have two sources of gases: the wall outlet and E cylinders attached to the machine itself. The cylinders are color coded and usually left shut off, being saved for use in an emergency.

A full green E cylinder of O_2 will have a pressure of 2000 psi and contain about 625 liters of O_2. Since the O_2 is a compressed gas, the volume in the tank will correlate linearly with the pressure on the gauge. Therefore, a pressure of 1000 psi means the O_2 tank has about 312 liters of gas left. At a flow of 2 L/min, there is enough O_2 in the tank to last 156 minutes, or about 2.5 hours.

A full blue E cylinder of N_2O will have a pressure of 750 psi and contain about 1590 liters of N_2O. Nitrous oxide, being a compressed liquid, acts differently than the compressed gas in the O_2 tank. The pressure in the N_2O tank will stay at 750 psi until all of the liquid has been vaporized, and only then will the pressure in the tank begin to fall. At this point there will be about 400 liters of N_2O left. Since the N_2O tank in the question shows a pressure of 750 psi, we cannot tell how much N_2O remains by looking at the pressure gauge, and therefore cannot predict how long we can supply this gas (see figure below).

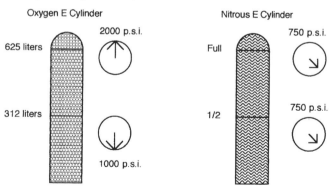

As oxygen is used, pressure in the tank decreases. In the nitrous oxide tank, the pressure remains constant until the tank is nearly empty.

17. What noninvasive method can be used to monitor pCO_2 in an anesthetized patient?
Capnography is the most commonly used method to estimate pCO_2 in the operating room and has become a standard for confirming successful endotracheal intubation and monitoring ventilation. A small amount of gas is continuously sampled from the anesthetic circuit. The instrument, whose

methods of analysis include infrared and mass spectrometry, then generates a numerical value for the pCO_2 of the gas sampled and an associated wave form, called a capnogram (see figure below). This method of monitoring assumes that end tidal CO_2 equates with $PACO_2$ and $PaCO_2$.

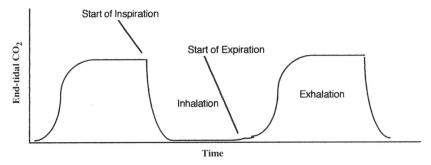

Normal capnogram waveform showing the inspiratory and expiratory phases.

18. What are the causes of a sudden decrease in end–tidal CO_2 in the anesthetized patient?

1. Low cardiac output
2. Pulmonary embolism
3. Venous-air embolism
4. Circuit leak or disconnection
5. Extubation
6. Obstruction of the airway or sampling tubing
7. Cardiac arrest

Anything that interrupts the perfusion of blood to the lungs or gas flow from the lungs will result in a decreased end–tidal CO_2. Beware of mechanical causes of decreased end–tidal CO_2, such as kinked tubing and disconnections.

BIBLIOGRAPHY

1. Barker SJ, Tremper KK: Physics applied to anesthesia. In Barash PG, Cullen BF, Stoelting RK (eds): Clinical Anesthesia. Philadelphia, J.B. Lippincott, 1992, pp 166–169.
2. Benumof JL: Conventional (laryngoscopic) orotracheal and nasotracheal intubation (single lumen type). In Benumof JL (ed): Clinical Procedures in Anesthesia and Intensive Care. Philadelphia, J.B. Lippincott, 1992, pp 115–148.
3. Brown M: ICU–critical care. In Barash PG, Cullen BF, Stoelting RK (eds): Clinical Anesthesia. Philadelphia, J.B. Lippincott, 1992, pp 1615–1618.
4. Carlson K, Jahr J: A historical overview and update on pulse oximetry. Anesthesiol Rev 20:173–181, 1993.
5. Foltz B, Benumof J: Mechanisms of hypoxemia and hypercapnia in the perioperative period. Crit Care Clin 3:269–286, 1987.
6. Ganong WF: Review of Medical Physiology. Norwalk, Appleton and Lange, 1987, pp 560–563.
7. Gilbert HC, Vender JS: Monitoring the anesthetized patient. In Barash PG, Cullen BF, Stoelting RK (eds): Clinical Anesthesia. Philadelphia, J.B. Lippincott, 1992, pp 737–741.
8. Kharash ED, Yeo KT, Kenny MA, et al: Atrial natriuretic factor may mediate the renal effects of PEEP ventilation. Anesthesiology 69:862, 1988.
9. Knill RL: Ventilatory responses to hypoxia and hypercarbia during halothane sedation and anesthesia in man. Anesthesiology 49:244–251, 1978.
10. Maarten JL: Does subanesthetic isoflurane affect the ventilatory response to acute isocapnic hypoxia in healthy volunteers? Anesthesiology 81:860–867, 1994.
11. Moyer GA, Rein P: Pre-oxygenation in the morbidly obese patient. Anesth Analg 65:S106, 1986.
12. Smith H, Lumb PD: Acid-base balance. In Barash PG, Cullen BF, Stoelting RK (eds): Clinical Anesthesia. Philadelphia, J.B. Lippincott, 1992, pp 245–249.
13. Stoelting R, Miller R: Basics of Anesthesia. New York, Churchill Livingstone, 1989, pp 15, 137–141, 452–454.
14. Weil WH, Bisera J, Trevino RP, et al: Cardiac output and end tidal carbon dioxide. Crit Care Med 13:907, 1985.
15. West JB: Respiratory Physiology—The Essentials. Baltimore, Williams & Wilkins, 1985, pp 51–52.
16. Wyche M, et al: Effects of continuous positive-pressure breathing on the functional residual capacity and arterial oxygenation during intra-abdominal operations. Anesthesiology 38:1,1973.

3. BLOOD GAS AND ACID-BASE ANALYSIS

Peter Sakas, M.D., and Matt Flaherty, M.D.

1. Why is arterial blood gas (ABG) analysis superior to noninvasive estimates of oxygenation and ventilation?

Pulse oximetry can readily and noninvasively measure oxygen saturation (SpO_2). Pulse oximetry, however, gives only an estimate of the arterial partial pressure of oxygen (PaO_2) when the oxyhemoglobin dissociation curve is not shifted and abnormal hemoglobin species, such as carboxyhemoglobin or methemoglobin, are not present. The oxyhemoglobin dissociation curve may shift in the presence of acidosis, alkalosis, hypothermia, hyperthermia, and altered 2,3-diphosphoglycerate, giving an inaccurate estimate of PaO_2. Saturation > 95% then may correlate with a wide range of PO_2 values. Even with a normal oxyhemoglobin dissociation curve of 70–100% SpO_2, the accuracy of most pulse oximeters is ± 2%; from 50–70% SpO_2, the accuracy is ± 3%, but below an SpO_2 of 50% there is little correlation. Also frequently used are noninvasive estimates of the arterial partial pressure of carbon dioxide (PCO_2), provided by **intraoperative end-tidal CO_2 monitoring** ($ETCO_2$). Correlation between arterial and $ETCO_2$ is usually close but may be distorted by interruptions in ventilation, chronic pulmonary disease, bronchospasm, and increased production of CO_2.

When these considerations are noted, SpO_2 and $ETCO_2$ may be good noninvasive estimates of PaO_2 and $PaCO_2$ in the patient who is well ventilated and has an unperturbed oxyhemoglobin dissociation curve. In the patient in whom there may be inadequate or inconsistent ventilation or physiologic compromise such that major changes in the oxyhemoglobin dissociation curve exist, ABG analysis may be required to quantitate the values of PaO_2 and $PaCO_2$ precisely. The ABG analysis also calculates the arterial pH, bicarbonate (HCO_3^-) and base excess, which further define the patient's condition. In these situations the possible complications of arterial puncture and the increased cost of ABG analysis are offset.

2. Why does an ABG sample require heparinization? How does this affect the sample?

The blood sample sent to the lab is drawn slowly through small tubes in a complex and expensive analyzer. The heparin is added to ensure that the blood does not clot in the machine's tubing, which would require expensive repair and cleaning. The effect of the heparin on the blood gas analysis is usually minimal. Heparin has an acidic moiety and can cause pH shifts and dilutional errors if the blood sample is a small volume relative to the heparin volume.

3. What are the normal ABG values at sea level?

Normal ABG Values

	SEA LEVEL (RANGE)	DENVER (ALT 5280 FT)
pH	7.40 (7.35–7.45 [± 2 SD])	NC
$PaCO_2$	40 mmHg (35–45 [± 2 SD])	34–38 mmHg
PaO_2	80–97 mmHg*	65–75 mmHg
HCO_3^-	24 mEq/L (22–26)	NC
SO_2	> 98%	92–94%
Base excess	0 mEq/L (−3–+3)	NC

NC = no change from sea-level value.
* PaO_2 varies with age and FiO_2.

4. Define the Henderson-Hasselbalch equation.

$$pH = 6.1 + \log (HCO_3^- / 0.03 \times PCO_2)$$

The Henderson-Hasselbalch equation describes the relationship between the plasma pH and the ratio of plasma PCO_2 and HCO_3^-. The equation really tells us that the primary determinant of the plasma pH is the ratio of PCO_2 to HCO_3^- and not the individual values alone. For example, a change in the PCO_2 may be accompanied by a change in the HCO_3^- such that the ratio of the two remains the same and the pH does not change.

5. Describe the major acid-base disorders and compensatory mechanisms seen when they are present.

Major Acid-Base Disorders and Compensatory Mechanisms

PRIMARY DISORDER	PRIMARY DISTURBANCE	PRIMARY COMPENSATION
Respiratory acidosis	↑ PCO_2	↑ HCO_3^-
Respiratory alkalosis	↓ PCO_2	↓ HCO_3^-
Metabolic acidosis	↓ HCO_3^-	Hyperventilation (↓ PCO_2)
Metabolic alkalosis	↑ HCO_3^-	Hypoventilation (↑ PCO_2)

The primary compensation (acute compensation) is generally achieved most rapidly through respiratory control of CO_2. Ultimately the renal system excretes acid or bicarbonate (chronic compensation) to reach the final response to the initial disturbance. Mixed disorders are common. Compensatory mechanisms never overcorrect for an acid-base disturbance; when ABG analysis reveals apparent overcorrection the presence of a mixed disorder should be suspected.

Rate of Compensatory Responses

PRIMARY DISORDER	PREDICTED RESPONSE
Respiratory acidosis	HCO_3^- increases 0.1/mmHg change in CO_2 (acute) HCO_3^- increases 0.25–0.55/mmHg change in CO_2 (chronic)
Respiratory alkalosis	HCO_3^- decreases 0.2–0.55/mmHg change in CO_2 (acute) HCO_3^- decreases 0.4–0.5/mmHg change in CO_2 (chronic)
Metabolic acidosis	$PaCO_2$ decreases 1–1.4/mEq HCO_3^- decrease
Metabolic alkalosis	$PaCO_2$ increases 0.4–0.9/mEq HCO_3^- increase

6. What are the major buffer systems of the body?

The bicarbonate-, phosphate-, and protein-buffering systems are the three major buffering systems. The **bicarbonate** system is primarily extracellular and the fastest to respond to pH imbalance, but it has less total capacity than intracelluar systems. Intracellular buffering is via the **phosphate** and **protein** systems. Intracellular buffering has a very large capacity, about 75% of the body's chemical buffering. Hydrogen ions are in dynamic equilibrium with all buffer systems of the body. CO_2 molecules also readily cross cell membranes and keep both intracellular and extracellular buffering systems in dynamic equilibrium. We commonly measure the status of the bicarbonate system because it exists in the plasma, in large quantities, and is readily measurable. Chemistry laboratories actually measure the total CO_2, a sum of all forms of CO_2 in the sample, such as bicarbonate, carbonic acid and dissolved CO_2 gas. The bicarbonate value reported on ABG analysis is calculated from a nomogram using the Henderson-Hasselbalch equation and the measured values for pH and $PaCO_2$.

7. Does the liver have a role in acid-base balance?

Metabolism of protein usually results in net production of acid. The liver metabolizes organic acids, such as lactate, which conserves plasma HCO_3^-. The result of hepatic lactate metabolism is

CO_2, which may eliminated by the lungs. Hepatic disease may lead to various acid-base disorders: respiratory alkalosis secondary to central nervous system stimulation; metabolic acidosis secondary to lactate accumulation or, commonly, coexisting renal disease; and mixed disorders due to combinations of these disorders.

8. How does the kidney influence acid-base balance?
The normal kidney maintains acid-base homeostasis by two mechanisms. Large amounts of bicarbonate (4500 mEq/day) are filtered at the glomerulus and then reclaimed prior to loss in the urine. The kidney also excretes acid when hydrogen ions combine with phosphate and ammonia and are excreted in the urine. Renal failure results in decreased clearance of inorganic acids. **Renal tubular acidosis** (RTA) results when either proximal tubular reabsorption of bicarbonate (RTA type II) or distal tubular ammonium ion excretion (RTA type I) is impaired.

9. What is the anion gap?
A major tool used in evaluating acid-base disorders, the anion gap is the calculated difference between the serum sodium concentration and the sum of serum chloride and bicarbonate:

$$Na - (Cl + HCO_3^-)$$

The plasma is actually electrically neutral, and the "gap" is composed of anions we do not usually measure. The normal anion gap is approximately 10 and normally ranges from 8–12. When an acid load is present, bicarbonate ions titrate the acid, and consequently, the bicarbonate concentration falls. This drop in HCO_3^- increases the calculated anion gap. Increases in the anion gap usually indicate that the HCO_3^- concentration is being decreased by a titratable acid, creating a condition known as an **anion gap metabolic acidosis**. Anion gap elevation can occur with elevated serum HCO_3^- concentrations in mixed acid-base disorders as well.

10. Name several causes of anion gap metabolic acidosis.
Increased acid production from any of the following sources:
- Ketoacidosis (diabetic, alcoholic, or starvation)
- Lactic acidosis (hypovolemia, hypotension, hypoxia, toxins, or enzyme defects)
- Toxins (salicylates, paraldehyde, methanol, or ethylene glycol)
- Hyperosmolar hyperosmotic nonketotic coma
- Uremic acidosis (acute or chronic renal failure)

11. Name several causes of non-anion gap acidosis.
Non-anion gap acidoses are usually due to loss of bicarbonate rather than the presence of acid. Potential causes include:
Renal tubular acidosis
Diarrhea
Ureteral diversions
Interstitial nephritis
Ureteral obstruction
Drugs (e.g., spironolactone, acetazolamide)

12. Describe lactic acidosis and its causes.
Lactic acid is formed by glycolysis and arises from many metabolic pathways. Hypoxia, hypotension, hypovolemia, and sepsis all can result in states of **low tissue oxygen delivery**. Cellular metabolism of carbohydrate (oxidative phosphorylation) requires O_2; when O_2 delivery fails, the cells rely on anaerobic metabolism, producing lactate. Less common causes of lactic acidosis include diabetic ketoacidosis, liver disease, cyanide poisoning, widespread malignancy, and alcohol consumption. If a blood sample is stored for a prolonged period, the cells continually metabolize glucose to lactate and may falsely elevate the lactate content of the sample.

13. When is it appropriate to administer bicarbonate?

Metabolic acidosis is commonly treated with sodium bicarbonate, although this is controversial. Bicarbonate combines with hydrogen ions and, in the presence of the enzyme carbonic anhydrase, becomes CO_2 and H_2O. Patients with adequate ventilation can eliminate the CO_2. However patients with inadequate ventilation only accumulate more CO_2, which can readily cross cell membranes and contribute to intracelluar acidosis, a theoretical concern. Bicarbonate administration is best reserved for patients with adequate ventilation and pH < 7.20 (the pH that begins to cause generalized enzymatic and metabolic dysfunction).

   Lactic acidosis may be due to tissue hypoperfusion, and therefore volume resuscitation and oxygenation should be addressed before attempting to correct the acidosis with bicarbonate infusion. There is no evidence that treatment of lactic acidosis with bicarbonate improves outcome.

   Bicarbonate has been shown to be useful in renal failure, other bicarbonate-wasting states, treatment of certain toxic ingestions (such as tricyclic antidepressant overdose), and hyperkalemia. The bicarbonate dose is calculated as follows:

$$BE \times 0.3 \times body\ wt = total\ base\ deficit$$

Where BE is the base deficit in mEq/L, 0.3 is the extracelluar water percentage, and body weight is in kg. The total base deficit, in mEq, is often corrected by approximately 50% and then reassessed with further ABG analysis.

14. What is a Clark electrode?

The Clark electrode, developed in 1956, measures the PO_2 in the blood sample. The oxygen electrode is based on the oxidation-reduction reaction of dissolved O_2 and water.

15. What is the Severinghaus electrode?

The Severinghaus electrode, developed in 1958, measures the PCO_2 in the blood sample.

16. Can anesthetics cause spurious readings by the Clark electrode?

Yes. In 1971 Severinghaus found that halothane caused upward drift of PaO_2 at the Clark electrode, although the clinical significance is minimal.

17. What factors determine the value of $PaCO_2$?

CO_2, a major product of cellular metabolism, is primarily produced in the mitochondria and eliminated through the lungs. A simple relationship can be assumed:

$$PaCO_2 = VCO_2/VA$$

where VCO_2 is total body CO_2 production, and VA is alveolar ventilation. **Hypocapnia**, defined as $PaCO_2$ < 35 mmHg at sea level, can be caused by decreased production (e.g., hypothermia, neuromuscular blockade) and/or increased elimination (e.g., overzealous mechanical ventilation, hypoxia or metabolic acidosis with compensatory hyperventilation, or pulmonary parenchymal disease that stimulates J-receptors and increases VA). **Hypercapnia,** defined as $PaCO_2$ > 45 mmHg at sea level, can be caused by increased production (e.g., light anesthesia, hyperthermia, shivering) or decreased elimination of CO_2 (e.g., hypoventilation, increased deadspace secondary to decreased cardiac output or pulmonary embolus, or rebreathing CO_2).

18. How does one determine if the PaO_2 value is "normal"?

First, determine the **alveolar PaO_2** via the alveolar gas equation:

$$PAO_2 = [(P_B-47)FiO_2] - PACO_2 \times 1.25$$

where P_B is barometric pressure, 47 is vapor pressure of water, and $PACO_2$ is the alveolar PCO_2, (substituted with $PaCO_2$ since they are in close approximation). The value of 1.25 is the respiratory quotient, which is an averaged value reflecting the amount of oxygen absorbed relative to the amount of CO_2 excreted. With a calculated PAO_2 and a known PaO_2 from the ABG the **alveolar–arterial oxygen gradient** (A–aDO_2 gradient) can be easily computed. For people ≤ 50 years old (breathing room air), the difference should be < 20 mmHg. A larger value indicates a deviation from normal oxygenation status due to intrinsic pulmonary parenchymal disease. Hypoxemia with a normal A–aDO$_2$ is due to hypoventilation. Age can decrease the PaO$_2$, so an approximation of normal PaO$_2$ (breathing room air at sea level) is:

$$\text{Age-adjusted PaO}_2 = 102 - [\text{age in yrs/3}]$$

19. What is the base excess or deficit?

Base excess or deficit is a calculated value that gives an estimation of "acid load." The pH is first titrated to 7.4, which negates the buffering effects of hemoglobin. The remaining value (difference of HCO$_3^-$ concentration from 24 mEq/L) represents the lack or excess of bicarbonate. Large negative values of base excess (i.e., deficit) represent metabolic acidosis, and large positive values indicate metabolic alkalosis.

20. What are the more common acid-base disorders seen in the postoperative period?

1. **Respiratory acidosis** is very common due to residual anesthetics and neuromuscular blocking agents, which blunt the response to rising PaCO$_2$.

2. **Metabolic acidosis** may occur when surgical blood loss or third-space losses are underappreciated and volume resuscitation is inadequate.

3. **Respiratory alkalosis** is also common due to pain or anxiety.

BIBLIOGRAPHY

1. Cissik JH, Salustro J, Patton OL, Louden JA: The effects of sodium heparin on arterial blood gas analysis. Cardiovasc Pulm 5:17–21, 1977.
2. Gal TJ: Monitoring the function of the respiratory system. In Lake CL (ed): Clinical Monitoring. Philadelphia, W.B. Saunders, 1990, pp 315–341.
3. Mizock BA, Falk JL: Lactic acidosis in critical illness. Crit Care Med 20:80–91, 1992.
4. Petty TL (ed): Intensive and Rehabilitative Respiratory Care, 2nd ed. Philadelphia, Lea & Febiger, 1974, p 68.
5. Schumaker PT, Cain SM: The concept of critical oxygen delivery. Intens Care Med 13:223–229, 1987.
6. Severinghaus JW, Naifeh KH: Accuracy of response of six oximeters to profound hypoxia. Anesthesiology 67:551–558, 1987.
7. Severinghaus JW, Weiskopf RB, Nishimura M, Bradley AF: Oxygen electrode errors due to polarographic reduction of halothane. J Appl Physiol 31:640–642, 1971.
8. Sorbini CA, Grassi V, Solinas E, Muiesan G: Arterial oxygen tension in relation to age in healthy subjects. Respiration 25:3–13, 1968.
9. Tremper KK, Barker SJ: Monitoring of oxygen. In Lake CL (ed): Clinical Monitoring. Philadelphia, W.B. Saunders, 1990, pp 283–313.
10. Vender JS, Gilbert HC: Blood gas monitoring. In Blitt CD, Hines RL (eds): Monitoring in Anesthesia and Critical Care Medicine, 3rd ed. New York, Churchill Livingstone, 1995, pp 407–421.

4. FLUIDS AND ELECTROLYTES

Fred M. Galloway, M.D.

1. Until the early 1960s, surgical patients were not given much intravenous fluid replacement in the perioperative period. Why? What brought about the dramatic change in fluid management?

Clinicians had investigated the observation that surgical patients excreted very little urine. It was assumed that something in the perioperative period—anesthetics, other drugs, or some factor such as surgical stress—interfered with renal function. They erroneously concluded that because patients did not excrete normal amounts of salt and water, they could not; thus such fluids were restricted.

By the early 1960s, numerous studies showed that surgical patients did not produce much urine because they were conserving salt and water. Although renal function was minimally impaired, patients could handle intravenous crystalloid and in fact needed far more than basal requirements. The use of balanced salt solutions and the new practice of central venous pressure (CVP) monitoring essentially eliminated the problems due to underhydration, such as hypovolemic shock and acute tubular necrosis.

2. Describe the functionally distinct compartments of body water, using a 70-kg patient for illustration.

Various authorities quote different percentages for the different body compartments, perhaps because they base composition on total body weight. Because people vary greatly in adipose content (a tissue with relatively low water content), basing body fluid compartments on lean, or ideal body weight (IBW), is advised.

The **total body water** (TBW) is 57% of the IBW (40 L).

The **intracellular fluid** (ICF) compartment comprises 35% of IBW or 63% of TBW (about 25 L). It is the principal potassium-containing space.

The **extracellular fluid** (ECF) compartment contains the remaining 15 L of TBW; it accounts for 22–24% of IBW and is subdivided into **interstitial fluid** (ISF) and **blood volume** (BV). The BV is 7% of an adult's IBW (about 5 L) and is composed primarily of plasma, plasma proteins, and formed blood elements, principally red blood cells. The plasma proteins generate a colloidal osmotic pressure, which is in part responsible for the distribution of water between the ISF and BV compartments.

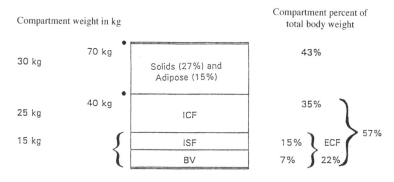

The compartments of body water based on 70-kg body weight.

3. Describe the dynamics of the distribution of fluids between the intravascular and interstitial fluid compartments.

The intravascular or blood volume and the interstitial fluid spaces (which make up the ECF) are in dynamic equilibrium, governed by hydrostatic and osmotic forces. Starling first described the microcirculation at the capillary level. The capillary hydrostatic pressure (Cp) at the arteriolar side causes an outward filtration of fluid, and the capillary osmotic pressure causes reabsorption on the venular side. A slight disequilibrium, as demonstrated below, produces a slight excess in the net filtration of fluid, which is subsequently returned to the circulation through lymphatics. Thus, intravenously administered crystalloid solutions distribute throughout the entire ECF compartment within minutes.

Forces determining outward filtration of ECF		Forces promoting reabsorption of ISF	
Mean capillary hydrostatic pressure (torr)	17.3	Plasma colloid osmotic pressure (torr)	28.0
Negative ISF pressure	3.0		
ISF colloid osmotic pressure	8.0		
TOTALS (torr)	28.3		28.0

4. Various methods have been used to calculate fluid requirements, including body surface area, caloric requirements, and body weight. Is there a common basis for fluid requirements?

Yes. Fluid requirements are most closely related to metabolic rate. Both caloric requirements and oxygen consumption are measures of metabolic rate. Caloric expenditure per kilogram declines with increasing body weight. Although the caloric expenditure per unit weight declines exponentially with increasing weight, the need for water is constant—about 1 ml per calorie. The following example determines the daily fluid requirement for a 40-kg person:

100 ml/kg/day for the first 10 kg	1000 ml
50 ml/kg/day for the second 10 kg	500 ml
20 ml/kg/day for the remaining 20 kg	400 ml
Daily fluid requirement for a 40-kg patient	1900 ml

The so-called "4-2-1 rule" for calculating hourly requirements is a derivation of this calculation. The factor in each step of the calculation is simply divided by 24. Hence, 4 ml/kg is the hourly requirement for the first 10 kg, 2 ml/kg for the second 10 kg, and 1 ml/kg for the remainder of the patient's weight.

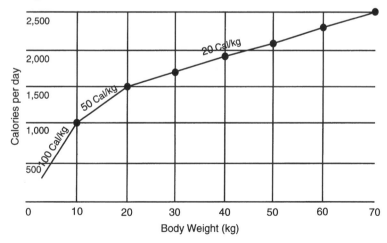

Reduction in daily caloric expenditure per kilogram with increasing body weight. (Adapted from Holliday MA, Segar WE: the maintenance need for water in parenteral fluid therapy. Pediatrics 19:823–832, 1957, with permission.)

5. Describe a proper preoperative evaluation of volume status.

Proper evaluation includes an interview with the patient, consideration of the clinical context, physical assessment, evaluation of vital signs and other hemodynamic measurements, assessment of urine output, and evaluation of selected laboratory values. An organized approach is helpful.

1. **History and clinical context**
   - NPO status—duration; volumes and composition of last ingested or administered fluids
   - History of vomiting, diarrhea, excessive diaphoresis, diabetes (mellitus or insipidus), alcohol ingestion
   - Review of medication, especially diuretic use
   - Bowel preparations may result in 2–4 liters of volume loss if not replaced
   - Have a high index of suspicion with certain conditions necessitating emergency operations and often accompanied by hypovolemia. Examples: ileus, peritonitis, bowel obstructions, gastrointestinal bleeding, burns, trauma, large bone and pelvic fractures, and febrile illnesses.
2. **Physical assessment**
   - Tailor the examination to the problem but always be thorough. Evaluate skin turgor, mucous membranes, capillary refill, edema (chronic—pitting edema; acute—periorbital and conjunctival edema), ascites, evidence of pleural effusions or pulmonary edema.
3. **Vital signs and hemodynamic measurements**
   - Pulse rate, pulse pressure, blood pressure, respiratory rate
   - Orthostatic changes in pulse and blood pressure
   - Central filling pressures—CVP, pulmonary artery and capillary wedge pressures as well as derived hemodynamic indices, such as cardiac output and index, mixed venous oxygen saturation, and oxygen delivery and consumption
4. **Urine output**
   - Oliguria, defined as < 0.5 ml/kg/hr, is a useful sign of inadequate fluid replacement or inadequate hemodynamics. An adequate urine output in an adult is 0.5–1.0 ml/kg/hr. Urine output in adults of > 1 ml/kg/hr may reflect overhydration in the absence of loop or osmotic diuretics. Alcohol or anesthetics also may alter urine output. Children should have a slightly more vigorous output; neonates should have an output of 2.0 ml/kg/hr.
5. **Laboratory determinations**
   - Useful laboratory values in the assessment of volume status include hemoglobin, hematocrit, electrolytes, blood urea nitrogen, creatinine, proteins, urine osmolality, specific gravity, and sodium concentration.

6. Describe the progression of signs and symptoms with unreplaced acute blood loss and their correlation with volume loss.

BLOOD VOLUME LOST	SIGNS AND SYMPTOMS
10%	Thirst Vasoconstriction—veins
20%	Sweating Mild-to-moderate increase in heart rate Slight drop in blood pressure Decreased urine output
30%	Tachycardia (–120 bpm plus) Moderate hypotension High degree of vasoconstriction Cool, clammy, and pale Anuria
40%	Severe hypotension and tachycardia Mental confusion
50%	Coma—near death

Note that blood pressure is not significantly affected until approximately 30% of blood volume is lost despite a decreasing cardiac output. Early compensatory mechanisms, including peripheral vasoconstriction and tachycardia, may mask significant volume loss.

7. Contrast the evolution and presentation of acute and chronic volume depletion.

Acute vs. Chronic Volume Depletion

% DECREASE IN INTRAVASCULAR OR ECF VOLUME	ACUTE VOLUME DECREASE	CHRONIC INTRAVASCULAR VOLUME DEPLETION
5–10	Mild resting tachycardia Thirst and salt craving common	Up to roughly 20% depletion is well tolerated, with blood pressure, pulse rate, and cardiac output near normal in the resting state until severely depleted. Patient then shows a progression of effects:
15	Tachycardia Orthostatic hypotension Cardiac output begins to drop Dry mucous membranes Poor skin turgor Oliguria	Deceased venous compliance Orthostatic hypotension—slowed response to normalize pressure
20	Moderate supine hypotension Heart rate > 120 bpm Reduced cardiac output Vasoconstriction, lethargy High degree of oliguria, sodium and water retention reflected in low urine sodium concentration and high osmolality (> 700 mOsm/kg)	Diminished activity Anorexia Decreased skin turgor Apathy Prerenal azotemia and elevated uric acid common Poor muscle tone Diminished deep tendon reflexes and sensation
25	Marked tachycardia and hypotension Low cardiac output High degree of vasoconstriction Poor tissue perfusion Anuria, obtunded state	Supine hypotension Cutaneous lividity Nausea and vomiting → ileus Stupor
30	Vascular collapse	Hypothermia

Chronic intravascular and extracellular fluid depletion seem to be well tolerated; blood pressure and cardiac output are well maintained until losses are severe. Fluid is drawn from the interstitial compartment and venous capacitance is reduced to support cardiac output. Renin and angiotensin release are stimulated. However, relatively small acute blood losses or the administration of most anesthetic agents may produce precipitous hypotension.

8. What are the goals in the resuscitation of hypovolemic patients? What is the preferred initial resuscitation fluid? How does it distribute?

The primary goal is the restoration of the microcirculation (tissue perfusion) and reversal of the hypovolemic state. These goals are accomplished only by restoring the extracellular fluid volume, both blood volume (BV) and interstitial fluid (ISF) compartments. The initial resuscitation fluid of choice is a balanced salt solution which will distribute quickly into both the BV and the ISF compartment. The initial distribution of crystalloid is approximately one-third intravascular and two-thirds interstitial. Because of passage into the ISF, blood loss must be replaced 3 to 1 with crystalloid solutions to be effective. Dilution of intravascular colloid osmotic pressure favors further significant passage of crystalloid into the ISF. It has been estimated that if two-thirds of a patient's blood volume were replaced with crystalloid solutions, the ratio of distribution between the ISF and BV would be approximately 10 to 1.

Initial resuscitation measures may result in a state of compensated shock, in which blood pressure appears normal, but diminished cardiac output persists, along with high systemic vascular resistance and tissue hypoperfusion. The patient remains somewhat tachycardic and anuric or oliguric and demonstrates a persistent metabolic acidosis with increased blood lactate levels. This situation cannot be ignored, for in patients with multiple injuries its persistence may predispose the patient to delayed sequelae of shock, such as multiple organ dysfunction and death.

Persisting indices of hypoperfusion, continued blood loss, and declining hematocrit (acceptable minimal levels depend on the age of the patient, coexisting disease, extent of injury, and expected future losses) suggest a need for blood transfusion. Transfusion therapy is covered in the chapters on hemotherapy and trauma.

9. What is meant by third-space losses? What are the effects of such losses?
The extracellular fluid (ECF) compartment is composed of the blood volume and interstitial fluid (ISF) volume. In certain clinical conditions, such as major intraabdominal operations, hemorrhagic shock, burns, and sepsis, patients develop fluid requirements that are not explained by externally measurable losses. Losses are internal, a temporary sequestration of ECF into a functionless third space, which does not participate in the dynamic fluid exchanges at the microcirculatory level. The volume of this internal loss is proportional to the degree of injury, and its composition is similar to plasma or ISF. The creation of the third space necessitates further fluid infusions to maintain intravascular volume, adequate cardiac output, and perfusion.

10. What are the determinants of perioperative fluid requirements?
1. **Basal requirements.** In the absence of catabolic states (e.g., starvation, burns, sepsis, fever), anesthetized patients are close to their basal metabolic rate; the same is true for fluid requirements (see question 4).

2. **Preoperative deficits** should be estimated (see question 5).

3. **Blood loss.** Estimates of blood loss are derived from measuring losses accumulating in suction canisters, observing or weighing blood loss on surgical sponges ("laps"), looking at the drapes, and being vigilant for occult blood loss (hidden in the drapes or lost on the floor).

4. **Third-space losses.** Minor operations with minimal tissue injury do not exhibit much third spacing. The third space requirements for major abdominal operations may be significant. For moderate surgical trauma (e.g., open cholecystectomy), estimate about 3 ml/kg/hr; for more extensive procedures, such as enteral resections, estimate 6–8 ml/kg/hr; and for major vascular resections (e.g., abdominal aortic aneurysms), estimate 10–20 ml/kg/hr.

5. **Transcellular fluid losses.** Estimate losses from transcellular fluids, such as ascites, pleural effusions, enteral fluids (e.g., gastric succor), and fistulas.

6. **Effects of anesthetic agents and technique.** Through a combination of sympathetic suppression, vasodilation, and myocardial depression, general anesthetics quickly unmask hypovolemia. Many patients with previously adequate filling pressures experience a significant decrease in blood pressure with the induction of anesthesia. Although occasionally administration of vasoactive substances is needed, patients often improve with fluid infusion.

During major conduction anesthesia (subarachnoid or epidural), the vasculature experiences a local anesthetic-induced loss of sympathetic tone. Decreases in blood pressure usually respond to modest fluid infusions, but sometimes pressors are required to support systemic pressures.

Clearly estimating perioperative fluid needs requires skill and vigilance. Frequently the best assessment of adequate volume status is satisfactory urine output (see question 5). Patients with impaired cardiac and renal function and patients undergoing extensive procedures with significant volume shifts may require CVP or PA catheter monitoring to assess adequately fluid and cardiovascular status.

11. What fluid and electrolyte disturbances are common in the perioperative period? Specify their cause.
1. **Hyponatremia** may be due to salt restriction in elderly patients, administration of hypotonic fluids, or absorption of sodium-poor irrigants, as during transurethral resection of the prostate (TURP) or when the uterus is distended to facilitate a surgical procedure. The inappropriate secretion of antidiuretic hormone (ADH) or excessive use of oxytocin (with ADH-like

properties) also may produce hyponatremia; other causes include diuretics, adrenal insufficiency, nephrotic syndrome, and congestive heart failure.

2. **Hypernatremia** tends to be less common than hyponatremia. It may be caused by dehydration, gastrointestinal losses, diabetes insipidus, and renal failure.

3. **Hypokalemia** is most commonly caused by diuretics; look for hypokalemia in patients receiving beta-adrenergic agonists.

4. **Hyperkalemia** may be drug-induced or iatrogenic; it also may be found in renal failure, diabetes mellitus, massive transfusion, and acidosis.

5. **Metabolic acidosis** is commonly seen in massive trauma or in extensive operations associated with massive fluid shifts.

6. **Hypocalcemia**—a decrease in ionized calcium—may be seen with rapid transfusion of citrated blood products.

12. When should hyponatremia be treated?

The rate at which hyponatremia develops and the presence of symptoms determine the aggressiveness of treatment. If hyponatremia has developed quickly, as during TURP, the patient may develop hypertension, bradycardia, confusion, apprehension, agitation, obtundation, or seizures; usually the sodium is found to be less than 125 mEq/L. The aggressiveness of treatment depends on the extent of symptoms. In the simplest cases, fluid restriction may be sufficient. More acutely ill patients may require diuresis or administration of hypertonic (3%) saline. Seizures require securing a protected airway, oxygenation, ventilation, and perhaps administration of anticonvulsants, although seizures are usually self-limited. Sodium bicarbonate provides 1 mEq of sodium/ml if a rapid sodium infusion is necessary.

13. How are body water and tonicity regulated?

The first mechanism involves release of ADH. ADH circulates unbound in plasma, has a half-life of roughly 20 minutes, and increases production of cyclic adenosine monophosphate (cAMP) in the distal collecting tubules of the kidney. The net effect increases tubular permeability to water and results in conservation of water and sodium and production of concentrated urine. Stimuli for the release of ADH include:

1. Osmoreceptors in the supraoptic nuclei of the hypothalamus have a mean osmotic threshold of 289 ± 2.3 mOsm/kg. Above this level, ADH release is stimulated.

2. A closely related mechanism for regulating body water and tonicity is the thirst reflex. Thirst center neurons are located in the lateral preoptic area of the hypothalamus, regulate conscious desire for water, and are activated by (1) an increase in plasma sodium of 2 mEq/L; (2) an increase in plasma osmolality of 4 mOsm/L; (3) an excessive loss of potassium from thirst center neurons; and (4) angiotensin II. Activation of the thirst center stimulates release of ADH.

3. Aortic baroreceptors and stretch receptors in the left atrium respond to intravascular volume and are sources of afferent innervation to the supraoptic neurons. Stretch receptors also give neural input to the sympathetic nervous system.

4. The effects of aldosterone on the renal tubules fine tune serum sodium levels (see question 23).

14. What is the difference between osmolarity and osmolality? Is there a difference between osmolality and tonicity? How is the osmolality of blood determined?

In casual discussion, osmolarity and osmolality often are used interchangeably, but in fact they are different. Osmolarity is defined as the number of osmoles of solute per liter of solution; osmolality is the number of osmoles of solute per kilogram of solvent. Osmolality of blood may be higher than tonicity if the blood contains substances to which cells are permeable (such as urea or alcohol), which contribute to osmotic pressure but not to tonicity. Osmolality is measured by determining the freezing point depression of the aqueous solution; the freezing point is lowered by 1.86° Celsius per osmol of solute. Osmolality can be estimated by the following equation:

Osmolality = 1.86 [Na in mEq/L] + [glucose in mg/dl] ÷ 18 + [BUN in mg/dl] ÷ 2.8.

15. Discuss the synthesis of antidiuretic hormone.

ADH, or vasopressin, is an octapeptide synthesized in the supraoptic and paraventricular nuclei of the hypothalamus. It is transported attached to carrier proteins (known as neurophysines) down the pituitary stalk in secretory granules along the axons of the cells of origin into the posterior pituitary gland (neurohypophysis), where it is stored and released into the capillaries of the neurohypophysis in response to stimuli from the hypothalamus. ADH-producing neurons receive efferent innervation form osmoreceptors and baroreceptors.

16. List conditions that stimulate and inhibit release of ADH.

Conditions that Stimulate and Inhibit Release of ADH

	STIMULATE	INHIBIT
Normal physiologic states	Hyperosmolality Hypovolemia Upright position Beta-adrenergic stimulation Pain Emotional stress Cholinergic stimulation	Hypoosmolality Hypervolemia Supine position Alpha-adrenergic stimulation
Abnormal physiologic states	Hemorrhagic shock Hyperthermia Increased intracranial pressure Head injury Positive airway pressure	Excessive water intake Hypothermia
Medications	Morphine Nicotine Barbiturates Tricyclic antidepressants Vincristine Cyclophosphamide Chlorpropamide	Ethanol Atropine Phenytoin Reserpine Glucocorticoids Chlorpromazine
Result	Low urine output Concentrated urine	High urine output Dilute urine

17. What is diabetes insipidus?

Diabetes insipidus (DI) is caused by a deficiency of ADH synthesis, impaired release of ADH from the neurohypophysis (neurogenic DI), or renal resistance to ADH (nephrogenic DI). The result is excretion of large volumes of dilute urine, which, if untreated leads to dehydration and hyperosmolality of body fluids. The usual test for DI is cautious fluid restriction. The inability to decrease and concentrate urine suggests the diagnosis, which may be confirmed by plasma ADH measurements. Administration of aqueous vasopressin tests the response of the renal tubule. Comparison of plasma and urine osmolality is useful; if the osmolality of plasma continues to exceed that of urine after mild fluid restriction, the diagnosis of DI is suggested.

18. Discuss the alternative treatments for DI.

Available preparations of ADH include pitressin tannate in oil, administered every 24–48 hours; aqueous pitressin, 5–10 units IV or IM every 4–6 hours; synthetic lysine vasopressin nasal spray (Diodid), 2 units 4 times/day; and 1-deamino-8-D-arginine vasopressin (DDAVP), 10–20 units intranasally every 12–24 hours. Incomplete DI may respond to thiazide diuretics, chlorpropamide (which potentiates endogenous ADH), carbamazepine, or clofibrate.

Because the patient is losing water, administration of isotonic solutions may cause hypernatremia; in addition, excessive vasopressin causes water intoxication. Management during surgery may require a continuous infusion of aqueous vasopressin of 100–200 mU/hr after a bolus of 100–200 mU. Measurement of plasma osmolality (or estimation from serum levels of sodium, glucose, and blood urea nitrogen) as well as urine output and osmolality is indicated when vasopressin is infused.

19. List causes of diabetes insipidus.
Vasopressin deficiency (neurogenic DI)
  Familial (autosomal dominant)
  Acquired
    Idiopathic
    Trauma (craniofacial and basilar skull fractures)
    Tumor (craniopharyngioma, lymphoma, metastasis)
    Granuloma (sarcoidosis, histiocytosis)
    Infections (meningitis, encephalitis)
    Vascular (Sheehan's syndrome, cerebral aneurysm, cardiopulmonary bypass)
    Hypoxic brain damage
Vasopressin insensitivity (nephrogenic DI)
  Familial (X-linked recessive)
  Acquired
    Infections (pyelonephritis)
    Post-renal obstruction (prostatic, ureteral)
    Hematologic (sickle-cell disease and trait)
    Infiltrative (amyloidosis)
    Polycystic kidney disease
    Hypokalemia, hypercalcemia
    Sarcoidosis
    Medications (lithium, demeclocycline, methoxyflurane)

20. Define the syndrome of inappropriate antidiuretic hormone release (SIADH). What is the primary therapy?
Hypotonicity due to the nonosmotic release of ADH, which inhibits renal excretion of water, typifies SIADH. Three criteria must be met to establish the diagnosis of SIADH: (1) the patient must be euvolemic or hypervolemic; (2) the urine must be inappropriately concentrated (plasma osmolality <280 mOsm/kg, urine osmolality >100 mOsm/kg); and (3) renal, cardiac, hepatic, adrenal, and thyroid function must be normal.

    The primary therapy for SIADH is water restriction. Postoperative SIADH is usually a temporary phenomenon and resolves spontaneously. Chronic SIADH may require the addition of demeclocycline, which blocks the ADH-mediated water resorption in the collecting ducts of the kidney.

21. What disorders are associated with SIADH?
CNS events are frequent causes, including acute intracranial hypertension, trauma, tumors, meningitis, and subarachnoid hemorrhage. Pulmonary causes are also common, including tuberculosis, pneumonia, asthma, bronchiectasis, hypoxemia, hypercarbia, and positive pressure ventilation. Malignancies may produce ADH-like compounds. Adrenal insufficiency and hypothyroidism also have been associated with SIADH.

22. Body fluid tonicity controls the intracellular (ICF) volume. What controls the extracellular fluid (ECF) volume?
The mechanisms that control blood volume simultaneously control the entire ECF volume, because the interstitial and intravascular volume are in dynamic equilibrium. Such mechanisms include the renal responses to changes in blood pressure (altering the glomerular filtration rate), the atrial volume receptors and aortic baroreceptors (modulating sympathetic nervous system activ-

ity and ADH release), and the renin-angiotensin-aldosterone system. Thus, intravascular volume and blood pressure are the primary regulators of sodium balance and excretion.

23. What is aldosterone? What stimulates its release? What are its actions?

Aldosterone, a mineralocorticoid, is the hormone responsible for the precise control of sodium excretion. A decrease in systemic or renal arterial blood pressure, as well as hypovolemia or hyponatremia, leads to release of renin from the juxtaglomerular cells of the kidney. Angiotensinogen, produced in the liver, is converted by renin to angiotensin I. In the blood stream angiotensin I is converted to angiotensin II, and the zona glomerulosa of the adrenal cortex is then stimulated to release aldosterone. An additional effect of angiotensin II is vasoconstriction. Aldosterone acts on the distal renal tubules and cortical collecting ducts, promoting sodium retention. Besides hyponatremia and hypovolemia, stimuli for aldosterone release include hyperkalemia, increased levels of adrenocorticotropic hormone (ACTH), and surgical procedures.

24. What are the clinical implications of disturbances in sodium balance and tonicity?

Hypotonicity, hyponatremia, severe hyperosmolar states, and failure to maintain an adequate blood volume may be life-threatening or produce irreversible neurologic and other end-organ damage. Therefore, it is mandatory to monitor fluid intake, urine output, serum sodium levels (and serum glucose in diabetic patients) during any major surgical procedure.

25. A 45-year-old patient scheduled for an elective cholecystectomy takes furosemide for hypertension. Preoperative laboratory tests are normal except for a potassium level of 3.0 mEq/L. What are the risks of proceeding? Why not give the patient enough potassium to restore the serum level to normal?

Hypokalemia favors the development of serious cardiac arrhythmias, especially in patients with ischemic heart disease or preexisting cardiac arrhythmias and patients receiving digitalis. Acute hypokalemia is probably more serious than chronic hypokalemia. The total body deficit of potassium, primarily an intracellular cation, is not well reflected by serum concentrations. A patient with a serum potassium of 3.0 mEq/L may have a total body deficit in excess of 400 mEq.

Historically, standard anesthetic practice was to consider even modest hypokalemia as a contraindication to elective procedures. However, sufficient data have been gathered that suggest

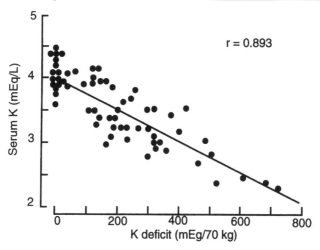

The relationship between serum and total body potassium (K). A 0.27-mEq/L reduction in the serum concentration is equivalent to 100-mEq total K deficit. (From Sterns RH, et al: Internal potassium balance and the control of plasma potassium concentration. Medicine 60:339, 1981, with permission.)

that patients without the above risk factors who are not undergoing major thoracic, vascular or cardiac procedures can tolerate modest hypokalemia (possibly as low as 2.8 mEq/L) without sequelae.

As mentioned, serum potassium levels do not reflect true body deficits. Attempts at rapid correction of serum potassium levels poorly address the extent of the problem and are more dangerous than modest hypokalemia. In fact, rapid attempts to correct hypokalemia have resulted in cardiac arrest.

26. A 48-year-old hypertensive patient with chronic renal failure requires an arteriovenous fistula for hemodialysis and is scheduled for a general anesthetic. Potassium is measured as 7.0 mEq/L. What are the risks of proceeding? How can life-threatening hyperkalemia be treated?

Hyperkalemia may produce ventricular arrhythmias, beginning with premature ventricular contractions and progressing to ventricular tachycardia and fibrillation. Hypoventilation and acidosis worsen hyperkalemia, as does the administration of succinylcholine and potassium-containing fluids or medications. Many anesthesiologists believe that hyperkalemia > 5.9 mEq/L should be corrected before elective procedures. Patients with chronic renal failure are normally dialyzed.

Emergent treatment of hyperkalemia consists of three mechanisms. Immediate, direct reversal of cardiotoxicity is accomplished by administration of calcium chloride. Potassium can then be quickly shifted intracellularly as a temporizing maneuver to decrease the serum level by hyperventilation, beta-adrenergic stimulation (e.g., beta-agonist nebulizer), sodium bicarbonate, and insulin and glucose. Removal of potassium from the body—the definitive treatment (and time-consuming)—can be accomplished by diuretics, Kayexalate, and dialysis. One should always consider hyperkalemia when a patient with renal failure suffers cardiac arrest.

BIBLIOGRAPHY

1. Barash PG, Cullen BF, Stoelting RK (eds): Clinical Anesthesia, 2nd ed. Philadelphia, J.B. Lippincott, 1992.
2. Goldmann DR, Brown FH, Guarniere DM (eds): Perioperative Medicine: The Medical Care of the Surgical Patient, 2nd ed. New York, McGraw-Hill, 1994.
3. Guyton AC (ed): Textbook of Medical Physiology, 8th ed. Philadelphia, W.B. Saunders, 1991.
4. Hirsch IA, Tomlinson DL, Slogoff S, Keats AS: The overstated risk of preoperative hypokalemia. Anesth Analg 67:131-136, 1988.
5. Holliday MA, Segar WE: The maintenance need for water in parenteral fluid therapy. Pediatrics 19:823–832, 1957.
6. Katz J, Benumof JL, Kadis LB (eds): Anesthesia and Uncommon Diseases, 3rd ed. Philadelphia, W.B. Saunders, 1990.
7. Kokko JP, Tannen RL (eds): Fluids and Electrolytes, 2nd ed. Philadelphia, W.B. Saunders, 1990.
8. Miller RD (ed): Anesthesia, 4th ed. New York, Churchill Livingstone, 1994.
9. Schwartz SI (ed): Principles of Surgery, 5th ed. New York, McGraw-Hill, 1989.
10. Sterns RH, Cox M, Feig PU, Singer IS: Internal potassium balance and the control of the plasma potassium concentration. Medicine 60:339, 1981.
11. Stoelting RK (ed): Pharmacology and Physiology in Anesthetic Practice. Philadelphia, J.B. Lippincott, 1987.
12. Vitez TS, Soper LE, Wong KC, Soper P: Chronic hypokalemia and intraoperative dysrhythmias. Anesthesiology 63:130-133, 1985.

5. HEMOTHERAPY

Jeremy J. Katz, M.D.

1. What is the average human blood volume?

In a 70-kg man, total body water comprises about 60% of body mass or about 42 L of fluid. This is divided between the intracellular compartment (40% of body mass or 28 L) and the extracellular compartment (20% of body mass or 14 L). The extracellular compartment is divided into the interstitial space (15.7% of body mass or 11 L) and plasma volume (4.3% of body mass or 3 L). The total intravascular blood volume is comprised of approximately 3 L of plasma plus 2 L of red cells for a total volume of about 5 L (see figure). Total body water volumes vary with age, sex, weight, and body habitus. The estimated total blood volume (EBV) of an average adult male is about 75 ml/kg and that of the average female about 65 ml/kg. Females have a greater percentage of adipose tissue which is less vascular compared to other tissues.

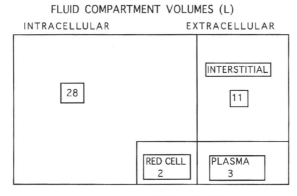

FLUID COMPARTMENT VOLUMES (L)

TOTAL BLOOD VOLUME = 5L

Volumes (L) of different body compartments (in a 70-kg male).

2. Are particular types of surgery associated with blood transfusion?

The need for blood transfusion can be anticipated during major vascular surgery, cardiopulmonary bypass, liver transplantation, hepatectomy, multiple trauma, radical prostatectomy, spinal surgery, total hip replacement, and craniofacial reconstruction, to name a few.

3. How is blood loss estimated?

There is no absolutely reliable way to estimate blood loss. Sometimes vast differences of opinion exist between surgeons and anesthesiologists in the estimation of blood loss. Close attention should be directed to observing blood suctioned from the surgical field and that lost into surgical sponges and drapes. During cases with extensive third space fluid loss and major fluid resuscitation, estimation of blood loss becomes even more difficult and serial hematocrits should be drawn. One way of estimating an "acceptable" blood loss prior to considering transfusion is as follows (illustrated with an example of a 60-kg man with a preoperative hematocrit of 42%):

- estimate total blood volume (TBV)

  TBV (ml) = weight (kg) × EBV (ml/kg)

  [TBV = 60 kg × 75 ml/kg = 4500 ml]

- estimate red blood cell volume (RBCV) at preoperative hematocrit ($RBCV_p$)

$$RBCV_p \text{ (ml)} = TBV \text{ (ml)} \times \frac{\text{preoperative hematocrit}}{100}$$

[$RBCV_p$ (ml) = 4500 ml $\times$ 0.42 = 1890 ml]

- estimate RBCV at hematocrit of 30% ($RBCV_{30}$)

$RBCV_{30}$ (ml) = TBV $\times$ 0.3

[$RBCV_{30}$ (ml) = 4500 $\times$ 0.3 = 1500 ml]

- allowable RBCV (ml) loss to reduce hematocrit to 30% = $RBCV_p - RBCV_{30}$

RBCV loss (ml) = 1890 ml – 1500 ml = 390 ml

- Then acceptable blood loss to reduce hematocrit to 30% (ml) = RBCV $\times \frac{100}{30}$

Allowing for conversion of red cell volume to blood volume at hematocrit of 30:
[acceptable blood loss = 390 ml $\times$ 3 = 1070 ml]

4. Is there a relationship between hematocrit and blood flow?

A reduction in hematocrit decreases blood viscosity. This effect is most profound in the postcapillary venules, which have the lowest mean flow velocity in the circulatory system. The lowered hematocrit improves tissue blood flow but at the expense of decreased oxygen-carrying capacity. The optimal hematocrit for tissue oxygen delivery is believed to be 30%.

5. What are the physiologic adaptations to acute normovolemic anemia?

During surgery, acute blood loss is usually replaced with crystalline solutions, and this, combined with the mobilization of interstitial and intracellular fluid that occurs, results in acute normovolemic hemodilution. Compensatory changes include increased cardiac output, redistribution of blood to the tissues that are oxygen supply-dependent (such as the heart and brain), and increased oxygen extraction. The increase in cardiac output is due to factors such as reduced blood viscosity, increased venomotor tone and venous return, and increased sympathetic nervous system activity. Similar changes occur in response to hemorrhagic shock, but the compensatory changes may be overwhelmed in severe or prolonged shock.

6. What is an acceptable preoperative hematocrit?

There is still no definitive answer. Elective surgery has been successfully performed in patients with preoperative hemoglobin levels as low as 6 g/dl, provided blood loss is kept to less than 500 ml. Clinical studies have also shown no increased morbidity or mortality in patients with perioperative anemia with hematocrits of 20–22%. There is no evidence that anemia increases the frequency or severity of postoperative infection or prolongs recovery in surgical patients.

The situation differs in patients with coexisting systemic disease, particularly impaired cardiac function. The myocardium, compared to other tissues, extracts by far the largest percentage of delivered oxygen and is most susceptible to a reduction in oxygen delivery. Less healthy patients demonstrate myocardial ischemia at a higher level of hemoglobin compared to more healthy patients.

7. What are current criteria for perioperative red cell transfusion?

It is unrealistic to expect that a specific number or value such as hematocrit or oxygen delivery can be applied to all situations as a "trigger" for transfusion. In the context of anemia and hypovolemia, there is a minimum hemoglobin value for each individual below which organ impairment is likely to occur. According to the Consensus Conference on Perioperative Red Blood Cell Transfusion, rigid adherence to the transfusion criterion of a hemoglobin concentration of less than 100 g/L is no longer acceptable.

The decision to transfuse a specific patient should combine good clinical judgment with laboratory data. Considerations include the duration of anemia, intravascular volume status, the extent of the operation, the probability of massive blood loss, and the presence of coexisting systemic disease, particularly cardiac disease. In the absence of cardiovascular instability, perioperative transfusion should be considered at these hematocrit values:

	Hematocrit
Healthy patients	18%
Patients with well-compensated systemic disease	24%
Patients with symptomatic cardiac disease	30%

8. What can be done to try to minimize intraoperative blood loss?

Rigorous hemostasis and avoidance of intraoperative hypertension are useful. Deliberate hypotension with anesthetic drugs or vasodilators is also effective. Regional anesthesia has been shown to reduce intraoperative blood loss, particularly in orthopedic surgery and craniofacial surgery.

9. For what is donor blood screened?

Donated blood is tested for blood group antigens and infectious disease markers. ABO and Rh antigen status are determined, and an antibody screen is performed to detect any unexpected red cell antibodies.

Infectious disease markers tested for include:
- Syphilis
- Viral hepatitis:
  Hepatitis B: hepatitis B surface antigen and antibody to hepatitis B core antigen assays
  Hepatitis C: antibody to hepatitis C virus assay
  Alanine aminotransferase: measured as a surrogate marker of nonspecific liver infection
- Retroviruses:
  Human immunodeficiency virus: antibodies to HIV-1 and HIV-2 assays
  Human T-cell lymphotropic virus-type I/II: antibody to HTLV-I/II assay

10. What types of red cell products are available?

- Red blood cells:
  —a unit with citrate, phosphate, dextrose-adenine (CPDA-1) anticoagulant has a volume of 300 ml with a hematocrit of about 65–80%; addition of additive solutions reduces the hematocrit to approximately 55%;
  —indicated for increasing oxygen-carrying capacity and volume expansion for significant hemorrhage.
- Red blood cells deglycerolized:
  —stored in the frozen state;
  —indicated for prolonged storage of rare red cells.
- Leukocyte-reduced red blood cells:
  —indicated for patients with a history of previous febrile transfusion reactions.
- Washed red blood cells:
  —useful in patients who have had previous severe allergic reactions.
- Whole blood:
  —rarely used;
  —obtained only with increasing difficulty; packed red cells are transfused in cases of less severe blood loss preserving plasma and other components for other patients;
  —indicated only for symptomatic deficit in oxygen-carrying capacity together with hypovolemia of sufficient degree to be associated with shock;
  —the usual unit contains about 500 ml of anticoagulated blood with a hematocrit of 35%–40%.

Federal regulation determines the duration of blood storage and requires that at least 70% of transfused red blood cells survive 24 hours after transfusion. Whole blood or red cells may be stored for 35 days with the anticoagulant preservative solution CPDA-1, and for 42 days when AS-1 (Adsol) or AS-3 (Nutrice) are added.

11. How should red blood cells be administered?
Suitable diluents include normal saline and isosmolar non-calcium-containing solutions, but the safest practice is to use only normal saline. Saline dilution will facilitate infusion and minimize hemolysis. Hypotonic solutions such as 5% dextrose should not be used to avoid hemolysis or cell clumping, and calcium-containing solutions should also be avoided to prevent clot formation.

A standard blood administration set with a pore size of 170 μm is recommended for infusion of red cell components. If only 1 or 2 units of blood are slowly administered to normothermic adult patients, warming of blood is not necessary. Warming is appropriate with rapid transfusion of large amounts of cold blood in pediatric patients and those recipients with potent cold agglutinins.

12. What happens when a type and screen is ordered?
The patient's blood is **typed** for ABO and Rh group and then **screened** for antibodies. The patient's red cells are tested against standardized commercially available anti-A and anti-B reagents for determination of the patient's ABO type. The patient's serum is also incubated with group A and B red blood cells to demonstrate the presence of the corresponding isoagglutinins.

The antibody screen has three phases and performance takes about 45 minutes. The patient's serum is tested against specially selected red cells containing all relevant blood group antigens for detection of clinically significant antibodies.

The donor's serum is also screened for unexpected antibodies to prevent their introduction into the recipient.

13. What is the difference between a type and screen and crossmatch?
In 1984 the Food and Drug Administration modified standards and regulations to permit blood to be released for transfusion without a crossmatch, provided certain criteria are met.

If blood is needed for transfusion and the antibody screen is negative, only an "abbreviated" partial crossmatch is done. The patient's serum and red cells from selected donor units are mixed and spun for 15 seconds—testing only for ABO and Rh type. Units can be released within approximately 5 minutes. A full crossmatch is usually performed after the blood is released.

If blood is needed for transfusion and the antibody screen is positive, then a crossmatch is necessary, requiring about 45 minutes for completion. Instead of the patient's serum being tested against commercially available red cells containing known antigens, the serum is tested against red cells from selected donor units. In addition to verifying ABO and Rh compatibility, the crossmatch detects more unique antibodies.

Degree of Crossmatch	Chance of Compatible Transfusion
ABO-Rh type only	99.8%
ABO-Rh type + antibody screen	99.94%
ABO-Rh type + antibody screen + crossmatch	99.95%

14. What type of blood should be used in an emergency situation?
Urgent need for blood may require incomplete compatibility testing. If time does not allow for complete crossmatching, the following may be transfused:
- type-specific, partially crossmatched
- type-specific, uncrossmatched
- type O, Rh negative, uncrossmatched.

Type O blood lacks both A and B antigens and cannot be hemolyzed by anti-A or anti-B antibodies in the recipient's serum. The use of O red blood cells, which contain a small volume of plasma and are almost free of hemolytic antibodies, is preferred to that of whole blood.

The patient may be switched back to type-specific blood even after transfusion of up to 10 units of type O red blood cells. When 2 or more units of type O, Rh-negative, noncrossmatched blood have been transfused, the patient should not be transfused with his or her type-specific blood until the blood bank has determined that the levels of transfused anti-A and anti-B antibodies have fallen to levels low enough to permit the transfusion.

Clerical or management system errors are the most frequent causes of ABO-incompatible transfusions. Each unit of blood should be checked prior to transfusion by two individuals to verify that the patient's name and identification number are the same as those on the blood unit. Expiration date, ABO, and Rh type should also be checked and the unit inspected for evidence of bacterial contamination such as discoloration, bubbles, and clots.

15. What are some of the complications of massive blood transfusion?
Massive transfusion is defined as the acute administration of more than one blood volume within several hours. Complications include:
- Coagulopathy due to:
    dilutional thrombocytopenia
    lack of coagulation factors V ad VIII (labile factors)
    DIC—associated with hypoperfusion or hemolytic reaction
- Metabolic problems (related to blood storage):
    hyperkalemia
    citrate toxicity
    acidosis
    impaired oxygen-carrying capacity (due to reduced 2,3,DPG concentration)
    hypothermia

16. By how much will transfusion of a unit of red cells increase the hematocrit?
Red cell units have a volume of about 310 ml of blood, plus anticoagulant and preservative. The hematocrit varies from 55–80%, depending on the method of preparation. One unit of red cells will increase the hematocrit by 3% and the hemoglobin by 1 g/dl in the average adult.

17. What are the risks of transfusion of infectious agents?
Human hepatitis viruses are the most frequently transmitted infectious agents. Before the introduction of testing for antibodies for hepatitis C virus, the frequency of transmission of hepatitis was believed to be 3% per transfusion episode. The risk of transmission of hepatitis C is currently estimated at 1:100 or less per unit and that of human immunodeficiency virus between 1:250,000 and 1:500,000 per unit. Bacteria, spirochetes, and parasites may also be transmitted.

18. What type of transfusion reactions may occur?
- Hemolytic transfusion reactions
- Allergic reactions
- Febrile nonhemolytic transfusion reactions

19. How is a hemolytic transfusion reaction managed?
Most hemolytic transfusion reactions are caused by anti-A or anti-B antibodies during an ABO incompatible transfusion. They may occur immediately (during or shortly after a transfusion) or later (5–7 days after transfusion).

Clinical manifestations include fever, chills, chest, flank and back pain, hypotension, nausea, flushing, diffuse bleeding, oliguria or anuria, and hemoglobinuria. General anesthesia may mask some of the clinical manifestations, and hypotension, hemoglobinuria, and diffuse bleeding may be the only visible signs.

When a reaction occurs, the following should be done:
- Stop the transfusion immediately and remove the blood tubing.
- Alert the blood bank and send a recipient and donor blood specimen for compatibility testing.

- Treat hypotension aggressively with IV fluids and pressor agents as needed.
- Maintain urine output.
  —Treat initially with IV fluid and mannitol. Use diuretics and renal-dose dopamine if urine output is not maintained.
- Massive hemolysis can release potassium—monitor potassium levels.
- DIC may occur—the best treatment is identifying and treating the underlying cause.
- Check urine and plasma hemoglobin levels.
- Verify hemolysis with direct antiglobulin (Coombs) test, bilirubin, and plasma haptoglobin levels.
- Perform baseline coagulation studies—PT, PTT, platelet count, fibrinogen level.

20. What alternatives are there to homologous blood transfusion?

- Autologous transfusion—the collection and reinfusion of the patient's own blood
- Perioperative blood salvage—the collection and reinfusion of blood lost during and immediately after surgery
- Intraoperative isovolemic hemodilution—the reduction of hematocrit or hemoglobin by withdrawal of blood and the simultaneous volume replacement with cell-free substitutes
- Use of substitute products for replacement of plasma and blood volume

The primary goal is maintaining perfusion with adequate intravascular volume replacement. Provided therapy is appropriately monitored and fluids given at an appropriate rate, any solution will adequately restore volume status. Replacement solutions include various crystalloid and colloid products that do not provide additional oxygen-carrying capacity. Research is being carried out into the use of non-blood oxygen-carrying solutions, including stroma-free hemoglobin solutions, polymerized hemoglobin, and perfluorochemicals, but none is yet available for widespread clinical use.

Comparison of Various Replacement Solutions

Physiologic crystalloid solutions (replacement volume is about three times that of blood loss because of distribution to the extracellular space; has only a transient effect)

Normal saline:	Iso-osmotic, mild hypernatremia and hyperchloremia with large volumes
Balanced salt (e.g., Ringer's lactate):	Hypotonic, causes fewer electrolyte disturbances

Colloids (replacement volume equal to that of blood lost)

Albumin (5% or 25%):	Overhydration; pulmonary edema, particularly with use of 25% solution, due to absorption of interstitial fluid into the vascular compartment
Hetastarch (Hespan):	Affects coagulation—use moderate amounts < 20 ml/kg
Dextrans (40 or 70):	Potential for anaphylaxis, interference with platelet, red cell function, and blood crossmatching

21. Should all autologous blood be returned to the donor?

Autologous blood is the safest possible transfusion product, but its administration is not without hazards such as clerical handling errors or contamination at time of collection. Less stringent indications for transfusion may be applied, but blood should be given only when anemia is present, when significant blood loss has occurred, or when additional bleeding is expected.

BIBLIOGRAPHY

1. American Society of Anesthesiologists: Committee on Transfusion Medicine: Questions and Answers about Transfusion Practices. Park Ridge, IL, American Society of Anesthesiologists, 1992, pp 1–44.
2. Christopherson R, Frank S: Low postoperative hematocrit is associated with cardiac ischemia in high-risk patients. Anesthesiology 75:A99, 1991.
3. Consensus Conference: Perioperative red blood cell transfusion. JAMA 260:2700–2703, 1988.

4. Cosby HT: Perioperative hemotherapy. I. Indications for blood component transfusion. Can J Anaesth 39:695–707, 1992.
5. Delima LGR, Wynands JE: Oxygen transport. Can J Anaesth 40:R81–86, 1993.
6. Irving GA: Perioperative blood and blood component therapy. Can J Anaesth 39:1105–1115, 1992.
7. Leone BJ, Spahn DR: Anemia, hemodilution and oxygen delivery. Anesth Analg 75:651–653, 1992.
8. Managing fluid, electrolytes and blood loss. In Longnecker DE, Murphy FL (eds): Introduction to Anesthesia. Philadelphia, W.B. Saunders, 1992, pp 166–167.
9. Mesmer KM: Hemodilution. Surg Clin North Am 55:659–678, 1975.
10. Miller RD: Transfusion therapy. In Miller RD (ed): Anesthesia. New York, Churchill Livingstone, 1994, pp 1619–1646.
11. Ramsay JG: Methods of reducing blood loss and non-blood substitutes. Can J Anaesth 38:595–612, 1991.
12. Rose D, Coutsoftides T: Intraoperative normovolemic hemodilution. J Surg Res 31:375–381, 1981.
13. Stehling L, Zauder HL: How low can we go? Is there a way to know? Transfusion 30:1–3, 1990.
14. Tremper KT: Techniques and solutions to avoid homologous blood transfusions. Refresher Courses in Anesthesiology. The American Society of Anesthesiologists, Inc. Philadelphia, J.B. Lippincott, 1994, pp 251–262.
15. Transfusion Alert. Use of Autologous Blood. NIH Publication No. 89-3038. U.S. Department of Health and Human Services, 1989, pp 1–16.
16. Welch HG, Meehan KR, Goodnough LT: Prudent strategies for elective red blood cell transfusion. Ann Intern Med 116:393–402, 1992.

6. COAGULATION

Jeremy J. Katz, M.D.

1. How does one identify the patient at risk for bleeding?

The most important factor is an accurate medical history. Questions about medications, including anticoagulants, nonsteroidal antiinflammatory agents, and aspirin; excessive or abnormal bleeding; and medical conditions known to be associated with bleeding disorders identify most at-risk patients. Platelet disorders usually present with petechial hemorrhages of the mucous membranes and skin, whereas clotting factor disorders have a more pronounced clinical picture with spontaneous intramuscular, joint, gastrointestinal, and intracranial hemorrhages. Inherited disorders usually present early in life with a positive family history. Previous major surgery without transfusion indicates the absence of an inherited coagulation disorder.

2. How useful are clotting function screening tests?

Prothrombin time (PT) and partial thromboplastin time (PTT), although useful in screening patients with a history of bleeding, have not been shown to have any value as screening tests in asymptomatic patients. Likewise, the routine use of bleeding times to assess platelet function in patients taking aspirin may have little value because of the small correlation between bleeding times and clinical hemorrhage.

3. What are the main components of the hemostatic mechanism?

The four main components of the hemostatic response are vascular reactivity, platelet activity, coagulation, and fibrinolysis. When ruptured, the microvascular system undergoes local reflex vasoconstriction. Simultaneous dilatation of adjacent arterioles diverts local blood flow from the bleeding site. Interaction between the blood vessels and platelets results in the temporary cessation of bleeding by the formation of a platelet plug. Coagulation is the organization of the platelet plug by fibrin formation. Fibrinolysis is the removal of fibrin to reestablish normal blood flow.

4. What is the function of the vascular endothelium?

Normally the vascular endothelium prevents blood from coagulating by secreting coagulation inhibitors such as:
- Glycocalyx, a mucopolysaccharide that prevents the interaction of platelets and coagulation proteins with collagen;
- Adenosine diphosphatase (ADPase), which decreases platelet adhesion by inactivating adenosine diphosphate (ADP);
- Prostacyclin (PGI2), a potent vasodilator and platelet aggregation inhibitor; and
- Protein C, which activates plasminogen and furthers fibrinolysis.

If endothelial integrity is broken, the collagen exposed in the subendothelial layers begins the coagulation process by allowing platelet adherence and activation.

5. How do platelets function in the coagulation process?

The platelet membrane enables physical interaction between the vascular endothelium and platelets. It also makes possible platelet interaction with the protein coagulation cascade. The platelet phospholipid, platelet factor 3 (PF3), limits coagulation to the site of platelet aggregation. Activated platelets also release the contents of their granules, including thromboxane A2 and ADP. Thromboxane A2 causes blood vessel constriction and increases ADP release, resulting in additional platelet aggregation and activation.

6. What is an acceptable preoperative platelet count?

A normal platelet count is 150,000–440,000/mm^3. Thrombocytopenia is defined as a count of <150,000/mm^3. Intraoperative bleeding can be severe with counts of 40,000–70,000/mm^3, and spontaneous bleeding usually occurs at counts < 20,000/mm^3. The minimal recommended platelet count before surgery is 75,000/mm^3. Although prophylactic preoperative platelet transfusion is generally advocated to treat preexisting thrombocytopenia, the methods of evaluating clinical need are imprecise.

Qualitative differences in platelet function make it unwise to rely on platelet number as the sole criterion for transfusion. Thrombocytopenic patients with accelerated destruction but active production of platelets have relatively less bleeding than patients with hypoplastic disorders at a given platelet count.

Assessment of preoperative platelet function is further complicated by lack of correlation between bleeding time or any other test of platelet function and a tendency to increased intraoperative bleeding. However, normal bleeding times range from 4–9 minutes, and a bleeding time >1½ times normal (>15 min) is considered significantly abnormal.

7. List the causes of platelet abnormalities.

1. **Quantitative platelet disorders**—thrombocytopenia
   • Dilution after massive blood transfusion
   • Decreased platelet production due to malignant infiltration (aplastic anemia, multiple myeloma), drugs (chemotherapy, cytotoxic drugs, ethanol, hydrochlorothiazide), radiation exposure, or bone marrow depression after viral infection
   • Increased peripheral destruction due to hypersplenism, disseminated intravascular coagulation (DIC), extensive tissue and vascular damage after extensive burns, or immune mechanisms (idiopathic thrombocytopenic purpura, drugs such as heparin, autoimmune diseases)
2. **Qualitative platelet disorders**
   • Inherited (e.g., von Willebrand disease)
   • Acquired (uremia; cirrhosis, particularly after ethanol; drugs, such as aspirin, nonsteroidal antiinflammatory agents)

8. How does aspirin act as an anticoagulant?

Primary hemostasis is controlled by the balance between the opposing actions of two prostaglandins, thromboxane A2 and prostacyclin. Depending on the dose, salicylates produce a differential effect on prostaglandin synthesis in platelets and vascular endothelial cells. Lower doses preferentially inhibit platelet cyclooxygenase, impeding thromboxane A2 production and inhibiting platelet aggregation. The effect begins within 2 hours of ingestion. Platelets lack a cell nucleus and cannot produce protein. Aspirin effect therefore lasts for the entire life of the platelet (7–10 days). Nonsteroidal antiinflammatory drugs have a similar but more transient effect than aspirin, lasting for only 1–3 days after cessation of use.

9. Discuss the intrinsic and extrinsic coagulation pathways.

The coagulation cascade requires sequential activation of inactive procoagulant molecules into active cleavage enzymes or serine proteases. Factors V and VIII are the labile factors that serve as cofactors in the cascade. The process of coagulation requires the presence of a phospholipid surface. The intrinsic pathway of coagulation occurs within the blood vessel with platelet phospholipid (PF3) as a catalyst. The extrinsic pathway occurs outside the blood vessel, beginning with the release of tissue thromboplastin (tissue phospholipid) from injured tissues. The phospholipid surface provides a site for the interaction of a complex reaction consisting of the phospholipid surface, calcium, and the activated substrate procoagulant clotting factor. Traditionally, the extrinsic and intrinsic pathways have been considered separate pathways that merge after the formation of activated factor X. In reality they have interrelated steps. The classic two-pathway concept is still useful for the interpretation of in vitro coagulation tests.

10. Discuss factor VIII.

Factor VIII is a large plasma protein complex of two noncovalently bound factors, von Willibrand factor (factor VIII:vWF) and factor VIII antigen, which has anticoagulant activity. The manufacture of each is under separate genetic control. Factor VIII:vWF is necessary both for platelet adhesion and formation of the definitive hemostatic plug through regulation and release of factor VIII antigen. In von Willebrand disease there is a decrease of both factor VIII antigen and factor VIII:vWF.

11. How is coagulation localized?

A number of processes regulate coagulation and confine clotting to sites of vascular damage:
- Rapid blood flow dilutes coagulation factors below coagulation threshold levels.
- Activated coagulation factors are preferentially cleared by the liver and reticuloendothelial system.
- Natural anticoagulants exist in the blood: (1) antithrombin III is a plasma protease inhibitor that serves as a protease scavenger and (2) protein C and its cofactor protein S inactivate the active cofactor forms of factors VIII and V.
- Activation of the fibrinolytic system digests fibrin both to prevent and to reopen thrombotic occlusion. Fibrinolysis is mediated primarily by plasmin, which is generated from plasminogen. Tissue plasminogen activator (tPA), which is released from endothelial cells, is the most important activator of plasminogen.

12. How does vitamin K deficiency affect coagulation?

Four clotting factors (II, VII, IX, and X) are synthesized by the liver. Each factor undergoes a final vitamin K–dependent enzymatic reaction that adds a carboxyl moiety to each factor. This moiety enables the factors to bind via calcium to the phospholipid surface. Without vitamin K the factors are produced but are not functional. The extrinsic pathway is affected first by vitamin K deficiency or liver dysfunction because the factor with the shortest half-life is factor VII, found only in the extrinsic pathway. With further deficiency both extrinsic and intrinsic pathways are affected.

The warfarinlike drugs compete with vitamin K for binding sites on the hepatocyte. Administration of subcutaneous vitamin K reverses the functional deficiency in 6–24 hours. With active bleeding or in emergency surgery, fresh frozen plasma (FFP) can be administered for immediate hemostasis.

13. How does heparin act as an anticoagulant?

Heparin is a polyanionic mucopolysaccharide that accelerates the interaction between antithrombin III and the activated forms of factors II, X, XI , XI and XIII, effectively neutralizing each. The half-life of heparin's anticoagulant effect is about 90 minutes in a normothermic patient. Patients with reduced levels of antithrombin III are resistant to the effect of heparin. Heparin also may affect platelet function and number through an immunologically mediated mechanism, either acutely or after 5–10 days of exposure.

14. Describe the different coagulation tests.

The basic difference between the intrinsic and extrinsic pathways is the phospholipid surface on which the clotting factors interact before union at the common pathway. Either platelet phospholipid (for the intrinsic pathway) or tissue thromboplastin (for the extrinsic pathway) can be added to the patient's plasma, and the time taken for clot formation is measured. Less than 30% of normal factor activity is required for the tests to be sensitive to decreased levels. The tests are also prolonged in cases of decreased fibrinogen concentration (<100 mg/dl^{-1}) and dysfibrinogenemias.

Measurement of the intrinsic and common pathways
1. Partial thromboplastin time (PTT)
   • Partial thromboplastin is substituted for platelet phospholipid and eliminates platelet variability.
   • PTT measures the clotting ability of all factors in the intrinsic and common pathways except factor XIII.
   • Normal PTT is about 40–100 seconds; > 120 seconds is abnormal.
2. Activated PTT (aPTT)
   • An activator is added to the test tube before addition of partial thromboplastin.
   • Maximal activation of the contact factors (XII and XI) eliminates the lengthy natural contact activation phase and results in more consistent and reproducible results.
   • Normal aPTT is 25–35 seconds.
3. Activated clotting time (ACT)
   • Fresh whole blood (providing platelet phospholipid) is added to a test tube already containing an activator.
   • The automated ACT is widely used to monitor heparin therapy in the operating room.
   • Normal range is 90–120 seconds.

Measurement of the extrinsic and common pathways
1. Prothrombin time (PT)
   • Tissue thromboplastin is added to the patient's plasma.
   • Test varies in sensitivity and response to oral anticoagulant therapy whether measured as PT in seconds or simple PT ratio ($PT_{patient}/PT_{normal}$) (normal = the mean normal PT value of the laboratory test system).
   • Normal PT is 10–12 seconds.
2. International normalized ratio (INR)
   • Developed to improve the consistency of oral anticoagulant therapy.
   • Converts the PT ratio to a value that would have been obtained using a standard PT method.
   • INR is calculated as $(PT_{patient}/PT_{normal})^{ISI}$ (ISI is the international sensitivity index assigned to the test system).
   • The recommended therapeutic ranges for standard oral anticoagulant therapy and high-dose therapy, respectively, are INR values of 2.0–3.0 and 2.5–3.5.

15. How is fresh frozen plasma prepared?

Fresh frozen plasma (FFP) is the fluid portion of human blood that has been centrifuged, separated, and frozen within 6 hours of donation. It contains the labile and stable components of the coagulation, fibrinolytic, and complement systems. With appropriate storage and handling, the loss of labile factors V and VIII is less than 30%. FFP should be used within 24 hours of thawing. Only ABO-compatible plasma should be used, employing a standard 170-μm filter.

16. What are the current indications for transfusion of FFP?

The consensus conference on the use of FFP recognized five indications for the use of plasma:
1. Deficiencies of factors II, V, VII, IX, X and XI
2. Reversal of Coumadin effect
3. Pathologic hemorrhage in patients with massive transfusion (> 1 blood volume)
4. Antithrombin III deficiency
5. Immunodeficiencies

There is no justification for use of FFP as a volume expander or as prophylaxis against coagulopathy and untoward bleeding in either massive transfusion or cardiopulmonary bypass.

17. How is platelet concentrate prepared?

Platelet concentrate (PC) is obtained by centrifugation of fresh whole blood to produce supernatant plasma, which is centrifuged again to remove all but about 30–50 ml of plasma. Storage at room temperature preserves function but is limited to 5 days. Platelet concentrate contains 60–80% of the platelets in a unit of fresh whole blood. Single-donor units, obtained by apheresis from a single donor, contain the equivalent of 5-8 units of PC and are reserved for use in patients with platelet antibodies or to avoid the risk of HLA antibody formation. To achieve an increase in platelet count, transfusion should consist of 1 unit of PC for each 10 kg of body weight. The administration of 1 unit of PC should increase the platelet count by 5,000–8,000/mm^3. Administration of ABO-incompatible platelets is accepted practice. The use of a standard 170-μm filter is recommended.

18. What are the current indications for the use of platelets?

The consensus conference on platelet use recognized three indications for platelet transfusion:

1. Clinically significant bleeding in a patient with thrombocytopenia or platelet abnormality
2. Bleeding prophylaxis in patients with severe thrombocytopenia
3. Following massive transfusion with thrombocytopenia and clinically abnormal bleeding; the platelet count at which coagulopathy is demonstrated following transfusion varies but generally is < 100,000/mm^3.

19. How is cryoprecipitate obtained?

Cryoprecipitate is obtained from FFP that is thawed in a controlled way. It contains large quantities of factor VIII, von Willebrand factor, fibrinogen, fibronectin, and factor XIII. Cryoprecipitate can be heat-treated to inactivate human immunodeficiency virus. A single donor unit contains about 100 antihemophiliac units and 250 mg of fibrinogen. Units usually are pooled and should be given through a 170-μm filter.

20. What are the indications for use of cryoprecipitate?

Cryoprecipitate is used for treatment of hemophilia A, von Willebrand disease, and factor XIII deficiency. It is also used in patients following massive transfusion who may need additional factor VIII and fibrinogen.

21. What is DIC?

Disseminated intravascular coagulation (DIC) is not a disease entity but rather a manifestation of disease associated with various well-defined clinical entities:

- Obstetric conditions (amniotic fluid embolism, placental abruption, retained fetus syndrome, eclampsia, saline-induced abortion)
- Intravascular hemolysis (hemolytic transfusion syndromes, minor hemolysis, massive transfusion)
- Septicemia (gram-negative—endotoxin; gram-positive—mucopolysaccharides)
- Viremias (cytomegalovirus, hepatitis, varicella, HIV)
- Disseminated malignancy
- Leukemia
- Burns
- Crush injury and tissue necrosis
- Liver disease (obstructive jaundice, acute hepatic failure)
- Prosthetic devices (LeVeen shunt, aortic balloon)

DIC usually is seen in clinical circumstances in which the extrinsic or intrinsic coagulation pathway or both are activated by circulating phospholipid, leading to generation of thrombin, but the usual mechanisms preventing unbalanced thrombus formation are impaired. After systemic deposition of intravascular fibrin thrombi, consumption of factors V and VIII, and loss of platelets, the resulting circulating level of clotting factors and platelets represents a balance between depletion and production. The fibrinolytic system is activated, and plasmin begins to cleave fibrinogen and fibrin into fibrinogen and fibrin degradation products (FDPs). Recognizing and understanding the syndrome are made difficult by the occurrence of both acute and chronic forms and by a clinical spectrum varying from diffuse thrombosis to diffuse bleeding or both.

22. What tests are used for the diagnosis of DIC?

There is no one pathognomonic test for diagnosis of DIC. In acute DIC, the prothrombin time is elevated in about 75% of patients, whereas PTT is prolonged in 50–60%. Platelet count is typically greatly reduced. Hypofibrinogenemia is common. The D-dimer test is a newer diagnostic test. The D-dimer is a neoantigen formed by the action of thrombin in converting fibrinogen to cross-linked fibrin. It is specific for fibrin degradation products formed from the digestion of cross-linked fibrin by plasmin. In 85–100% of patients, FDPs are elevated. Elevated levels are not diagnostic of DIC but indicate the presence of plasmin and plasmin degradation of fibrinogen or fibrin.

23. Describe the treatment of DIC.

The treatment of DIC is confusing and controversial. The triggering process should be identified and treated accordingly. If bleeding continues, heparin is used to stop the consumption process before administration of specific coagulation products. If these measures fail, specific blood components may be depleted and should be replaced after identification. If bleeding still continues, antifibrinolytic therapy with epsilon aminocaproic acid should be considered, but only if the intravascular coagulation process is shown to have stopped and residual fibrinolysis to continue.

BIBLIOGRAPHY

 1. Bick RL, Scates SM: Disseminated intravascular coagulation. Lab Med 23:161–165, 1992.
 2. Consensus Conference: Fresh frozen plasma: Indications and risks. JAMA 253:551–553, 1985.
 3. Consensus Conference: Platelet transfusion therapy. JAMA 257:1777–1780, 1985.
 4. Cosby HT: Perioperative haemotherapy: I. Indications for blood component transfusion. Can J Anaesth 39:695–707, 1992.
 5. Ellison N: Hemostasis and hemotherapy. In Barash PG, Cullen BF, Stoelting (eds): Clinical Anesthesia. Philadelphia, J.B. Lippincott, 1992, pp 251–264.
 6. Hardy J, Belisle S, Robitaille D: Blood products: When to use them and how to avoid them. Can J Anaesth 41:R52–61, 1994.
 7. Irving GA: Perioperative blood and blood component therapy. Can J Anaesth 39:1105–1115, 1992.
 8. McLaren ID, Crider BA: Monitoring the coagulation system. Anesthesiol Clin North Am 12:211–236, 1994.
 9. Petrovich C: Perioperative evaluation of coagulation. In Refresher Courses in Anesthesiology. Philadelphia, J.B. Lippincott,1992, pp 169–190.
10. Spiess BD: Coagulation function in the operating room. Anesthesiol Clin North Am 481–499, 1990.
11. Stehling L: Indications for perioperative blood transfusion in 1990. Can J. Anaesth 38:601–604, 1991.
12. Tuman KJ: Coagulation and the anesthesiologist. In Review Course Lectures. Cleveland, International Anesthesia Research Society, 1995, pp 82–88.

7. AIRWAY MANAGEMENT

G. Samuel Baker, M.D., and James Duke, M.D.

1. Why is airway management important?

To maintain homeostasis within the human organism, all tissues require oxygen. Although tissues require a surprisingly small oxygen tension (on the order of a few millimeters of pressure), it is essential that delivery be reliable and constant. Hence, maintaining a patent airway and ventilation is paramount. Perhaps because of anatomic abnormalities, acute or chronic illness, or a surgical, diagnostic, or therapeutic procedure, the airway or ventilation may be insufficient to deliver a reliable and constant supply of oxygen to the tissue level. In such instances airway management becomes important. Although achieving a satisfactory airway and maintaining adequate ventilation go hand in hand, airway management during surgical procedures is the focus of this chapter.

2. List several indications for endotracheal intubation.

Indications in the operating room include (1) the need to deliver positive pressure ventilation; (2) protection of the respiratory tract from aspiration of gastric contents; (3) surgical procedures about the head and neck in which the anesthesiologist is unable to support the airway manually; (4) general anesthesia in nonsupine positions in which it is impossible to support the airway; (5) most situations in which neuromuscular paralysis has been instituted; (6) surgical procedures within the chest, abdomen, or cranium; (7) procedures in which intracranial hypertension must be treated; and (8) protection of a healthy lung from a diseased lung to ensure its continued performance (e.g., hemoptysis, empyema, pulmonary abscess). Nonoperative indications include (1) profound disturbances in consciousness with the inability to protect the airway, (2) tracheobronchial toilet, and (3) severe pulmonary and multisystem injury associated with respiratory failure (e.g., severe sepsis, airway obstruction, hypoxemia, and hypercarbia of various etiologies).

Objective measures that suggest the need to intubate include a respiratory rate > 35 breaths per minute, vital capacity < 15 ml/kg in adults and 10 ml/kg in children, inability to generate a negative inspiratory force of 20 mmHg, PaO_2 < 70 mmHg on 40% oxygen, alveolar-arterial (A-a) gradient > 350 mmHg on 100% O_2, $PaCO_2$ > 55 mmHg (except in chronic retainers), and dead space (Vd/Vt) > 0.6.

3. How is the airway assessed?

A patient's airway is assessed by historical interview and physical examination and occasionally through inspection of radiographs, pulmonary function tests, and direct fiberoptic examination. Patients should be questioned about adverse events related to previous episodes that required airway management. For instance, were they informed by an anesthesiologist that they had an unexpectedly difficult airway management problem (i.e., "difficult to ventilate, difficult to intubate")? Have they had a tracheostomy or other surgery about the face and neck? Have they sustained significant burns to these areas? Do they have obstructive sleep apnea or temporomandibular joint (TMJ) dysfunction? Unfortunately, patients and family often gloss over the difficulties that other health care providers have experienced in airway management, because such difficulties rarely if ever manifest in activities of daily living. Close review of the patient chart, particularly anesthetic records, is often helpful.

Physical examination is the single most reliable method of detecting and anticipating difficulties in airway management. First, a general assessment of the patient is indicated. Is the patient able to sit and talk without becoming breathless? Is the patient pale or cyanotic, cachectic or acutely ill? Is the patient receiving chronic oxygen therapy? Is the patient markedly obese or scarred, particularly about the chest and neck? Review the vital signs, particularly pulse oximetry (SpO_2) values.

A **focused exam of the airway** follows. Examine the mouth and oral cavity, noting the extent and symmetry of opening (three fingerbreadths is optimal), the health of the teeth (loose, missing, or cracked teeth should be documented), and the presence of dental appliances. Prominent buck teeth may interfere with the use of a laryngoscope. The size of the tongue is noted (large tongues rarely make airway management impossible, only more difficult), as is the arch of the palate (high arched palates have been associated with difficulty in visualizing the larynx).

The appearance of the **posterior pharynx** may predict difficulty in laryngoscopy and visualization of the larynx. Mallampati has classified patients in classes I–IV based on the visualized structures (a diagram of the visualized structures may be found in the chapter on preoperative evaluation). Visualization of fewer structures (particularly class III and IV) was associated with difficult laryngeal exposure. With the patient sitting erect, mouth fully open, and tongue protruding, grading is based on visualization of the following structures:

Class I: Pharyngeal pillars, entire palate, and uvula visible.

Class II: Pharyngeal pillars and soft palate visible, visualization of uvula obstructed by tongue.

Class III: Soft palate visible but pharyngeal pillars and uvula not visualized.

Class IV: Only hard palate visible with soft palate, pillars, and uvula not visualized.

After examination of the oral cavity is completed, attention is directed at the **size of the mandible and quality of TMJ function**. A short mandibular body (three fingerbreadths) as measured from the mental process to the prominence of the thyroid cartilage (thyromental distance) suggests difficulty in visualizing the larynx. Patients with TMJ dysfunction may have asymmetry or limitations in opening the mouth as well as popping or clicking. Manipulation of the jaw in preparation for laryngoscopy may worsen symptoms postoperatively. Curiously, some patients with TMJ dysfunction have greater difficulty with opening the mouth after general anesthesia and neuromuscular paralysis than when they are awake and cooperative.

Finally, the **anatomy of the neck** is inspected. Again, evidence of prior surgeries (especially tracheostomy) or significant burns is noted. Does the patient have abnormal masses (e.g., hematoma, abscess or cellulitis, lymphadenopathy, goiter, tumor, soft tissue swelling) or tracheal deviation? A short or thick neck may prove problematic. Is the patient especially obese, or does the patient have large breasts (as often in late pregnancy), which may make use of a laryngoscope difficult?

It is also important to have the patient demonstrate the **range of motion of the head and neck**. Preparation for laryngoscopy requires extension of the neck to facilitate visualization. Elderly patients and patients with cervical fusions may have marked limitation of motion. Furthermore, patients with cervical spine disease (disk disease or cervical instability, as in rheumatoid arthritis) may develop neurologic symptoms with motion of the neck. Such problems should be noted and incorporated into the airway management plan. Radiologic views of the neck in flexion and extension also may reveal worrisome cervical instability.

Particularly in patients with **pathology of the head and neck** (such as laryngeal cancer), it is valuable to know the results of indirect laryngoscopy or direct fiberoptic nasolaryngoscopy, which is often performed by otolaryngologists in the course of evaluating such patients. Finally, if history suggests dynamic airway obstruction (as in intrathoracic or extrathoracic masses), **pulmonary function tests**, including flow-volume loops (as discussed in the chapter on pulmonary function testing), may alert the clinician to the potential for loss of airway once paralytic agents are administered. Anatomic differences between adult and pediatric airways are discussed in the chapter on pediatric anesthesia.

4. Discuss the anatomy of the larynx.
The larynx, located in adults at cervical levels 4–6, protects the entrance of the respiratory tract as well as allows phonation. It is composed of **three unpaired cartilages** (thyroid, cricoid, and epiglottis) and **three paired cartilages** (arytenoid, corniculate, and cuneiform). The thyroid

cartilage is the largest and most prominent, forming the anterior and lateral walls. The cricoid cartilage is shaped like a signet ring, faces posteriorly, and is the only complete cartilaginous ring of the laryngotracheal tree. The cricothyroid membrane connects these structures anteriorly. The epiglottis extends superiorly into the hypopharynx and covers the entrance of the larynx during swallowing. The corniculate and cuneiform pairs of cartilages are relatively small and do not figure prominently in the laryngoscopic appearance of the larynx or in its function. The arytenoid cartilages articulate upon the posterior aspect of the larynx and are the posterior attachments of the vocal ligaments (or cords). Identification of the arytenoid cartilages may be important during laryngoscopy. In a patient with an "anterior" airway, the arytenoids may be the only visible structures. Finally, the vocal cords attach anteriorly to the thyroid cartilage.

The **innervation of the larynx** consists of the superior laryngeal and recurrent laryngeal nerves, both of which are branches of the vagus nerve. The superior laryngeal nerves decussate into internal and external branches. The internal branches provide sensory innervation of the larynx above the vocal cords, whereas the external branches provide motor innervation to the cricothyroid muscle, a tensor of the vocal cords. The recurrent laryngeal nerves provide sensory innervation below the level of the cords and motor innervation of the posterior cricoarytenoid muscles, the only abductors of the vocal cords. The glossopharyngeal or ninth cranial nerve provides sensory innervation to the vallecula (the space anterior to the epiglottis, a point of contact for curved, Macintosh laryngoscope blades) and the base of the tongue.

Laryngoscopy and endotracheal intubation are **potent noxious stimuli** because of the rich innervation of these structures. The procedures produce marked autonomic discharge. Strategies must be developed to abolish such profound stimulating effects, particularly in patients with coronary artery disease or systemic or intracranial hypertension and patients in whom awake intubation is planned.

Arteries that supply the larynx include the superior laryngeal (a branch of the superior thyroid artery) and inferior laryngeal (a branch of the inferior thyroid) arteries. Venous drainage follows the same pattern as the arteries; there is also ample lymphatic drainage.

5. Discuss the various instruments available to facilitate airway management, especially endotracheal intubation.

The devices, adjuncts, and tubes developed to facilitate airway management and intubation are a tribute to the ingenuity of many individuals; they are also a testament to the anticipated and unexpected difficulties that arise, if not frequently, at least with regularity. The devices described below are divided roughly into those that enhance oxygenation, those which maintain the airway without endotracheal intubation, those that are associated with direct laryngoscopy and intubation, and those that are used for a difficult or awake intubation.

Oxygen supplementation is always a priority when patients are sedated or anesthetized, when the airway is compromised, or when disease processes make tissue oxygenation problematic. Devices range from nasal cannulas, face tents, and simple masks to masks with reservoirs and masks that can be used to deliver positive pressure ventilation. Their limitation is the concentration of oxygen that can be delivered effectively. The limitations and advantages of many such devices are discussed in detail in the chapter on respiratory therapy.

Devices that help to maintain a patent airway short of endotracheal intubation include oral airways, nasal airways, and laryngeal mask airways. **Oral airways** are usually constructed of hard plastic; they are available in numerous sizes and shaped to curve behind the tongue, lifting it off the posterior pharynx. The importance of these simple devices cannot be overstated, because the tongue is the most frequent cause of airway obstruction, particularly in obtunded patients. Oral airways, which tend to be poorly tolerated in awake, semiconscious, and lightly anesthetized patients, are best inserted under direct visualization, using depressors to manipulate the tongue. Blindly inserting the airway upside down and turning it 180° once it is in the mouth may push the tongue against the posterior pharynx or traumatize oral structures. **Nasal airways** ("trumpets") can be gently inserted down the nasal passages into the nasopharynx and are better tolerated than oral airways in awake or lightly anesthetized patients.

Laryngeal mask airways (LMAs) are useful in maintaining an airway during anesthesia when endotracheal intubation may not be desired (e.g., asthmatic patients, Luciano Pavarotti). In appropriately chosen patients (with difficult airways but no high risk for aspiration), LMAs may prove a successful management strategy. Fiberoptic endotracheal intubation through an LMA also may be performed; all the while the patient is oxygenated and ventilated. LMAs come in various adult and pediatric sizes. They are poorly tolerated in unanesthetized patients.

Laryngoscopes are left-handed tools designed to facilitate visualization of the larynx. The handles are designed for a number of different battery sizes. Some handles are short and work best for patients with obese, thick chests or large breasts.

Laryngoscope blades also come in various styles and sizes. The most commonly used blades include the curved Macintosh (no. 3 or 4) and the straight Miller blades (no. 2 or 3). The curved blades are inserted into the vallecula, immediately anterior to the epiglottis, which is literally flipped out of the visual axis to expose the laryngeal opening. The Miller blade is inserted past the epiglottis, which is simply lifted out of the way of laryngeal viewing. Clinicians usually have a favorite blade, but facility in the use of both is needed. Many agree that in difficult airways, when the larynx is situated anterior to the visual axis or the epiglottis is particularly long or floppy, the straight blade frequently affords improved visualization. An incandescent bulb at the end of the laryngoscope may be the source of illumination, or fiberoptic cables may transmit very bright, high-quality illumination from a light source in the handle.

Endotracheal tubes come in a multitude of sizes and shapes. They are commonly manufactured from polyvinyl chloride, with a radiopaque line from top to bottom, standard size connectors for anesthesia circuits or self-inflating resuscitation bags, a high-volume, low-pressure cuff and pilot balloon, and a hole in the beveled, distal end (the Murphy eye). Internal diameter ranges from 2.0–10.0 mm in half millimeter increments. Endotracheal tubes may be reinforced with wire, designed with laser applications in mind, or unusually shaped so that they are directed away from the surgical site (oral or nasal Rae tubes). A recently developed product, the Lita tube, has an injection port and orifices about the endotracheal cuff for instillation of local anesthetic to the airway, providing local anesthesia, which improves tolerance of the endotracheal tube. The Lita tube may be advantageous when testing of surgical repairs (ventral hernias) or increases in intracranial or intraocular pressure secondary to coughing or bucking are undesirable. Double-lumen endotracheal tubes are designed so that one lung may be isolated from the other to facilitate surgery within a hemithorax or to provide differential ventilation to the lungs.

6. What devices and maneuvers are available for patients who are difficult to intubate?

A few available devices that are not often used by clinicians skilled in intubation and fiberoptic endoscopy include the esophageal obturator and combitube. Although they usually can be found in "difficult airway" carts, they find little if any use within most hospital settings.

When inserted into an endotracheal tube, **light wands** may be useful for blind intubation of the trachea. The technique is termed "blind" because the laryngeal opening is not seen directly. When light is well transilluminated through the neck (the jack-o'-lantern effect), the end of the endotracheal tube is at the entrance of the larynx, and the tube can be threaded off the wand and into the trachea in a blind fashion. **Gum elastic bougies** are flexible, somewhat malleable stylets with an anteriorly directed, bent tip that may be useful for intubating a tracheal opening anterior to the visual axis.

Fiberoptic endoscopy is commonly used to facilitate difficult intubations (when visualization with regular laryngoscopes proves impossible). The endoscope is introduced into the nose or mouth of a sedated patient with a topically anesthetized airway or an unconscious, anesthetized patient. Anatomic structures are identified, and the larynx and trachea are entered under direct visualization.

Finally, the trachea may be intubated using a **retrograde technique**. In simplistic terms, a long Seldinger-type wire is introduced through a catheter that punctures the cricothyroid membrane. The wire is directed superiorly and brought out through the nose or mouth, and an endotracheal tube is threaded over the wire and lowered into the trachea.

7. Describe rapid-sequence induction (RSI). Which patients are best managed in this fashion?

It is easiest to appreciate the distinctions of RSI if an induction under non–rapid-sequence conditions is understood. Ordinarily the patient has fasted for at least 6–8 hours and is not at risk for a full stomach and gastric aspiration. The patient is preoxygenated, and an agent is administered to render the patient unconscious. Once it is established that the patient can be satisfactorily mask-ventilated, a muscle relaxant is administered. The patient is then mask-ventilated until complete paralysis is ensured by electrical nerve stimulation. Laryngoscopy and endotracheal intubation are undertaken, and the case proceeds.

In contrast, RSI is undertaken in patients who are thought to have an airway that can be quickly intubated and controlled with direct laryngoscopy but who are at risk for pulmonary aspiration of gastric contents. Aspiration is a serious anesthetic complication with significant potential morbidity (see chapter 45). Patients with full stomachs are thought to be at risk; other risk factors include pregnancy, diabetes, pain, opioid analgesics, recent traumatic injury, intoxication, and pathologic involvement of the gastrointestinal tract, such as small bowel obstruction. Patients at risk for full stomach should be premedicated with agents that reduce the acidity and volume of gastric contents, such as histamine-2 receptor blockers (ranitidine, cimetidine), nonparticulate antacids (Bicitra or Alka-Seltzer), and gastrokinetics, when appropriate (metaclopramide).

The goal of RSI is to secure and control the airway rapidly. The patient is preoxygenated. An induction agent is administered, followed quickly by a rapid-acting relaxant (either succinylcholine or rocuronium) in high doses. Simultaneously an assistant applies pressure to the cricoid cartilage (the only complete cartilaginous ring of the respiratory tract), which closes off the esophagus and prevents entry of regurgitated gastric contents into the trachea and lungs. Known as the Sellick maneuver, such pressure is maintained until the airway is protected by tracheal intubation.

8. Describe the indications for an awake intubation.

If the physical exam leaves in question the ability to ventilate and intubate adequately once the patient is anesthetized and paralyzed, serious consideration should be given to awake intubation. Patients with a previous history of difficult intubation, acute processes that compromise the airway (e.g., soft-tissue infections of the head and neck, hematomas), mandibular fractures or other significant facial deformities, morbid obesity, or cancer involving the larynx are prudent candidates for awake intubation.

9. How is awake intubation performed?

A frank discussion with the patient is necessary. The anticipated difficulty of airway management and the risks of proceeding with anesthesia without previously securing a competent airway are conveyed in clear terms. Compassion and concern for patient safety are priorities.

Preparation of the operative suite is also important. Topical local anesthetics, intravenous sedatives, a selection of oral and nasal airways and endotracheal tubes, suction, a fiberoptic endoscope, and other airway adjuncts should be readily available. The anesthesiologist should formulate a plan for achieving awake intubation and consider a back-up plan as well. A surgeon capable of creating a surgical airway should be at bedside when loss of airway is a real possibility.

In preparing the patient, intramuscular administration of glycopyrrolate, 0.2–0.4 mg 30 minutes before the procedure, is useful to reduce secretions. Many clinicians also administer nebulized lidocaine to provide topical anesthesia of the entire airway.

Once the patient arrives in the operating suite, standard anesthetic monitors (ECG, noninvasive blood pressure, pulse oximetry) are applied and supplemental oxygen is administered. The patient is sedated with an appropriate agents (e.g., opioid, benzodiazepine, droperidol, propofol). The choice depends on the clinician's experience and preference as well as patient considerations. Of highest importance, the level of sedation is titrated so that the patient is not rendered obtunded, apneic, or unable to protect the airway.

As sedation is titrated, the route of intubation may be oral or nasal, depending on surgical needs and patient factors. Many anesthesiologists prefer the nasal route, because fiberoptic visualization of the larynx is thought to be easier; again, this is a matter of preference. If nasal intubation is planned, nasal and nasopharyngeal mucosa must be anesthetized; vasoconstrictor substances are applied to prevent epistaxis. Often nasal trumpets with lidocaine ointment are inserted gently; large trumpets are used in sequence to dilate the nasal passages. Simultaneously the tongue, posterior pharynx, and hypopharynx are topically anesthetized with anesthetic sprays. Once the tongue is anesthetized, it is often possible to perform gentle laryngoscopy, spraying tissues deeper and deeper into the hypopharynx until the larynx is visualized. It is inappropriate to introduce an endotracheal tube until the trachea is also anesthetized. Often a transtracheal injection of lidocaine is performed via needle puncture of the cricothyroid membrane; it is also possible to introduce lidocaine into the trachea via a channel of the fiberoptic laryngoscope. Nerve blocks are also useful to provide topical anesthesia (see question 10).

Once an adequate level of sedation and topical anesthesia is achieved, the endotracheal tube is loaded on the fiberoptic endoscope. The endoscope is gently lowered into the chosen passage; with practiced skill, the endoscope is directed past the epiglottis, through the larynx, and down the trachea, visualizing tracheal rings and carina. The endotracheal tube is passed into the trachea, and the endoscope is removed; the endotracheal tube is connected to the anesthesia circuit, and breath sounds and end-tidal carbon dioxide are confirmed. The patient may then be fully anesthetized by intravenous agents or administration of volatile anesthetic.

Useful Medications for Awake Intubations

PURPOSE	MEDICATION	DOSE	ROUTE	COMMENTS
Antisialagogue	Glycopyrrolate	0.2–0.4 mg	IV or IM	Give 30 minutes before intubation
Sedation*	Midazolam	1–2 mg	IV	Amnestic
	Fentanyl	50–250 μg	IV	Analgesic
	Droperidol	1.25–2.5 mg	IV	Neuroleptic
Topical anesthesia	Cocaine	40–160 mg	Intranasal	Good anesthetic and vasoconstrictor; may produce coronary vasospasm
	1% Phenylephrine/ 4% Lidocaine	1–2 ml 2–4 ml	Intranasal	Vasoconstrictor and local anesthetic
	2% Viscous lidocaine	5–20 ml	Oral	"Swish and swallow"
	Cetacaine spray	2–4 sprays	Oral	Contains benzocaine; excessive use may produce methemoglobinemia
	1% Lidocaine	2–3 ml	Airway blocks	Aspirate before injection
	4% Lidocaine	2–3 ml	Transtracheal	Aspirate before injection

* All sedatives should be slowly titrated to effect. Excessive doses may produce respiratory depression, hypoxemia, and carbon dioxide retention. Suggested doses are for otherwise healthy, approximately 70-kg patients.

10. Are nerve blocks useful when awake intubation is planned?

The glossopharyngeal nerve, which provides sensory innervation to the base of the tongue and the vallecula, may be blocked by transmucosal local anesthetic injection of the tonsillar pillars. The superior laryngeal nerve provides sensory innervation of the larynx above the vocal cords and may be blocked by injection just below the greater cornu of the hyoid. Care must be taken to aspirate before injection, because this is carotid territory. An intravascular injection of local anesthetic into the carotid is likely to produce seizures at a minimum, if not respiratory arrest and vascular collapse. Many clinicians are reluctant to block the superior laryngeal nerves *and* to perform a transtracheal block in patients with a full stomach, because all protective airway reflexes are lost. Such patients are unable to protect themselves from aspiration if gastric contents are regurgitated.

11. The patient has been anesthetized and paralyzed, but the airway is difficult to intubate. Is there an organized approach to handling this problem?

The patient who is difficult to ventilate and difficult to intubate is quite possibly the most serious problem faced by anesthesiologists. Organs that consume practically all of the oxygen delivered to them (the heart and particularly the brain) are at risk for profound and irreversible ischemic injury with relatively brief (5 minutes or so) interruptions in oxygen supply.

It is always wise to consider the merits of regional anesthesia (local anesthetic infiltration of the operative area, nerve blocks, and spinal or epidural anesthesia) to avoid a known or suspected difficult airway. Although a thorough history and physical exam are likely to identify the majority of patients with difficult airways, unanticipated problems occasionally present. Only through preplanning and practiced algorithms are such situations managed optimally. The American Society of Anesthesiologists has prepared a difficult airway algorithm (see following page) to assist the clinician. Key features include anticipating the likelihood of difficult intubation or ventilation. The relative merits of different management options (surgical vs. nonsurgical airway, awake vs. postinduction intubation, spontaneous ventilation vs. assisted ventilation) are weighed. Once these decisions have been made, primary and alternative strategies are laid out to assist in stepwise management, especially if the patient continues to be difficult to ventilate or intubate. This algorithm deserves close and repeated inspection before the anesthesiologist attempts to manage such problems. This is no time for heroism; if intubation or ventilation is difficult, call for help!

12. Transtracheal ventilation is mentioned in the difficult airway algorithm. Describe the technique and its limitations.

Transtracheal ventilation is a nonsurgical technique perhaps best described as a temporizing measure if mask ventilation and oxygenation become inadequate. A catheter (12- or 14-gauge) is connected to a jet-type (Sanders) ventilator, which in turn is connected to an oxygen source capable of delivering gas at a pressure around 50 psi, and inserted into the trachea through the cricothyroid membrane. The gas is delivered intermittently by a hand-held actuator. The duration of ventilation is best assessed by watching the rise and fall of the chest; an inspiratory to expiratory ratio of 1:4 seconds is recommended. Usually oxygenation improves rapidly; however, patients frequently cannot expire fully, perhaps because of airway obstruction, and carbon dioxide retention may limit the duration of the technique's usefulness. An additional risk is barotrauma secondary to high pressures. However, transtracheal ventilation is an effective temporizing measure, allowing team members time to catch *their* breath and to develop and implement further strategies (usually a surgical airway at this point).

13. Define criteria for extubation.

The patient should be awake and responsive with stable vital signs, good grip, and sustained head lift. Adequate reversal of neuromuscular blockade must be established. In equivocal situations, negative inspiratory force should exceed 20 mmHg and vital capacity should exceed 15 ml/kg.

14. The patient has been delivered to the postanesthetic care unit (PACU). The pulse oximeter is attached, and oxygen saturations are noted to be in the upper 80s. Chest wall movement does not appear to be adequate. How should the patient be managed?

As in cardiopulmonary resuscitation (CPR) the ABCs (airway, breathing, and circulation) are fundamental in managing such situations. When the ABCs are so familiar that they are second nature, the clinician may think more deeply about the problem at hand while stabilizing the patient. Assessment, treatment, and reassessment are continuous.

Successful management requires an increase in inspired oxygen concentration. Assess the patient in general (mental status, color, other vital signs) while establishing a patent airway, if needed. A chin lift or jaw thrust may be necessary. Suction the patient's airway, and inspect for foreign bodies. Is the trachea in midline? Are neck masses or swelling problematic? Once the airway appears patent, assess adequacy of ventilation by inspecting and auscultating the chest,

DIFFICULT AIRWAY ALGORITHM†

1. Assess the likelihood and clinical impact of basic management problems:
   A. Difficult intubation
   B. Difficult ventilation
   C. Difficulty with patient cooperation or consent
2. Consider the relative merits and feasibility of basic management choices:
   A. Nonsurgical vs. surgical technique for initial approach to intubation
   B. Awake intubation vs. intubation attempts after induction of general anesthesia
   C. Preservation of spontaneous ventilation vs. ablation of spontaneous ventilation
3. Develop primary and alternative strategies:

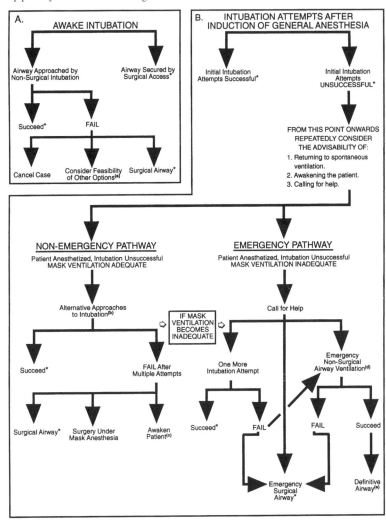

* CONFIRM INTUBATION WITH EXHALED CO_2

(a) Other options include (but are not limited to): surgery under mask anesthesia, surgery under local anesthesia infiltration or regional nerve blockade, or intubation attempts after induction of general anesthesia.

(b) Alternative approaches to difficult intubation include (but are not limited to): use of different laryngoscope blades, awake intubation, blind oral or nasal intubation, fiberoptic intubation, intubating stylet or tube changer, light wand, retrograde intubation, and surgical airway access.

(c) See awake intubation.

(d) Options for emergency nonsurgical airway ventilation include (but are not limited to): transtracheal jet ventilation, laryngeal mask ventilation, or esophageal-tracheal combitube ventilation.

(e) Options for establishing a definitive airway include (but are not limited to): returning to awake state with spontaneous ventilation, tracheotomy, or endotracheal intubation.

† Reproduced with permission of the American Society of Anesthesiologists.

observing for normal, symmetric rise and fall. Is respiration paradoxical? Does the abdomen distend and the chest retract with inspiration, suggesting airway obstruction or inadequate reversal of neuromuscular blockade? Auscultate breath sounds, checking for symmetry, wheezing, and other adventitious sounds. Palpate pulses and listen to the heart, because circulatory depression may be associated with oxygen desaturation. Assess the patient's strength by hand grip and sustained head lift. Insufficient strength suggests the need to assess neuromuscular blockade through electrical stimulation. Abnormal findings at any point in the physical exam should be addressed.

15. The patient develops stridorous breath sounds. Describe the likely cause and the appropriate management.
A likely cause of stridorous breath sounds in the early postextubation period is laryngospasm, although other causes of upper airway obstruction (e.g., postextubation croup, expanding hematomas, soft tissue swelling) should be excluded. Laryngospasm may be precipitated by extubation during light planes of anesthesia; secretions falling on the vocal cords or insertion of an oral airway also may produce laryngospasm. If laryngospasm is incomplete, the patient will have stridorous breath sounds. However, if laryngospasm is complete, little if any air movement is possible and breath sounds will be totally absent.

The treatment for laryngospasm is to support ventilation. Call for an assistant, provide a jaw thrust, and assist the patient's inspiratory efforts with positive pressure ventilation, using 100% oxygen. If this approach proves unsatisfactory, administer succinylcholine, 0.15–0.30 mg/kg (about 10–20 mg in adults), to relax the vocal cords. If the patient continues to experience difficulty with ventilation, reintubation with approximately 100 mg of succinylcholine may be necessary. Once intubation is completed and breath sounds have been verified (as well as end-tidal CO_2, if available), the patient should receive assisted ventilation. It may be wise to sedate the patient. When reextubation is attempted in the near future, laryngospasm may recur.

If stridorous breath sounds are due to laryngeal edema, administration of nebulized racemic epinephrine and intravenous steroids may be indicated; reintubation may be necessary if oxygenation continues to deteriorate.

16. The patient is diagnosed and treated for laryngospasm, which resolves. Oxygenation is still not optimal, and chest auscultation reveals bilateral rales. What is the most likely cause?
Although congestive heart failure, fluid overload, adult respiratory distress syndrome, and aspiration of gastric contents need to be considered, negative pressure pulmonary edema (NPPE) is the likely cause. NPPE results from generation of markedly negative intrapleural pressures when the patient inspires against a closed or obstructed glottis. Whereas intrapleural pressures vary between –5 and –10 cm H_2O during a normal respiratory cycle, inspiration against a closed glottis may generate between –50 and –100 cm H_2O pressure. Such increased pressures increase venous return into the thorax and pulmonary vasculature, thereby increasing transcapillary hydrostatic pressure gradients and producing pulmonary edema. Cardiac effects include right ventricular distention, leftward shift of the interventricular septum, and decreased left ventricular compliance, which increases left ventricular end-diastolic pressure and thus pulmonary microvascular resistance.

In addition to its association with laryngospasm, NPPE has been noted with supraglottitis, aspiration, upper airway tumors and foreign bodies, bronchospasm, croup, airway trauma, and strangulation as well as after difficult airway management. Patients who are intubated with small endotracheal tubes and spontaneously breathing also may be at risk. The onset of edema has been noted from 3–150 minutes after the inciting event.

Once the airway obstruction is relieved, treatment is supportive. The pulmonary edema usually resolves between 12 and 24 hours. Continue oxygen therapy; continuous positive airway pressure (CPAP) and mechanical ventilation with PEEP may occasionally be needed, depending on the severity of gas exchange impairment.

BIBLIOGRAPHY

1. American Society of Anesthesiologists' Task Force on Management of the Difficult Airway: Practice Guidelines for Management of the Difficult Airway. Anesthesiology 78:597–602, 1993.
2. Benumof JL: Management of the difficult adult airway. Anesthesiology 75:1087–1110, 1991.
3. Birmingham PK, Cheney FW, Ward RJ: Esophageal intubation: a review of detection techniques. Anesth Analg 65:886–891, 1986.
4. Bogdomoff DL, Stone DJ: Emergency management of the airway outside of the operating room. Can J Anaesth 39:1069–1089, 1992.
5. Geffin B: Anesthesia and the "problem upper airway." Int Anesth Clin 28:106-114, 1990.
6. Malampati RS, Gatt SP, Gugino LD et al.: A clinical sign to predict difficult tracheal intubation: a prospective study. Can Anesth Soc J 32:429–435, 1985.
7. McCullough TM, Bishop MJ: Complications of translaryngeal intubation. Clin Chest Med 12:507–521, 1991.
8. Miller KA, Harkin CD, Bailey PL: Postoperative tracheal extubation. Anesth Analg 80:149–172, 1995.
9. Salem MR, Mathrebhotham M, Dennett EJ: Difficult intubation. N Engl J Med 295:879–881, 1976.
10. Salem MR, Wong AY, Mani M, Sellick BA: Efficiency of cricoid pressure in preventing gastric inflation during bag-mask ventilation in pediatric patients. Anesthesiology 40:96–98, 1974.
11. Stone DJ, Bogdonaff DL: Airway considerations in the management of patients requiring long term endotracheal intubation. Anesth Analg 74:276–287, 1992.

II. Pharmacology

8. VOLATILE ANESTHETICS

Stephan O. Fiedler, M.D.

1. What are the properties of an ideal anesthetic gas?

An ideal anesthetic gas would have a predictable action and rapid onset of induction and emergence; provide muscle relaxation, cardiostability, and bronchodilation; not trigger malignant hyperthermia or other significant side effects (such as nausea and vomiting); be inflammable; undergo no transformation within the body; and allow easy estimation of concentration at the site of action.

2. What is the chemical composition of the more common anesthetic gases? Why do we no longer use the older ones?

Molecular structure of contemporary gaseous anesthetics.

Many older anesthetic agents had unfortunate properties and side effects such as flammability (cyclopropane and fluroxene), slow induction (methoxyflurane), hepatotoxicity (chloroform and fluroxene), and nephrotoxicity (methoxyflurane).

3. How are the potencies of anesthetic gases compared?

The potency of anesthetic gases is compared using **minimal alveolar concentration** (MAC), which is the concentration at one atmosphere that abolishes motor response to a painful stimulus (namely, surgical incision) in 50% of patients. MAC appears to be consistent across species lines and was found to correlate with median effective dose (ED_{50}), the inspired dose of anesthetic that prevents movement in 50% of mice in response to tail clamping. The measurement of MAC assumes that alveolar concentration reflects directly the partial pressure of the anesthetic at its site of action as well as equilibration between the sites.

4. What other uses does MAC have?

MAC allows us not only to predict the required anesthetic dose for a patient but to compare the effects of other factors on MAC itself. The highest MACs are found in infants at term to 6 months of age and decrease with both increasing age and prematurity. For every Celsius degree drop in body temperature, MAC decreases approximately 2–5%. The following formula illustrates that at increasing altitudes (with lower barometric pressures), a fixed anesthetic concentration results in a lower partial pressure of anesthetic:

$$\text{Partial pressure} = \text{concentration} \times \text{barometric pressure}$$

Thus, a higher concentration of volatile anesthetic needs to be administered to achieve the same effect observed at a lower concentration at one atmosphere of barometric pressure.

Hyponatremia, opioids, barbiturates, calcium channel blockers, and pregnancy are known to decrease MAC. Factors that do not affect MAC include hypocarbia, hypercarbia, gender, thyroid function, and hyperkalemia.

Because MAC relates solely to units of anesthetic requirements rather than units of concentration among agents, it is also additive; that is, 0.7 MAC isoflurane plus 0.3 MAC nitrous oxide is equipotent to 1.0 MAC isoflurane. However, dose-dependent effects on organ systems are not comparable in terms of equivalent MACs or equivalent anesthetic gas concentrations.

5. Define partition coefficient. Which partition coefficients are important?

A partition coefficient describes the distribution of a given agent at equilibrium between two substances at the same temperature, pressure, and volume. Thus the blood:gas coefficient describes the distribution of anesthetic between blood and gas at the same partial pressure. A higher blood:gas coefficient correlates with a greater concentration of anesthetic in blood (i.e., a higher solubility). Therefore, a greater amount of anesthetic is taken into the blood, which acts as a reservoir for the agent, rendering it unavailable at the site of action and thus slowing the rate of induction.

Other important partition coefficients include brain:blood, fat:blood, liver:blood, and muscle:blood. Except for fat:blood, these coefficients are close to one (equally distributed). Fat has partition coefficients for different volatile agents of 30–60; that is, anesthetics continue to be taken into fat for quite some time after equilibration with other tissues.

Compared with equilibration between inspired and alveolar gas partial pressures, equilibration is relatively quick between alveolar and arterial gas tension as well as between arterial and brain anesthetic partial pressure. Thus alveolar concentration ultimately is the principal factor in determining onset of action.

Physical Properties of Contemporary Anesthetic Gases

	ISOFLURANE	DESFLURANE	ENFLURANE	HALOTHANE	NITROUS OXIDE	SEVOFLURANE
Molecular weight	184.5	168	184.5	197.5	44	200
Boiling point (C)	48.5	23.5	56.5	50.2	−88	58.5
Vapor pressure (mmHg)	238	664	175	241	39,000	160
Partition coefficients (at 37° C)						
Blood:gas	1.4	0.42	1.91	2.3	0.47	0.69
Brain:blood	2.6	1.2	1.4	2.9	1.7	1.7
Fat:blood	45	27	36	60	2.3	48
Oil:gas	90.8	18.7	98.5	224	1.4	47.2
MAC (% of 1 atm)	1.15	6.0	1.7	.77	104	1.7

6. What physical properties of the anesthetic are related to potency? Who first noted the correlation?

No one physical property of a volatile anesthetic best predicts potency of the gas. However, increasing lipid solubility (oil:gas partition coefficient) appears to correlate with potency. At the turn of the century Meyer and Overton independently observed that an increasing oil:gas partition coefficient correlated with anesthetic potency. Thus they believed that anesthesia was somehow created through incorporation of lipophilic anesthetics into the lipid membrane.

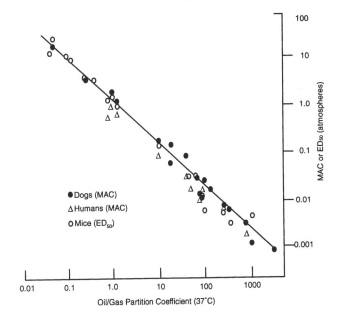

Correlation of MAC in mammals and lipid solubility. (From Miller RD (ed): Anesthesia. New York, Churchill Livingstone, 1994, pp 67–156, with permission.)

7. What other theories address the mechanism of anesthesia?

Two other theories of anesthetic action include a specific receptor theory for anesthetics and modification of neurotransmission at receptors for gamma-aminobutyric acid (GABA), a naturally occurring neuroinhibitor. The Meyer-Overton lipid solubility theory dominated for nearly half a century before it was modified. Franks and Lieb found that an amphophilic solvent (octanol) correlated better with potency than lipophilicity and concluded that the anesthetic site must contain both polar and nonpolar sites. Modifications of Meyer and Overton's membrane expansion theories include the **excessive volume theory,** in which anesthesia is created when apolar cell membrane components and amphiphillic anesthetics synergistically create a larger cell volume than the sum of the two volumes together. In the **critical volume hypothesis**, anesthesia results when the cell volume at the anesthetic site reaches a critical size. Both theories rely on the effects of membrane expansion on and at ion channels.

8. Increasing alveolar concentration is obviously important for rapid induction of anesthesia. What other factors influence speed of induction?

In simple terms, factors that increase alveolar concentration of anesthetic gas speed onset of anesthesia, whereas factors that decrease alveolar concentration slow onset. Inhalation of increasing concentrations of anesthetic increases alveolar concentration of anesthetic, whereas a high-flow breathing circuit ensures that the same concentration of gases from the vaporizer is delivered to the patient. For the more highly soluble agents, an increase in minute ventilation increases the total amount of anesthetic delivered to the alveoli and taken into the pulmonary circulation. This effect is less dramatic with less soluble anesthetics, because alveolar concentrations rise and approach inspired concentrations more rapidly. However, as mentioned previously, an increase in solubility (increasing blood:gas coefficient) increases the required amount of anesthetic because of the reservoir effect of blood. Similarly, an increase in cardiac output slows induction by decreasing anesthetic partial pressure at the alveolus, in this case by increasing uptake. Again, this effect is most notable for the more highly soluble agents, larger amounts of which are taken into the blood.

Another mechanism involves the gradient between alveolar partial pressure and pulmonary artery (venous return) partial pressure, which sets up a diffusion gradient that also determines the rate of uptake. Thus if the partial pressure of anesthesia in the pulmonary artery and veins is nearly equal, alveolar partial pressure rises more rapidly.

9. What is the second gas effect?
The second gas effect usually refers to nitrous oxide in combination with a volatile anesthetic. Because nitrous oxide is insoluble in blood, its rapid absorption from alveoli causes an abrupt rise in the alveolar concentration of the other more potent volatile anesthetic. Even at high concentrations (70%) of nitrous oxide, this effect accounts for only a small increase in concentration of volatile anesthetic within the first few minutes of anesthesia. In theory, this phenomenon should speed the onset of induction through two mechanisms discussed earlier: increasing alveolar concentration of anesthetic (known as the concentration effect) and increasing ventilation by increasing flow.

10. Why can nitrous oxide be dangerous if administered to patients with pneumothorax? Are there other conditions in which nitrous oxide should be avoided?
Although nitrous oxide has a low blood:gas partition coefficient, it is 20 times more soluble than nitrogen (which comprises 79% of atmospheric gases). Thus, nitrous oxide can diffuse 20 times faster into closed spaces than it can be removed, resulting either in expansion of pneumothorax, bowel gas, and air embolism or in an increase in pressure within noncompliant cavities such as the cranium or middle ear.

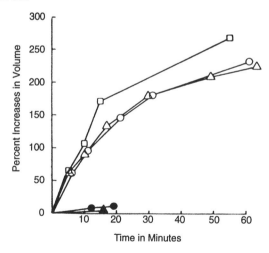

Expansion of a pneumothorax when breathing oxygen (filled figures) vs .75% nitrous oxide (open figures). (From Eger EI II, Saidman LJ: Hazards of nitrous oxide anesthesia in bowel obstruction and pneumothorax. Anesthesiology 26:61–68, 1965, with permission.)

11. Describe the ventilatory effects of the volatile anesthetics.
Many of the effects and responses of the pulmonary system were quantified with spontaneously breathing human volunteers. Delivery of anesthetic gases results in a dose-dependent depression of ventilation mediated directly through medullary centers and indirectly through effects on intercostal muscle function. Minute volume decreases secondary to reductions in tidal volume, although rate appears generally to increase in a dose-dependent fashion. Ventilatory drive in

response to hypoxia can be easily abolished at one MAC and attenuated at lower concentrations. The ventilatory response to hypercarbia also is attenuated by increasing MAC in a dose-dependent fashion.

12. What effects do volatile anesthetics have on hypoxic pulmonary vasoconstriction? On airway caliber? On mucociliary function?

Hypoxic pulmonary vasoconstriction (HPV) is a locally mediated response of the pulmonary vasculature to decreased alveolar oxygen tension and serves to match ventilation to perfusion. The vast majority of whole and isolated animal preparation studies confirm that addition of inhalational anesthetics decreases this response. Human studies with isolated single-lung ventilation (one lung ventilated with oxygen, the other with nitrogen) followed by lung perfusion scan demonstrated that inhalational agents attenuated the HPV response. Other studies of humans undergoing one-lung ventilation have not been able to confirm these results. Attenuation of HPV has been found to be dose-related in rats. Unfortunately, the effects of atelectasis during single-lung ventilation, lateral positioning, and inherent lung disease make it difficult to attribute HPV attenuation solely to anesthetic gases.

All volatile anesthetics appear to decrease **airway resistance** by a direct relaxing effect on bronchial smooth muscle and by decreasing the bronchoconstricting effect of hypocapnia. The bronchoconstricting effects of histamine release also appear to be decreased when an inhalational anesthetic is administered.

Mucociliary clearance appears to be diminished by volatile anesthetics, principally through interference with ciliary beat frequency. The effects of dry inhaled gases, positive pressure ventilation, and high inspired oxygen content also contribute to ciliary impairment.

13. What effects do volatile anesthetics have on the circulation?

In contrast to the pulmonary effects, circulatory effects are best measured with controlled ventilation.

Circulatory Effects of Contemporary Anesthetic Gases

	ISOFLURANE/ DESFLURANE	HALOTHANE	ENFLURANE	NITROUS OXIDE
Cardiac output	0	–*	–*	+
Heart rate	++/0	0	++*	+
Blood pressure	––*	–*	––*	0
Stroke volume	–*	–*	––*	–
Contractility	––*	–––*	––*	–*
Systemic vascular resistance	––	0	–	0
Pulmonary vascular resistance	0	0	0	+
Coronary blood flow	+	0	0	0
Cerebral blood flow	+	+++	+	0
Muscle blood flow	+	–	0	0
Catecholamine levels	0	0	0	0

* = dose-dependent, ++ = large increase, + = increase, 0 = no change, – = decrease, – – = large decrease.

14. Which anesthetic agent is associated with the greatest frequency of cardiac dysrhythmias?

Although volatile agents have a negative chronotropic effect on the heart, halothane has been shown to increase the sensitivity of the myocardium to epinephrine, resulting in more frequent premature ventricular contractions and tachydysrhythmias. The mechanism may be related to the prolongation of conduction through the His-Purkinje system, which facilitates the reentrant phenomenon, and alpha-1 adrenergic receptor stimulation within the heart. Compared with adults, children undergoing halothane anesthesia appear to be relatively resistant to this sensitizing effect, although halothane has been shown to have a cholinergic, vagally induced bradycardic effect in children.

15. Discuss the biotransformation of volatile anesthetics and its significance.
It was initially believed that inhalational anesthetics were inert and underwent no transformation. For the most part, oxidative metabolism occurs within the liver via the cytochrome P-450 system, but metabolism also occurs to a lesser extent in the kidneys, lungs, and gastrointestinal tract. Desflurane and isoflurane undergo virtually no metabolism, whereas halothane is more than 20% metabolized by the liver. Under hypoxic conditions, halothane may undergo reductive metabolism, producing metabolites that may cause hepatic necrosis.

Fluoride is another potentially toxic product of anesthetic metabolism. Fluoride-associated renal dysfunction has been linked with the use of methoxyflurane and greatly contributed to the withdrawal of methoxyflurane from the market. The small amount of fluoride produced by other agents has not been implicated in renal dysfunction. Another rare entity, halothane hepatitis, may be related to the above hypoxic model, but it is more likely secondary to an autoimmune hypersensitivity reaction.

16. Which anesthetic agent has been shown to be teratogenic in animals?
Nitrous oxide, administered to pregnant rats in concentrations greater than 50% for over 24 hrs, has been shown to increase skeletal abnormalities. The mechanism is believed to be related to the inhibition of methionine synthesis, which is necessary for DNA synthesis; the mechanism also may be secondary to the physiologic effects of impaired uterine blood flow by nitrous oxide. Although direct effects have not been seen in humans, it may be prudent to limit the use of nitrous oxide in pregnant women during the first trimester.

Several surveys have attempted to quantify the relative risk of operating room personal exposure to nonscavenged anesthetic gases. Pregnant women were found to have a 30% increased risk of spontaneous abortion and a 20% increased risk for congenital abnormalities. However, responder bias and failure to control for other exposure hazards may account for some of these findings.

BIBLIOGRAPHY

 1. Albrecht RF, Miletich DJ: Speculations on the molecular nature of anesthesia. Gen Pharmacol 19:339–346, 1988.
 2. Atlee JL, Bosnjak ZJ: Mechanisms for cardiac dysrhythmias during anesthesia. Anesthesiology 72: 347–374, 1990.
 3. Barash PG, Cullen BF, Stoetling RK (ed): Clinical Anesthesia. Philadelphia, J.B. Lippincott, 1992, pp 439–480.
 4. Bjertnaes LJ: Hypoxia-induced pulmonary vasoconstriction in man: Inhibition due to diethyl ether and halothane anesthesia. Acta Anaesthesiol Scand 22: 570–588, 1978.
 5. Eger EI II: Isoflurane (Forane): A Compendium and Reference. Madison, WI, Anaquest, 1986.
 6. Eger EI II (ed): MAC, Anesthetic Uptake, and Action. Baltimore, Williams & Wilkins, 1974.
 7. Eger EI II, Saidman LJ: Hazards of nitrous oxide anesthesia in bowel obstruction and pneumothorax. Anesthesiology 26: 61–68, 1965.
 8. Epstein RM, Rackow H, Salanitre E, Wolf GL: Influence of the concentration effect on the uptake of anesthetic mixtures: The second gas effect. Anesthesiology 25:364–371, 1964.
 9. Miller RD (ed): Anesthesia. New York, Churchill Livingstone, 1994, pp 67–156.
10. Quasha AL, Eger EI II, Tinker JH: Determination and applications of MAC. Anesthesiology 53: 315–334,1980.

9. INTRAVENOUS INDUCTION AGENTS

Gladstone C. McDowell II, M.D.

1. What is an intravenous (IV) induction agent?
An IV induction agent is an intravenously injected drug used to induce unconsciousness at the onset of general anesthesia but allows rapid recovery after termination of its effect.

2. How do IV induction agents work?
Of the multiple theories proposed, perhaps the most widely accepted is that they enhance the transmission of gamma aminobutyric acid, thereby interfering with transmembrane electrical activity.

3. Describe the properties of an ideal induction agent.
1. The drug should be water soluble and stable in aqueous solution with chemical stability and IV fluid compatibility.

2. The onset of anesthesia should be rapid (within 1 arm-brain circulation time) without unwanted movement or unpredictable cardiovascular or neurologic side effects.

3. The drug should possess anticonvulsant, antiemetic, analgesic and amnestic properties.

4. Recovery from anesthesia should be rapid and predictable (dose-related).

5. There should be no impairment of renal or hepatic function, steroid synthesis, or teratogenicity.

No ideal intravenous induction drug exists, but many agents possess most of the desired physical and pharmacologic properties. With increasing age, the total volume of distribution increases and elimination clearance decreases, resulting in longer-lasting drug effects. Older patients are more sensitive to intravenous anesthetics and dose reductions may be required. Dosage calculation for induction should be based on estimates of lean body mass.

4. What are the different classes of intravenous induction agents?
Barbiturates—thiopental (Pentothal), methohexital (Brevital), thiamylal (Surital)
Alkylphenol—propofol (Diprivan)
Etomidate (Amidate)
Phencyclidine—ketamine (Ketalar , Ketaject)
Benzodiazepines—midazolam (Versed), diazepam (Valium), lorazepam (Ativan)
Opioids—fentanyl (Sublimaze), sufentanil (Sufenta), alfentanil (Alfenta)

5. What are the properties and side effects of barbiturates?
Barbiturates are derived from barbituric acid; only the shorter acting drugs have clinical use in anesthesia. They produce a dose-dependent CNS depression with hypnosis and amnesia. The rapidity of the onset of action (1 arm-brain circulation time with maximal effect within 1 minute) reflects lipid solubility. The actions of the long- and medium-acting drugs are terminated by metabolism; the shorter-acting drugs are redistributed from the central compartment. The most commonly used barbiturates are thiopental (Pentothal), methohexital (Brevital) and thiamylal (Surital).

Sodium thiopental (Pentothal), the prototypical barbiturate, is a thiobarbiturate usually prepared as a 2.5% solution; it is stable up to 1 week if refrigerated. It has a pH of 10.5 and can be irritating when injected intravenously. The usual IV induction dose of 3–6 mg/kg produces a loss of consciousness within 15 seconds and recovery within 5–10 minutes. It is 99% metabolized by liver (10–15% per hour), with less than 1% excreted unchanged by the kidneys. The elimination half-life is long (6–12 hours) and may contribute to slow recovery and "hangover" sensation.

Approximately 28–30% may be detectable in the body after 24 hours. Because of known accumulation with repeated doses, thiopental is not used to maintain anesthesia. Studies in healthy volunteers demonstrate impairment of driving skills for up to 8 hours.

Methohexital (Brevital) is usually prepared as a 1% solution and is slightly less lipid soluble and less ionized at physiologic pH than thiopental. With induction doses of 1–2 mg/kg, loss of consciousness and recovery rates are similar to thiopental. However, the clearance rate for methohexital is 3–4 times faster with an elimination half life of 2–4 hours. Reconstituted solutions of methohexital are stable up to 6 weeks. Full recovery from the CNS effects is significantly more rapid than with thiopental.

Thiamylal (Surital) is usually reconstituted as a 2% solution with an induction dose of 3–5 mg/kg. Thiamylal is less commonly used, but studies indicate no significant difference in potency, side effects, or recovery time compared with thiopental.

Barbiturates may cause myoclonus; hiccoughing may occur during induction but is usually brief and self-limiting. Respiratory depression depends on the rate of infusion. Cardiovascular depression (hypotension due to direct myocardial depression and tachycardia from venodilation) occurs often in elderly or volume-depleted patients and appears to be dose-related.

6. What are the properties and side effects of propofol?

Propofol (Diprivan), chemically described as an alkylphenol (2,6 diisopropylphenol), is an IV sedative-hypnotic agent used for induction and maintenance of anesthesia as well as sedation. It is a hydrophobic liquid at room temperature and is formulated in a white soybean oil-egg yolk lecithin emulsion (essentially Intralipid 10%). It is highly lipophilic (volume of distribution [Vd] = 2.8 L/kg), which enhances its ability to cross the blood-brain barrier.

Induction doses of 2–2.5 mg/kg produce loss of consciousness in less than 1 minute and last 4–6 minutes. Propofol is cleared rapidly by both redistribution to fatty tissues and rapid clearance via the liver to inactive metabolites that are eliminated by the kidneys. The rapidity of induction is comparable to methohexital and thiopental, but several studies have demonstrated more rapid awakening and discharge from the postanesthetic care unit with propofol. Patients tend to have less residual cloudiness and psychomotor impairment than with barbiturates. The incidence of postoperative nausea and emesis is significantly less. Pain on injection appears to occur in 38–90% of patients and is more pronounced in the small veins of the dorsum of the hand vs. the veins in the arm. The pain appears to be due to the drug itself and not to the rate of injection or lipid emulsion. The addition of 40 mg of lidocaine to the solution or pretreatment with a small amount of opioid, or 20-40 mg of lidocaine, may ameliorate the discomfort. During induction with propofol, rapid arterial and venous vasodilation and mild negative inotropic effects cause a decrease in blood pressure of 20–30%. The decrease is usually most profound in patients who are hypovolemic and may be reduced by a slow rate of infusion and preinduction volume-loading.

7. What are the properties and side effects of etomidate?

Etomidate (Amidate) is a carboxylated imidazole compound dissolved in 35% propylene glycol; it is structurally unrelated to any of the other IV anesthetic agents. The usual induction dosage of 0.2–0.4 mg/kg IV provides rapid loss of consciousness, which lasts 3–12 minutes. The duration of CNS depression is dose-dependent, and recovery of psychomotor function is equivalent to that of thiopental. The short duration of action appears to result from redistribution and rapid hepatic metabolism to inactive carboxylic acid metabolites that are excreted in the urine. Etomidate is cleared 5 times faster than thiopental, and the elimination half-life is shorter (2–5 hours).

Venoirritation with rapid infusion is possible, because etomidate is a weak base dissolved in propylene glycol. Prior IV administration of lidocaine, 40 mg, or fentanyl, 50 µg, may help. Myoclonus during induction may occur secondary to disinhibition of subcortical neuronal activity. Pretreatment with an opioid may blunt this effect. The incidence of nausea and emesis is fairly high, and prophylaxis with an antiemetic is recommended.

8. What are the properties and side effects of ketamine?
Ketamine (Ketalar, Ketaject) is a phencyclidine (PCP) derivative available as a racemic mixture of two isomers; it was released in 1970 for induction of anesthesia. It is 10 times more lipid-soluble than thiopental and produces rapid CNS depression with hypnosis (within 30 seconds), sedation, amnesia, and analgesia. The anesthetic induction doses are 1–2 mg/kg IV, with effects lasting 5–10 minutes, or 10 mg/kg IM, which acts in 3–5 minutes and lasts 20–30 minutes. A stun dose of 4 mg/kg IM is sometimes administered to uncooperative patients (e.g., mentally retarded children) to facilitate intravenous catheter insertion or other procedures.

Ketamine is rapidly redistributed to muscle and fat and metabolized in the liver to a weakly active metabolite, norketamine. Clearance depends on hepatic blood flow, and the elimination half-life is approximately 3 hours. Ketamine is unique in that it stimulates the cardiovascular system, increasing heart rate, blood pressure, and cardiac output; such effects are not dose-dependent. In addition, ketamine tends to provide bronchial smooth muscle relaxation, which may be beneficial in patients with reactive airway disease or bronchospasm.

Ketamine has a high incidence of disturbing "bad trips" or emergence reactions commonly described as vivid dreaming, out-of-body sensation, and illusions. Salivary gland secretions are increased, and pretreatment with an antisialagogue such as glycopyrrolate is recommended. Ketamine also may interact with tricyclic antidepressants, resulting in hypertension and cardiac dysrhythmias. Ketamine increases intracranial pressure and cerebral metabolism and is contraindicated in patients with intracranial mass lesions or already elevated intracranial pressure.

9. What are the properties and side effects of benzodiazepines?
The three benzodiazepines most commonly used in clinical anesthesia are **midazolam** (Versed), **diazepam** (Valium), and **lorazepam** (Ativan). Midazolam is the most commonly used as a premedicant-sedative or for induction of anesthesia. Midazolam is a water-soluble, highly lipophilic imidazobenzodiazepine derivative with sedative-hypnotic and amnestic (antegrade) properties. Because of its lipid solubility, midazolam causes the least venoirritation of all benzodiazepines. Onset of action is rapid; an IV induction dose of 0.15–0.2 mg/kg results in loss of consciousness within 60–90 seconds. Tissue distribution peripherally contributes to termination of action; hepatic metabolism plays a smaller role. The elimination half-life is rapid at 2.5 hours. However, in elderly or obese patients, clearance and elimination half-lives may be prolonged, requiring dosage adjustments. Recovery of cognitive function is slower after use of induction doses compared with propofol, methohexital, or etomidate. Benzodiazepines are covered in greater detail in chapter 11.

The major side effects of diazepam and lorazepam are venoirritation and thrombophlebitis secondary to the use of organic solvents; both compounds are water-insoluble. Prolonged postoperative amnesia, sedation, and rare cases of significant respiratory depression may occur with all benzodiazepines.

10. Can the adverse affects of benzodiazepines be reversed?
Flumazenil (Romazicon) is the first specific benzodiazepine antagonist available for clinical use. Flumazenil, an imidazobenzodiazepine with minimal antagonistic effects, is a competitive antagonist for the benzodiazepine receptor. The recommended dose of 0.2 mg IV should produce a rapid reliable reversal of sedation, unconsciousness, and respiratory depression. If reversal is not achieved within 45 seconds, an additional dose of 0.2 mg may be administered at 60-second intervals to a maximum of 1 mg. Higher doses are often required to reverse lorazepam compared with diazepam or midazolam. Because of flumazenil's short half-life of 60 minutes (compared with midazolam [1.7–2.5 hours], diazepam [26–50 hours], and lorazepam [11–22 hours]), resedation from the longer-acting benzodiazepines may occur.

11. What are the properties and side effects of the opioid IV induction agents?
Fentanyl (Sublimaze) is 100 times as potent as morphine. When used in anesthetic doses of 30–100 μg/kg, it has a rapid onset of action of 1–2 minutes with peak effect within 4–5 minutes.

Fentanyl causes minimal histamine release and results in minimal cardiovascular changes when used alone for induction.

Sufentanil, a structural analog of fentanyl, is 5–7 times more potent and has a more rapid onset of effect. The elimination half-life of 2–3 hours is slightly shorter than that of fentanyl and produces more rapid awakening and less residual, postoperative respiratory depression. Induction doses range from 5–13 μg/kg.

Alfentanil (Alfenta) is a fentanyl analog which is one-fifth to one-third as potent as fentanyl. Because of its decreased lipid solubility, it tends to have a more rapid onset of action and a shorter duration of effect. Its effects are similar to those of fentanyl. Because of its shorter duration of action, it tends to be used more in outpatient anesthesia, although the incidence of nausea and vomiting limits its efficacy in this setting.

All opioids may produce dose-dependent respiratory and CNS depression (fentanyl < sufentanil < alfentanil). Postoperative nausea and emesis may occur with all opioids via stimulation of the chemoreceptor trigger zone in the medulla. Opioids have been suspected to cause spasm of the sphincter of Oddi, resulting in high common bile duct pressures, and should be used judiciously in patients with gallbladder disease (particularly if intraoperative cholangiograms are necessary). Muscle rigidity often accompanies induction doses of all opiates but appears to be of greater magnitude and duration with alfentanil. Recent clinical studies have found that pretreatment with midazolam, 2–5 mg 1 minute before induction, may diminish this effect. Alternatively, pretreatment with small doses of a nondepolarizing muscle relaxant may attenuate the rigidity and allow mask ventilation.

12. Which are the best agents for outpatient anesthesia?

Propofol is rapidly becoming the most desirable IV agent in outpatient anesthesia because of rapid induction and recovery. The lower incidence of nausea and emesis and the prompt return of cognitive function facilitate a shorter stay in the postanesthesia care unit and increase patient satisfaction. Midazolam is used less often because of its slower recovery profile but in combination with nitrous oxide and fentanyl, sufentanil, or alfentanil may be of use for brief procedures. With the recent availability of flumazenil, which promptly reverses much of the residual benzodiazepine sedative effects, usage may be increased. Alfentanil has been used because of its rapid onset of action and ability to maintain anesthesia via continuous infusion with prompt awakening after discontinuance. The higher incidence of postoperative nausea and emesis may be diminished if used in conjunction with an antiemetic and/or propofol.

13. Which IV anesthetics are recommended for use in major trauma or other hypovolemic cases?

Ketamine is recommended for patients who are acutely hypovolemic because of its cardiostimulatory effect of increasing heart rate and peripheral vasoconstriction. However, chronically or critically ill patients who have depleted endogenous catecholamines may be unable to respond to the sympathomimetic action of ketamine. In this scenario, the unchecked direct myocardial depressant effect of ketamine may produce even more profound hypotension. Etomidate also may be as an induction agent because of its cardiovascular stability.

14. Which agents may be used in combination with other IV drugs to maintain anesthesia?

Propofol is perhaps the most commonly used agent for total IV anesthesia in combination with an opioid (alfentanil or sufentanil); delivery via the new easily programmable, computerized pumps provides safe, effective total intravenous anesthesia (TIVA). Recently, ketamine has been combined with these agents, because its sympathomimetic properties provide more stable hemodynamics.

15. Which induction agents reduce and which increase intracranial pressure (ICP)?

Etomidate, thiopental, propofol, and fentanyl reduce ICP secondary to a decrease in cerebral blood flow and cerebral metabolic consumption of oxygen. Ketamine increases cerebral blood flow, ICP, and cerebral metabolism.

16. Which IV induction agents are used for pediatric anesthesia?

The majority of pediatric cases are performed with inhalational mask induction to avoid the anxiety of preoperative needle placement. If an IV agent is required, it is usually started after the patient is asleep. However, in patients with an IV in situ or in whom the magnitude of the procedure requires preoperative venous access, it is used for induction.

Thiopental is the most frequently used intravenous induction agent in children. Children generally require larger doses, and the recommended dose is 5–6 mg/kg, with neonates requiring 7–8 mg/kg.

Thiamylal is used in dosages similar to thiopental.

Methohexital has been used in dosages ranging from 1–2.5 mg/kg IV. Venoirritation is common, making this a less favorable agent in the pediatric population. The higher dose range may cause musculoskeletal hyperactivity and hiccups.

Propofol has a 10-year history of use for IV induction. In general the induction dose (2.5–3.5 mg) is 50% higher than for adults, with the higher dose required for infants.

Ketamine (1–2 mg/kg) has utility in children with significant cardiovascular disease or severe reactive airway disease. Avoid using this agent in children with Wolff-Parkinson-White syndrome, as the resultant tachycardia can precipitate arrhythmias.

Midazolam is rarely used, as it offers little advantage over the other agents.

BIBLIOGRAPHY

1. Barley PL, Stanley TH: Intravenous opioid anesthetics. In Miller RD (ed): Anesthesia, 4th ed. New York, Churchill Livingstone, 1994, pp 291–387.
2. Chittleborough MC, et al: Double-blind comparison of patient recovery after induction with propofol or thiopental for day-case general anesthesia. Anesth Intens Care 20:169–173, 1992.
3. Fragen RJ, Avram MJ: Barbiturates. In Miller RD (ed): Anesthesia, 4th ed. New York, Churchill Livingstone, 1994, pp 229–246.
4. Fragen RJ, Avram MJ: Non-opioid intravenous anesthetics. In Barash PG, Cullen BF, Stoelting RK (eds): Clinical Anesthesia, 2nd ed. Philadelphia, J.B. Lippincott, 1992, pp 385–412.
5. Gregory GA: Pediatric Anesthesia, 3rd ed. New York, Churchill Livingstone, 1994, pp 547–549.
6. Reves JG, Glass PSA: Non-barbiturate intravenous anesthesia. In Miller RD (ed.): Anesthesia, 4th ed. New York, Churchill Livingstone, 1994, pp 247–289.
7. Smith I, White PF, et al: Propofol: An update on its clinical use. Anesthesiology 81:1005–1043, 1994.
8. Twersky RS: The pharmacology of anesthetics used for ambulatory surgery. ASA Refresher Courses in Anesthesiology 21:159–175, 1993.

10. OPIOIDS

John Alden Hatheway, M.D.

1. What are opioids?
Opioids, a class of drugs derived from the poppy (*Papaver somniferum*), are used primarily for analgesia but have several other actions as well. Opioids interact with several types of receptors, both peripherally and centrally. Opium, the Greek word for juice, contains more than 20 different alkaloids, all of which belong to one of two classes—phenanthrenes or benzylisoquinolones. Morphine, codeine, and thebaine are the primary phenanthrenes, whereas papaverine and noscapine are the principal benzylisoquinolines. Opioids are either natural (from the poppy), derived from modifying the natural compound (semisynthetic), or completely manufactured (synthetic). The term opioid refers to all drugs, synthetic and natural, that have morphinelike actions, including antagonistic actions.

2. When were opioids first used?
Opium was first mentioned by Theophrastus in the third century B.C. It was used commonly by Arabian physicians, and the Arabs were responsible for introducing the drug to the Orient. Although opium was used for both medicinal and recreational purposes for thousands of years, it was not until the early 1800s that specific opioid compounds were isolated.

3. Name the commonly used opioids, their trade names, half-lives, equivalent morphine dose, and class.

Commonly Used Opioids

OPIOID	TRADE NAME	HALF-LIFE (hr)	EQUIVALENT MORPHINE DOSE (mg) IM/IV	EQUIVALENT MORPHINE DOSE (mg) PO	OPIOID CLASS
Morphine	Morphine sulfate Duramorph	2	10	60	Agonist
Levorphanol	Levo-Dromoran	12–16	2	4	Agonist
Fentanyl	Sublimaze	3–4	0.1	—	Agonist
Sufentanil	Sufenta	2–3	0.01–0.02	—	Agonist
Meperidine	Demerol	3–4	75–100	300	Agonist
Alfentanil	Alfenta	1–1.5	0.5–1	—	Agonist
Codeine	Tylenol 3	2–4	130	200	Agonist
Hydrocodone	Vicodin	4	—	30	Agonist
Oxycodone	Rixocodone, Roxicet, Percocet, Percodan, Tylox	—	15	30	Agonist
Hydromorphone	Dilaudid	2–3	1.2	7.5	Agonist
Methadone	Dolophine	15–40	10	20	Agonist
Naloxone	Narcan	1	—	—	Antagonist
Nalbuphine	Nubain	4–6	10	—	Partial agonist
Pentazocine	Talwin	4–6	50–60	180	Partial agonist

IM = intramuscularly, IV = intravenously, PO = orally.

4. What were the first natural opioids to be used medicinally?
Morphine was the first natural opioid to be isolated in 1803. Codeine and papaverine were introduced in 1832 and 1848, respectively. The introduction of the syringe in 1845 and the hollow needle in 1855 led to the parenteral use of morphine in the mid 19th century.

5. When were opioids first described as surgical anesthetics?
In the early 20th century morphine was used for surgical anesthesia. However, its use fell into disfavor after several deaths were attributed to respiratory depression; these reports predated the introduction of mechanical ventilation.

6. What was the first synthetic opioid introduced?
Meperidine was introduced in 1938.

7. Define the term narcotic.
Narcotic is derived from the Greek word for stupor. For many years narcotic referred to drugs with morphinelike action. Currently, however, the word refers to any drug that can cause dependence; therefore, the term is no longer specific for opioids.

8. Where do opioids act?
Because opioids are similar in structure and exhibit stereospecificity, a receptor site was sought. The opioid nalorphine antagonizes morphine yet produces analgesia. This provides evidence not only for specific opioid receptors but possibly for more than one receptor type. In the 1970s three distinct opioid receptors were identified: mu, kappa, and sigma. The mu receptor has been subdivided into Mu_1 and Mu_2. The sigma receptor is not specific for opioids and therefore is no longer considered an opioid receptor. Recently a delta and an epsilon receptor have been described.

9. Describe the prototype ligand and action of each receptor.
    1. **Mu:** Morphine is the prototype exogenous ligand.
       • **Mu_1:** The main action at this receptor is analgesia; the endogenous ligands are enkephalins.
       • **Mu_2:** Respiratory depression, bradycardia, physical dependence, euphoria, and ileus are elicited by binding at this receptor. No endogenous ligands have been identified.
    2. **Delta:** This receptor modulates the activity at the Mu receptor. It has the highest selectivity for the endogenous enkephalins, but opioid drugs still bind. It is thought that mu and delta receptors exist together as a complex.
    3. **Kappa:** Ketocyclazocine and dynorphin are the prototype exogenous and endogenous ligands, respectively. Analgesia, sedation, dysphoria, and psychomimetic effects are produced by this receptor. Binding to the kappa receptor inhibits release of vasopressin and thus promotes diuresis. Pure kappa agonists do not produce respiratory depression.
    4. **Sigma:** N-allylnormetazocine is the prototype exogenous ligand. This receptor is not a pure opiate binding site; many other types of compounds bind at the sigma receptor. Only levorotatory opioid isomers have opioid activity. The sigma receptor binds primarily dextrorotatory compounds. Naloxone does not antagonize sigma receptor effects. Dysphoria, hypertonia, tachycardia, tachypnea, and mydriasis are the principal effects of the sigma receptor.

10. How can one take advantage of the multiple opioid receptors to provide more appropriate analgesia?
By synthesizing opioids with specificity for one or more receptor types, more specific analgesia can be provided. For instance, meptazinol is an example of a synthetic opioid that is fairly specific for the mu1 receptor site; it provides supraspinal analgesia without ventilatory depression. Unfortunately, at higher doses meptazinol acts at the sigma receptor to produce dysphoria.

11. Are there any endogenous opioids?

Yes. The realization of specific receptors for substances derived from the poppy sparked research for possible endogenous opioids or endorphins. Endorphins are derived from one of three precursor molecules:

1. Proenkephalin
2. Proopiomelanocortin
3. Prodynorphin

These opioids are believed to function as part of an endogenous pain suppression system. Of interest, proopiomelanocortin is also the precursor for adrenocorticotropic hormone and α- and β-melanocyte–stimulating hormone.

12. Do opioids have a place in regional anesthesia?

Because opioid receptors exist in the spinal cord, opioids can be used intrathecally or epidurally for perioperative analgesia. Neuraxial opioids alone do not provide appropriate conditions for surgical anesthesia, but they decrease minimal alveolar concentration (MAC) for inhalational agents. Neuraxial opioids also may be used for postoperative pain management; unlike neuraxial local anesthetics, they do not affect the sympathetic nervous system, skeletal muscle tone, or proprioreception. For instance, epidural morphine infusion provides similar analgesia to 0.5% bupivacaine but with a longer duration of action and a decreased incidence of hypotension. Compared with parenteral opioids, spinal opioids have the advantage of (1) increased potency, (2) decreased daily dose requirements, (3) decreased CNS depression, (4) decreased incidence of ileus, and (5) decreased potential for abuse.

13. What are the side effects of neuraxial opioids?

Pruritus	Nausea and vomiting
Urinary retention	Ventilatory and circulatory depression

14. Explain the mechanism of spinal (epidural or intrathecal) opioids.

Opioids that are injected into the epidural or intrathecal space bind to receptors in the dorsal horn of the spinal cord; more specifically, in the substantia gelatinosa. This area of the spinal cord processes afferent pain information and contains mu, delta, and kappa receptors. Mu_1 and delta receptors, when activated, decrease somatic pain. Both kappa and mu_1 receptors inhibit visceral pain. Kappa receptor activation is thought to inhibit release of substance P through blockade of calcium entrance into neurons. Mu and delta receptor activation is thought to cause hyperpolarization of the neuron through increased potassium conductance.

15. How does one choose a specific opioid for postoperative spinal analgesia?

Selection of a specific opioid is based on lipid solubility. Lipophilic opioids readily diffuse through the spinal membranes and spinal cord to produce rapid onset. Hydrophilic opioids traverse these tissues much more slowly and hence have delayed onset compared with lipophilic agents. However, the more lipophilic an opioid, the more likely that it will be absorbed by vasculature and fat; thus lipophilic agents have a shorter duration of action than hydrophilic agents. Metabolism does not affect duration of action of spinally injected opioids. The spinal duration of action of lipophilic agents is limited by systemic absorption, whereas the spinal duration of action of hydrophilic agents is limited by absorption in rostral arachnoid granulations. Hydrophilic agents remain longer in the cerebrospinal fluid and slowly migrate to higher levels in the spinal canal. Therefore, a lipophilic opioid such as fentanyl or sufentanil is appropriate for procedures at the level of opioid injection, whereas a hydrophilic agent such as morphine is appropriate when the opioid is injected at a distance from the surgical stimulus. Side effects of spinal opioids are also related to lipid solubility. The more lipid-soluble agents are absorbed readily by local vasculature, rapidly reach significant intravenous concentrations, and may cause the usual parenteral side effects. Because hydrophilic agents may spread as far rostral as the brainstem, they may depress the respiratory center several hours after injection. In fact, morphine may cause respiratory depression soon after injection (through systemic absorption) or several hours later (through rostral spread).

16. What is the effect of combining low-dose local anesthetics with opioids during postoperative infusion?
The combination provides an additive analgesic effect; analgesia is greater than with either agent alone. This method allows lower dosage of both agents and hence decreased side effects associated with each drug.

17. Describe the onset, duration, and elimination times for the commonly administered opioids, morphine and fentanyl.
The onset of action is much shorter for fentanyl than for morphine. The effects of fentanyl may be seen as early as 30 seconds after IV administration, whereas initial effects of morphine take place within a few minutes; the effect of morphine peaks at 10–15 minutes after IV administration. Duration of action is also significantly shorter for fentanyl than for morphine. Fentanyl (185–219 min) has a longer elimination half-life than morphine (114 min).

18. Explain how fentanyl can have a shorter duration of action but a longer elimination half-life than morphine.
Fentanyl is much more lipid-soluble than morphine. Therefore, fentanyl is rapidly redistributed to other tissues, such as fat and skeletal muscle, after initial distribution to vessel-rich tissues. Secondly, 75% of a fentanyl dose is absorbed by the lung—a phenomenon referred to as the pulmonary first-pass effect. Thus, the duration of action of fentanyl is not dictated by elimination but by redistribution and first-pass effect. After redistribution, fentanyl is slowly released into the plasma and hence made available to the liver for clearance. Molecular size, ionization, lipid solubility, protein binding, and elimination determine the onset and duration of action of a particular opioid.

19. What percentage of an intravenously administered dose of morphine has entered the CNS at the time of peak plasma concentrations? Why?
Morphine is poorly lipid soluble, primarily ionized at physiologic pH, partially protein bound, and is rapidly converted to glucuronide metabolites.

20. Explain why patients with renal failure may have a prolonged ventilatory depressant effect with morphine.
Morphine is metabolized by the liver to morphine-3-glucuronide (75–85%) and morphine-6-glucuronide (5–10%). Both compounds are excreted by the kidney. Morphine-6-glucuronide is an active metabolite that accumulates with renal failure. Therefore, in patients with tenuous renal function, morphine should be used carefully.

21. Is analgesia more prominent if an opioid is administered before or after the painful stimulus?
Analgesia is more potent when the opioid is given before the painful stimulus. In fact, opioid administration before a painful stimulus decreases the amount of postoperative pain medication.

22. Describe the cardiovascular effects of opioid agonists.
Opioids are considered to be cardiac-stable drugs. In fact, opioids are often used alone for cardiac anesthesia because of their hemodynamic stability. However, important cardiovascular implications must be kept in mind. Opioids may cause a dose-dependent bradycardia. This effect is most likely secondary to direct, central stimulation of the vagal nucleus. An anticholinergic may be used to block or reverse this effect. The one exception to this rule is tachycardia caused by meperidine. Because the structure of meperidine resembles that of atropine, it may elicit atropinelike effects. Some opioids cause the release of histamine, which in turn may cause vasodilation and hypotension.

23. What commonly used opioid agonist is the only one known to cause direct myocardial depression at clinically useful doses?
Meperidine may cause a negative ionotropic effect at doses of 2–2.5 mg/kg. Other opioids induce a negative ionotropic affect at doses much higher than those used clinically. Although meperidine is rarely used in clinical anesthesia, it is commonly used for postoperative pain relief.

24. Which opioids are known to stimulate the release of histamine?
Morphine, codeine, and demerol stimulate release of histamine, which causes vasodilatation and hence may lead to hypotension. Fentanyl, sufentanil, and alfentanil do not stimulate histamine release.

25. Describe the typical breathing pattern elicited by opioids.
Opioids initially decrease the rate of breathing without affecting the tidal volume. Higher doses decrease the tidal volume, and even higher doses produce apnea. This pattern contrasts with the rapid, shallow breathing common to inhalational agents. Opioids also cause an irregular pattern of breathing.

26. Explain the effect of opioids on the central ventilatory centers with respect to the arterial content of carbon dioxide.
Opioids shift the carbon dioxide response curve to the right; that is, it takes a higher concentration of carbon dioxide in the blood to stimulate ventilation in a patient treated with opioids. This concept is important in clinical anesthesia and must be remembered when a patient awakens from a general anesthetic that includes opioids.

27. Is it true that opioids should not be used during procedures involving the biliary tract?
No. Opioids have been reported to cause biliary smooth muscle spasm, but the incidence is low and variable with different opioids. Traditionally, meperidine is thought to cause the least amount of biliary tract spasm. Theoretically, opioid-induced biliary spasm may mimic a common bile duct stone and confuse intraoperative cholangiography. In doubtful cases, naloxone (an opioid antagonist), glucagon, nitroglycerin, or atropine may be given to reverse the spasm. Naloxone may prove problematic if it is given in sufficient doses to reverse analgesia. Of interest, in an awake patient the opioid-induced epigastric pain associated with biliary tract disease may be confused with angina pectoris. Naloxone relieves biliary spasm but does not relieve angina pectoris. Nitroglycerin relieves both types of discomfort and hence is not helpful in determining the cause of the discomfort.

28. Name the opioid antagonist most commonly used in clinical anesthesia.
Naloxone is the pure antagonist used to treat opioid overdose and to reverse opioid-induced ventilatory depression. Naloxone binds to the mu receptor and competitively antagonizes the opioid.

29. What are the main side effects of naloxone?
By reversing the ventilatory depressant effects of opioids with naloxone, one also reverses the analgesia. Abrupt reversal of analgesia is thought to cause a catecholamine surge, which explains the tachycardia, hypertension, pulmonary edema, and cardiac dysrhythmias sometimes seen with use of naloxone. To avoid the abrupt reversal of analgesia, naloxone should be administered in doses of about 40 μg (0.1 ml), repeated in a few minutes if necessary. Naloxone also may be administered by infusion.

Because naloxone has a short duration of action, it often is necessary to repeat the dosage or to give a continuous infusion to avoid further depression of ventilation. A longer-acting pure mu antagonist, nalmefene hydrochloride, has recently been introduced. In contrast to naloxone, which has a half-life of about 1 hour, nalmefene has a half-life of 11 hours. Clinical use of nalmefene to date has been minimal, and its benefit awaits further use. Naloxone also may cause nausea and vomiting. Anecdotally, naloxone has been reported to increase myocardial contractility and survival in hypovolemic shock.

30. What are opioid agonist-antagonists?
This term was originally applied to a class of opioids that appeared to cause an antagonist action at the mu receptor as well as an agonist action at the kappa receptor. However, subsequent research revealed that many of the drugs in fact produce partial agonist actions at more than one receptor. A partial agonist is defined as a ligand that has the capacity to produce a less than maximal effect when bound to a receptor. The antagonist action appears when a pure agonist is present at high concentration and the partial agonist is added. When the partial agonist is added, it displaces the pure agonist and lessens the overall opioid effect. However, if a partial agonist is added to a small concentration of pure agonist, the overall opioid effect is increased, because not all of the opioid receptors are bound; hence the partial agonist provides an additive effect. Therefore, the term agonist-antagonist is not entirely accurate. Partial agonist at multiple receptors is more descriptive.

31. What is the advantage of using a partial agonist as an antagonist if naloxone is readily available?
As mentioned earlier, naloxone reverses not only respiratory depression but also analgesia. Evidence suggests that partial opioid agonists do not reverse analgesia to the same degree as naloxone. Furthermore, some partial agonists do not cause the unfavorable cardiac and pulmonary side effects of naloxone. More research is needed to determine whether partial agonists are more efficacious in selected cases.

32. What are the proposed advantages of opioid partial agonists?
Opioid partial agonists produce a ceiling effect for respiratory depression, have a lower potential for abuse, and may cause fewer side effects. At commonly used doses, however, partial agonists produce similar respiratory depressant effects as pure agonists. In addition, surgical patients are at low risk for developing addiction because of the short period of use. Thus two of the potential advantages may be irrelevant. However, decreased potential for abuse may be an important advantage in dealing with chronic pain.

CONTROVERSY

33. Can opioids act peripherally?
Research has shown that local injection of opioids into an inflamed site produces analgesia. The doses were far smaller than an effective parenteral dose. Of interest, peripheral opioid action seems to be present only in conjunction with inflammation. It is thought that during inflammation the usual protective barrier or perineurium is disrupted, allowing access to opioid-binding sites on peripheral nerves. Human studies are currently under way; some of the results have been favorable.

BIBLIOGRAPHY

1. Bovill JG: Pharmacokinetics and pharmacodynamics of opioid agonists. Anesth Pharm Rev 2:122–134, 1993.
2. Bowdle TA: Partial agonist and agonist-antagonist opioids: Basic pharmacology and clinical applications. Anesth Pharm Rev 2:135–151, 1993.
3. Jaffe JH, Martin WR: Opioid analgesics and antagonists. In Gilman AG, Rall TW, Nies AS, Taylor P (eds): Goodman and Gilman's the Pharmacological Basis of Therapeutics. New York, Pergamon Press, 1990, pp 485–521.
4. Murphy M: Opioids. In Barash PG, Cullen BF, Stoelting RK (eds): Clinical Anesthesia. Philadelphia, J.B. Lippincott, 1989, pp 413–438.
5. Pleuvry BJ: The endogenous opioid system. Anesth Pharm Rev 2:114–121, 1993.
6. Stein C: Morphine-A "local analgesic." Pain Clin Updates 3:1–4, 1995.
7. Stein C: The control of pain in peripheral tissue by opioids. N Engl J Med 332:1685–1690, 1995.
8. Stoelting RK: Pharmacology and Physiology in Anesthetic Practice. Philadelphia, J.B. Lippincott, 1991, pp 70–101.

11. BENZODIAZEPINES AND OTHER AMNESTICS

Gene Winkelmann, M.D.

1. What drugs are commonly used as amnestics in the practice of anesthesiology?

Benzodiazepines are commonly used in anesthetic practice and include lorazepam, diazepam, and midazolam. Benzodiazepines contain a benzene ring connected to a seven-membered diazepine ring.

2. Where do benzodiazepines exert their amnestic effect?

Benzodiazepine receptors, which are found on postsynaptic nerve endings in the central nervous system (CNS), are part of the gamma-amino butyric acid (GABA) receptor complex. GABA is the primary inhibitory neurotransmitter of the CNS. The GABA receptor complex is composed of two alpha subunits and two beta subunits. The alpha subunits are the binding sites for benzodiazepines. The beta subunits are the binding sites for GABA. A chloride ion channel is located in the center of the GABA receptor complex.

3. What is the mechanism of action of benzodiazepines?

Benzodiazepines produce their effects by enhancing the binding of GABA to its receptor. GABA activates the chloride ion channel, allowing chloride ions to enter the neuron. The flow of chloride ions into the neuron hyperpolarizes and inhibits the neuron.

4. What are the clinical effects of benzodiazepines?

Benzodiazepines produce anxiolysis, sedation, amnesia, suppression of seizure activity, and in high enough doses, unconsciousness and respiratory depression. The effects depend on the dose. At low concentrations, benzodiazepines produce only anxiolysis. Higher concentrations produce anxiolysis, sedation, and anterograde amnesia; patients will remain conscious but will not remember events during this type of sedation. At still higher concentrations, benzodiazepines produce unconsciousness.

A complete general anesthetic provides unconsciousness, amnesia, analgesia, control of the autonomic nervous system, and sometimes muscular relaxation. Benzodiazepines in low doses may be administered to supplement inhaled or intravenous anesthetics to ensure amnesia. Benzodiazepines in high doses may be used as part of a general anesthetic technique because of their ability to produce unconsciousness and amnesia. Benzodiazepines are not complete anesthetics because they lack particular analgesic properties, and they should not be used alone to produce general anesthesia.

5. What are some of the important differences between midazolam, lorazepam and diazepam?

All three benzodiazepines have different potency, duration of action, and elimination half-times. The onset and duration of action of a single bolus of benzodiazepine depend on its lipid solubility. Onset of action is a function of rapid distribution to vessel-rich groups, particularly the brain. Awakening depends on redistribution to other body tissues. Midazolam is the most lipid soluble of the three, and, as a result, has a rapid onset and a relatively short duration of action. Awakening following an induction dose of midazolam of 0.15 mg/kg occurs at about 17 minutes. The induction dose of diazepam is 0.5 mg/kg and onset is slightly slower than that of midazolam. Initial recovery times for diazepam are similar to those of midazolam. Lorazepam is the least lipid soluble of the three, resulting in a slow onset of action and a long duration of action. The long elimination half-lives of diazepam and lorazepam may lead to prolonged sedation and delayed awakening. In addition, diazepam has two active metabolites that can produce sedation 6–8 hours after its initial administration.

Comparison of Benzodiazepines

DRUG	RELATIVE POTENCY	EQUIVALENT DOSAGES	ELIMINATION HALF-LIFE	INDUCTION DOSE
Diazepam	1	10 mg	21–37 hours	0.3–0.5 mg/kg
Midazolam	3	3.3 mg	1–4 hours	0.1–0.2 mg/kg
Lorazepam	5	2 mg	10–20 hours	0.1 mg/kg*

*Infrequently used for induction.

6. How do benzodiazapines differ in their amnestic properties?
Lorazepam is a more powerful amnestic agent than is diazepam. Midazolam is also a powerful amnestic agent, but its duration of action is much shorter than that of diazepam. The duration of anterograde amnesia produced by benzodiazepines is dose-related and often parallels the degree of sedation. A 4–mg dose of lorazepam produces about 6 hours of anterograde amnesia. Benzodiazepines are not considered to provide retrograde amnesia.

7. Describe some unique properties of midazolam.
Midazolam is both water and lipid soluble. Commercially prepared, midazolam is highly water soluble. Upon entrance into the blood stream, the pH of blood modifies the structure of midazolam into one that is highly lipid soluble. This unique property of midazolam improves patient comfort when administered by the intravenous (IV) or intramuscular (IM) route and eliminates the need for an organic solvent like propylene glycol. Both diazepam and lorazepam are insoluble in water and are dissolved in propylene glycol. Injection of diazepam or lorazepam by the IV or IM route may be painful and can cause venoirritation and thrombophlebitis.

8. How are benzodiazepines metabolized?
Benzodiazepines are metabolized in the liver by hepatic microsomal oxidation or glucuronidation. Metabolism may be impaired in the elderly and in patients with liver disease. Diazepam has two active metabolites that may prolong the sedative effects of this drug. Lorazepam has no active metabolites and midazolam has a metabolite with minimal activity.

9. What are the clinical uses for benzodiazepines?
Benzodiazepines are used in anesthesia for
1. Preoperative medication
2. Intravenous sedation
3. Induction of anesthesia
4. Maintenance of anesthesia
5. Suppression of seizure activity

Amnesia, anxiolysis, and sedation are properties that make benzodiazepines excellent preoperative medications.

10. What are the respiratory side effects of benzodiazepines?
When given in sufficient doses, all benzodiazepines produce respiratory depression. When benzodiazepines are combined with opioids, their respiratory depressant effects are synergistic.

11. Are there any cardiovascular effects from benzodiazepines?
Induction doses of benzodiazepines produce minimal decreases in blood pressure (BP), cardiac output (CO), and systemic vascular resistance (SVR). Benzodiazepines do not produce direct cardiovascular effects. The combination of opioids and benzodiazepines is associated with

decreases in BP, CO, and SVR that may be due to decreased sympathetic outflow from the CNS. The combination of benzodiazepines and nitrous oxide produces minimal cardiac changes.

12. What are the dosage recommendations for benzodiazepines?

Sedation (anxiolysis, amnesia, and elevation of the local anesthetic seizure threshold)

Titrate to effect with endpoints being adequate sedation or dysarthria. Diazepam (5–10 mg) or midazolam (1–2.5 mg) administered IV is useful for sedation during regional anesthesia. Midazolam has a more rapid onset and greater degree of amnesia than diazepam. Lorazepam is slower in onset and longer lasting than midazolam or diazepam. A dose of 2 mg of lorazepam is frequently used for preoperative sedation in cardiovascular procedures.

Treatment of seizures

The efficacy of benzodiazepines as anticonvulsants, especially diazepam, is consistent with the ability of these drugs to enhance the inhibitory effects of GABA, especially in the limbic system. Indeed, diazepam, 0.1 mg/kg IV, is effective in abolishing seizure activity produced by local anesthetics, alcohol withdrawal, and status epilepticus.

Induction and maintenance of anesthesia

Midazolam is the benzodiazepine of choice for anesthetic induction (fast onset, lack of venous complications). An induction dose of midazolam produces about 2 hours of anterograde amnesia. Delayed awakening is a potential disadvantage of administering a benzodiazepine, especially diazepam and lorazepam, for the induction of anesthesia. The slow onset and prolonged duration of action of lorazepam limit its usefulness for preoperative medication or induction of anesthesia when rapid awakening at the end of surgery is desirable.

13. Is there an antagonist for benzodiazepines?

Flumazenil is a competitive antagonist and will reverse unconsciousness, sedation, respiratory depression, and anxiolysis produced by benzodiazepines. Its effect is dose-dependent and influenced by plasma benzodiazepine levels. The onset of flumazenil is rapid, with the peak effect occurring in about 1 to 3 minutes. Flumazenil is given in increments of 0.2 mg IV until respiratory depression or sedation is reversed. A maximum total dosage of 3 mg is recommended for the reversal of benzodiazepines.

14. Are there any side effects to the use of flumazenil?

Resedation is a possible side effect. The elimination half-life of flumazenil is 1 hour. In comparison, the shortest elimination half-life for the benzodiazepine agonists is 2–3 hours (midazolam). Thus, the potential for resedation is possible following the administration of flumazenil; however, this is more likely to occur with benzodiazepines that have longer half-lives (diazepam and lorazepam). When resedation is likely, the patient should be closely monitored. Resedation can be treated with repeated doses or a continuous infusion (0.5–1 µg/kg/min) of flumazenil.

15. Describe the amnestic effects of scopolamine.

Scopolamine is an anticholinergic agent with amnestic properties. Scopolamine, 0.4 mg IM, is frequently combined with morphine, 0.1–0.15 mg/kg IM, to produce sedation and amnesia. Scopolamine is also synergistic with the benzodiazepines. However, scopolamine is not as effective an amnestic as benzodiazepines and may not reliably produce amnesia in all patients. Scopolamine may help ensure amnesia in patients who are hemodynamically unstable and who cannot tolerate administration of other anesthetics.

16. Are other anticholinergic drugs effective as amnestics?

Other anticholinergic drugs (atropine and glycopyrrolate) are not effective as amnestics. Atropine produces minimal CNS effects at clinically useful doses. Atropine and scopolamine are tertiary amines that are capable of crossing the blood–brain barrier. Glycopyrrolate is a quaternary ammonium compound that does not cross the blood–brain barrier. Glycopyrrolate does not have CNS effects.

17. What are the side effects of scopolamine?
Tachycardia
Relaxation of the lower esophageal sphincter
Mydriasis and cycloplegia
Elevation of body temperature
Delirium and central anticholinergic syndrome
Drying of airway secretions
Bronchodilation

18. What is central anticholinergic syndrome (CAS)? How is it treated?
CAS can be produced by scopolamine or atropine. It manifests as confusion, restlessness, or prolonged somnolence after anesthesia and is more likely to occur with scopolamine than atropine. Hypoxia, hypotension and pain should be ruled out as the cause of the patient's symptoms. Elderly patients are especially susceptible to the development of CNS toxicity from anticholinergic drugs.

CAS is caused by blockade of muscarinic cholinergic receptors in the CNS. The treatment for CAS is physostigmine, a tertiary amine anticholinesterase drug, administered IV in 15–60 µg increments, up to a total dose of 1–2 mg.

BIBLIOGRAPHY

1. Corssen G, Reves JG, Stanley TH: Intravenous Anesthesia and Analgesia. Philadelphia, Lea & Febiger, 1988, pp 219–255.
2. Reeves GJ, Glass PSA, Lubarsky DA: Nonbarbiturate intravenous anesthetics. In Miller RD (ed): Anesthesia, 4th ed. New York, Churchill Livingstone, 1994, pp 248–259.
3. Stoelting RK: Pharmacology and Physiology in Anesthetic Practice. Philadelphia, J.B. Lippincott, 1991, pp 118–133, 242–251.
4. Wood M: Intravenous anesthetic agents. In Wood M, Wood Alastair JJ (eds): Drugs and Anesthesia, Pharmacology for Anesthesiologists, 2nd ed. Baltimore, Willliams & Wilkins, 1990, pp 196–206.

12. NEUROMUSCULAR BLOCKING AGENTS

David Hudson, C.R.N.A., and Doug Warnecke, C.R.N.A.

1. What are neuromuscular blocking agents (NMBs)?

NMBs, commonly called muscle relaxants, are drugs that interrupt transmission at the neuromuscular junction. These drugs provide skeletal muscle relaxation and, consequently, can be used to facilitate tracheal intubation, assist with mechanical ventilation, and optimize surgical conditions. Occasionally, they may be used to reduce the metabolic demands of breathing; in the management of status epilepticus (though they do not diminish CNS activity), status asthmaticus, or tetanus; and to facilitate the treatment of raised intracranial pressure.

These drugs are very dangerous and inhibit the function of all skeletal muscle, including the diaphragm, and must be administered only by personnel skilled in airway management. NMBs should never be given without preparation to maintain the airway and ventilation. The concomitant use of sedative-hypnotic or amnestic drugs is indicated, because NMBs alone achieve complete paralysis while allowing the patient complete recall.

2. How are impulses transmitted at the neuromuscular junction?

The neuromuscular junction consists of a prejunctional motor nerve ending and a postsynaptic receptor area on the skeletal muscle membrane. As the impulse arrives at the nerve ending, an influx of calcium causes the release of acetylcholine. Acetylcholine binds to the nicotinic cholinergic receptors located on the postsynaptic membrane. Receptor pores are opened and extracellular ions move down their concentration gradient, causing the transmembrane potential to decrease, with subsequent action potential propagation along the muscle fiber, leading to muscle contraction. The rapid hydrolysis of acetylcholine by acetylcholinesterase (true cholinesterase) and return of normal ionic gradients return the neuromuscular junction and muscle to a nondepolarized, resting state.

3. How are NMBs classified?

These drugs are classified into two groups according to their actions at the neuromuscular junction:

1. **Depolarizing NMB** (succinylcholine): Succinylcholine mimics the action of acetylcholine by depolarizing the postsynaptic membrane at the neuromuscular junction. Because the postsynaptic receptor is occupied and depolarized, acetylcholine has no effect.

2. **Nondepolarizing NMBs**: These agents act by competitive blockade of the postsynaptic membrane, so that acetylcholine is blocked from the receptors and cannot have a depolarizing effect.

4. Describe the mechanism of action of succinylcholine.

Succinylcholine (SCH) is the only depolarizing agent to be used widely in clinical anesthetic practice. The depolarizing agent mimics the action of acetylcholine. However, because SCH is hydrolyzed by plasma cholinesterase, (pseudocholinesterase), which is present only in the plasma and not at the neuromuscular junction, the length of blockade is directly related to the rate of diffusion of SCH away from the neuromuscular junction. Consequently, the resultant depolarization is prolonged. Depolarization gradually diminishes, but relaxation persists as long as SCH is present at the postsynaptic receptor.

5. What are the indications for using succinylcholine?

In clinical situations in which the patient has a full stomach and is at risk for regurgitation and aspiration when anesthetized, rapid paralysis and airway control are priorities. Such situations include diabetes mellitus, hiatal hernia, obesity, pregnancy, severe pain, and trauma.

SCH provides the most rapid onset of any NMB currently available. In addition, the duration of blockade induced by SCH is only 5–10 minutes. Respiratory muscle function returns quickly should the patient prove difficult to intubate (see question 11).

6. If succinylcholine works so rapidly and predictably, why not use it all the time?

SCH does indeed work rapidly and predictably and has been in clinical use for decades. This extended clinical use has provided ample time to ascertain its drawbacks and dangers.

1. Its duration of action can be unpredictably prolonged in the presence of pseudo-cholinesterase deficiency (seen in liver disease, pregnancy, malnutrition and malignancies).

2. SCH stimulates all cholinergic receptors—nicotinic in the autonomic ganglia and, especially important, the muscarinic receptors in the sinus node. All types of arrhythmias can be seen, especially bradycardia.

3. Hyperkalemia may result in situations where there is a proliferation of extrajunctional receptors. Extrajunctional receptors are not normally present and are suppressed by normal neural activity. However, any condition that decreases motor nerve activity causes a proliferation of extrajunctional receptors (e.g., burns, muscular dystrophies, prolonged immobility, spinal cord injuries, upper and lower motor neuron disease, and closed head injuries). Depolarization of such receptors by SCH may lead to massive release of intracellular potassium and resultant hyperkalemia, predisposing to malignant ventricular arrhythmias.

4. SCH can trigger malignant hyperthermia and should be avoided when family or previous anesthetic history suggests the likelihood of this disease.

5. In cases of increased intracranial pressure (ICP) or open eye injury, SCH administration may produce increases in intraocular pressure (IOP) and ICP. (However, the modest increases in IOP and ICP should be weighed against the risk of aspiration in these patients, and its careful use may be warranted.)

6. SCH increases intragastric pressure, although the increase in lower esophageal sphincter (LES) tone is greater and there is no increased risk of aspiration unless the patient has an incompetent LES.

7. After prolonged exposure to SCH (7–10 mg/kg), the neuromuscular blockade changes in character and resembles a nondepolarizing block. This is known as a phase II, or desensitization, blockade.

7. What questions should an anesthesiologist ask to ascertain if a patient is at risk for succinylcholine administration?

1. Has the patient or any family member had a fever or unexplained death during a previous anesthesia?

2. Has the patient or any family member ever felt weak after a previous anesthesia or needed a breathing machine after a routine surgical problem?

3. Has the patient or any family member had a "crisis" under anesthesia that was unexplained by any known medical problems?

4. Has the patient or any family member ever had a fever or severe myalgias after exercise?

8. What is plasma cholinesterase (pseudocholinesterase)?

Plasma cholinesterase is produced in the liver and metabolizes SCH as well as ester anesthetics and mivacurium, a nondepolarizing NMB. A reduced quantity of plasma cholinesterase, such as occurs with liver disease, pregnancy, malignancies, malnutrition, collagen vascular disease, and hypothyroidism, may prolong the duration of blockade with SCH.

9. Explain the importance of a dibucaine number.

Plasma cholinesterase can have qualitative as well as quantitative effects, the most common being **dibucaine-resistant cholinesterase deficiency**. Dibucaine inhibits normal plasma cholinesterase by 80%, while atypical plasma cholinesterase is inhibited only by 20%. A patient with normal SCH metabolism will have a dibucaine number of 80. If a patient has a dibucaine number of

40–60, then that patient is heterozygous for this atypical plasma cholinesterase and will have a moderately prolonged block with SCH. If a patient has a dibucaine number of 20, the patient is homozygous for atypical plasma cholinesterase and will have a very prolonged block with SCH.

It is important to remember that a dibucaine number is a qualitative, and not quantitative, measurement. Consequently, a patient may a dibucaine number of 80 but have prolonged blockade with SCH related to decreased levels of normal plasma cholinesterase.

10. My patient woke up beautifully after a "textbook" anesthesia but complained of pain all over. What went wrong?

The only NMB commonly used that causes myalgia is SCH. The incidence of muscle pains following the use of this agent ranges from 10–70%. It occurs more frequently in muscular individuals and patients ambulatory soon after surgery. Though the incidence of myalgias does not appear related to fasciculations, the frequency of myalgias has been shown to decrease with administration of small doses of nondepolarizing NMBs, such as atracurium, 0.025 mg/kg.

11. How are nondepolarizing NMBs classified?

Neuromuscular Relaxants: Doses, Onset of Action, and Duration

RELAXANT	ED95 (MG/KG)	INTUBATING DOSE (MG/KG)	ONSET AFTER INTUBATING DOSE (MIN)	DURATION (MIN)*
Short-acting				
Succinylcholine†	0.3	1.0	0.75	5–10
Mivacurium	0.08	0.2	1.0–1.5	15–20
Rocuronium	0.3	0.6	2–3	30
Rocuronium	—	1.2	1.0	60
Intermediate-acting				
Vecuronium	0.05	0.15–0.2	1.5	60
Vecuronium	—	0.3–0.4	1.0	90–120
Atracurium	0.23	0.7–0.8	1.0–1.5	45–60
Long-acting				
Pancuronium	0.07	0.08–0.12	4–5	90
Pipecuronium	0.05	0.07–0.85	3–5	80–90
Doxacurium	0.025	0.05–0.08	3–5	90–120

*Duration measured as return of twitch to 25% of control. ED95 = dose expected to reduce twitch height by 95%.

All competitive antagonists at the neuromuscular junction, including nondepolarizing relaxants, are usually classified by their duration of action (short-, intermediate-, and long-acting), as noted in the table. The times listed are only approximate, as there is a tremendous variation between patients. The best course of action is to titrate whenever possible.

Trends in the development of new nondepolarizing NMBs focus on (1) the development of longer-acting agents free of side-effects and (2) development of a relaxant with quick onset and short duration like SCH without its side effects. A recently released nondepolarizing NMB, rocuronium, seems to have met the challenge of equaling the rapid onset of SCH, though at doses of 1.2 mg/kg, rocuronium's duration of action equals that of the intermediate-acting nondepolarizing NMBs.

12. Describe the breakdown and elimination of nondepolarizing NMBs.

Atracurium is unique in that it undergoes spontaneous breakdown at physiologic temperatures and pH (Hoffmann elimination) as well as ester hydrolysis, and thus it is ideal for use in patients with compromised hepatic or renal function. Mivacurium, like SCH, is metabolized by pseudo-cholinesterase.

Aminosteroid relaxants (pancuronium, vecuronium, pipecuronium, and rocuronium) are deacetylated in the liver, and their action may be prolonged in the presence of hepatic dysfunction. Vecuronium and rocuronium also have significant biliary excretion, and their action may be prolonged with extrahepatic biliary obstruction.

Relaxants with significant renal excretion include tubocurarine, metocurine, doxacurium, pancuronium, and pipecuronium.

13. Do other drugs affect the actions of neuromuscular blockers?

Medications that Potentiate Nondepolarizing Relaxants

All volatile agents	Hexamethonium
Local anesthetics	Trimethaphan
Beta blockers	Immunosuppressants
Calcium channel blockers	High-dose benzodiazepines
Aminoglycosides	Dantrolene
Polymixins	Magnesium
Linosamines	

A variety of drugs interfere with nondepolarizing muscle relaxants. Inhalational anesthetics produce CNS depression and a general decrease in neuronal activity. Other drugs interfere at the level of the neuromuscular junction. Local anesthetics decrease propagation of the action potential. Certain antibiotics, such as neomycin and streptomycin, inhibit the formation of acetylcholine. Drugs such as magnesium and lithium inhibit the release of acetylcholine at the nerve terminal.

The duration of effect of SCH can be prolonged by a multitude of drug interactions, the most common being the inhibition of plasma cholinesterase activity. Echothiophate eye drops and organophosphate pesticides fall into this category.

14. Describe the most common side effects of nondepolarizing NMBs. Which drugs are associated with them?

Histamine release is most significant with *d*-tubocurarine but is also noted with mivacurium, atracurium, and doxacurium. The amount of histamine released is frequently dose-related. **Tachycardia** is usually a side effect of pancuronium (due to ganglionic stimulation and vagolysis).

15. Is it possible to reverse the effects of the nondepolarizing NMBs?

Just as competition at the receptor sites of the neuromuscular junction allows the relaxant to overcome the effects of acetylcholine, medications that increase the amount of acetylcholine at the neuromuscular junction facilitate reversal of relaxation. Reversal agents are **acetylcholinesterase inhibitors**, and include neostigmine, pyridostigmine, and edrophonium. These drugs inhibit the enzyme that breaks down acetylcholine, making more of this neurotransmitter available at each receptor. Physostigmine, another acetylcholinesterase inhibitor, crosses the blood-brain barrier and is not used for reversal of muscle relaxants. Pyridostigimine is used in the management of patients affected with myasthenia gravis. The acetylcholinesterase inhibitors possess positively charged quaternary ammonium groups, are water-soluble, and are renally excreted.

NMB Reversal Agents

DRUG	DOSE (MG/KG)	ONSET (MIN)	DURATION (MIN)
Edrophonium	0.5–1.0	2	45–60
Neostigmine	0.035–0.07	7	60–90
Pyridostigmine	0.15–0.25	11	60–120

16. NMB reversal agents cause an increase in available acetylcholine. Is this a problem?
It is important to remember that the muscarinic effects of these drugs at cholinergic receptors in the heart must be blocked by atropine or glycopyrrolate to prevent bradycardia. The degree of bradycardia may be significant. Even asystole has been noted. The most common doses used for this purpose are 0.01 mg/kg of atropine and 0.005-0.015 mg/kg of glycopyrrolate.

To prevent bradycardias associated with the anticholinesterases it is important to administer an anticholinergic with a similar onset of action. Atropine is administered with edrophonium and glycopyrrolate with neostigmine.

17. The heart is a muscle. Do muscle relaxants decrease contraction of the myocardium?
The NMBs have their primary effect at nicotinic cholinergic receptor sites. The myocardium is a muscle with nerve transmission accomplished via adrenergic receptors using norepinephrine as the transmitter. Consequently, muscle relaxants have no effect on cardiac contractility. NMBs also have no effect on smooth muscle.

18. How do we make muscle relaxants work faster if we need to secure the airway sooner?
By overwhelming the sites of action (receptors in the neuromuscular junction), one can provide a competitive advantage for the blocking drug over acetylcholine. This is exactly what is done with the standard intubating dose of a nondepolarizing relaxant. The usual intubating dose (see question 11) is approximately three times the ED95 (the dose expected to show 95% reduction in twitch height on electrical stimulation). For relaxants with cardiovascular stability, further increases in initial dose can provide some decrease in onset time without producing side effects. However, with the exception of the nondepolarizing NMB rocuronium, it is very difficult to decrease the onset time to that of SCH. For drugs with side effects such as histamine release, increases in dose usually increase side effects as well.

Another method of decreasing onset time is the **priming technique**. By giving one-third of the ED95 at 3 minutes before the intubating dose, one can decrease onset time by as much as 1 minute. However, sensitivity to the paralyzing effects of these agents varies greatly among patients, and some patients may become totally paralyzed with a priming dose. Other patients may experience distressing diplopia, dysphagia, or the sensation of not being able to take a deep breath. For this reason, the practice of administering "priming" doses of relaxants is discouraged by many anesthesiologists. Once relaxants are administered at any dose, the caregiver should be in the position to assist ventilations.

BIBLIOGRAPHY

1. Bevan DR, Bevan JC, Donati F: Muscle Relaxants in Clinical Anesthesia. Chicago, Year Book Medical Publishers, 1988.
2. Hunter JM: New neuromuscular blocking drugs. N Engl J Med 332:1691–1699, 1995.
3. Lebowitz DW, Ramsey FM: Muscle Relaxants. In Barash PG, Cullen BF, Stoelting RK (eds): Clinical Anesthesia. Philadelphia, J.B. Lippincott, 1992, pp 339–370.
4. Miller RD, Savarese JA: Muscle relaxants. In Miller RD (ed): Anesthesia, 4th ed. New York, Churchill Livingstone, 1994.

13. LOCAL ANESTHETICS

Kevin Fitzpatrick, M.D.

1. What role do local anesthetics play in the practice of anesthesiology?

Local anesthetics enable anesthetists to eliminate pain perception without inducing unconsciousness. For example, a catheter placed in the lumbar epidural space of a pregnant woman can alleviate the pain of labor and delivery. Even if she must be brought to the operating room for a cesarean section, she can be comfortable, awake, and alert, and thus share in the birth of her baby.

Alternatively, local anesthetics may be administered directly into the sheath containing the brachial plexus (nerve roots C5, C6, C7, C8, T1), providing complete anesthesia to the upper extremities and shoulders from 1 to 12 hours or more.

Local anesthetics are also used for selective blocks of the lower extremities, cervical and celiac plexuses, and for areas of the body innervated by the lumbar, thoracic, and cervical spinal cord.

Finally, local anesthetics are useful as adjuncts to general anesthesia (in the unconscious patient) and in the management of acute and chronic pain.

2. How are local anesthetics classified? (see figure)

Esters

Esters are local anesthetics whose intermediate chain forms an *ester* link between the aromatic and amine groups. Commonly used esters include: procaine, chloroprocaine, cocaine, and tetracaine.

Amides

Amides are local anesthetics with an *amide* link between the aromatic and amine groups. Commonly used amide anesthetics include: lidocaine, bupivacaine, mepivacaine, and etidocaine.

AROMATIC GROUP — INTERMEDIATE CHAIN — N ⟨ C_nH_n / C_nH_n ⟩ AMINE GROUP

3. How can the name of the local anesthetic identify it as an amide?

Amide local anesthetics contain an "**i**" in the drug name followed by the "**caine**," as in lido-caine or etido-caine.

4. How are local anesthetics metabolized?

Esters undergo hydrolysis by pseudocholinesterases found principally in plasma.

Amides undergo biotransformation in the liver via aromatic hydroxylation, N-dealkylation, and amide hydrolysis.

5. How are impulses conducted in nerve cells?

Transmission of impulses depends upon the electrical gradient across the nerve membrane which, in turn, depends upon the movement of sodium (Na^+) and potassium (K^+) ions. Application of a stimulus of sufficient intensity leads to a change in membrane potential (from –90mV to –60mV), subsequent depolarization of the nerve, and propagation of the impulse.

Depolarization is due to inflow of Na^+ ions from the extracellular to the intracellular space.
Repolarization is due to outflow of K^+ ions from the intracellular to the extracellular space.

The Na^+–K^+ pump then restores equilibrium in the nerve membrane after completion of the action potential.

6. What is the mechanism of action of local anesthetics?
The cascade of events (see figure):
 1. Diffusion of the unionized (base) form across the nerve sheath and membrane.
 2. Re-equilibration between the base and cationic forms in the axoplasm.
 3. Binding of the cation to a receptor site inside of the Na^+ channel, resulting in its blockade and consequent inhibition of Na^+ conductance.

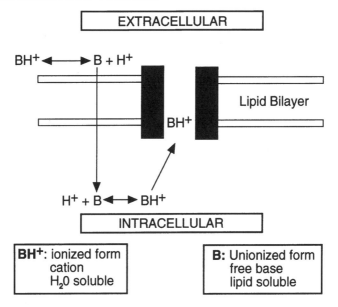

7. Your patient states he was told he is "allergic" to Novocain, which he received for a tooth extraction. Should you avoid using local anesthetics in this patient?
Probably not. Novocain is the trade name for procaine, an ester local anesthetic. Esters are derivatives of *para*-aminobenzoic acid (PABA), reactions to which, although rare, do occur. A thorough history will reveal whether or not the patient experienced the symptoms of a true allergic reaction—hives, wheezing, tachycardia, shock. Symptoms of palpitations and nervousness may represent a response to a local anesthetic additive, like epinephrine, **not** an allergic reaction.

Additionally, the patient may be describing the sequelae of an accidental intravascular injection or overdose of local anesthetic (see #17). If a true allergy is suspected, another class of local anesthetic may be used, as cross-reactivity between local anesthetics is rare indeed. If the offending allergen remains unidentified, skin testing followed by a subcutaneous challenge injection may be warranted, but is not without hazard.

8. What determines local anesthetic potency?
Lipid solubility: the higher the solubility, the greater the potency. Because bupivacaine and tetracaine are very lipid soluble, they are potent local anesthetics (see table, next page).

AGENT	LIPID SOLUBILITY	RELATIVE POTENCY	PROTEIN BINDING (%)	DURATION	PKA	ONSET TIME
Procaine	<1	1	5	Short	8.9	Slow
2-Chloroprocaine	>1	2	–	Short	9.1	Very quick
Mepivacaine	1	2	75	Medium	7.6	Quick
Lidocaine	4	4	65	Medium	7.7	Quick
Bupivacaine	28	16	95	Long	8.1	Moderate
Tetracaine	80	16	85	Long	8.6	Slow
Etidocaine	140	16	95	Long	7.7	Quick
Ropivacaine	*	?16	94	Long	8.1	Moderate

* Not established.

9. What determines local anesthetic duration of action?

Protein binding: the greater the protein binding, the longer the duration of action. Because bupivacaine, tetracaine, and etidocaine are all highly protein bound, they are long-acting local anesthetics (see table above).

10. What determines local anesthetic onset time?

Degree of ionization: the closer the pKa of the local anesthetic is to tissue pH, the more rapid the onset time. pKa is defined as the pH at which the ionized and unionized forms exist in equal concentrations (see figure). Because all local anesthetics are weak bases, those whose pKa lies near physiologic pH (7.4) will have more molecules in the unionized, lipid-soluble form. Recall from the previous figure that it is the unionized form that must cross the axonal membrane in order to initiate neural blockade (see table above).

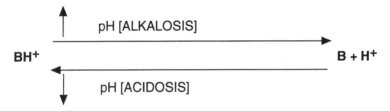

11. How does the onset of anesthesia proceed in a peripheral nerve block?

Conduction blockade proceeds from the outermost (mantle) to the innermost (core) nerve bundles. Generally speaking, mantle fibers innervate **proximal** nerves and core fibers innervate **distal** nerves.

12. You performed an ankle block on your patient who required amputation of his great toe for a nonhealing foot ulcer. You know your technique was impeccable, yet, the moment the incision was made, the patient screamed in agony. What happened?

First, never let the surgeon cut into the patient before confirming the adequacy of the block! A gentle pinch with a small clamp should suffice. Second, since the local tissue pH surrounding the infected toe is likely to be <7.4, much of the anesthetic injected near this area will remain in its ionized form and be unable to cross the neuronal membrane. Local infiltration anesthesia near infected tissue suffers from the same limitations. However, a more proximal peripheral nerve block or spinal anesthetic is likely to be effective.

13. What is ion trapping? What is its significance with regard to obstetric anesthesia?

Ion trapping refers to the accumulation of the ionized form of a local anesthetic in acidic environments due to a pH gradient between the ionized and unionized forms. This type of gradient can certainly exist between a mother and an asphyxiated (acidotic, hypercarbic) fetus, and may lead to the accumulation of local anesthetic in fetal blood. This accumulation may adversely affect the fetal circulatory system response to asphyxia.

14. Your surgical colleague informs you of her intention to infiltrate a patient's surgical incision at the conclusion of the operative procedure. She is going to use 0.25% bupivacaine (Marcaine), and asks you how many milliliters she may safely inject into the wound site. What is your response?

DRUG	MAXIMUM DOSE (MG/KG)
Procaine	7
Chloroprocaine	8–9
Tetracaine	1.5 (topical)
Lidocaine	5 or 7 (w/epinephrine)
Mepivacaine	5
Bupivacaine	2.5
Etidocaine	5

The maximum dosages listed in the table above are based on subcutaneous administration and apply only to single-shot injections. Continuous infusions of local anesthetic, as might occur over several hours during epidural anesthesia for labor and delivery, allow for a greater total dose of anesthetic before toxic plasma levels are reached.

Maximum dose of bupivacaine: 2 mg/kg
Patient weight: 70 kg
0.25% bupivacaine = 2.5 mg bupivacaine per ml of solution
Maximum total dose of bupivacaine for this patient: 2 mg/kg × 70 kg = 140 mg
Maximum total mls 0.25% bupivacaine allowable: 140 mg/(2.5 mg/ml) = 56 ml.

15. Why are epinephrine and phenylephrine often added to local anesthetics?
These drugs cause local tissue vasoconstriction, limiting uptake of the local anesthetic into the vasculature and thus prolonging its effects and reducing its toxic potential (see #17).

16. When are vasoconstrictor additives contraindicated?
1. Unstable angina pectoris
2. Cardiac dysrhythmia
3. Peripheral nerve blocks to fingers, toes, and penis (areas without collateral blood flow)

17. How does a patient become toxic from local anesthetics? What are the clinical manifestations of local anesthetic toxicity?
Systemic toxicity is due to elevated plasma levels of local anesthetic. It is usually a manifestation of overdose or inadvertent subarachnoid or intravascular injection. Toxicity involves the cardiovascular and central nervous systems. Because the CNS is generally more sensitive to the toxic effects of local anesthetics, it is usually affected first. The manifestations are presented below in chronologic order.

CNS
• Lightheadedness, tinnitus, perioral numbness, confusion
• Muscle twitching, auditory and visual hallucinations
• Tonic-clonic seizure, unconsciousness, respiratory arrest

Cardiac
• Hypertension, tachycardia
• Decreased contractility and cardiac output, hypotension
• Sinus bradycardia, ventricular dysrhythmias, circulatory arrest

18. What anatomic approach in the performance of a regional anesthetic is associated with the greatest degree of systemic vascular absorption of local anesthetic?

Intercostal nerve block > caudal > epidural > brachial plexus > sciatic-femoral > subcutaneous. Because the intercostal nerves are surrounded by a rich vascular supply, local anesthetics injected into this area will be more rapidly absorbed, thus increasing the likelihood of achieving toxic levels.

19. Is there an easy way to remember important data about lidocaine?

Yes. Because lidocaine is one of the safest and most commonly used local anesthetics, it is useful to commit to memory certain information about this drug. Its molecular weight is 234, protein binding 56%, and pKa 7.8 (2, 3, 4, 5, 6, 7, 8).

20. What is ropivacaine and what are its potential applications?

Ropivacaine is a new amide local anesthetic that is structurally and behaviorally similar to bupivacaine. Like bupivacaine, it is highly protein bound and has a lengthy duration of action. It is, however, less cardiotoxic.

Ropivacaine is capable of providing differential blockade. In other words, it is possible to separate its sensory and motor anesthetic properties. With ropivacaine, one may provide sensory anesthesia without a significant degree of motor blockade. These characteristics may make ropivacaine an ideal anesthetic for use in obstetric anesthesia.

BIBLIOGRAPHY

1. Covino BG: Pharmacology of local anesthetics. Rational Drug Therapy 21(8):1–9, 1987.
2. Covino BG: Toxicity of local anesthetics. Adv Anesth 3:37–65, 1986.
3. Datta S: Pharmacology of local anesthetics. ASA Refresher Course 21:241–254, 1993.
4. deJong RH: Local Anesthetics. St. Louis, Mosby, 1994.
5. Ellis JS: Local anesthetics. In Kirby RR, Gravenstein N (eds): Clinical Anesthesia Practice. Philadelphia, W.B. Saunders, 1994, pp 621–639.
6. Feldman HS, Arthur GR, Covino BG: Comparative systemic toxicity of convulsant and superconvulsant doses of intravenous ropivacaine, bupivacaine, and lidocaine in conscious dogs. Anesth Analg 69:794–801, 1989.
7. Finster M, Halston DH, Pedersen H: Perinatal pharmacology. In Schnider SM, Levinson G (eds): Anesthesia for Obstetrics, 3rd ed. Baltimore, Williams & Wilkins, 1993, pp 71–79.
8. Rowlongson JC: Toxicity of local anesthetic additives. Reg Anesth 18:453–460, 1993.
9. Schneider M, Ettlin T, Kaufmann M, et al: Transient neurologic toxicity after hyperbaric subarachnoid anesthesia with 5% lidocaine. Anesth Analg 76:1154–1157, 1993.
10. Stoelting RK, Miller RD: Local anesthetics. In Basics of Anesthesia, 3rd ed. New York, Churchill Livingstone, 1994, pp 73–82.
11. Tucker GT: Pharmacokinetics of local anesthetics. Br J Anaesth 58:717, 1986.

14. INOTROPES AND VASOACTIVE DRUGS

Robert F. Bossard, M.D., and Charles W. Whitten, M.D.

1. Why are cardiovascular drugs used clinically?

All of the components of cardiac output and organ perfusion, including preload (end-diastolic volume), afterload (vascular tone), inotropy, heart rate, and even myocardial oxygen supply and demand can be impacted with available cardiovascular drugs. An underlying concept is the Frank-Starling principle, which states that increased myocardial fiber length, or "preload," improves contractility up to a point of ultimate decompensation.

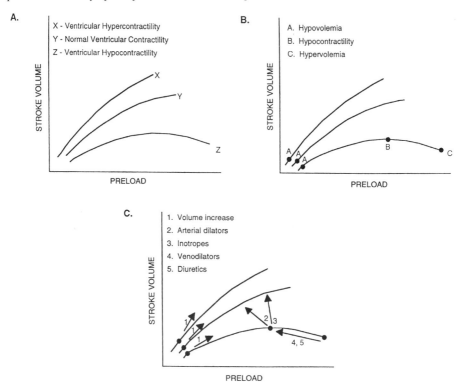

Hemodynamic parameters, intravascular volume, and cardiovascular drugs interact to affect cardiac function and stroke volume. *A*, Classic Frank-Starling relation shows how stroke volume varies with varying preload. *B*, Causes of low stroke volume include hypovolemia, hypocontractility, and hypervolemia. *C*, Various therapeutic maneuvers can be applied to increase stroke volume, depending on the existent ventricular contractility and the volume status of the patient. (Adapted from Bossard RF, Goshi GP, Whitten CW: Perioperative fluid therapy in geriatric patients. In Smith RB, Gurkowski MA, Bracken CA (eds): Anesthesia and Pain Control in the Geriatric Patient. New York, McGraw-Hill, 1995.)

2. Discuss the use and limitations of drugs that alter vascular tone.

Preload can be altered with drugs that dilate or constrict vascular beds, most importantly the venous or capacitance vessels. In addition, arterial dilators effectively shift failing myocardium to an improved contractility curve, due to decreased impedence to ventricular ejection. However, the intrinsic inotropic state is not specifically improved by vasodilators, in contrast to the effect of positive inotropic agents. The beneficial effects of arterial vasodilators are limited by their lesser but parallel effect on venous capacitance, which decreases ventricular preload. Maintenance of preload with volume infusion is an important consideration when using vasodilators.

3. Describe the actions of cardiovascular drugs as agonists and antagonists.
A cardiovascular drug is either an agonist or antagonist. An **agonist** interacts with a receptor, most commonly on the cell surface and causes a change in the receptor, thus initiating a cascade of intercellular events that culminates in a specific clinical effect. An **antagonist**, on the other hand, blocks the cell surface receptor, thereby preventing the unwanted action of an agonist.

4. What are some commonly used sympathomimetic amines? What is their site of action?
Sympathomimetic Amines Useful In Heart Failure

Catecholamines	Noncatecholamines
Epinephrine	Ephedrine
Norepinephrine	Metaraminol
Isoproterenol	Phenylephrine
Dopamine	Methoxamine
Dobutamine	
Dopexamine	

Adapted from Kaplan JA, Griffin AV: The treatment of perioperative left ventricular failure. In Kaplan JA (ed): Cardiac Anesthesia. Philadelphia, W.B. Saunders.

Most cardiovascular drugs currently used for increasing inotropy or vascular tone, particularly in the acute setting, are sympathomimetic amines, all of which have β-phenylethylamine as a parent compound. Sympathomimetic amines can be classified as either catecholamines or noncatecholamines based on the presence or absence in their structure of a catecholamine moiety, which simply means that the benzene ring has hydroxyl groups substituted at the 3 and 4 positions. Sympathomimetics exert their actions via adrenergic receptors.

5. How are adrenergic receptors classified? What physiologic functions do they subserve?
Adrenergic receptors (ARs) are divided into alpha (α) and beta (β) types, which are further divided into subtypes. Classically, those pertinent to the cardiovascular system include α_1, α_2, β_1, and β_2 subtypes, although modern genetic techniques have led to the identification and cloning of new subtypes. A classification of the AR subtypes from a historical perspective, as well as their cardiovascular and bronchial effects, is delineated in the following figure.

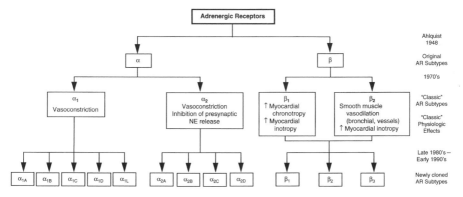

History of adrenergic receptor (AR) subtypes. (NE = norepinephrine). (Adapted from Schwinn DA: Cardiac pharmacology. In Estafanous FG, Barash PG, Reves JG (eds): Cardiac Anesthesia: Principles and Practice. Philadelphia, J.B. Lippincott, 1994, p 26.)

6. How selective are the cardiovascular drugs that act upon adrenergic receptors?
Most AR agonists and antagonists presently in clinical use are not very subtype-selective. An example is dopamine, which activates dopamine receptors as well as all AR subtypes, depending on the dose used (see question 28).

7. Describe the determinants of myocardial oxygen demand (MVO_2) and supply.
Myocardial oxygen supply is dependent upon both the oxygen content of arterial blood and coronary perfusion, the latter of which is influenced by heart rate (slower heart rate increases diastolic time, during which left ventricular subendocardial coronary perfusion occurs), diastolic blood pressure (which determines coronary perfusion pressure), and coronary blood flow (regulated by local metabolic effects, autoregulation, and coronary vascular tone). MVO_2 depends upon preload, afterload, inotropy, and heart rate. An increase in preload (increased ventricular diameter) or inotropy increases MVO_2. A decrease in afterload decreases impedence to ventricular ejection and therefore decreases MVO_2. In general, a decrease in heart rate decreases MVO_2 while improving myocardial oxygen supply (unless supply becomes compromised by decreased cardiac output), whereas increased heart rate has the opposite effect.

8. Name the common types of chronic preoperative medications encountered in patients with cardiovascular disease.
1. Digitalis
2. Diuretics
3. Coronary vasodilators (nitrates)
4. β-Adrenergic receptor antagonists
5. Calcium channel blockers
6. Angiotensin-converting enzyme inhibitors

9. Which of these are used to treat angina?
The three major groups of anti-ischemic agents, which form the backbone of therapy for angina, are nitrates, β-adrenergic antagonists, and calcium channel blockers.

10. What are the general goals of inotropic support and the characteristics of the ideal inotrope?
1. Increase cardiac output by improving myocardial contractility.
2. Decrease ventricular diameter, wall tension, and therefore MVO_2
3. Optimize tissue perfusion and blood pressure
4. Decrease pulmonary vascular resistance and cor pulmonale
   A perfect inotrope would achieve these goals without tachycardia, arrhythmias, hypertension, or increased myocardial oxygen consumption.

11. What is the mechanism of action of digitalis?
Abnormal intracellular calcium kinetics is a major factor in ventricular failure of various etiologies. Digitalis binds to the alpha-subunit of sarcolemmal sodium-potassium adenosine triphosphatase (Na-K ATPase), completely inhibiting transport processes and thereby increasing intracellular Na and Ca. Increased intracellular Na makes available intracellular Ca more accessible to contractile proteins and also indirectly elevates intracellular Ca levels by decreasing Ca efflux via Na-Ca exchange. Ca interacts with troponin C, the regulatory protein closely associated with myosin, to increase cross-bridging between actin and myosin myofilaments, thus inducing excitation-contraction coupling. Strength of contraction is proportional to the number of Ca binding sites on tropomyosin that are occupied.

12. What are the advantageous effects of digitalis in patients with congestive heart failure?
As inotropy is increased by digitalis, end-systolic volume and pressure are decreased. The decrease in heart size decreases myocardial wall tension, MVO_2, and angina. In addition, digitalis

decreases systemic vascular resistance and venomotor tone in patients with congestive heart failure (CHF), again with a salutary impact on MVO_2. In fact, doses of digitalis which show positive results in the treatment of chronic CHF may not produce significant inotropism, suggesting that the benefit comes from modification of reflex responses to heart failure.

13. Discuss factors which predispose to digitalis toxicity.
  • Advanced age
  • Hypothyroidism
  • Hypoxia
  • Hypomagnesemia
  • Hypokalemia
  • Hypocalcemia
  • Drugs (such as propranolol, amiodarone, verapamil, or quinidine)

14. What are the manifestations of digitalis toxicity?
Cardiac manifestations result from two mechanisms: enhanced automaticity, almost always junctional or ventricular in origin, and atrioventricular block. Extracardiac symptoms are primarily neurally related and protean in their manifestations, ranging from nausea, vomiting, and diarrhea to confusion, delerium, and convulsions.

15. How is digitalis toxicity managed?
Management of digitalis toxicity includes discontinuation of the drug and normalization of electrolyte derangements. In serious cases, digoxin-immune antibodies can be given. Treatment of serious digitalis-induced arrhythmias may necessitate administration of lidocaine, procainamide, phenytoin, propranolol, or even direct-current countershock. Although countershock itself may result in fatal arrhythmias in this setting, this problem is minimized by use of the lowest amount of energy which is efficacious and administration of lidocaine to suppress ventricular arrhythmias.

16. Is digitalis useful as an inotrope intraoperatively?
Because of its narrow therapeutic ratio and adverse interactions with fluid and electrolyte shifts, digitalis is rarely used intraoperatively as an inotrope.

17. What are the role and physiologic effect(s) of diuretics in the treatment of congestive heart failure?
CHF results in renal hypoperfusion, stimulating the kidney to retain salt and water and thus increasing cardiac preload. Diuretics inhibit solute reabsorption, decreasing congestion. Because cardiac output is often also decreased secondary to decreased preload, diuretic therapy must be carefully monitored. Furosemide can decrease ventricular filling pressures by the additional mechanism of direct vasodilation and increased venous capacitance. Ethacrynic acid, furosemide, and bumetanide increase renal blood flow via decreased renal vascular resistance. On the other hand, thiazide diuretics, although otherwise generally efficacious in CHF, slightly increase renal vascular resistance.

18. What are the mechanism and site(s) of action of nitrovasodilators?
Nitrates such as nitroglycerin and sodium nitroprusside penetrate the vascular endothelium and act as substrates for the formation of nitric oxide (formerly known as endothelium-derived relaxing factor). Nitric oxide binds to the enzyme guanyl cyclase, stimulating the formation of cyclic guanine monophosphate (cGMP), which acts as a second messenger producing relaxation of vascular smooth muscle. Whereas sodium nitroprusside acts primarily on the arterial vasculature, nitroglycerin has its most prominent effect on venous capacitance vessels, although this distinction blurs at higher doses.

19. Describe the antianginal effect(s) of nitrates.
Beneficial effects of nitroglycerin and other nitrates in anginal therapy result from platelet effects, a reduction in MVO_2, and improved coronary perfusion. Platelet aggregation is inhibited by release of nitric oxide and increased formation of cyclic guanosine monophosphate. Venodilation reduces venous return, ventricular filling pressures, wall tension, and MVO_2 and improves subendocardial and collateral blood flow. Also, coronary artery spasm is ameliorated, and dilation of epicardial coronary arteries, coronary collaterals, and atherosclerotic stenotic coronary segments occurs.

20. What are the beneficial effects of β-adrenergic receptor antagonists in patients with congestive heart failure? Why should they *not* be withheld before surgery?
β-Adrenergic receptor (β-AR) antagonists (such as metoprolol) reduce MVO_2 by lowering heart rate, systemic blood pressure, and myocardial contractility. Slower heart rates also augment diastolic function and improve myocardial oxygen delivery. β-ARs, down-regulated by CHF, are normalized by β-AR antagonists. Withholding these antagonists preoperatively exposes an upregulated pool of receptors to the predictable perioperative surge in endogenous catecholamines, resulting in tachycardia, positive inotropy, worsened myocardial oxygen balance, and increased incidence of myocardial ishemia and infarction.

21. What are the important interactions of calcium channel blockers with anesthetic agents and other drugs?
Calcium channel blockers (CCBs) can exaggerate the cardiovascular-depressant effects of volatile and narcotic anesthetics. Nevertheless, as with β-AR antagonists, these drugs should not be withheld preoperatively. Muscle relaxants are potentiated by CCBs. Caution should be used when administering β-AR antagonists, particularly intravenously, in the presence of CCBs because of additive effects.

22. How can the hemodynamic and electrophysiologic effects of CCBs be antagonized?
Increasing extracellular Ca ion concentration augments ion flux across unblocked slow Ca channels, thereby antagonizing the effects of CCBs. Hemodynamic effects (negative inotropic and vasodilatory) are impacted more in this way than electrophysiologic effects (negative chronotropic and dromotropic). Both hemodynamic and electrophysiologic effects can be antagonized with catecholamines, which increase the number of Ca channels that can be activated. Atropine may reverse sinoatrial and atrioventricular rhythm disturbances. In addition, both amrinone and glucagon, separately or in combination, have been used successfully in the treatment of hypotension and myocardial depression secondary to CCB overdose. Glucagon is known to stimulate adenyl cyclase via nonadrenergic mechanisms.

23. What are the hemodynamic effects of volatile inhaled agents?
In general, these agents produce dose-dependent decreases in blood pressure secondary to myocardial depression and vasodilation, but the profile of each agent is somewhat different. Halothane and enflurane act principally to decrease myocardial contractility and cardiac output, whereas isoflurane and desflurane primarily decrease systemic vascular resistance and therefore tend to support cardiac output. Nevertheless, in a patient with cardiomyopathy, isoflurane and desflurane can result in significant myocardial depression and a critical decrease in cardiac output. During cardiopulmonary bypass, for example, the perfusionist will usually discontinue administration of any volatile agent (isoflurane is commonly in use) for 10 minutes or so before termination of bypass to avoid the myocardial depressive effects of the agent during subsequent emergence from bypass.

24. What cardiovascular drugs are used acutely for hemodynamic control in the perioperative setting?
Efficacious inotropic agents include the sympathomimetic amines, both catecholamines and noncatecholamines. Other inotropes used include phosphodiesterase III (PDE III) inhibitors

(sometimes referred to as inodilators because of their dual impact on both myocardial contractility ["ino-"] and vascular tone ["-dilator"]), calcium chloride, thyroid hormone (less commonly), and glucose-insulin-potassium infusions (rarely). Vasodilators, including the newly available CCB nicardipine, and β-AR antagonists, especially the cardioselective $β_1$ antagonist esmolol, are effective. Labetalol is a unique drug that conveys nonselective β-AR and selective $α_1$-AR antagonistic properties in a 7:1 potency ratio with intravenous administration.

25. What intracellular intermediary, or second messenger, is involved in the actions of sympathomimetic amines and PDE III inhibitors?
Cyclic adenosine monophosphate (cAMP). Both classes of drugs increase intracellular cAMP concentrations, albeit via different mechanisms. β-AR stimulation by sympathomimetics activates sarcolemmal adenyl cyclase, resulting in the generation of increased cAMP from adenosine triphosphate, whereas PDE III inhibitors decrease the breakdown of cAMP.

26. How does increased intracellular cAMP affect the myocyte? What are the corresponding effects on myocardial function?
Increased intracellular cAMP activates protein kinases, which phosphorylate proteins in the sarcolemma, sarcoplasmic reticulum (SR), and tropomyosin complex, increasing Ca influx via Ca channels and also amplifying the effect of Ca on contractile elements. In addition, increased protein phosphorylation in the SR and tropomyosin complex, respectively, improves diastolic relaxation (or so-called lusitropy) by stimulating reuptake of Ca into the SR and dissociation of contractile elements. Therefore, β-AR agonists and PDE III inhibitors improve both systolic (increased inotropy and chronotropy) and diastolic (enhanced lusitropy) function.

27. What is the result of combining a β-adrenergic agonist with a phosphodiesterase III inhibitor?
An additive or synergistic effect results due to the influence of PDE III inhibitors distal to the β-receptor.

28. Describe the hemodynamic profiles of the naturally occurring endogenous catecholamines.
The effects of a low-dose infusion of **epinephrine** (1–2 μg/min) are primarily limited to stimulation of $β_1$- and $β_2$-ARs in the heart and peripheral vasculature, resulting in positive chronotropy, dromotropy, and inotropy, increased automaticity, and vasodilation. Moderate-dose infusion (2–10 μg/min) generates greater α-AR effects and vasoconstriction, and high-dose infusion results in such prominent vasoconstriction that many of the β-AR effects are blocked.

Hemodynamic Dose-Response Relationship of Epinephrine

1–2 μg/min	Primarily β-stimulation
2–10 μg/min	Mixed α- and β-stimulation
10–20 μg/min	Primarily α-stimulation

The potency of **norepinephrine** in stimulating β-ARs is similar to that of epinephrine, but it results in significant α-AR stimulation at much lower doses. **Dopamine** stimulates specific postjunctional dopaminergic receptors in renal, mesenteric, and coronary arterial beds to produce vasodilation. These dopaminergic effects occur at lower doses (0.5–1.0 μg/kg/min), becoming maximal at 2–3 μg/kg/min. At intermediate doses (2–6 μg/kg/min), $β_1$-AR stimulation is evident. Beginning at doses of about 10 μg/kg/min (but as low as 5 μg/kg/min), α-AR stimulation is seen which at higher doses overcomes dopaminergic effects, producing vasoconstriction.

29. What are the hemodynamic profiles of the available synthetic catecholamines?
Isoproterenol is the most potent $β_1$- and $β_2$-AR agonist, but possesses no α-AR stimulating properties. Therefore, isoproterenol increases heart rate, automaticity, and contractility and also

produces marked dilation of both venous capacitance vessels and arterial vessels. **Dobutamine** acts principally on β-ARs, impacting β_1-ARs in a relatively selective fashion. In addition, it has a mild indirect α_1-AR stimulating effect that is secondary to prevention of norepinephrine uptake at adrenergic nerve terminals and is offset by slightly more potent β_2-AR stimulation. Generally, at clinical doses, minimal increases in heart rate, positive inotropy, increased cardiac output, and minimal or modest decreases in systemic and pulmonary vascular resistance occur. Because of the indirect α_1-AR stimulating effect, patients concurrently receiving β-AR antagonists can exhibit marked increases in systemic vascular resistance without improvement in cardiac output. In addition, an occasional patient will display a significant increase in heart rate in a dose-related manner.

30. Which characteristics of β-adrenergic agonists limit their effectiveness?
  • Positive chronotropic and arrhythmogenic effects (primarily with epinephrine and isoproterenol and less commonly with dobutamine)
  • Vasoconstriction secondary to α_1-AR activation (with norepinephrine and higher-dose epinephrine and dopamine)
  • Vasodilation due to stimulation of vascular β_2-AR receptors (with isoproterenol and, less commonly, dobutamine)

31. How may the side effects and limitations of β-adrenergic agonists be minimized?
Side effects can be minimized by appropriate dosage adjustments or use of combinations of agents. In modern practice, PDE III inhibitors have assumed a prominent role in this regard (see questions 32 and 34). Often, dopamine is added to infusions of one of the other catecholamines to improve renal perfusion and to minimize the dosage requirement of the first agent. A traditional example of combination therapy is the use of phentolamine (Regitine) with norepinephrine (Levophed) to minimize the vasoconstrictive effects of the latter. Other agents to consider include lidocaine (for antiarrhythmogenic effects), nitroglycerin, and sodium nitroprusside.

32. Discuss the hemodynamic profile of the phosphodiesterase inhibitors amrinone and milrinone.
Amrinone and milrinone are approximately as potent in increasing cardiac output as the milder β-AR agonists dopamine and dobutamine. Inotropy is increased, and lusitropy is improved. In addition to direct myocardial effects, prominent vasodilation is produced, and in fact it is difficult to separate out the relative contributions of vasodilation and inotropic effects in increasing cardiac output. Overall hemodynamic effects are intermediate between those of dobutamine and sodium nitroprusside. Both venous and arterial vasodilation occur, which decreases right and left ventricular filling pressures, pulmonary and systemic vascular resistance, pulmonary artery pressure, and mean arterial pressure. Right ventricular dynamics are particularly favorably impacted. Coronary vessels are dilated. In patients with severe CHF, MVO_2 is actually decreased, presumably because of the prominent vasodilatory effects. Compared to the effects seen with the β-AR agonists, heart rate is unchanged or modestly increased, and significant proarrhythmia is less problematic.

33. What untoward effects can result from use of a phosphodiesterase III inhibitor? How are these minimized?
Because the vasodilatory effects of PDE III inhibitors are profound, concurrent use of a vasoconstrictor (such as epinephrine, norepinephrine, or even phenylephrine) may be needed. This is particularly true after cardiopulmonary bypass, when systemic vascular resistance is typically very low in response to anesthesia, hemodilution, and rewarming. In addition, prolonged infusion of amrinone, but not milrinone, sometimes causes significant thrombocytopenia, which is thought to result from nonimmune-mediated peripheral platelet destruction. Furthermore, milrinone has a significantly shorter half-life, making it more titratable, and therefore milrinone has supplanted amrinone as the PDE III inhibitor of choice.

34. Discuss advantageous characteristics of the phosphodiesterase inhibitors.
In addition to positive inotropy and lusitropy, vasodilation, and a relative lack of significant tachyarrhythmias, PDE III inhibitors have other advantages. In patients in CHF with down-regulation of β-ARs, PDE III inhibitors can transiently restore $β_1$-AR function by decreasing cAMP breakdown. PDE III inhibitors potentiate the action of β-AR agonists, permitting a decrease in the dose and undesirable side effects (especially vasoconstriction) of these agents. PDE III inhibitors may help reduce myocardial ischemia by several mechanisms, including:

    1. Dilation of coronary arteries and arterial conduits, including the internal mammary artery and especially the gastroepiploic artery;

    2. Improved coronary collateral circulation;

    3. Attenuation of platelet aggregation and thromboxane activity; and

    4. Decreased MVO_2.

In fact, preliminary evidence suggests a potential decrease in the incidence of myocardial infarction after coronary artery bypass in amrinone-treated patients compared to dobutamine-treated patients. In addition, by reducing leukocyte aggregation, PDE III inhibitors may play a role in reducing reperfusion injury after cardiopulmonary bypass.

35. What are the hemodynamic effects of intravenously administered calcium chloride?
In patients with normal or increased serum Ca levels, an intravenous $CaCl_2$ bolus produces a transient increase in systemic vascular resistance. In patients who are profoundly hypocalcemic, exogenous $CaCl_2$ may generate a significant inotropic response.

36. What is the role of calcium chloride used after cardiopulmonary bypass?
Traditionally, a $CaCl_2$ bolus has been routinely administered at termination of cardiopulmonary bypass (CPB) to enhance cardiovascular performance. This practice has been challenged recently for several reasons. First, patients are generally only mildly hyopocalcemic immediately after CPB. Predictably, therefore, experimental evidence indicates that increases in cardiac output and blood pressure secondary to serial $CaCl_2$ boluses (3 mg/kg) after CPB are not related to improvements in myocardial performance. Secondly, exogenous $CaCl_2$ may actually attenuate myocardial response to effects of B-AR agonists, possibly via an adverse interaction at the β-AR complex. Thirdly, actual tissue injury may result involving intracellular Ca overload, myocardial necrosis, and even pancreatic injury. Nevertheless, administration of a $CaCl_2$ bolus, usually 1 gm, after a period of reperfusion and just prior to termination of CPB continues to be common practice, in part to antagonize the transient presence of hyperkalemia due to potassium cardioplegia.

37. Can β-adrenergic abnormalities occur secondary to myocardial dysfunction?
Desensitization of the myocardial β-AR-guanine nucleotide protein–adenyl cyclase (β-AGA) system occurs secondary to cardiomyopathies of multiple etiologies, including coronary artery disease, pulmonary hypertension, and idiopathic causes. Even aging results in a significant decrease in β-AGA responsiveness. Potential abnormalities of the β-AGA system include: (1) reduced number of ARs (down-regulation); (2) uncoupling of the AR from the guanine nucleotide protein (G protein); (3) increased activity of the inhibitory G protein; (4) decreased catalytic activity of the adenyl cyclase subunit; and (5) sequestration or internalization of ARs (i.e., redistribution of ARs from the cell surface into the intracellular milieu).

38. What role do catecholamines play in the pathophysiology of β-adrenergic abnormalities?
One of the known mechanisms of β-AGA desenitization is exposure to elevated catecholamine levels. Teleologically, β-AGA desensitization may be a protective mechanism in the face of elevated catecholamine levels, as occurs in patients with CHF. Myocardial β-AGA desensitization during and after CPB has been well documented. During aortic cross-clamping, intrinsic release of norepinephrine and epinephrine has been demonstrated from cold, anoxic, isolated myocardium. Subsequently, during the rewarming phase of CPB, the heart is reperfused with blood containing levels of catecholamines which are profoundly elevated as a result of the stress

response to CPB. β-AGA desensitization has obvious important implications regarding weaning from CPB. A similar, more protracted desensitization process occurs in potential heart transplant recipients receiving chronic dobutamine infusions.

39. What preoperative indicators predict the need for inotropic support after cardiopulmonary bypass?
Preoperative factors that help predict which patients will require exogenous inotropes to separate successfully from CPB include impaired global ventricular function, regional wall motion abnormalities, and depressed ejection fraction. Ejection fraction is a particularly robust indicator. Older age, cardiac enlargement, female sex, and higher left ventricular end-diastolic pressures before and after radiographic contrast-injection are also predictive.

40. Can intraoperative indicators predict the need for inotropic support after cardiopulmonary bypass?
The hemodynamic response to anesthetics before CPB gives an indication of cardiac reserve. A judgment can sometimes be made by the surgeon as to the quality of myocardial preservation during aortic cross-clamping, as well as the adequacy of revascularization or valvular repair. The length of aortic cross-clamp time is particularly important, with cross-clamp times > 120 minutes (90 min based on some data) correlating directly with adverse outcomes, particularly reversible global ventricular dysfunction (myocardial stunning). Increased length of CPB (> 150 min) is predictive, especially (and seemingly paradoxically) when the preoperative left ventricular ejection fraction is > 0.45. During partial separation from CPB, as occurs after discontinuance of the left ventricular vent, it is helpful to observe the arterial waveform for the presence or absence of brisk left ventricular ejection in conjunction with observation of the pulmonary artery pressure. If the pulmonary artery pressure subsequently rises with little discernible left ventricular ejection, pharmacologic support will most likely be needed. Similarly, although only the right ventricle and a portion of the right atrium and left ventricle are visible through a sternotomy, direct visualization of the anterior surface of the beating heart just prior to separation from CPB can be informative.

41. What inotropes or combinations are best employed after cardiopulmonary bypass?
There are no definitive scientific data favoring the choice of one inotrope over another. In many cases, regional preferences prevail and may be based on philosophical or teleological considerations. For example, one very prominent expert has recently opined that epinephrine is the first-line inotrope of choice due to its titratable potency and, moreover, because it is a naturally evolved substance that has enabled man to "run from the saber-toothed tiber." Commonly, **dobutamine** is chosen as a first-line agent because of its relatively low potency (and therefore lesser impact on MVO$_2$) and its hemodynamic profile (decreased impedence to left and right ventricular ejection). In the event of failed therapy with dobutamine (persistent low cardiac output or "failed wean" from CPB), therapy can be supplemented with other inotropes, such as epinephrine or a PDE III inhibitor, for their additive effects. On the other hand, clinicians favoring PDE III inhibitors as a first-line agent cite its specific advantages, which have already been discussed. Selection of an inotrope should occasion consideration of the underlying pathophysiology. For example, in the presence of significant pulmonary hypertension or cor pulmonale, strong consideration may be given to the use of a PDE III inhibitor, which in the opinion of many clinicians is the inotrope of choice in such a scenario.

42. Can ephedrine be used to advantage after cardiopulmonary bypass?
Ephedrine, a mixed direct- and indirect-acting nonselective α- and β-AR agonist, is transiently effective in supporting blood pressure and cardiac output after CPB and has a reasonable margin of safety, despite its propensity to generate tachycardia (although in general, heart rates > 100 are poorly tolerated and tend to result in ischemia). Tachyphylaxis limits the utility of ephedrine to one or two doses.

43. Are thyroid hormones active as inotropic agents?

CPB results in a significant decrease in serum levels of triiodothyronine (T3), thyroxine (T4), and thyroid-stimulating hormone (TSH) that persists for several days. In addition, a "euthyroid sick syndrome" has been demonstrated after CPB. In studies involving small numbers of normothyroid patients undergoing CPB, Novitsky and colleagues investigated the effect of T3 administration and found a decreased need for inotropic therapy in patients with impaired preoperative ventricular function and an improvement in stroke volume, cardiac output, and systemic and pulmonary vascular resistance in all patients. T4 has been reported to immediately enhance cardiac activity in patients with preexisting hypothyroidism.

44. What mechanisms of action account for the inotropic effect of thyroid hormone?

Thyroid hormone has chronic actions requiring time for protein synthesis, such as alterations of nuclear synthetic machinery, structural changes in the myosin isozyme, and increased expression of β-adrenergic receptors. In addition, more immediate augmentation of contractility occurs secondary to an increase in mitochondrial respiratory rate and ATP production, enhanced function of sarcolemmal Ca-ATPase, and augmented Na entry into myocytes. Elevated intracellular Na levels increase intracellular Ca concentration and activity (see question 11).

45. In which patient population(s) undergoing heart surgery is use of thyroid hormone indicated?

Although the use of thyroid hormone is certainly indicated in patients with preexisting hypothyroidism, there are at present minimal data confirming its efficacy in euthyroid patients. One common use of thyroid hormone currently is after cardiac transplantation. These patients are severely ill and more likely to exhibit the euthyroid sick syndrome.

46. How do glucose-insulin-potassium (GIK) infusions improve myocardial function?

GIK infusion preoperatively increases myocardial glycogen, which is important in preserving myocardium during surgery, and increases glucose utilization and ATP production, which is associated with improved myocardial performance and tolerance of ischemia. Furthermore, administration of GIK following cardiac surgery decreases the need for inotropic support. Mechanistically, the benefit of GIK may accrue from its favorable impact on the state of perioperative insulin resistance, thereby decreasing myocardial uptake of free fatty acids, increasing carbohydrate metabolism, and decreasing myocardial oxygen expenditure.

47. What potential problems are associated with GIK therapy?

Resultant hypokalemia can result in arrhythmias, and hyperglycemia can be detrimental in the presence of neurologic ischemia. Although not demonstrated in humans, experimental evidence in animals shows that insulin can increase Ca binding to myocardial receptors and Ca-actin-myosin ATPase activity to cause myocardial contractures and myocardial ischemia. Preliminary clinical evidence regarding metabolic support with GIK therapy for myocardial ischemia in humans is favorable.

BIBLIOGRAPHY

1. Bohm M, La Rosee K, Schwinger RH, Erdmann E: Evidence for reduction of norepinephrine uptake sites in the failing human heart. J Am Coll Cardiol 25:146–153, 1995.
2. Butterworth JF: Use of amrinone in cardiac surgery patients. J Cardiothorac Vasc Anesth 7(2 Suppl 1):1–7, 1993.
3. Cheng DC, Asokumar B, Nakagawa T: Amrinone therapy for severe pulmonary hypertension and biventricular failure after complicated valvular heart surgery. Chest 104:1618–20, 1993.
4. Clark RE: Cardiopulmonary bypass and thyroid hormone metabolism. Ann Thorac Surg 56:S35–S42, 1993.
5. Feldman AM: Modulation of adrenergic receptors and G-transduction proteins in failing human ventricular myocardium. Circulation 87(5 Suppl 4):IV27–IV34, 1993.
6. Levy JH, Bailey JM: Amrinone: Its effect on vascular resistance and capacitance in human subjects. Chest 105:62–64, 1994.

7. Levy JH, Salmenpera MT, Bailey JM, Ramsay JG: Postoperative circulatory control. In Kaplan JA (ed): Cardiac Anesthesia. Philadelphia, W.B. Saunders, 1993, pp 1168–1193.
8. Merin RG: Positive inotropic drugs and ventricular function. In Waltier DC (ed): Ventricular Function. Baltimore, Williams & Wilkins, 1995, pp 181–212.
9. Novitsky D: Heart transplantation, euthyroid sick syndrome, and triiodothyronine replacement. J Heart Lung Transplant 11(4 Pt 2): S196–S198, 1992.
10. Reves JG: Pharmacology of vasoactive drugs. In Thomas SJ, Kramer JL (eds): Manual of Cardiac Anesthesia. New York, Churchill Livingstone, 1993, pp 315–335.
11. Royster RL: Myocardial dysfunction following cardiopulmonary bypass: Recovery patterns, predictors of inotropic need, theoretical concepts of inotropic administration. J Cardiothorac Vasc Anesth 7(4 Suppl 2):19–25, 1993.
12. Schwinn DA: Cardiac pharmacology. In Estafanous FG, Barash PG, Reves JG: Cardiac Anesthesia: Principles and Practice. Philadelphia, J.B. Lippincott, 1994, pp 21–60.
13. Svedjeholm R, Hakanson E, Vanhanen I: Rationale for metabolic support with amino acids and glucose-insulin-potasssium (GIK) in cardiac surgery. Ann Thorac Surg 59(2 Suppl):S15–S22, 1995.
14. Whitten CW, Latson TW, Klein KW, et al: Anesthetic management of a hypothyroid cardiac surgical patient. J Cardiothorac Anesth 5:156–159, 1991.
15. Zaloga GP, Prielipp RC, Butterworth JF, Royster RL: Pharmacologic cardiovascular support. Crit Care Clin 9 (2) 335–362, 1993.

III. Preparing for Anesthesia

15. THE PREOPERATIVE EVALUATION

Philip A. Role, M.D., and Frederick M. Galloway, M.D.

1. What are the goals of the preoperative evaluation?

The preoperative evaluation consists of gathering information on the patient and formulating an anesthetic plan. The overall objective is reduction of perioperative morbidity and mortality.

Ideally, the preoperative evaluation is done by the person who will administer the anesthesia. The anesthesiologist should review the surgical diagnosis, organ systems involved, and planned procedure. Through interview, physical exam and review of pertinent current and past medical records, the patient's physical and mental status are determined. All recent medications are recorded and a thorough drug allergy history is taken. The patient should be questioned about use of cigarettes, alcohol, and illicit drugs. The patient's prior anesthetic experience is of particular interest—specifically, if there has been a history of any anesthetic complications, problems with intubation, delayed emergence, malignant hyperthermia, prolonged neuromuscular blockade, or postoperative nausea and vomiting. From this evaluation, the anesthesiologist decides if any preoperative tests or consultations are indicated and then formulates an anesthetic care plan.

Informed consent is the communication of this anesthetic plan, in terms the patient understands, and covers everything from premedication, preoperative procedures, and intraoperative management, through the recovery room and postoperative pain control. The alternatives, potential complications, and risks versus benefits are discussed, and the patient's questions are answered. If the interview is done by someone other than the person who will administer the anesthesia, the patient should be informed of this and told that the anesthesiologist will have all this information.

Done well, the preoperative evaluation establishes a trusting doctor–patient relationship that significantly diminishes patient anxiety and measurably influences postoperative recovery and outcome.

2. What is the American Society of Anesthesiologists' (ASA) physical status classification?

The ASA classification was created in 1940 for the purposes of statistical studies and hospital records. It is useful both for outcome comparisons and as a convenient means of communicating the physical status of a patient among anesthesiologists. Unfortunately, it is imprecise, and a patient often may be placed in different classes by different anesthesiologists. Also the higher ASA class only roughly predicts anesthetic risk. The five classes, as last modified in 1961, are:

Class 1—Healthy patient, no medical problems
Class 2—Mild systemic disease
Class 3—Severe systemic disease, but not incapacitating
Class 4—Severe systemic disease that is a constant threat to life
Class 5—Moribund, not expected to live 24 hours irrespective of operation

An *e* is added to the status number to designate an emergency operation. An organ donor is usually designated as a Class 6.

3. Describe the two key features of the airway examination.

Current practice includes evaluation of both the oropharynx and mental space. The **oropharynx** is examined with the patient in the sitting position, with the neck extended, tongue out, and phonating. The four classes of oropharynx, originally described by Mallampati, are grouped according to visualized structures:

   Class I—Soft palate, fauces, uvula, anterior and posterior tonsillar pillars
   Class II—Soft palate fauces, uvula
   Class III—Soft palate, base of uvula
   Class IV—Soft palate only

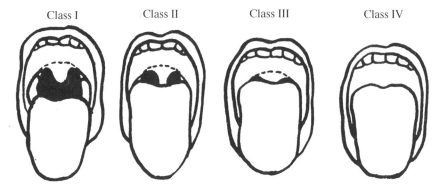

Class I   Class II   Class III   Class IV

Mallampati classification of the oropharynx. (From Benumof JL: Management of the difficult airway. Anesthesiology 75:1087–1110, 1991; adapted from Mallampati SR, et al: A clinical sign to predict difficult tracheal intubation: a prospective study. Can Anaesth Soc J 32:429–434, 1985.)

The **mental space** is the distance from the thyroid cartilage to the inside of the mentum, measured while the patient sits with the neck in the sniff position.

Mallampati found a correlation between higher oropharyngeal class and decreased glottic exposure at laryngoscopy. Benumof more recently demonstrated that higher oropharyngeal class, *combined with* a mental space < 2 fingerbreadths, better predicted increased difficulty with intubation. Other features on exam that increase the likelihood of difficult intubation include diminished neck extension, decreased tissue compliance, large tongue, overbite and/or large teeth, narrow high-arched palate, decreased temporomandibular joint mobility, and short thick neck.

4. How long should a patient fast before surgery?

In recent years, feelings concerning the traditional 12-hour fast have changed, because it has been found that this fast does not always ensure an empty stomach and needlessly results in dehydration and stress for the patient. Current guidelines for adults with no risk factors for aspiration (*see* question #4) include: no solid food for at least eight hours, unrestricted clear liquids up to two hours before surgery, and oral preoperative medications up to 1-2 hours before anesthesia with sips of water.

   Current fasting guidelines for pediatric patients are:

   1. Clear liquids up to 2 hours preoperatively in newborns ≤ 6 months.

   2. Solid foods, including milk, up to 4 hours preoperatively in newborns ≤ 6 months up to 6 hours in children 6 months to 3 years; and up to 8 hours in children > 3 years.

5. Which patients are at higher risk for aspiration?

Higher-risk patients are those with any degree of gastrointestinal obstruction, a history of gastroesophageal reflux, diabetes (gastroparesis), recent solid-food intake, abdominal distention (obesity, ascites), depressed consciousness, or recent opioid administration (decreased gastric emptying). In addition, naso-oropharyngeal or upper gastrointestinal bleeding, airway trauma, and emergency surgery are high-risk settings.

A pregnant patient undergoing emergency cesarean section presents a good example of **multiple risk factors**: full stomach, gastroesophagel reflux, abdominal distention, gestational diabetes, and difficult airway. A classic situation for **aspiration** involves a patient with a difficult airway in whom mask ventilation has led to insufflation of the stomach, and the anesthesiologist is struggling with laryngoscopy, insufficient depth of anesthesia, and muscle relaxation.

6. A trauma patient has just arrived in the operating room for emergency surgery. What are the bare essentials of your preoperative evaluation?
Remember your basic ABCs:

A Airway
B Breathing
C Circulation

If the patient is not already intubated, the airway evaluation in a trauma case includes checking the cervical spine status and checking for airway or facial injuries. Determine the oxygen saturation, respiratory rate, effort, and symmetry of breath sounds. Assess the current hemodynamic status, estimated blood loss, urine output, fluid and blood resuscitation and response to therapy.

Determine the level of consciousness and whether there are any focal neurologic deficits. An altered level of consciousness may be due to head trauma, pretrauma alcohol or drug ingestion, and/or metabolic derangements. Check the primary and associated injuries. The mechanism of injury, blunt vs. penetrating, is as significant as the site. Maintain a high index of suspicion for unappreciated additional injuries. If time and condition permit, ask about allergies, medications, major medicial problems, and previous anesthesia history.

7. What particular medical and anesthetic problems are associated with obesity?
Obesity is defined as excess body weight > 20% over the predicted ideal body weight. Obese patients have a higher incidence of diabetes, hypertension, and cardiovascular disease. There is a higher incidence of difficulty with both mask ventilation and intubation. They have a decreased functional residual capacity, increased O_2 consumption and CO_2 production, and often, diminished ventilation ranging from mild ventilation/perfusion mismatch to actual obesity-hypoventilation and obstructive sleep apnea (pickwickian syndrome). These changes result in more rapid apneic desaturation. If the patients are pickwickian, they may have pulmonary hypertension with or without right ventricular failure. Increased intra-abdominal pressure is associated with hiatal hernia and reflux. Because of their higher gastric volume and lower pH, obese patients are at greater risk for aspiration. Pharmacokinetics for many drugs and anesthetic agents are altered in them. Finally, regional anesthesia is more difficult and more often unsuccessful.

8. Which conditions identified at preoperative evaluation most commonly result in changes in the anesthetic care plan?
In a study at the University of Florida, care plans were altered in 20% of *all* patients (including 15% of ASA class I and II patients) due to conditions identified at the preoperative evaluation. The most common conditions resulting in changes were gastric reflux, insulin-dependent diabetes mellitus, asthma, and suspected difficult airway. These findings indicate that it is preferable in all patients, whenever possible, to do the preoperative evaluation before the day of surgery.

9. What are the appropriate preoperative laboratory tests? Which patients should have an electrocardiogram? Chest radiography?
Preoperative testing should be tailored to the individual patient and the specific surgical procedure. Indiscriminate batteries of tests have a low yield for detecting unsuspected disease and can result in false-positives that add additional costs and risks to the patient, as well as increase the medicolegal risks for the physician. Studies looking at the risks/benefits of different tests have yielded the following recommendations:

Recommended Preoperative Tests for Asymptomatic Patients

| AGE | ASYMPTOMATIC PATIENTS | | INDIVIDUALS NOT RECEIVING GENERAL OR MAJOR CONDUCTION ANESTHESIA | |
	Men	Women	Sedative-Hypnotics for Monitored Anesthesia	Peripheral or IV Nerve Block
6 mo–40 yr	None	Hct ? Pregnancy test	None	None
40–50 yr	ECG	Hct ? Pregnancy test	None	None
50–64 yr	ECG	Hgb/Hct ? Pregnancy test ECG	Hct*	None
65–74yr	Hgb or Hct ECG BUN Glucose	Hgb/Hct ECG BUN Glucose	Hct* ECG*	Hct*
	Hgb/Hct ECG BUN Glucose ? Chest x-ray	Hgb/Hct ECG BUN Glucose ? Chest x-ray	Hct ECG* BUN* Glucose*	Hct* ECG*

* Or substitute test measured within the previous 6 months, or for an electrocardiogram (ECG), within 1 year.
Hct, hematocrit; Hgb, hemoglobin; BUN, blood urea nitrogen.
From Roizen MF: Preoperative assessment: What is necessary to do? In 45th Annual Refresher Course Lectures and Clinical Update Program. San Francisco, ASA, 1994; with permission.

Additional Preoperative Testing for Patients with Underlying Medical Conditions
or Procedures with Blood Loss

| PREOPERATIVE CONDITION | HEMOGLOBIN | | WBC | PT/ PTT | PLATELETS/ BT | ELECTRO-LYTES | CR/ BUN | BLOOD GLUCOSE | AST/ APASE | X-RAY | ECG |
	M	F									
Procedure with blood loss*	X	X									
Neonates	X	X									
Age											
<40		X									
40–49		X										m
50–64		X									X
65–74		X					X	X		±	X
≥ 75		X					X	X		±	X
Cardiovascular disease							X			X	X
Pulmonary disease										X	X
Malignancy	X	X	*LK	*LK						X	
Radiation therapy			X							X	X
Hepatic disease									X		
Exposure to hepatitis									X		
Renal disease	X	X				X	X				

Table continued on following page.

Additional Preoperative Testing for Patients with Underlying Medical Conditions or Procedures with Blood Loss (Continued)

PREOPERATIVE CONDITION	HEMOGLOBIN M	HEMOGLOBIN F	WBC	PT/ PTT	PLATELETS/ BT	ELECTRO-LYTES	Cr/ BUN	BLOOD GLUCOSE	AST/ APase	X-RAY	ECG
Bleeding disorder				X	X						
Diabetes						X	X	X			X
Smoking ≥ 20 pack/yr	X	X								X	
Use of											
Diuretics						X	X				
Digoxin						X	X				X
Steroids						X		X			
Anticoagulants	X	X		X							
CNS disease			X			X	X	X			X

* Also obtain blood typing and screening for unexpected antibodies.
Not all diseases are included in this table. The physician's judgment is needed regarding patients with diseases not listed.
Symbols: ± = perhaps obtain; LK = obtain for leukemias only; X = obtain; m = obtain for men only
Abbreviations: WBC, white blood cell count; PT, prothrombin time; PTT, partial thromboplastin time; BT, bleeding time; Cr/BUN, creatine or blood urea nitrogen; AST/APase, serum aspartate aminotransferase (SGOT) and alkaline phosphatase.

10. What is the generally accepted minimum hematocrit for elective surgery?

There *is not* a specific minimum; it depends on the clinical setting. The hemoglobin or hematocrit is just one component of oxygen delivery. O_2 delivery is a function of the hematocrit, cardiac output, and arterial O_2 saturation, and blood viscosity (inversely related to the hematocrit). One also must consider medical conditions that place certain organs at increased risk for inadequate oxygenation, such as coronary atherosclerosis, cerebral insufficiency, or renovascular disease. Finally, the potential blood loss and O_2 demands associated with the proposed surgical procedure must be considered.

If there is cardiovascular stability in a volume-resuscitated ASA class I–II patient with minimal anticipated blood loss, a hematocrit down to 18% is acceptable before transfusion. A patient with well-compensated systemic disease (ASA class III) in the same setting should tolerate a hematocrit as low as 24%. In a patient with coronary disease or other significant vascular insufficiency, the hematocrit should be kept > 30%. In the setting of trauma and potential multiorgan failure, keep the hematocrit > 35%.

11. Which patients should have pulmonary function tests (PFTs)?

Because PFTs are relatively insensitive and expensive, they are not recommended routinely for smokers or other patients with underlying lung disease. In most cases, the history, auscultation, and chest radiograph are adequate to formulate the anesthetic plan. In patients undergoing lung resection, PFTs in combination with a ventilation/perfusion lung scan help determine perioperative management and predict outcome. A predicted *postoperative* FEV_1 of < 800 ml is a contraindication to pulmonary resection.

PFTs may be useful sometimes in patients with symptomatic lung disease who are having upper abdominal procedures or otherwise prolonged and/or extensive surgery, in whom they can serve as a predictive device or to monitor the response of the patient's pulmonary condition to preoperative treatment. Flow volume loops can help distinguish fixed airway obstruction from variable extrathoracic or intrathoracic obstruction that has implications for anesthetic management. In variable intrathoracic obstruction, neuromuscular blockade or positive pressure ventilation can worsen obstruction.

12. When are preoperative consultations with other specialists indicated?
Preoperative consultations fall into two general categories:

   1. Those cases that need more information or expertise to establish and/or quantify a diagnosis that has implications for the anesthetic management; or

   2. Patients in whom the diagnosis is known, but further evaluation and treatment are needed to optimize their medical condition prior to surgery.

An example of the first type of referral would be asking a cardiologist to evaluate a 50-year-old man with recent onset of exertional chest pain.

Referring patients with poorly controlled diabetes, hypertension, or asthma to an internist is a good example of the second type of consultation.

13. What benefits can be derived from preoperative cigarette cessation? How long prior to surgery must the patient quit to realize these benefits?
Carbon monoxide (CO) from cigarette smoking diminishes oxygen delivery to tissues. Nicotine increases heart rate and can cause peripheral vasoconstriction. Within 12–24 hours of discontinuing cigarettes, CO and nicotine levels return to normal. Bronchotracheal ciliary function improves within 2–3 days of cessation, and sputum volume decreases to normal levels within about 2 weeks. However, studies have not demonstrated a significant decrease in postoperative respiratory morbidity until after 6–8 weeks of abstinence.

14. Are there any risks associated with quitting cigarettes?
Following cessation, some smokers will have an initial *increase* in sputum production, and others may have new onset or exacerbation of existing reactive airways disease. Although the risk of *arterial* thrombosis decreases with cessation, there may be an increase in risk of deep venous thrombosis. There are also possible short-term negative effects of the irritability and anxiety associated with nicotine withdrawal.

15. What are Goldman's criteria of cardiac risks associated with noncardiac surgery?
In a 1977 prospective study of 1001 patients over age 40 who were undergoing surgery, Goldman et al. identified nine independent risk factors for life-threatening and/or fatal cardiac complications of noncardiac surgery. Through multivariate discriminant analysis, they assigned relative risk (RR) "points" to each variable and then categorized patients into four risk classes by their total points (cardiac risk index) to determine their risk of postoperative cardiac complications post-op. Although improvements in perioperative care in recent years have diminished the predictive value of the index for class I and II patients, Goldman classes III and IV continue to represent a high-risk cohort.

Nine Independent Risk Factors for Life-Threatening and/or Fatal Cardiac Complications of Noncardiac Surgery

RISK FACTORS	RELATIVE RISK POINTS
1. Preoperative third heart sound or jugular venous distention	11
2. Myocardial infarction in the preceding six months	10
3. More than 5 premature ventricular contractions per minute documented at any time before operation	7
4. Rhythm other than sinus or presence of premature atrial contractions on preoperative ECG	7
5. Age over 70	5
6. Intraperitoneal, intrathoracic or aortic operation	3
7. Emergency operation	4
8. Important valvular aortic stenosis	3
9. Poor general medical condition	3

Goldman Classification for Cardiac Risk in Noncardiac Surgery

CLASS	TOTAL POINTS (POSSIBLE 53)	NO OR MINIMAL CARDIAC COMPLICATIONS	LIFE-THREATENING CARDIAC COMPLICATIONS	CARDIAC DEATH
I	0–5	99%	0.7%	0.2%
II	6–12	93%	5%	2%
III	13–25	86%	11%	2%
IV	> 25	22%	22%	56%

16. How would you approach the preoperative evaluation of a patient with chest pain?

Myocardial infarction, occurring perioperatively, carries a mortality of up to 50%. It is therefore imperative to identify ischemic heart disease before surgery so that steps can be taken to prevent infarction.

The **history** is the most important diagnostic tool. Ask the patient to describe his or her chest pain. Determine the frequency, character, location, duration, and any radiation of the pain. If the chest pain occurs with exertion, quantify the amount required to precipitate the pain. Ask about associated symptoms of dyspnea, palpitations, or lightheadedness. If the patient has a prior history of infarction, how long ago was it and have there been any subsequent revascularization procedures? What are the patient's current cardiac medications?

On **physical examination** check the heart rate and blood pressure. Are there any arrhythmias? Are the blood pressures symmetrical in the upper extremities? Look for peripheral edema, jugular venous elevation, and a third heart sound.

The ECG might be completely normal or show arrhythmias, evidence of prior infarction, or ongoing ischemia. Compare it with a previous tracing whenever possible. Check the patient's records and/or contact his or her cardiologist for results of other tests, such as echocardiograms, treadmill ECGs, or cardiac catheterizations. Echocardiograms can be useful in delineating the nature and extent of any ventricular dysfunction as well as any associated valvular problems. Exercise ECG is a noninvasive and cost-effective test that identifies ischemic heart disease (IHD) with reasonable sensitivity and specificity as well as measures the hemodynamic threshold of the patient's ischemia (blood pressure × heart rate). The sensitivity and specificity of exercise testing can be enhanced with the addition of thallium radioisotope imaging. In patients who are unable to exercise, thallium redistribution in ischemic areas of myocardium can be elicited pharmacologically with coronary vasodilators (dipyridamole or adenosine) or with agents that increase myocardial O_2 demand (dobutamine). Cardiac catheterization is the "gold standard" for evaluating coronary flow, extent of myocardium at risk, and ventricular function.

The results of these tests help the anesthesiologist decide what types of monitoring are required intraoperatively and what anesthetic agents to use. Cardiology consultation is indicated if a patient has a history suggestive of IHD and has not been adequately evaluated or if a patient with known IHD has had a change in clinical status or requires optimization of their medical management. Also certain asymptomatic individuals, such as diabetics (especially those with autonomic neuropathy), hypertensives with left ventricular hypertrophy, and patients scheduled for vascular surgery, are at high risk for associated IHD and warrant preoperative cardiology evaluation.

17. In the evaluation of a patient's coagulation status, what are the key features in the history? What constitutes the basic laboratory evaluation?

The anesthesiologist should *always* ask about **abnormal bleeding** or **bruising**, medical conditions or medications associated with increased bleeding, family history of excessive bleeding, or unusual bleeding with prior surgery. If there is a positive response to any of these, further questioning is indicated: Is there epistaxis, hematuria, or menorrhagia? These would suggest a problem with primary hemostasis indicative of impaired platelet function and/or thrombocytopenia. Hematuria may also occur with a coagulopathy.

Gingival bleeding could be due to primary gum disease, uremia, or thrombocytopenia. Petechiae suggest quantitative or qualitative platelet abnormalities or impaired vascular integrity. Gastrointestinal bleeding may be due to abnormal primary hemostasis, coagulopathy, or fibrinolysis. A history of severe, life-threatening bleeding, bleeding into deep tissue planes, muscles, or the retroperitoneal space, and, especially, spontaneous ecchymoses or hemarthrosis, usually is due to a defect in the coagulation pathway. Initial bleeding that stops and then spontaneously recurs also suggests a coagulopathy.

The **basic laboratory** evaluation includes platelet count, bleeding time, prothrombin time (PT), partial thromboplastin time (PTT), and thrombin time. The minimal number of normally functioning platelets to prevent surgical bleeding is 50,000/mm³. It is important to note that both the PT and PTT require about a 60–80% *loss* of coagulation activity before becoming abnormal, but patients with smaller decreases in function can still have significant surgical bleeding. Therefore the history is still very important.

18. Can a patient with a prosthetic heart valve who is taking anticoagulants undergo a spinal or epidural anesthetic? What about a patient with osteoarthritis on aspirin?
Regional anesthesia in a patient on anticoagulation should be done only when the benefits/risks outweigh those associated with alternative techniques. In a patient with a prosthetic valve, discontinuation of anticoagulants carries a real risk of valvular thrombosis and/or embolic phenomena. Therefore, the timing is critical to achieve a coagulation "window" short enough to avoid pathologic thrombosis and long enough to avoid neuraxial bleeding. Oral anticoagulants should be stopped 3–5 days prior to surgery, and the patient simultaneously started on intravenous heparin. The heparin is stopped 4–6 hours before the spinal or epidural and not resumed for at least 1 hour to avoid epidural hematoma. If there is a possibility of surgical bleeding, the delay should be at least 12 hours before resuming heparin.

Unless there is a history of actual bleeding or bruising, patients receiving antiplatelet medications (aspirin or other nonsteroidal anti-inflammatory drugs) can safely have epidural or spinal anesthesia.

19. Discuss the preoperative evaluation of a diabetic patient.
How long has the patient had diabetes mellitus? How good is the glycemic control? Patients with frequent insulin reactions and episodes of ketoacidosis (i.e., "brittle" diabeties) are more likely to be metabolically unstable perioperatively. Diabetics with a long history of poor control are also more likely to have end-organ disease. Specifically, the anesthesiologist should look for evidence of coronary disease (often "silent"), hypertension, autonomic neuropathy (check for orthostatic changes in vital signs), renal insufficiency, cardiomyopathy, and gastroparesis (ask about reflux and early satiety). Find out what medications the patient takes for the diabetes, the most recent dose, and current blood sugar. Some diabetics may have diminished neck extension due to atlanto-occipital involvement with the stiff joint syndrome.

Serious preoperative metabolic derangements are seen more often in insulin-dependent diabetics, especially in the setting of trauma or infection. Look for high or low glucose levels, electrolyte abnormalities, ketoacidosis, hypovolemia, and hyperosmolarity.

Preoperative testing should include, at a minimum, glucose, electrolytes, BUN, creatinine, urinalysis, and ECG. Additional lab work might include arterial blood gas, ketones, osmolarity, calcium, phosphorus, and magnesium.

20. What are the anesthetic implications of chronic alcohol consumption? What should an alcoholic's preoperative evaluation include?
With an estimated 18 million alcoholics in America, an anesthesiologist can expect to encounter this problem frequently during preoperative evaluations. Alcoholism is a multisystem disease. Increased CNS tolerance to volatile anesthetics and induction agents is observed. Perioperative withdrawal seizures or delerium tremens can occur. Some alcoholics exhibit paradoxical excitation when given sedatives and hypnotics. Peripheral neuropathy may be present with implications

for the use of regional anesthesia. Cardiovascular features include an increased incidence of hypertension and possible presence of alcoholic cardiomyopathy (associated with congestive heart failure, arrhythmias, and enhanced sensitivity to the cardiodepressant effects of volatile anesthetics). Gastrointestinal problems include gastritis, bleeding, hepatitis, and pancreatitis.

Chronic alcohol exposure leads to increased hepatic metabolic activity with increased tolerance of local anesthetics, sedatives, analgesics, and some neuromuscular blockers. Conversely, once liver function becomes impaired, one observes *increased* drug effect, as well as coagulopathy, and possible esophageal varices. Metabolic/nutritional abnormalities include thiamine deficiency, hypophosphatemia, hypomagnesemia, and hypocalcemia. Finally, the alcoholic may have leukopenia and anemia, and in the presence of liver disease, in addition to coagulopathy, they may have thrombocytopenia and a predisposition to disseminated intravascular coagulation.

The diagnosis of alcoholism is often missed because denial is a prominent feature. The brief **CAGE** questionnaire may be more informative than simply asking the patient "how much do you drink?"

C   Do you occasionally cut down on your alcohol intake?
A   Are you annoyed when people criticize your drinking?
G   Do you feel guilty at times about your drinking?
E   Do you ever take an "eye opener" in the morning?

Determine the quantity and frequency of consumption and most recent alcohol intake. Ask about withdrawal symptoms and prior abstinence phenomena. Look for signs of early withdrawal (tremor, agitation, confusion, increased heart rate), stigmata of liver disease (spider angiomata, palmar erythema, jaundice, ascites, gynecomastia, enlarged parotids and lacrimals, abnormal coagulation), and check for hypertension and cardiomyopathy. If a regional technique is planned, document any preexisting neuropathy. Laboratory evaluation should include a complete blood count, platelet count, electrolytes, BUN, creatinine, glucose, liver enzymes, albumin, bilirubin, coagulation tests, calcium, magnesium, and phosphorus. A preoperative ECG is indicated.

If alcohol is noted on the patient's breath, or there is other reason to suspect recent ingestion, an alcohol level should be checked. If the surgery is emergent, the patient should be treated as having a "full stomach." If the surgery is elective, delay the procedure.

21. What are the anesthetic implications of acute alcohol intoxication?

Alcohol is involved in more than 50% of automobile accidents, 67% of homicides, and 35% of suicides. It is the leading killer of persons in the 15–45-year age group. Therefore, many patients presenting for emergency surgery will be intoxicated.

All of these patients are considered as having "full stomachs." Many are dehydrated due to inhibition of antidiuretic hormone (ADH) by alcohol. This, in conjunction with their vasodilation, make them prone to hypotension. Some are hypothermic. Because they are already partially "anesthetized," MAC is decreased, and alcohol works synergistically with the cardiorespiratory depressant effects of sedatives and narcotics. One should not automatically attribute an altered level of consciousness to inebriation, but keep a high index of suspicion for associated head injury and/or metabolic derangements (lactic acidosis, alcoholic ketoacidosis, hypoglycemia). Laboratory workup includes a blood alcohol level, drug screen (polydrug consumption is common), complete blood count, electrolytes, glucose, liver function tests, coagulation tests, ECG, calcium, phosphorus, and magnesium.

Most acutely intoxicated patients are *chronic* alcoholics, and therefore all the anesthetic implications outlined in question #20 are also applicable.

22. Which medical conditions should be looked for in the preoperative evaluation of an obstetric patient?

Although most pregnant patients are young and healthy, it is still very important, whenever possible, to do the same careful medical history and preoperative examination. However, some potential problems are unique to the gravid patient. Gestational **diabetes mellitus** is common, and any preexisting diabetes may be exacerbated. **Reactive airways disease** may worsen during pregnancy. The hemodynamic changes of pregnancy, specifically the increased intravascular volume and the demand for a higher cardiac output, may decompensate some forms of **valvular heart disease**, particularly mitral stenosis. **Preeclampsia** is seen in 5–10% of pregnancies. The presence of placenta previa, abruptio placentae, prior cesarian section, fetal prematurity (is the patient on a tocolytic?), abnormal fetal presentation, fetal distress, or multiple gestations all have important implications for the anesthetic management. The weight increase, enlarged breasts, and pharyngolaryngeal edema associated with pregnancy (and especially preeclampsia) can turn a normal airway into a difficult airway.

23. In an obstetric emergency, what is the minimal information needed?
Too frequently, the anesthesiologist may first meet the obstetric patient en route to a "stat" cesarean delivery. The minimal information to be obtained in this setting would include the indication for the cesarean (prior cesarean delivery?), allergies, time of last oral intake, medical illnesses before and during the pregnancy, current medications, prior anesthetic complications, fetal status, and the parturient's vital signs, airway, and general medical condition.

CONTROVERSY

24. A 3-year-old child comes in for an elective tonsillectomy. His mother reports that for the last 3 days, he has had a runny nose and postnasal drip. Should you postpone surgery?
Viral upper respiratory tract infection (URI) alters the quality and quantity of airway secretions and increases airway reflexes to mechanical, chemical, or irritant stimulation. Some clinical studies have shown associated intraoperative and postoperative bronchospasm, laryngospasm, and hypoxia. There is evidence that the risk of pulmonary complications may remain high for at least 2 weeks, and possibly 6–7 weeks, after a URI. Infants have a greater risk than older children, and intubation probably confers additional risk. An editorial in *Anesthesiology* in 1991 recommended avoiding anesthesia whenever possible for at least several weeks after a URI.

However, as a practical matter, young children can average 5–8 URIs per year, mostly from fall through spring. If a 4–7-week symptom-free interval were rigorously followed, an elective surgery might be postponed indefinitely. Therefore, most anesthesiologists distinguish chronic nasal discharge from uncomplicated URI from that associated with more severe URI with or without lower respiratory tract infection (LRI). Chronic nasal discharge is usually noninfectious in origin and caused by allergy or vasomotor rhinitis. An uncomplicated URI is characterized by sore or scratchy throat, laryngitis, sneezing, rhinorrhea, congestion, malaise, nonproductive cough, and fever < 38° C. More severe URI or LRI may include severe nasopharyngitis, purulent sputum, high fever, deep cough, and associated auscultatory findings of wheezes or rales.

It is generally agreed that chronic nasal discharge poses no significant anesthesia risk. In contrast, children with severe URI or LRI almost always have their elective surgery postponed. Probably *most* anesthesiologists will proceed to surgery with a child with a resolving uncomplicated URI, unless the child has a history of asthma or other significant pulmonary disease.

BIBLIOGRAPHY

1. Abrams KJ: Preanesthetic assessment of the multiple trauma victim. Anesthesiol Clin North Am 8:811–827 1990.
2. Ammon JR: Perioperative management of the diabetic patient. In 45th Annual Refresher Course Lectures and Clinical Update Program. San Francisco, ASA, 1994.
3. Benumof JL: Management of the difficult airway. Anesthesiology 75:1087–1110, 1991.
4. Betts EK: In the real world. In Wetchler BV (ed): Anesthesia for Ambulatory Surgery, 2nd ed. Philadelphia, J.B. Lippincott, 1991, pp 506–508.
5. Bishop MJ: The patient with respiratory disease: Evaluation, preparation and timing of surgery. In 44th Annual Refresher Course Lectures and Clinical Update Program. Washington, DC, ASA, 1993.
6. Buckley FP: Anesthetizing the morbidly obese patient. In 44th Annual Refresher Course Lectures and Clinical Update Program. Washington, DC, ASA, 1993.

7. Cote CJ: Changing concepts in preoperative medication and "NPO" status of the pediatric patient. In 44th Annual Refresher Course Lectures and Clinical Update Program, Washington, DC, ASA, 1993.

8. Fiamengo SA: Alcoholism. In Yao FF, Artusio JF (eds): Anesthesiology, 3rd ed. Philadelphia, J.B. Lippincott, 1993, pp 693–707.

9. Fleisher LA: Preoperative evaluation of the cardiac patient undergoing noncardiac surgery. In 45th Annual Refresher Course Lectures and Clinical Update Program. San Francisco, ASA, 1994.

10. Fong J: Preanesthetic assessment of the patient with coagulopathies. Anesthesiol Clin North Am 8:727–739, 1990.

11. Frost EA, Siedel MR: Preanesthetic assessment of the drug abuse patient. Anesthesiol Clin North Am 8:829–833, 1990.

12. Gibbs CP, Modell JH: Management of aspiration pneumonitis. In Miller R (ed): Anesthesia, 3rd ed. Philadelphia, W.B. Saunders, 1990, pp 1437–1459.

13. Gibby GL, Gravenstein JS, Layon AJ, Jackson KI: How often does the preoperative interview change anesthetic management [abstract]? Anesthesiology 77:A1134,1992.

14. Goldman L: Multifactorial index of cardiac risk in noncardiac surgical procedures. N Engl J Med 287:843–850, 1977.

15. Goldman L: Cardiac risks and complications of noncardiac surgery. Ann Intern Med 98:504–513, 1983.

16. Horlocker TT,Wedel D: Anticoagulants, antiplatelet therapy, and neuraxis blockade. Anesthesiol Clin North Am 10:1–11, 1992.

17. Hurford WE: Evaluating the patient before anesthesia: specific considerations with pulmonary disease. In Fireston LL, Lebowitz PW, Cook CE (eds): Clinical Anesthesia Procedures of the Massachusetts General Hospital, 3rd ed. Boston, Little, Brown & Co., 1988.

18. Jacoby DB, Hirshman CA: General anesthesia in patients with viral respiratory infections: An unsound sleep [editorial]? Anesthesiology 74:969–972, 1991.

19. Jones GA: Preanesthetic Assessment of the Patient with Endocrine Disease. Anesthesiol Clin North Am 8:697–711, 1990.

20. Levine E: Physiologic effects of acute anemia: Implications for a reduced transfusion trigger. Transfusion 30:11–13, 1990.

21. Lewis M, Keramati S, Benumof JL, Berry CB: What is the best way to determine oropharyngeal classification and mandibular space length to predict difficult laryngoscopy? Anesthesiology 81:69–75,1994.

22. Mallampati SR: A clinical sign to predict difficult tracheal intubation: A prospective study. Can Anaesth Soc J 32:429–434, 1985.

23. Pawlowski J: Evaluating the patient before anesthesia; specific considerations with cardiac disease. In Fireston LL, Lebowitz PW, Cook CE (eds): Clinical Anesthesia Procedures of the Massachusetts General Hospital, 2nd ed. Boston, Little, Brown and Co., 1988, pp 15–19.

24. Pearce AC, Jones RM: Smoking and anesthesia: preoperative abstinence and perioperative morbidity. Anesthesiology 61: 576–584, 1984.

25. Petrovitch CT: Perioperative evaluation of coagulation. In 45th Annual Refresher Course Lectures and Clinical Update Program. San Francisco, ASA, 1994.

26. Roizen MF: Preoperative assessment: What is necessary to do? In 45th Annual Refresher Course Lectures and Clinical Update Program. San Francisco, ASA, 1994.

27. Schwalbe SS: Preanesthetic assessment of the obstetric patient. Anesthesiol Clin North Am 8:741–758, 1990.

28. Stehling L, Zauder HL: How low can we go? Is there a way to know [editorial]? Transfusion 30:1, 1990.

29. Stoelting RK: "NPO" and Aspiration Pneumonitis—Changing Perspectives. In 45th Annual Refresher Course Lectures and Clinical Update Program. San Francisco, ASA, 1994.

30. Tait AR, Knight PR: Upper respiratory infection. In Bready LL Smith RB (eds): Decision Making in Anesthesiology, 2nd ed. St. Louis, Mosby, 1992, pp 76–77.

31. Tremper KK, Techniques and solutions to avoid homologous blood transfusions. In 45th Annual Refresher Course Lectures and Update Program. San Francisco, ASA, 1994, pp 251–262.

32. Yao FF, Savarese JJ: Morbid obesity. In Yao FF, Artusio JF (eds): Anesthesiology, 3rd ed. Philadelphia, J.B. Lippincott, 1993, pp 751–766.

33. Zibrak JD, O'Donnell CR, Marton K: Indications for pulmonary function testing: Ann Intern Med 112: 763–771, 1990.

16. PREOPERATIVE MEDICATION

Jeff Nabonsal, M.D.

1. List the possible reasons to use premedication.
Patient comfort
  • Anxiolysis
  • Sedation
  • Amnesia
  • Analgesia
Decrease in gastric volume and increase gastric pH
Decrease in airway secretions
Decrease in incidence of nausea and vomiting
Decrease in autonomic responses (both sympathetic and parasympathetic)
Prophylaxis against allergic reactions
Continued therapy for concurrent disease
Prevention of infection

2. List the most commonly used preoperative medications with the appropriate dose.

Common Preoperative Medications: Dosage, Route, and Indications

DRUG	DOSE*	ROUTE	INDICATIONS
Midazolam	0.5–2 mg doses	Intravenous (IV)	Sedation, amnesia
	0.05–0.1 mg/kg	Intramuscular (IM)	Sedation, amnesia
	0.5–1.0 mg/kg	Oral (PO)	Sedation, amnesia
	(maximum: 20 mg)	(for pediatric patients)	
	0.2–0.3 mg/kg	Intranasal	Sedation, amnesia
Diazepam	5–20 mg	PO	Sedation, amnesia
Methohexital	25 mg/kg	Rectal (PR)	Pediatric sedative
Ketamine	1–2 mg/kg	IM, IV, or PO	Sedation, analgesia
Morphine	0.1–0.2 mg/kg	IM or IV	Analgesia, sedation
Droperidol	5–100 µg/kg	IV	Neuroleptic
Atropine	5–20 µg/kg	IM or IV	Vagolytic
Glycopyrrolate	2–5 µg/kg	IM or IV	Antisialagogue
Scopolamine	5–8 µg/kg	IM or IV	Sedation, amnesia
Ranitidine	1–3 mg/kg	PO or IV	H2 blockade
Cimetidine	2–4 mg/kg	IM, IV, or PO	H2 blockade
Metoclopramide	0.1–0.25 mg/kg	IM, IV, or PO	Prophylaxis for
Antacids (nonpar- ticulate)	30 ml	PO (for adults)	aspiration

* Assume 70 kg if not in mg/kg.

3. What factors should always be considered in premedicating patients?
Physical status (as defined by the American
  Society for Anesthesiologists [ASA])
Age and weight
Levels of anxiety and pain
Previous history of drug use or abuse
Previous nausea and vomiting related
  to anesthesia
Allergies
Inpatient vs. outpatient
Planned surgical procedure

4. Describe factors that limit ones ability to give depressant medications preoperatively.
Patients at the extremes of age
Head injuries or altered mental status
Minimal cardiac or pulmonary reserve
Hypovolemia
Full stomachs

5. What is meant by psychological preparation? How should a patient ideally present in the operating suite for an elective procedure?
Psychological preparation begins with a reassuring preoperative interview by an anesthesiologist in which anticipated events are explained and all the patients questions are answered. Ideally, for elective operations the patients should be anxiety-free, sedated, easily arousable, and cooperative.

6. Why are gastric volumes and pH a concern for the anesthesiologist? How can they be altered by premedication?
Approximately 40–80% of patients scheduled for elective surgery are at risk of developing aspiration pneumonitis secondary to the presence of a gastric volume > 25 ml and a gastric pH < 2.5 (Mendelson's syndrome). Preanesthetic treatment that reduces gastric volume and increases pH is expected to reduce the incidence and severity of aspiration.

Nonparticulate liquid antacids raise gastric pH and are effective immediately; however, the H2 blockers need to be given approximately 8 hours before induction of anesthesia to obtain full benefit. Metoclopramide increases gastric motility and relaxes the gastroduodenal sphincter, thereby promoting gastric emptying. Metoclopramide also functions centrally as an antiemetic. Metoclopramide acts within 1–4 minutes if given intravenously and within 30–60 minutes if given orally.

7. Name factors that make the drugs described in question 6 an important consideration.
Pregnancy — Trauma
Obesity — Diabetes mellitus
Opiate use — Difficult airway
Pain — Ileus or obstruction
Alcohol — Increased intraabdominal pressure

8. Describe the most common side effects when opiates are used as a premedication.
Pruritus — Histamine release
Nausea and vomiting — Delayed gastric emptying
Respiratory depression — Stiff chest syndrome
Orthostatic hypotension — Sphincter of Oddi spasm

9. Describe the reasons for choosing an anticholinergic agent as a premedication. Name the three most commonly used anticholinergics.
Anticholinergic premedication is not mandatory and should be tailored to the patient's needs. Reasons for use include vagolytic and antisialogogue effects as well as sedation, amnesia, and antiemetic effects. The three most commonly used anticholinergics are atropine, scopolamine, and glycopyrrolate. The antisialogogue effect is of utmost importance in managing fiberoptic intubations. Decreased secretions improve visualization and topicalization with local anesthesia. Vagolytic effects also may decrease airway responsiveness.

10. Show the relative potencies of the three most commonly used anticholinergic agents and their effects.

Effects of Commonly Used Anticholinergic Agents

	ATROPINE	SCOPOLAMINE	GLYCOPYRROLATE
Tachycardia	+++	+	++
Antisialogogue effect	+	+++	++
Sedation, amnesia	+	+++	0
Central nervous system toxicity	+	++	0
Lower esophageal sphincter relaxation	++	++	++

0 = none, + = mild, ++ = moderate, +++ = marked.

11. List some side effects of anticholinergic medications.
Side effects seen with anticholinergics include:
CNS toxicity
Decrease in lower esophageal sphincter tone
Mydriasis and cycloplegia
Increase in physiologic dead space
Prevention of sweating
Hyperthermia

12. Explain why glycopyrrolate has no side effects on the central nervous system.
Glycopyrrolate has no CNS side effects because it is a positively charged quaternary amine, and hence does not cross the blood–brain barrier (BBB). Tertiary amines are neutrally charged and cross the BBB, thus affecting the CNS.

13. A patient in the preoperative holding area is delirious after receiving only 0.4 mg of scopolamine as a premedication. What is the cause of the delirium? Describe its management.
The most likely cause of the delirium is central anticholinergic crisis. The reversal agents for anticholinergics include neostigmine, pyridostigmine, and physostigmine. Physostigmine (Antilirium) is the only acetylcholinesterase inhibitor that crosses the BBB and therefore is the only agent that treats central anticholinergic crisis. The dose of physostigmine is 1 mg, given slowly; the dose may be repeated after 15 minutes.

14. When is it mandatory to use a premedication specifically directed at attenuating sympathetic nervous system (SNS) responses? What options are available?
Patients with known hypertension may develop a marked rise in blood pressure after or during laryngoscopy or intubation. Patients with known coronary artery disease may poorly tolerate the tachycardia associated with instrumentation of a lightly anesthetized airway. Such patients may benefit from premedication that attenuates SNS responses.

   Drug regimens that may have beneficial effect on the SNS include clonidine, beta blockers, and high-dose opioids, which cannot be given as a premedication because of respiratory depression. Clonidine is a centrally alpha-2 agonist that attenuates blood pressure and heart rate responses to noxious stimuli and reduces inhaled or injected anesthetic requirements by 40% when given as an oral premedication at 5 μg/kg. Clonidine may produce significant bradycardia or hypotension when combined with beta blockers or calcium channel blockers and may cause marked sedation and drowsiness postoperatively.

15. Describe the medications available for prophylaxis against allergic reactions.
H1 blockers (diphenhydramine) and H2 blockers (ranitidine and cimetidine), along with corticosteroids, can be used as prophylaxis against allergic reactions; however, the efficacy is unproved.

16. Why is premedication particularly important in pediatric patients?
Premedication in children is particularly important because children may be difficult to prepare psychologically for the operating suite. Separation from parents and fear of needles may cause great anxiety. Consequently, many children are given oral sedation before induction of anesthesia. Children also have a high vagal tone that responds to laryngoscopy paradoxically with bradycardia as opposed to the tachycardia usually seen in adults. For this reason, immediately before laryngoscopy small children often receive an anticholinergic, given IM or IV once the child is anesthetized.

17. At what age and stage of development do children begin to require sedation?
Children begin to require sedation at approximately 6 months of age, because this is the age at which they develop separation anxiety. Before 6 months of age most children do not respond negatively to separation from their parents.

18. Does preoperative medication of a pregnant woman involve special consideration?
Most procedures are not done electively in pregnant women; however, the need to perform anesthetics in this population is not uncommon.

Psychological preparation can make a big difference. Benzodiazepines and nitrous oxide are the only two commonly used anesthetic drugs that have been implicated as teratogenic during the first trimester. Opioids are considered relatively safe, but because most drugs are listed as pregnancy class C (not tested in pregnant women), attempts are usually made to minimize all preoperative/intraoperative medications. Ideally, one administers regional anesthesia, whenever possible, with only a vocal premedicant. Many pregnant women agree to this plan when the anesthesiologist explains concerns for the unborn fetus.

19. Name the antiemetic that has caused patients to cancel elective surgery when given preoperatively.
Droperidol, a butyrophenone, is a dopamine antagonist that is a potent antiemetic drug. It may make patients extremely dysphoric and frightened to the point that they cancel surgery. This phenomenon is usually seen when the drug is given alone; however, it has also seen in patients given fentanyl with droperidol (Innovar). The author recommends a good benzodiazepine base before using droperidol whenever possible.

20. Describe the management of a morbidly obese patient with a difficult airway preoperatively. Assume that the patient is otherwise healthy.
A morbidly obese patient is considered a full stomach. Therefore, H2 blockers given the evening before and the morning of surgery, preoperative metoclopramide, and oral nonparticulate antacids are in order.

Glycopyrrolate is useful for planned fiberoptic bronchoscopy. It improves visualization by drying secretions, increases the effectiveness of the topical anesthesia, and decreases airway responsiveness.

Sedation with narcotics, benzodiazepines, and droperidol should be judiciously titrated, using supplemental oxygen and close observation to ensure an awake, appropriately responding patient who can protect his or her own airway.

BIBLIOGRAPHY

1. Beecher HK: Preanesthetic medication. JAMA 157:242, 1955.
2. Reves JG, Fragen RJ, Vinick HR, et al: Midazolam: Pharmacology and uses. Anesthesiology 62:310, 1985.
3. Lee CM, Yeakel AE: Patient refusal of surgery following Innovar premedication. Anesth Analg 54:224, 1975.
4. Manchikanti L, Grow JB, Collvier JA et al: Sodium citrate and metoclopramide in outpatient anesthesia for prophylaxis against aspiration pneumonitis. Anesthesiology 63:378, 1985.
5. Manchikanti L, Kraus JW, Edds SP: Cimetidine and related drugs in anesthesia. Anesth Analg 61:595, 1982.
6. Mirakhur RK: Anticholinergic drugs. Br J Anaesth 51:671, 1979.

17. THE ANESTHESIA MACHINE

Robert W. Phelps, Ph.D., M.D.

1. What is an anesthesia machine?

A more modern and correct name for an anesthesia machine is an **anesthesia delivery system**. The job of the first anesthesia machines was to supply a mixture of anesthetizing and life-sustaining gases to the patient. A modern anesthesia delivery system not only delivers anesthetic gases, vapors, and oxygen, but also it provides a number of basic monitoring functions and the ability to ventilate the patient automatically. It is virtually impossible to purchase a gas machine today without integrated vaporizers, airway pressure, flow and oxygen monitors, and an automatic ventilator.

2. What is the purpose of an anesthesia machine?

The most important purpose is to help the anesthesiologist keep the patient alive, safe, and adequately anesthetized.

3. Are there different kinds of anesthesia machines?

Anesthesia machines used to be available in many different varieties from many different manufacturers. Today, anesthesia machines have become much more standardized, and currently there are two major manufacturers in the United States: **Dräger** and **Ohmeda**. Although there are many differences between the machines manufactured by each of the two companies, there are also many similarities, some initiated by user demands, others by governmental and industrial standards.

4. One of the primary determinants of gas delivery is plumbing. Simplify the plumbing of an anesthesia machine to create an overview of its essential interconnections.

Leaving out the safety features and monitors, the anesthesia machine is divided into three sections.

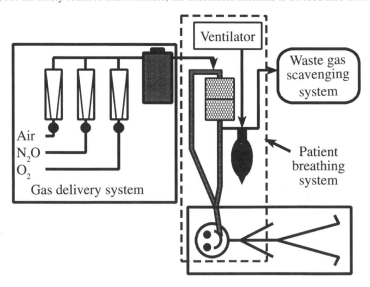

Three main subsystems of an anesthesia machine: gas delivery, patient breathing circuit (which includes the absorber and ventilator), and scavenger.

1. A **gas mixer**, or gas delivery system, which supplies at its outlet a defined mixture of gas chosen by the user.

2. The **patient breathing system**, including the patient breathing circuit, absorber head, ventilator, and sometimes gas pressure and flow monitors.

3. A **scavenger system**, which collects excess gas from the patient and the gas supply section itself and expels the gas outside the hospital to reduce the exposure of operating room personnel to anesthetic gases.

5. Are the three gases, air, oxygen (O_2), and nitrous oxide (N_2O), standardly available on all anesthesia machines?

This combination of gases is probably the most common, but other combinations are also found. O_2 and N_2O are available on almost every anesthesia machine. The third gas may be absent or may be a number of other gases, including helium (He), heliox (a mixture of He and O_2), carbon dioxide (CO_2), or nitrogen (N_2). If the third gas does not contain O_2 (as do air and heliox), it is possible to deliver a (dangerous) hypoxic mixture to the patient.

6. Where do the gases come from?

Usually the gas source for anesthesia machines in hospitals is from a central supply of gas, called the wall or pipeline supply, that is piped into the operating room. An emergency supply of gases is stored in tanks attached to the anesthesia machine. These tanks should be checked daily to ensure they contain an adequate backup supply in case of a pipeline failure.

7. What is a "regulator" and how does it control the release of gas from the tanks?

The gas in the supply tanks is pressurized to approximately 2200 psig. (The abbreviation "psig" stands for pressure-per-square-inch-gauge.) The difference between this and absolute pressure, psi, is the background or atmospheric pressure. Gauges are usually calibrated to read 0 at atmospheric pressure, so their actual reading reflects the pressure above atmospheric pressure.) The "works" of the anesthesia machine requires gas at approximately 50 psig, roughly the pressure of the gas from the wall supply. A regulator is used to reduce the pressure. The regulator is designed so that the pressure at its outlet is constant regardless of the starting pressure and the flow rate of gas. There is a separate regulator for each gas supplied by tanks, and the regulators are adjusted so that the resulting pressure is slightly below the usual wall pressure. The wall gas and tank supply are then connected with a check valve. This check valve selects the gas source with the highest pressure for use by the machine. Thus, under normal circumstances, the wall supply is used preferentially and the tank supply only if the wall supply fails.

8. You installed a new tank of N_2O and your pressure gauge reads only about 750 psig. Is the pressure in the N_2O tank different from the pressures of other gases?

At room temperature, N_2O condenses into a liquid at 747 psig. Air and O_2 are compressed gases in their tanks if they are at room temperature, but N_2O is a liquid. The pressure in the tank stays the same until most of the N_2O is released because of the gas/liquid interface. N_2O E-cylinders (those on the back of the machine) hold the equivalent of about 1600 L of gas, whereas E-cylinders of O_2 and air hold only about 600 L.

9. List the uses of O_2 in an anesthesia machine.

- Provides all or part of the fresh gas flow
- Provides gas for the O_2 flush
- Powers the low O_2 alarm (Ohmeda)
- Is used, along with N_2O, by the Dräger ORM and ORMC to prevent delivery of hypoxic mixtures of gas to the patient
- Powers the "fail-safe" valves
- Powers the ventilator

10. How can one be sure that when the O_2 valve is turned on, the anesthesia machine really delivers O_2?

1. All wall supply gas connectors are keyed so that only the O_2 supply hose can be plugged into the O_2 connector on the wall, the N_2O hose into the N_2O outlet, and so on. This is known as a Diameter-Index-Safety-System (DISS) and by other similar proprietary names. Several manufacturers make such systems, but they are usually all from one manufacturer (and should be) throughout a particular hospital.

2. The gas cylinders are keyed using a Pin-Index-Safety-System (PISS—no kidding, that's what it's called!) so that only the correct tank can be attached to the corresponding yolk on the anesthesia machine.

3. All anesthesia machines are required to have an O_2 monitoring device attached to it that monitors the O_2 concentration in the gas going to the patient. These devices have alarms that indicate when the delivered O_2 concentration is below a set value.

11. In addition to the distinctions described previously, what other ways are gases distinguished to help prevent human error?
First, the **O_2 flow knob** is distinctively fluted. Knobs for other gases are knurled. Second, a **color code** exists such that each gas knob, flowmeter, tank, and wall attachment bears the corresponding color for its associated gas. In the United States, O_2 is green, air is yellow, and N_2O is blue. International standards differ from the standards in many countries, including the United States. Note that in Germany, the color for O_2 is blue and its flowmeter is always on the left. Thus it is easy for O_2 and N_2O to be confused by someone giving anesthesia in these two countries.

12. How does the hospital piped gas supply compare to the use of tank gas?
The only real differences between the two gas sources are the pressure supplied and the volume of gas available. Wall gases are, for practical purposes, infinite in volume availability (everyone knows this until someone forgets to refill the main hospital tank). Wall gas pressures are typically about 55 psig. Tank pressure is generally regulated by the first-stage regulator to 45 psig. The anesthesia machine preferentially chooses the source with the highest pressure. As long as everything is working correctly, the wall supply is used rather than the tank supply.

13. Is one gas supply preferable to the other? Why?
The wall supply is preferable because it is available in greater volumes and is cheaper. This preserves the tank supply for use only in emergency situations.

14. There are two flowmeters for each gas on an anesthesia machine. Couldn't you safely get away with only one, making the machine less expensive?
Two flowmeters are used on many modern anesthesia machines to increase the range of flows over which an accurate measurement can be obtained. The flow tubes in anesthesia machines are always placed in series (which is not necessarily true on other equipment using flowmeters) so that all the gas flows through both tubes. You can read the flow from either tube, whichever tube is calibrated for the appropriate flow range. To measure flows accurately in the ranges used for low flow or even closed-circuit anesthesia (200 to 1000 ml/min) to nonrebreathing flows (6 L/min and higher), two flow tubes are essential.

15. Why are the flowmeters for air, O_2, and N_2O arranged in the order they are in?
Part of the reason the flow tubes are arranged in the order they are in is because of a U.S. government standard, part is for safety reasons, and part is determined by the manufacturers' conventions. In the United States, according to government (NIOSH) standards, the O_2 flowmeter must always be on the right. Requiring the O_2 knob to be in the same relative position on all anesthesia machines decreases the risk of the anesthesiologist turning the wrong knob if he or she uses different machines from time to time. There is also an issue of mechanical safety—in this case, the

O_2 should enter the common manifold closest to the gas egress side. That way, most leaks will tend to lose gases selectively other than O_2.

16. Can flowmeters be arranged in a different order?
Convention has resulted in some differences. Ohmeda has the N_2O flowmeter located in the center position, and Dräger has N_2O positioned on the left. Theoretically, you could order your machine with the flowmeters in any order as long as the O_2 was on the right, but the company might not accept your order.

17. All anesthesia machines are required to have "fail-safe" valves to prevent gas administration when no O_2 is present. Have there been any new developments in this area?
"Fail-safe" valves are a somewhat archaic method of providing a necessary, although not a truly "fail-safe," safety feature. The Ohmeda fail-safe device cuts off the flow of all other gases when the O_2 pressure falls below 25 psig. The figure shows how the flows of O_2 and N_2O change as O_2 pressure is lost. Note that O_2 flow does not start to fall in Ohmeda machines until the pressure reaches 16 psig because of the second-stage O_2 regulator (part of their Link-25 system). On Dräger machines, the O_2 flow falls proportionally with supplied O_2 pressure because of Dräger's Oxygen Failure Protection Device (OFPD). The proportional decrease begins at full working pressure because Dräger machines have no second-stage regulator.

Output when oxygen pressure is lost

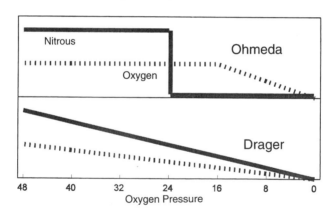

Effect of fail-safe device and OFPD.

18. Is there a distinctive alarm to warn of an O_2 supply failure?
When O_2 pressure fails, Ohmeda warns of the failure using a reed whistle, which is powered by an internal reserve tank of O_2 that refills every time the machine is turned on. Dräger's O_2 failure alarm is similar to Dräger's other alarms, but the final beep is of a different pitch. Dräger continues to warn the user of the O_2 failure every 30 seconds, but unfortunately it is often mistaken for Dräger's other alarms and frequently ignored. Ohmeda's distinctive whistle occurs only once.

19. Would it be safer to leave the tank O_2 supply on your machine turned on so that if the pipeline O_2 failed, the machine would automatically switch immediately to the backup tank supply?
No, for two reasons. **First**, assume that all equipment is functioning properly. The only disadvantage to leaving the tank on is that if a failure in wall O_2 should occur, your machine will use

gas from the tank. You may not know it until the machine (and tank) is totally out of O_2 and the low O_2 pressure alarm begins to sound. At this point, you must really scramble to find O_2 quickly.

The **second reason** allows for equipment failure—there are two parts to the explanation. (1) When no gas is flowing, it is possible for pressure to be maintained in the gauge despite a leak where the tank is connected to the yolk. Thus it is possible to have a full indication on the pressure gauge and an empty tank. If the tank is off, it cannot leak. This is why all O_2 pressure should be bled down during the preoperative check. (2) If wall O_2 pressure drops too low, the tank could be drained supplying the anesthesia machine rather than saving tank O_2 for emergencies. A second check valve prevents the tank O_2 from entering the wall supply plumbing should the wall supply fail. If this valve fails, one's tank could, for the short period until the tank empties, backfill the hospital system, helping to supply O_2 to ward patients.

20. How long can you continue to deliver O_2 when the wall supply fails?

The E-cylinders that supply O_2 to most anesthesia machines hold approximately 600 L when full. If the ventilator is not in use (remember that O_2 powers the ventilator), the O_2 flowmeter indicates how much O_2 is being used. With a flow of O_2 of 2 L/min, there is approximately 300 minutes (or 5 hours) of O_2 available. If the ventilator is in use, the additional gas required for this purpose is equal to the minute volume on Ohmeda ventilators. The amount of O_2 used by Dräger ventilators may be either higher or lower than the minute volume, depending on the settings of the ventilator. In either case, the length of time the tank supply will last will be significantly decreased below the previously estimated 5 hours (for a full tank).

* ⚔ 21. Sometimes your North American Dräger anesthesia machine alarms when you accidentally try to administer a hypoxic mixture of N_2O and O_2 and sometimes it does not. Is there a malfunction in the machine?

The flows of all gases are controlled by the settings of their individual valves. These valves are of a specific type called needle valves. The gas that flows through the valve then enters the corresponding flowmeter so the user can see how much of each gas is flowing. The flow of N_2O is also limited by the oxygen ratio monitor controller (ORMC) valve if there is an attempt by the user to deliver too much N_2O relative to the flow of O_2. The ORMC limits the flow of N_2O so that the ratio of N_2O to O_2 can never exceed 75%:25%. North American Dräger machines have a switch that controls whether the machine can deliver only N_2O and O_2, or all gases. The table shows the effect of each position of the switch. With regard to this question, you probably had the switch in different positions at different times, and the position of the switch explains the apparent occasional failure of the ORMC alarm.

Dräger Gas Selector Switch Setting

"$O_2 + N_2O$" MODE	"ALL GASES" MODE
ORMC alarms enabled	ORMC alarms disabled
Minimum O_2 flow enabled	Minimum O_2 flow disabled
Third gas disabled at its OFPD	Third gas enabled

⚔ 22. Ohmeda anesthesia machines do not have such a switch. Why is it necessary to have a switch to select "all gases" or "N_2O/O_2"?

It is not necessary. The switch is present for historical reasons. Early anesthesia machines did nothing to prevent delivery of hypoxic mixtures. When Dräger first developed the Oxygen Ratio Monitor (ORM, not the ORMC), addition of a third gas that did not contain O_2 could easily make

---

* This symbol symbolizes victory in the understanding of previous material. The material in this question is considered to be more esoteric and/or difficult and can be skipped on first reading.

the ORM inaccurate and possibly result in delivery of hypoxic mixtures to the patient. Therefore, Dräger chose to allow delivery of either N_2O or a third gas (along with O_2, of course). At that time, the third gas was frequently CO_2 or helium, and the forced choice made some sense. When the third gas is air (which by definition is not hypoxic), such a choice makes little sense. Because of pressure from users, although they insisted on retaining the switch, Dräger changed its function so it selected between all gases and only N_2O and O_2.

23. How does the ORM and ORMC work?

The **ORM** was originally developed as an alarm to warn the anesthesiologist that he or she was attempting to deliver a hypoxic mixture. It compared the pressure distal to the O_2 needle valve with the corresponding pressure of N_2O. By monitoring the pressure distal to the flow valve, pressure is proportional to flow, and thus a comparison of pressures was equivalent to a comparison of flows. This comparison is accomplished by linking two diaphragms with a rod (see figure). Mounted on the rod is an electrical contact, which, when the rod moved, could engage an electrical contact, thus powering an alarm. Because the alarm might be incorrect when a third gas is added, the engineers decided simply to disable the alarm when flow of a third gas was allowed. The **ORMC** added an additional "slave" valve to the N_2O gas path, which limited the flow of that gas via a feedback mechanism so that it became impossible to deliver more than 75% N_2O. This limitation occurs whether or not an audible alarm is permitted by the setting of the N_2O/O_2–all gas switch.

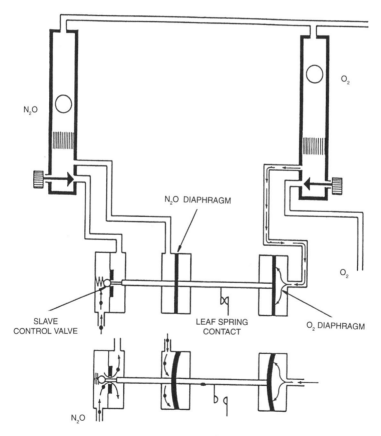

Oxygen ratio monitor controller (ORMC). Dräger's device for preventing delivery of hypoxic mixtures.

24. Ohmeda machines accomplish the same task with their Link-25 system. How does the Link-25 device work?

Ohmeda controls the relative flows of O_2 and N_2O mechanically (see figure). First the pressures of the two gases are carefully regulated with second-stage regulators to 14 and 26 psig. Then two gears with 29 teeth (O_2) and 14 teeth (N_2O) are coupled with a chain. The O_2 gear engages only when an attempt is made to deliver greater than 75% N_2O. At that time, any attempt to deliver more N_2O causes the O_2 knob also to increase at a ratio of 14:29. Similarly an attempt to decrease O_2 delivery also decreases delivery of N_2O. The pressure ratio and gear ratio compensate for various flow rates and the density and viscosity of the two gases.

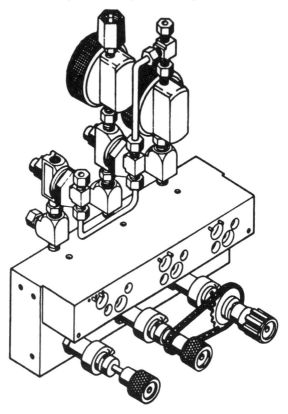

The Ohmeda Link-25 proportioning system.

25. At an altitude of 7000 ft, you have to administer significantly more desflurane than you would expect given the published minimum alveolar concentration (MAC) of that agent. A similar problem does not occur with other agents. Explain.

Conventional vaporizers (including the Dräger 19.1 and Ohmeda TEC 3, 4, and 5) are coincidentally "altitude compensated." The altitude compensation occurs because the diverting valve is functionally located at the outlet of the vaporizer, a variation in design that minimizes the pumping and pressurizing effects. The output of these vaporizers is a constant partial pressure of agent with altitude, not a constant volume percent. The desflurane vaporizer (Ohmeda TEC 6) does not divert a portion of the fresh gas flow through a vaporizing chamber but rather adds vapor to the gas flow to produce a true volume percent output. Because it is the number of molecules of agent (the partial pressure) that anesthetizes the patient, conventional vaporizers provide the same anesthetizing power at altitude. The TEC 6 delivers the set volume percent regardless of altitude, which represents a partial pressure (anesthetizing power) 24% less than the same concentration at sea level. Thus, one must deliver a correspondingly higher percentage of desflurane to achieve MAC at 7000 ft.

26. Can the O_2 flush valve be used to perform jet ventilation instead of purchasing a separate apparatus?

Most anesthesia machines have an internal "pop-off" valve, which limits the maximum pressure that can be delivered via the fresh gas outlet. The actual pressure limit varies with the age and brand of machine, so without testing an individual machine, it is not possible to know for sure exactly what maximum pressure can be delivered. As a rule of thumb, however, most current Ohmeda machines pop off at about 3 to 5 psig and Dräger machines at 18 psig. Effective jet ventilation usually requires between 30 and 50 psig.

27. Compare the performance of "closed circuit" anesthesia using a Dräger ventilator and an Ohmeda 7000 series ventilator.

On both Ohmeda and Dräger anesthesia machines, the ventilator exhaust valve opens only when the bellows is completely full and the pressure inside the bellows exceeds the pressure in the clear bellows chamber by approximately 2.5 cm H_2O. If the bellows never reach the top, the exhaust valve never opens and circuit is closed. Because the Dräger anesthesia ventilator's tidal volume is controlled by a mechanical stop, it is difficult to ensure that the circuit stays closed and at the same time ensure continued delivery of the desired tidal volume.

The Ohmeda bellows always starts its inspiratory excursions from the top and proceeds down a distance appropriate for the requested tidal volume. It is possible to deliver the same tidal volume from different starting points of the bellows. For example, if the bellows starts at 200 ml from the top, a tidal volume of 1000 ml can be delivered if the bellows descends to 1200 ml. If the fresh gas flow is adjusted to maintain the end expiration position below the top of the bellows enclosure but high enough so the set tidal volume can be delivered, the circuit will remain closed.

28. A patient with malignant hyperthermia needs to be anesthetized. Does the service technician need to remove the vaporizers from the anesthesia machine?

Ohmeda vaporizers are easily removed simply by releasing a latch and lifting the vaporizer from the machine. On the Dräger anesthesia machines, it is necessary to remove two Allen screws to release the vaporizers. Then unless the vaporizer is being replaced by a second one, it is necessary to install a bypass block to the empty vaporizer slot. These tasks are easily accomplished by anyone capable of manipulating an Allen wrench, but Dräger's recommendations are that their vaporizers be changed only by authorized service personnel.

29. One of your O_2 flow tubes broke. Until you can get replacement, can you put one of the air flowmeters in its place as long as you remember not to turn on the air?

If you remove one of the flow tubes, there will be a leak in the gas collecting manifold unless the hole the tube inserts into is plugged. Remember, the needle valve is located at the inlet of the flow tube, so shutting off the air valve prevents air from entering the (removed) tube fitting. The fitting at which gas exits the tube, however, allows gas from the other flow tubes to flow backwards through this opening. You must also remember that flowmeters, also known as Thorp tubes, must be calibrated individually for each gas because the flow characteristics through the tubes varies depending on the density and viscosity of the gas. Finally, each tube must be mated with its own float, and the calibration of each tube and float pair are unique. Using a tube calibrated for air to measure O_2 provides inaccurate flow readings.

30. Is the airway pressure measured in different places in the Ohmeda versus the Dräger absorber?

Dräger measures the pressure in the absorber canister both for the reading of the pressure gauge and for the reading from the remote pressure waveform and disconnect sensor. This assumes, which is indeed the case when there is no disconnect or obstruction to gas flow, that the pressure throughout the breathing circuit is the same. **Ohmeda** senses the pressure on the patient's side of both the inspiratory and expiratory valves. The expiratory pressure is used, among other things, by the ventilator to detect disconnects. The inspiratory pressure may better reflect actual airway pressures, especially in the face of partial tubing kinks, and is the pressure displayed on the pressure gauge on the absorber head.

31. What is the best way to add positive end-expiratory pressure (PEEP) to the patient breathing circuit?

A version of PEEP can be simulated on an anesthesia machine by controlled inhibition of expiration. Several ways of accomplishing this have been devised and are in common use. In anesthesia, two methods predominate, but neither is ideal. The first is by inserting a PEEP valve in the expiratory limb of the anesthesia breathing circuit. These devices use either gravity to hold a marble in the air path or are spring loaded so gravity is immaterial. They prevent expiration until the airway pressure exceeds the set PEEP pressure, usually 5 or 10 cm H_2O. The second way is to place a functionally similar valve in the scavenging limb of the breathing circuit and/or ventilator. This results in the entire breathing circuit being pressurized, not just the expiratory limb, but the result is the same. This is not true PEEP because small perturbations in lung volumes (such as a partial inspiration) eliminate the PEEP temporarily.

32. How can fresh gas flow change the minute volume?

The fresh gas continues to flow into the inspiratory limb of the patient breathing circuit continuously. During inspiration, this gas is added to the gas already going to the patient from the breathing bag or ventilator. The amount of gas added to the patient's tidal volume is simply the amount of fresh gas that enters during the inspiratory portion of the breathing cycle. For example, with a respiratory rate of 10, each ventilatory cycle is 6 seconds long (60 divided by 10). If the I:E ratio is 1:2, 2 seconds of each cycle is the inspiratory (I) portion and 4 seconds is the expiratory (E) portion. The fresh gas flowing during these 2 seconds of the inspiratory cycle is what is added to each tidal volume. At a fresh gas flow rate of 6 L/m, 100 ml flows each second, and the tidal volume would be increased by 200 ml because of this fresh gas flow.

33. Why does the patient's breathing bag always become empty on the Dräger anesthesia machine when the ventilator is used?

Both Ohmeda and Dräger anesthesia machines have a switch that allows the anesthesiologist to choose whether the ventilator or the bag and pop-off (automatic pressure limiting or APL) valve are connected to the breathing circuit. If the switch is in the bag position, the ventilator bellows is disconnected from the breathing circuit. In the ventilator position, the bag and APL valve are disconnected from the circuit, but they are still connected to the scavenger. The bag on the Dräger machine becomes empty because of a difference in the way the APL valve functions on the two machines. The Ohmeda APL valve is spring loaded. For gas to escape from the circuit, a minimum pressure difference must occur across the valve to force it open. The amount of pressure required is a function of the adjustment of the valve control itself. The Dräger APL valve is a simple variable orifice valve. That is, it always allows gas to flow if any pressure difference at all exists—the flow of gas through the valve is a function of how open the valve is and what the pressure difference is across the valve. Closed scavengers can produce a small negative pressure on the distal side of the APL valve. This negative pressure is too small to open the Ohmeda APL but can slowly suck gas from the isolated breathing bag of the Dräger machine.

34. What is a scavenger?

Except in a closed circuit situation, gas is always entering and leaving the anesthesia breathing circuit. The exhaust gas is a mixture of expired gas from the patient and excess fresh gas that exceeded the patient's needs but nevertheless contains anesthetic agent. To reduce exposure of operating room personnel to trace amounts of anesthetic agents, it is considered necessary and appropriate to capture and expel this "contaminated" gas from the operating room environment. The device used to transfer this gas safely from the breathing circuit into the hospital vacuum system (or other exhaust system) is called a scavenger. Because of the periodicity of breathing, gas exits the breathing circuit in puffs. The scavenger provides a reservoir for the exhaust gas until the exhaust or vacuum system, which works at a constant flow rate, can dispose of the gas. The scavenger must also prevent excess suction or an occlusion from affecting the patient breathing circuit. It does this by providing both positive and negative relief valves. Thus, if the vacuum system fails or is adjusted to too low a rate, back pressure exits through a positive pressure relief valve. (Granted it contaminates the operating room, but that problem is minimal compared to blowing the patient's lungs up like a balloon.) If the vacuum is adjusted too high, a negative pressure relief valve allows room air to mix with the exhaust gas, preventing buildup of more than a 2.5 mmHg suction at the breathing circuit.

35. Do you need an O₂ monitor on your machine if you have an end tidal anesthesia gas monitor that includes the measurement of end tidal (or inspired) O₂?

No, however, for historical reasons, it has become routine to monitor O_2 with a polarographic or galvanic (fuel cell) sensor located on the absorber head. Some administrators believe that the use of these older sensors is required, but the standards require only that O_2 be monitored. The fact is that monitoring O_2 at the patient's airway is probably safer and more representative of what is actually delivered to the patient.

36. What is more important, your anesthesia machine or your family?

It depends. Excluding time spent asleep (and maybe even counting that time), you will spend more time next to your anesthesia machine than you will spend next to anything or anyone until you retire. It is essential you make the anesthesia machine your friend. Unfortunately, there are certain things your anesthesia machine cannot do for you that your family can. Therefore, understand your anesthesia machine but do not spend any more time with it than you have to. Spend as much time as you can playing with and loving your family.

BIBLIOGRAPHY

1. Bowie E, Huffman LM: The Anesthesia Machine: Essentials for Understanding. Madison, WI, BOC Health Care, 1985.
2. Cicman J, Himmelwright C, Skibo V, Yoder J: Operating Principles of Narkomed Anesthesia Systems. Telford, PA, North American Dräger, 1993.
3. Eisenkraft JB: The anesthesia machine. In Ehrenwerth J, Eisenkraft JB (eds): Anesthesia Equipment: Principles and Applications. St. Louis, Mosby, 1993, pp 27–56.
4. Petty CP: The Anesthesia Machine. New York, Churchill Livingstone, 1987.

18. ANESTHESIA CIRCUITS

Steven J. Luke, M.D.

1. What are the different types of anesthesia circuits?
Breathing circuits are usually classified as open, semiopen, semiclosed, or closed. Variable features of each type include a source of fresh gas, corrugated tubing, one-way valves, active or passive carbon dioxide scavenging and elimination, rebreathing of exhaled gases, and a pressure relief valve (pop-off).

2. Give an example of an open circuit.
An open circuit is the method by which the first true anesthetics were given 150 years ago. The "circuit" consists simply of a bit of cloth saturated with ether or chloroform and held over the patient's face. The patient breathes the vapors and becomes anesthetized. The depth of anesthesia was controlled by the amount of liquid anesthetic on the cloth; hence, it took a great deal of trial and error to become good at the technique. Later, the cloth was placed over wire-mesh face masks designed to fit the patient's face. Face masks of the same style are still used, albeit without the wire mesh.

3. Give an example of a semiopen circuit.
The various semiopen circuits were fully described by Mapleson and are commonly known as the Mapleson A, B, C, D, E and F circuits. All have in common a source of fresh gas, corrugated tubing (corrugated tubing is more resistant to kinking), and a pop-off or adjustable pressure limiting valve. Differences among the circuits include the location of the pop-off valve and fresh gas input and whether or not a gas reservoir bag is present. Advantages of the Mapleson series are simplicity of design, ability to change the depth of anesthesia rapidly, portability, and lack of rebreathing of exhaled gases (provided fresh gas flow is adequate). Disadvantages include lack of conservation of heat and moisture, limited ability to scavenge waste gases, and high requirements for fresh gas flow. The Mapleson series is the most commonly used anesthetic delivery system in Great Britain.

4. Give an example of a semiclosed circuit.
The prototypical semiclosed circuit is the circle system, which is found in most operating rooms in the United States. Every semiclosed system contains an inspiratory limb, expiratory limb, unidirectional valves, carbon dioxide absorber, gas reservoir bag, and a pop-off valve on the expiratory limb. Advantages of a circle system include conservation of heat and moisture, ability to use low flows of fresh gas (thereby conserving volatile anesthetic and the ozone layer), and the ability to scavenge waste gases. Disadvantages include a complex design with approximately 10 connections, each of which has the potential for failure; a large, bulky design that limits portability; and rebreathing of exhaled gases.

5. Give an example of a closed circuit.
In closed breathing systems the inflow of fresh gas into a circle system is low enough to allow closure of the overflow valve and all carbon dioxide (CO_2) is eliminated by the absorber. Closed-circuit anesthesia is a tedious theoretical exercise that appears every year on the in-training/board examination, although few people use it on a regular basis in the operating room. A full discussion of this complex subject can be found in most standard textbooks.

6. Draw the Mapleson A, B, C, D, E and F circuits.

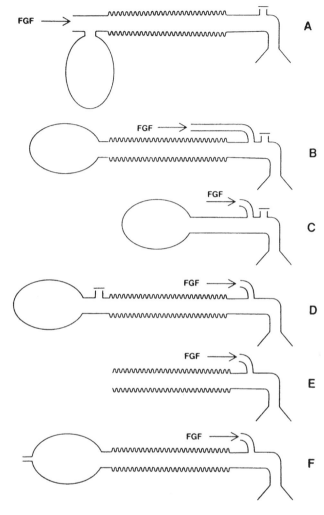

FGF = fresh gas flow. (From Willis BA, Pender JW, Mapleson WW: Rebreathing in a T-piece: Volunteer and theoretical studies of the Jackson-Rees modification of Ayre's T-piece during spontaneous respiration. Br J Anaesth 47:1239–1246, 1975, with permission.)

7. What are the fresh gas flow requirements for each Mapleson circuit to prevent re-breathing of CO_2?

A: Spontaneous breathing—equal to patient's minute volume
Controlled ventilation—3x minute ventilation

B: No common clinical use, but requires twice the patient's minute volume

C: No common clinical use, requires but twice the patient's minute volume

D: Spontaneous breathing—2x minute ventilation
Controlled ventilation—70–80 ml · kg^{-1} · min^{-1} or ml/kg/min

E: Spontaneous breathing–3x minute ventilation
Controlled ventilation—unable to use this circuit for controlled ventilation

F: Twice the minute volume is needed for both controlled and spontaneous ventilation

8. Rank the Mapleson circuits in order of efficiency for controlled and spontaneous ventilation.

Controlled: D > B > C > A (<u>D</u>ead <u>B</u>odies <u>C</u>an't <u>A</u>rgue)

Spontaneous: A > D > C > B (<u>A</u>ll <u>D</u>ogs <u>C</u>an <u>B</u>ite)

9. What are the other names for the Mapleson circuits ?

The Mapleson A circuit is known as the Magill circuit, named for Sir Ivan Whiteside Magill (1888–1986), who introduced endotracheal intubation and Magill's forceps and first described and used circuit A. If the fresh gas flow tubing of a Mapleson D circuit travels within the corrugated tubing, the circuit becomes a Bain circuit. This design was first used by Sir Robert Macintosh (of laryngoscope fame) and E.A. Pask during the Second World War to test the buoyant qualities of life jackets with unconscious persons. Pask allowed himself to be anesthetized using the Bain circuit and was then tossed into choppy water on several occasions. Because he did not drown, the life jacket design was deemed a success. The Mapleson E circuit is known as the Ayre's T-piece and was used primarily for pediatric anesthesia years ago; now it is used for weaning patients from mechanical ventilation and is often incorrectly referred to as a "T-bar." The Mapleson F circuit is known as the Jackson-Rees modification of the Ayre's T-piece.

10. Draw a circle system.

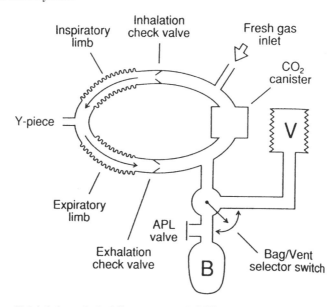

From Andrews JJ: Inhaled anesthetic delivery systems. In Miller RD (ed): Anesthesia, 4th ed. New York, Churchill Livingstone, 1994, pp 185–228, with permission.

11. How can one check for leaks in a circle system?

One should close the pop-off valve, occlude the Y-piece, and press the oxygen flush valve until the pressure is 30 cm H_2O. The pressure will not decline if there are no leaks. One should then open the pop-off valve to ensure that it is in working order. In addition, one should check the function of the unidirectional valves by breathing down each limb individually, making sure that one cannot inhale from the expiratory limb or exhale down the inspiratory limb. These tests, however, do not substitute for the negative pressure test recommended by Ohmeda and Drager for leaks in the machine proximal to the common gas outlet. To perform this test, a no-flow state is first achieved by turning off the machine. The hose connected to the fresh gas outlet is then removed, and the leak detector device (essentially a suction bulb) is attached. After all of the gas is removed from the machine, a flowmeter is opened, and the suction bulb is compressed until it stays flat. If the bulb does not reinflate in 30 seconds, the flowmeter is considered safe. The remaining flowmeters and vaporizers are tested individually in the same way. If all pass, the machine is safe for use. If the machine does not pass, it should be removed for service.

12. How does one detect a breathing circuit disconnection during delivery of an anesthetic?
Breath sounds are no longer detected with an esophageal or precordial stethoscope, and, if the parameters are properly set, the airway pressure monitor and tidal volume/minute volume monitor alarm will sound. The capnograph no longer detects carbon dioxide, and several minutes later the oxygen saturation begins to decline. To use these monitors most effectively, the alarm limits should be set appropriately for each patient. On the Ohmeda Modulus II machine using an Ohmeda 7000 series ventilator, the airway pressure threshold monitor is preset to alarm if the airway pressure does not exceed 6 cm H_2O. The pressure sensor is located on the patient's side of the expiratory valve. The Narkomed 2A machine has a selector switch giving either 8, 12, or 26 cm H_2O as options for the pressure threshold. The value closest to but below the patient's peak pressure should be chosen. The sensor is located either at the carbon dioxide absorber or at the Y-piece. These monitors have a rather limited ability to detect partial disconnection, because enough pressure can be developed in the circuit to exceed the alarm limits, with little or no gas delivered to the patient. The Narkomed 2B and 3 machines overcome this potential problem by using a fully adjustable airway pressure monitor. The threshold pressure alarm can and should be set within 5 cm H_2O of peak ventilatory pressure. For example, if the peak airway pressure is 22 cm H_2O, the alarm limit should be set at 17 cm H_2O. Thus the alarm will sound if the pressure in the circuit does not reach 17 cm H_2O and detect a complete or partial disconnection. When respiratory volume monitors are used, the alarm limits should be set slightly above and below the patient's values. Exhaled carbon dioxide is probably the best monitor to detect disconnections; a decrease or absence of carbon dioxide is sensitive though not specific for disconnection.

13. How is CO_2 eliminated from a circle system?
The exhaled gases pass through a canister containing a CO_2 absorbent such as soda lime or baralyme. Soda lime consists of calcium hydroxide [$Ca(OH)_2$] with lesser quantities of sodium hydroxide (NaOH) and potassium hydroxide (KOH), along with the amount of water necessary for proper activity. Baralyme consists of barium hydroxide [$Ba(OH)_2$], calcium hydroxide, and water of crystallization. Both soda lime and Baralyme react with CO_2 to form heat, water and calcium carbonate ($CaCO_3$). For the chemically inclined, the soda lime reactions are as follows:

$$CO_2 + H_2O \rightarrow H_2CO_3$$
$$H_2CO_3 + 2NaOH \rightarrow Na_2CO_3 + 2H_2O + Heat$$
$$Na_2CO_3 + Ca(OH)_2 \rightarrow CaCO_3 + 2NaOH$$

14. How much CO_2 can the absorbent neutralize? What factors affect its efficiency?
Soda lime is the most common absorber and at most can absorb 23 L of CO_2 per 100 gm of absorbent. However, the average absorber eliminates 10–15 L of CO_2 per 100 gm absorbent in a single-chamber system and 18–20 L of CO_2 in a dual-chamber system. Factors affecting efficiency include the size of the absorber canister (the patient's tidal volume should be accomodated entirely within the void space of the canister), the size of the absorbent granule (optimal size is 2.5 mm or between 4 and 8 mesh), and the presence or absence of channeling (loose packing allowing exhaled gases to bypass absorber granules in the canister).

15. How does one know when the absorbent has been exhausted?
A pH-sensitive dye added to the granule changes color in the presence of carbonic acid. The most common dye in the U.S. is ethyl violet, which is white when fresh and turns violet when the absorbent is exhausted. In the United Kingdom the most common dye indicator is mimosa 2, which

is initially pink and turns white when the absorbant is exhausted. Who said "two nations divided by a common language"?

BIBLIOGRAPHY

1. Andrews JJ: Inhaled anesthetic delivery systems. In Miller RD (ed): Anesthesia. New York, Churchill Livingstone, 1994, pp 185–228.
2. Atkinson RS, Rushman GB, Davies NJH: Lee's Synopsis of Anaesthesia, 11th Ed. Oxford, Butterworth-Heinemann, 1993, pp 97–126, 239–246.
3. Dorsch JA, Dorsch SE: Understanding Anesthesia Equipment. Baltimore, Williams & Wilkins, 1994, pp 149–224.
4. Morgan GE, Mikhail MS: Clinical Anesthesiology. Norwalk, CT, Appleton & Lange, 1992, pp 23–46, 696–720.
5. Willis BA, Pender JW, Mapleson WW: Rebreathing in a T-piece: Volunteer and theoretical studies of the Jackson-Rees modification of Ayre's T-piece during spontaneous respiration. Br J Anaesth 47:1239–1246, 1975.

19. ANESTHESIA VENTILATORS

Steven J. Luke, M.D.

1. How are ventilators classified?

Ventilators are classified according to their power source, drive mechanism, cycling mechanism, and bellows type. The ventilator may be conceived of as a replacement for squeezing the breathing bag. The power source is compressed gas, electricity, or both. The compressed gas comes from the hospital wall source, because large volumes of gas are needed for each ventilator cycle. The E cylinder would be emptied in short order if it were used to power the ventilator. For this reason the E cylinders attached to the anesthesia machine should not be used in preference to the wall source of oxygen when the patient is mechanically ventilated. Most ventilators use a double circuit pneumatic driving mechanism; that is, the gas used to drive the bellows is separate from the gas inside the bellows, which is given to the patient. Time cycling is used most commonly on current anesthesia ventilators. For example, if the ventilator is set to give 10 breaths per minute, each inhalation and exhalation cycle must take 6 seconds (60 sec/10 cycles = 6 sec/cycle). With an inspiratory to expiratory ratio of 1:2, exhalation is twice as long as inhalation; thus in a 6-second cycle exhalation is 4 seconds and inhalation is 2 seconds. All modern anesthesia ventilators use ascending bellows. Bellows are named according to their movement during exhalation.

2. Why is oxygen used to drive the bellows in a ventilator?

If there is a hole in the bellows, the driving gas will enter the bellows and dilute the gas mixture delivered to the patient. Use of oxygen reduces the potential for creating a hypoxic mixture.

3. Why are pressure-cycled ventilators no longer used?

In the past many anesthesia ventilators were pressure-cycled (e.g., the Bird ventilator). The machine delivered gas until a preset pressure was achieved and the gas flow stopped. This system could not compensate for changes in pulmonary compliance and might underventilate the patient if compliance worsened. Compliance is the ratio of the change in volume relative to the change in pressure. For example, if tidal volume is 1000 ml and peak pressure is 20 cm H_2O, compliance equals 50 ml/cm H_2O. If compliance fell to 25 ml/cm H_2O and peak pressure stayed at 20 cm H_2O, tidal volume would fall to 500 ml. Compliance may change quickly from standing to supine positions and from the awake to the anesthetized state. Obesity also decreases compliance, as do such pulmonic processes as adult respiratory distress syndrome (ARDS) and pulmonary contusion or infiltrate.

4. Why have descending bellows been abandonded in favor of ascending bellows?

If a circuit disconnection occurs when an ascending bellows is used, the bellows will not rise and refill during exhalation. The ventilator will be unable to deliver the next breath, and the alarm will sound. If a disconnection in the circuit occurs while a descending bellows is used, by gravity the bellows will continue to descend, giving the appearance of ventilating the patient. The ventilator will ventilate the room and not the patient. If the circuit were only partially disconnected, enough pressure might be generated to overcome the airway pressure threshold monitor alarm settings and hypoventilation could ensue.

5. How should one set the airway pressure threshold monitor?

See p. 121 for answer.

6. How should one set the respiratory volume monitor?

The alarm should be set slightly above and below the patient's values. For example, if one is monitoring tidal volume and the exhaled tidal volume is 600 ml, one may set the high value at

700 ml and the low value at 500 ml. If one is monitoring minute volume and the patient's minute volume is 5 L/min, one may set the high value to 6 L/min and the low value to 4 L/min.

7. How can one convert the ventilator on a Narkomed 2A anesthesia machine from time-cycled to pressure-cycled?
One should raise the bellows stop to the top of the chamber and adjust the driving pressure to achieve the desired peak inspiratory pressure. Thus the tidal volume delivered will depend on the patient's compliance. When it is time for the patient to resume spontaneous ventilation, the ventilator can be turned off and the descent of the bellows with each breath can be noted, giving the anesthesiologist some idea of spontaneous tidal volume. This method may be substituted if a respiratory volume monitor is not available.

8. What can one do if the bellows on a Narkomed 2A anesthesia machine fails to rise completely between each tidal volume?
One can convert to pressure-cycled ventilation as (see question 7) or increase the fresh gas flows. If the bellows fails to ascend completely, the machine should be removed from service at the conclusion of the case and repaired. If the situation is critical, the anesthesiologist can ventilate the patient by hand with a Jackson-Rees circuit or Ambu bag and portable oxygen tank while the machine is switched. A secondary source of oxygen and means of ventilation should be available at any anesthetizing location.

9. How does fresh gas flow rate contribute to tidal volume?
Let us assume that fresh gas flow is 6 L/min, the respiratory rate is set at 6 breaths/minute with an inspiratory to expiratory ratio of 1 to 2, and tidal volume is set to 1000 ml. Each breath cycle is then 10 seconds; thus each inspiration lasts 3.33 seconds, and each expiration lasts 6.66 seconds. Six liters/minute is equal to 100 ml/second, and 100 ml/second multiplied by 3.33 seconds is equal to 330 ml. The delivered tidal volume is thus 1330 ml.

10. Why are the delivered tidal volume and returned tidal volume sometimes not equal?
Anesthesia machine ventilators are not capable of compensating for poorly compliant lungs, and gases are compressible. When the lungs and chest become poorly compliant, a greater peak pressure is needed to maintain tidal volume. Because the compliance of the corrugated tubing does not change, it expands when exposed to higher pressures. Thus some of the tidal volume is compressed in the corrugated tubing and not delivered to the patient.

11. When using very low flows of fresh gas, why is there sometimes a discrepancy between inspired oxygen concentration and exhaled oxygen concentration?
Basal oxygen consumption in the adult human is approximately 3 ml/kg/min. In a 70-kg person oxygen consumption is therefore 210 ml/min. If one is providing low flow anesthesia with a total fresh gas flow of 1 L/min and only 350 ml/min is oxygen, the difference is due to the patient's oxygen consumption.

12. What are the desirable features of an ideal ventilator?
The ideal ventilator should have the following features: (1) maximal flow rate of 80 L/min, tidal volume of 50–1500 ml, rates up to 50/min and a variable inhalation-exhalation (I:E) ratio; (2) positive end-expiratory pressure (PEEP) when desired; (3) humidification of inspired gases; (4) nebulization of drugs; (5) design that is easy to clean and sterilize; (6) design that is adaptable to pediatric use; (7) monitoring of oxygen percentage in the gases delivered to the patient; (8) warning system and provision for manual ventilation in an emergency; (9) ability to compensate for tidal volume loss due to compression in the corrugated tubing; and (10) ability to use varying modes of mechanical ventilation.

13. What ventilator modes are commonly used in the intensive care unit?
- Controlled mechanical ventilation (CMV) provides a fixed tidal volume and rate and is used in patients with no ventilatory effort.
- Assist-control (AC) ventilation senses inspiratory effort and then delivers a set tidal volume and delivers a fixed minute volume if it does not sense patient effort.
- Intermittent mechanical ventilation (IMV) allows spontaneous ventilation while the patient is on the ventilator. Its best feature is reduction in mean airway pressure. With this mode the number of breaths per minute can be reduced over time in a weaning protocol.
- Synchronized intermittent mechanical ventilation (SIMV) times the mechanical breath to coincide with a spontaneous effort to prevent stacking of a mechanical breath on a spontaneous breath, which would result in a very large tidal volume.
- Pressure support ventilation (PSV) augments the tidal volume of spontaneously breathing patients and can greatly decrease the work of breathing. It is useful in a weaning protocol, because the amount of support may be decreased over time as the patient's strength increases.
- Inverse ratio ventilation (IRV) reverses I:E ratios to more than 1:1 (e.g., 2:1, 3:1). It is useful in patients with poor compliance, such as those with ARDS, and should improve oxygenation. It is still a controversial treatment modality.
- Airway pressure release ventilation (APRV) is a new mode of ventilation that periodically augments exhalation by reducing levels of continuous positive airway pressure. It is purported to reduce barotrauma and adverse hemodynamic effects.
- High-frequency ventilation (HFV) describes three different types of ventilation: (1) high-frequency positive-pressure ventilation (HFPPV) uses small tidal volumes at a rate of 60–120/minute; (2) high-frequency jet ventilation (HFJV) uses a small cannula injecting gas 80–300 times per minute and employs the Bernoulli effect to augment tidal volume; (3) high frequency oscillation (HFO) creates to-and-fro gas movement at rates of 600–3000 times per minute and probably works by gas diffusion.

14. What are the beneficial and adverse effects of PEEP?
Beneficial effects include an increase in functional residual capacity (FRC) by recruitment of partially closed alveoli, improvement in lung compliance, and correction of ventilation/perfusion abnormalities. The overall result is improved oxygenation. Adverse effects include barotrauma from high pressures, which may lead to pneumothorax, pneumomediastinum, pneumopericardium, subcutaneous emphysema, or pneumoperitoneum. PEEP raises intrathoracic pressure and may compromise venous return, leading to decreased cardiac output, but this usually occurs only with PEEP in excess of 10 cm H_2O. The rise in central venous pressure may result in a rise in intracranial pressure. PEEP also decreases renal and hepatic blood flow.

BIBLIOGRAPHY

1. Andrews JJ: Inhaled anesthetic delivery systems. In Miller RD (ed): Anesthesia. New York, Churchill Livingstone, 1994, pp 185–228.
2. Dorsch JA, Dorsch SE: Understanding Anesthesia Equipment. Baltimore, Williams & Wilkins, 1994, pp 255–280.
3. Atkinson RS, Rushman GB, Davies NJH: Lee's Synopsis of Anaesthesia, 11th ed. Oxford, Butterworth-Heinemann, 1993, pp 97–126, 239–246.
4. Morgan GE, Mikhail MS: Clinical Anesthesiology, Norwalk, Connecticut, Appleton & Lange, 1992, pp 23–46, 696–720.

20. VAPORIZERS

Matt Flaherty, M.D.

1. Give a simple definition of a vaporizer.

The anesthetic vaporizer changes stored liquid anesthetic into anesthetic vapor. The gas leaving the vaporizer contains a carefully controlled quantity of the anesthetic vapor.

2. What physical principles are involved in the process of vaporization?

The saturated vapor pressure of the volatile anesthetic, which varies with temperature, determines the concentration of vapor molecules above the liquid anesthetic. The heat of vaporization is the energy required to release molecules of a liquid into the gaseous phase. The liquid phase needs external heat during vaporization, or it will become cooler as molecules leave and enter the gaseous phase. Thermal conductivity is the ability of heat to flow through a substance. Vaporizers are constructed of metals with high thermal conductivity, allowing heat to flow from the vaporizer into anesthetic in the liquid phase, supplying energy for the heat of vaporization.

3. How are vaporizers classified?

Modern vaporizers are grouped by their function and features: regulation of vapor concentration, method of vaporization, temperature compensation, agent specificity, and location in or out of the breathing circuit.

4. Where is the vaporizer located?

In modern anesthetic systems the vaporizers are located downstream from the flowmeters. Fresh gas passes from the flowmeters to the vaporizer, then on to the common gas outlet. Freestanding vaporizers, added to anesthesia machines after the common gas outlet, are prone to a number of hazards, including tipping, increased resistance to gas flow, and increased output with use of the high-pressure oxygen flush.

5. Name some common vaporizers in use today.

The Ohmeda Tec 4, Tec 5, and Tec 6, and the Drager 19.1 are the most common vaporizers in the U.S. today.

6. What does variable bypass mean?

Fresh gas from the flowmeters enters the vaporizer and is divided into two streams. About 80% enters the bypass chamber and is not exposed to the volatile agent. The remaining gas enters the vaporizing chamber and becomes saturated with anesthetic. The concentration dial determines the amount of gas flow that enters each of the two streams. These then reunite near the vaporizer outlet. The fresh gas leaving the vaporizer contains a concentration of vapor as specified by the concentration dial.

7. What does temperature compensation mean?

During vaporization the liquid anesthetic will cool, drawing heat from the metal of the vaporizer, which draws heat from the operating room. As liquid anesthetic cools, the saturated vapor pressure decreases, as does vaporizer output. Temperature compensation means the vaporizer has mechanisms for adjusting the output regardless of cooling. The vaporizer is built of metals that have high thermal conductivity, allowing rapid heat transfer to the liquid anesthetic as it cools. The variable bypass mechanism will direct more gas flow to the vaporizing chamber as the vaporizer cools to compensate for decreased saturated vapor pressure.

8. What is the pumping effect?

Positive pressure can be transmitted back into the vaporizer during ventilation of the patient. The positive pressure can briefly cause gas to reverse flow within the vaporizer, allowing gas in the vaporizing chamber to enter the bypass chamber. The result of the pumping effect is increased vaporizer output beyond that indicated on the concentration dial. Modern vaporizers have mechanisms to compensate for the pumping effect.

9. How does altitude affect modern vaporizers?

The effect of the change in barometric pressure on volumes percent output can be calculated as follows: x' = x (p/p'), where x' is the output in volumes percent at the new altitude (p'), and x is the concentration output in volumes percent for the altitude (p), where the vaporizer is calibrated. Example: Consider a vaporizer calibrated at sea level (p = 760 torr), taken to Denver (p' = 630 torr), set to deliver 1% halothane vapor (x). The actual output (x') is 1%(760/630) = 1.2%. Remember that partial pressure of the vapor, and not the concentration in volumes percent, is the important factor in depth of anesthesia. Note that 1% at sea level (760 torr) is 7.6 torr, and that 1.2% at Denver (630 torr) is 7.6 torr, so regardless of altitude the clinical effect is unchanged.

10. What is the relationship of fresh gas inflow to vaporizer output?

Variable bypass vaporizers have less output than the concentration dial setting specified at very low (250 ml/min) and very high (15 L/min) gas flow rates.

11. What is the relationship of fresh gas composition to vaporizer output?

Most vaporizers are calibrated using 100% oxygen as the fresh gas. Changing to 100% nitrous oxide (which is never actually done) would decrease vaporizer output to about 10% less than the dial setting. This decrease is due to differences in viscosity between the two gases, changing the flow within the vaporizer.

12. What is a drawover vaporizer?

Drawover vaporizers are designed for use as part of the patient breathing circuit. These vaporizers are small, easily portable, and can typically vaporize any volatile anesthetic. Drawover vaporizers are used under severe economic limitations and battlefield conditions. Ambient air is often the fresh gas and is drawn through the vaporizer by the spontaneously breathing patient.

13. What is a copper kettle vaporizer?

This vaporizer is no longer manufactured. A measured amount of fresh gas bubbles up through liquid anesthetic and becomes completely saturated; this vapor then combines with additional fresh gas (calculated by the anesthesiologist) to form the final desired concentration. The copper kettle is not temperature compensated and can use multiple agents. Copper is used due to its high thermal conductivity.

14. What is a multiagent vaporizer?

Most vaporizers in use today are agent specific, meaning they are calibrated and designed for only one anesthetic agent. Multiagent vaporizers, such as the copper kettle, are capable of using any of the common volatile anesthetics. Because the anesthesiologist has to calculate the output, any anesthetic agent, knowing the vapor pressure, can be used. Some drawover vaporizers have different dial covers, each calibrated for a specific agent, and the dial must match the agent contained in the vaporizer. Multiagent vaporizers never use more than one agent at a time.

15. What happens if you put the wrong agent in a vaporizer calibrated for another agent?

The incorrect agent in an agent specific vaporizer will deliver either an overdose or underdose. The most important factor in determining the direction of error is the vapor pressure. If an agent with a high vapor pressure is put into a vaporizer meant for a less volatile agent, the output will be excessive. If an agent with a lower vapor pressure than the agent intended for the vaporizer is accidentally used, the anesthetic output will be lower than anticipated. Even if halothane and isoflurane, having similar vapor pressures, are interchanged, the outputs will still not be accurate. The use of isoflurane in a halothane vaporizer will give 25–50% more anesthetic output than the dial setting. The use of halothane in an isoflurane vaporizer will give less anesthetic output than the dial setting.

16. What is different about the desflurane vaporizer?
The Tec 6 vaporizer is a unique vaporizer designed for desflurane, which has a vapor pressure of 664 torr at 20°C. This vaporizer actively heats the liquid agent to 39°C. It was deemed necessary to provide active heating to consistently vaporize desflurane since it boils near room temperature, and small changes in the vaporizer temperature would cause large changes in saturated vapor pressure. Desflurane is less potent than other common agents and up to 18% volumes percent may be delivered. There are electronic alarms for low agent level, no agent output, and low battery. Desflurane boils at room temperature, and the bottles interlock with the vaporizer to prevent loss of agent while filling.

17. What happens if you tip a variable bypass vaporizer on its side?
Liquid anesthetic may spill from the vaporizing chamber to the bypass chamber, effectively creating two vaporizing chambers and increasing vaporizer output.

18. What prevents turning on two vaporizers simultaneously?
Most anesthesia machines have an interlock system or an interlocking manifold that allows only one vaporizer to be turned on at a time. This can be tested by attempting to turn on more than one agent. Improper use of the interlock systems or manifolds can cause gas and anesthetic agent leaks, or simultaneous administration of multiple agents. Ohmeda machines that have three attachment sites for vaporizers must have a vaporizer in the central position to activate the safety interlock mechanism.

19. What prevents filling the vaporizer with the wrong agent?
There are several key-type filling systems. A keyed filler top fits a specific bottle of anesthetic agent, which fits only a specific vaporizer. Funnel type or open filling port type vaporizers can easily be misfilled; only vigilance can prevent mistakes.

BIBLIOGRAPHY
1. Andrews JJ: Anesthesia Systems. In Barash PG, Cullen BF, Stoelting RK (eds): Clinical Anesthesia. Philadelphia, J.B. Lippincott, 1989, pp 516–522.
2. Bowie E, Huffman LM: The Anesthesia Machine: Essentials for Understanding. Madison, Ohmeda/BOC Health Care, 1985, pp 91–103.
3. Carter KB, Gray WM, Railton R, Richardson W: Long term performance of Tec vaporizers. Anaesthesia 43:1042–1046, 1988.
4. Coleshill GG: Safe vaporizers. Can J Anaesth 35:667–668, 1988.
5. Dorsch JA, Dorsch SE: Understanding Anesthesia Equipment: Construction, Care and Complications, 3rd ed. Baltimore, Williams & Wilkins, 1994, pp 91–148.
6. James MFM, White JF: Anesthetic considerations at moderate altitude. Anesth Analg 63:1097–1105,1984.
7. Lewis JJ, Hicks RG: Malfunction of vaporizers. Anesthesiology 27:324–325, 1966.
8. Tec 4 continuous flow vaporizer, operator's manual. Steeton, England, Ohmeda/BOC group, 1986.
9. Vapor 19.1, Operating Manual. Lubeck, Federal Republic of Germany, Dragerwerk, 1985.

21. PATIENT POSITIONING

James W. Rosher, M.D.

1. What is the goal of positioning a patient for surgery?

The goal of surgical positioning is to facilitate the surgeon's technical approach while balancing the risk to the patient. The anesthetized patient cannot make the clinician aware of compromised positions; therefore, the positioning of a patient for surgery is critical for a safe outcome. Proper positioning requires that the patient be securely placed on the operating table, padding all potential pressure areas, intravenous (IV) lines and catheters free flowing and accessible, endotracheal tube in proper position, ventilation and circulation uninterrupted, and general patient comfort and safety maintained for the duration of the surgery.

2. Describe the most common positions used in the operating room.

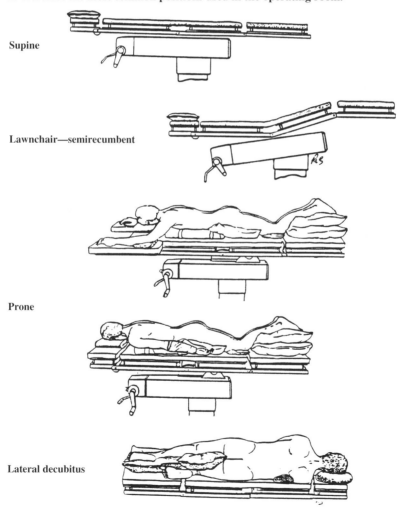

Supine

Lawnchair—semirecumbent

Prone

Lateral decubitus

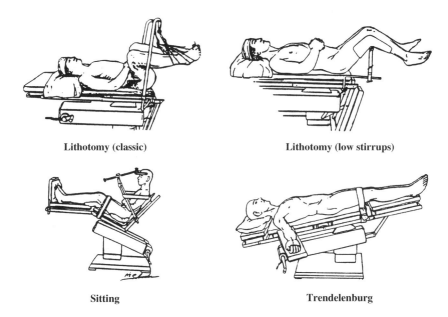

Lithotomy (classic)   Lithotomy (low stirrups)

Sitting   Trendelenburg

Figures on pages 129–130 are reprinted with permission from Martin JT: Positioning in Anesthesia and Surgery, 2nd ed. Philadelphia, W.B. Saunders, 1987.

3. What physiologic effects are related to change in body position?

Most physiologic changes associated with positioning are related to the gravitational effects on the cardiovascular and respiratory systems. The changes in position redistribute blood within the venous, arterial, and pulmonary vasculature, depending on the body position. Pulmonary mechanics also change with varying body positions. Changing from the erect to the supine position increases cardiac output secondary to increases in venous return and stroke volume. There is minimal change in blood pressure, because reflex stimulation of the parasympathetic nervous system produces decreases in heart rate and cardiac contractility. Cardiovascular changes are exaggerated by clinical situations resulting in increased abdominal girth, such as abdominal tumors, ascites, obesity, or pregnancy. The resulting decreased venous return and cardiac output may lead to hypotension in the supine position. The supine position results in decreased functional residual capacity and total lung capacity secondary to the abdominal contents impinging on the diaphragm. Anesthesia and muscular relaxation further diminish these lung volumes. Some improvement is achieved with positive pressure ventilation, but the diaphragm is not restored to the awake position. The Trendelenburg and lithotomy positions may result in further compression of the lung bases, resulting in further decreases in pulmonary compliance. Intracranial pressure increases are seen in these position as well secondary to increased central venous pressure and decreased cerebral drainage.

4. Name the advantages and disadvantages of the sitting position when used for a posterior fossa craniotomy.

Advantages
- Improved surgical exposure owing to decreased pooling of blood in the surgical field
- Optimal positioning for surgical exposure
- Decreased facial swelling
- Easy access to the endotracheal tube
- Ability to monitor the facial nerve easily when indicated by the surgical procedure

Disadvantages
- Possibility of venous air emboli (VAE)
- Hypotension
- Brainstem manipulations resulting in hemodynamic changes
- Risk of airway obstruction

The risk of VAE requires monitoring with transthoracic Doppler, right atrial catheters, transesophageal echocardiography, capnography, esophageal stethoscope, or mass spectroscopy to help detect or treat the VAE. The sensitivity in decreasing order of detection of VAE are

Transesophageal echocardiography	End-tidal carbon dioxide
Transthoracic Doppler	Right atrial catheter
End-tidal nitrogen	Esophageal stethoscope

The risk of hypotension may require invasive blood pressure monitoring with an arterial catheter. Care to level the arterial transducer at the external auditory meatus helps correlate the measured arterial pressure with the cerebral perfusion pressure. The sitting or head-up position decreases venous return and subsequently cardiac output. Cerebral blood flow is decreased approximately 20% in these patients and may lead to cerebral ischemia. Often these patients require elastic lower extremity stockings to decrease the venous pooling during surgery, improving blood return to the heart. Prevention of airway obstruction requires vigilance to prevent extreme flexion of the head and neck with resultant kinking of the endotracheal tube.

5. What specific concerns are associated with the prone position?

The anesthesiologist is in charge of controlling the patient's head during positioning. Avoid disconnecting or removing IV lines, Foley catheters, or endotracheal tubes while positioning. The prone position results in a cephalad displacement of the diaphragm. Chest rolls are important to prevent abdominal compression, which impairs diaphragmatic excursion and obstructs the aorta and inferior vena cava. Proper padding of all pressure points, including the face, eyes, ears, nose, arms, knees, hips, ankles, breasts, and genitalia, is necessary in this position. The patient should be free from pressure on the ECG electrodes, wires, and tubing.

6. A patient scheduled for a thoracotomy is being positioned in the lateral decubitus position. What special concerns should the operating room team be aware of in positioning this patient?

1. The dependent lung is underventilated and relatively overperfused. In contrast, the nondependent lung is overventilated owing to the increase in compliance. The resulting ventilation/perfusion inequality may result in unexpected hypoxia. Usually, changes in ventilation and perfusion are well tolerated, but in a compromised patient it may prove problematic.

2. All patients in the lateral position should have an axillary roll positioned to prevent compression of the dependent arm's neurovascular bundle. Checking the radial pulse or use of a pulse oximeter on the dependent hand may help to signal impending arterial compression. The arms are usually positioned perpendicular to the torso using a holding device known as an "airplane" or supported and padded with pillows.

3. Proper padding is essential in this position, especially facial structures, breasts, and genitalia. The dependent leg is usually flexed at the hip and knee with padding between the legs. The peroneal nerve at the head of the fibula is also at risk for compression. The head position should remain neutral to prevent stretching of the brachial plexus of the nondependent arm. Often a "bean bag" padding device is used to maintain the patient in a stable lateral position. ECG electrodes, wires, IV tubing, and Foley catheters should all be positioned so they are free and well padded.

7. In the pregnant patient, what is the most desirable position for an abdominal procedure?

The pregnant patient is susceptible to aortocaval compression secondary to the gravid uterus exerting pressure on these vascular structures, potentially decreasing the uteroplacental blood flow and return to the heart. The most favorable position is left uterine displacement by placing a pillow or wedge under the right hip.

8. Which surgical procedures employ the lithotomy position?
- Anal procedures (e.g., hemorrhoidectomy)
- Abdominoperineal procedures (e.g., colorectal procedures)
- Urologic and gynecologic procedures

Depending on the type of surgery, variations of the lithotomy position can be used, such as the classic lithotomy or the low stirrups position.

9. What are the most common complications occurring from the lithotomy position?
The nerves that supply the lower extremity are often damaged because of compression or stretching of the nerves from improper positioning or improper padding. The most common nerves injured are the common peroneal, sciatic, femoral, saphenous, and occasionally the obturator or posterior tibial nerve.

The **common peroneal nerve** may be injured when the head of the fibula (lateral aspect of the knee) is compressed against the leg support device or insufficiently padded. The **sciatic nerve** can be stretched by exaggerated flexion of the hips during positioning. The **femoral nerve** may become kinked under the inguinal ligament from extreme flexion and abduction of the thighs during positioning. The **saphenous nerve** may become injured when the medial tibial condyle is compressed by the leg supports. The **obturator nerve** may be stretched as it exits the obturator foramen during thigh flexion.

Other injuries that occur in the lithotomy position are dislocations of the hips, lower extremity tendon and ligament injuries, and low back discomfort. Occasionally at the end of a procedure, the fingers can be crushed or amputated when the leg section of the table is elevated.

10. Why is it important to move both legs at the same time when positioning patients in the lithotomy position?
The proper way to position a patient in the lithotomy position is to flex both legs at the hips and knees simultaneously, then position the legs in the stirrups. Special care should be taken to prevent extreme flexion of the knees or hips during movement, and a good rule is to avoid flexing the hips greater than 90 degrees. This technique helps prevent nerve injuries and hip dislocations. Proper padding of the ankles, knees, and stirrup braces helps reduce nerve compression injuries.

11. When is it advantageous to use the "lawnchair position"?
The "lawnchair position," a variant of the supine position, is often used for patient comfort, especially in prolonged procedures in which regional anesthesia is used. It is often the preferred position for head and neck procedures. Flexion of the knees and hips places the joints in a more anatomically neutral position. This position also facilitates breathing.

12. How long is it safe to keep an extremity tourniquet inflated and why?
The time limit for inflation of an extremity tourniquet is approximately 2–3 hours to prevent neurovascular complications. The tourniquet may be deflated to allow recirculation and then reinflated to ensure adequate perfusion to the limb.

13. What peripheral nerves are most commonly injured during surgery and why?
The **ulnar nerve** is the most frequently injured peripheral never because of its superficial location at the elbow. During surgical procedures, the ulnar nerve may be compressed between the patient and the surgical table. This can be prevented by proper padding of the medial aspect of the elbow.

The **brachial plexus** becomes stretched owing to abduction greater than 90 degrees or with improper head positioning. In all surgical positions, the arms should be properly secured and padded to prevent them from falling off the arm supports.

The **radial nerve** can become injured as a result of improper positioning of the noninvasive blood pressure cuff at the brachial aspect of the arm. It can also be injured by direct external compression of the radial nerve in the spiral groove on the lateral aspect of the humerus.

14. What areas of the body are prone to injury secondary to prolonged or improper positioning?

The eyes are vulnerable to injury by abrading the cornea or direct compression of the globe. The retinal artery can become compressed by external pressure, resulting in retinal ischemia and blindness. This can be prevented by padding around the orbits in the lateral decubitus and prone positions. Taping the eyes shut and use of eye lubricants decrease the incidence of corneal abrasion and prevent drying of the cornea.

Skin breakdown can occur owing to improper or prolonged positioning. Pressure on the scalp can result in alopecia. Bony prominences need to be well padded, especially the iliac crest, sacrum, and heels. Nasogastric and endotracheal tubes can produce pressure necrosis of the lips or nares. The face mask may decrease the skin perfusion over the bridge of the nose and should be repositioned frequently during general mask cases. The breast, nipples, scrotum, and male genitalia are susceptible to skin breakdown and require special positioning and padding.

15. Describe the features of the orthopedic fracture table.

The fracture table is designed to facilitate the manipulation of the extremity and to provide access to fluoroscopy of the fracture extremity. The table has a body section to support the head and thorax. A sacral plate is available for support of the pelvis with a well-padded perineal post to allow traction to be applied to the fractured extremity. Adjustable footplates allow for surgical manipulations while maintaining traction and stability.

16. How does the head position affect the position of the endotracheal tube with respect to the carina?

During laryngoscopy and intubation, the endotracheal tube should be placed to the proper depth and verified by auscultation. With patient movement, the head may be flexed or extended in relationship to its original position. A general rule is that the tip of the endotracheal tube follows the direction of the tip of the patient's nose. For example, if the patient's head is flexed, the tip of the endotracheal tube moves toward the carina. The endotracheal tube may enter a mainstem bronchus. If the head is extended, the tip of the endotracheal tube moves cephalad, possibly resulting in extubation. Always verify bilateral breath sounds after repositioning a patient.

BIBLIOGRAPHY

1. Anderton JM, Keen RI, Neave R: Positioning the Surgical Patient. London, Butterworths, 1988.
2. Cucchiara RF, Faust RJ: Patient positioning. In Miller R (ed): Anesthesia. New York, Churchill & Livingstone, 1994, pp 1057–1073.
3. Martin JT: The physiology of the patient's posture. In Collins V (ed): Principles of Anesthesiology. Philadelphia, Lea & Febiger, 1993, pp 163–173.
4. Martin JT: Complications of patient positioning. In Collins V (ed): Principles of Anesthesiology. Philadelphia, Lea & Febiger, 1993, pp 192–206.
5. Martin JT: Patient positioning. In Barash PG, Cullen BF, Stoelting RK (eds): Clinical Anesthesia. Philadelphia, J.B. Lippincott, 1992, pp 709–736.
6. Martin JT: Positioning in Anesthesia and Surgery. Philadelphia, W.B. Saunders, 1987.
7. Martin JT, Collins VJ: Technical aspects of patient positioning. In Collins V (ed): Principles of Anesthesiology. Philadelphia, Lea & Febiger, 1993, pp 174–191.
8. Stoelting RK, Miller R: Positioning. In Stoelting RK, Miller R (eds): Clinical Anesthesia. Philadelphia, J.B. Lippincott, 1992, pp 709–736.

22. INFUSION DEVICES

Judith Russell, L.P.N., C.A.T.S.

Electronic control devices for fluid and drug delivery have become increasingly popular within the past several years. Their use has progressed from critical care to routine intravenous lines. With the increase in administration of vasoactive and chemotherapy agents, the demand for sophisticated and accurate electronic delivery systems has led to the development of many different types of pumps.

1. Are there different modes of operation, or are all pumps the same?
All infusion devices measure fluid infusion electronically and can be classified according to simple criteria. There are two basic categories: devices that use positive pressure to deliver volume and devices that do not. In simpler terms, positive pressure pumps actively draw the solution out of a container, whereas gravity controllers depend on gravity to force solution delivery. Proper use of an electronic delivery system depends on the route of administration, frequency of therapy, and setting of care (inhouse vs. home care).

2. Describe the differences between the two categories.
   Controllers are basically electronic tubing clamps that depend on gravity, as mentioned, and traditionally have an electronic eye to count the drips as they are delivered. Thus, the opening and closing of the delivery tubing is synchronous with the counting of drips. This type of system is appropriate for a noncritical situation as well as for a nonviscous solution. One must bear in mind that drip sizes vary, and the volume given over time will vary accordingly. The maximal flow rate is affected by the height of the bag over the intravenous insertion site as well as the size of the angiocatheter. Straight-line gravity tubing is used with controllers, keeping the cost to the patient at a minimum. Most controllers use monitoring to signal completed volume, empty containers, and occlusions. Low battery alarms are also incorporated.
   Positive-pressure or volumetric devices apply a driving force that displaces a measured volume within a container. This mechanism pushes the fluid into the patient and provides a more accurate infusion method. Each cycle delivers a precise amount of solution and eliminates the variables of drip size and rate. The major benefit of volumetric devices is improved accuracy.
   Peristaltic delivery systems use either rotary cams or fingerlike projections to propel fluid through tubing. This manner of propulsion is similar to gastrointestinal action; hence the term peristaltic delivery. Peristaltic devices do not count drops; instead, they measure a fixed volume of fluid to be delivered. Because of constant massage, the diameter of the tubing changes, affecting the accuracy of delivery. Most systems, however, are accurate within ± 5–10% . To overcome this deficiency, more recent tubing includes silicone around the area of contact to the cams. Peristaltic systems use both dedicated and generic tubing and are appropriate for use in both critical care and routine settings. Examples include the Ivac pump and the newer Gemini pump.
   Volumetric cassette devices are designed to deliver a specific amount of volume at a set rate, measured in ml/hr. The requirement of a dedicated tubing set adds to the expense. Many hospitals purchase the pumps through an upcharge on the disposables, eliminating the upfront cost and passing it on to the patient. Volumetric cassette pumps require a two-cycle delivery sequence to administer fluids: (1) a filling cycle that fills the system with a precise amount and (2) a delivery cycle that infuses the solution. Volumetric pumps do not depend on gravity to infuse; they are extremely accurate and equipped with all necessary alarms. Because of their reliability, volumetric pumps are an excellent choice for fluid delivery in all clinical settings, delivering intravenous admixtures, solutions, and blood products. They are the workhorses of the pump industry, and are used more widely than any other pump. An example is the blue product line of Abbott Lifecare.

Single-channel delivery pumps are the early version of the positive-pressure devices. They use cassette tubing and a two-cycle method of delivery. The majority of single-channel pumps operate with a piston diaphragm design within the cassette. This chamber holds the selected volume to be delivered; infusion occurs when the chamber is compressed. All conventional measuring and alarms are included.

3. Is it possible to deliver multiple solutions through one pump?

Dual and multi-channel pumps, the newest variation on the market, infuse separate solutions through one specialty cassette. Each channel is controlled by individual programming; thus flow is concurrent. Computerized programming allows multiple infusions at independent rates. Standard alarms and delivery tracking are included, as well as more sophisticated record keeping, such as can be found on the OmniFlow 4000 Plus. Downloading to a printer is also available on some models.

Dual and multiline systems deliver fluids through multiple sets to separate sites. The cost increases with the number of solutions delivered, and flow is not concurrent.

A common feature to both systems is use of a single pump, which is an obvious advantage in a cluttered intensive care unit or during transfer of a critical care patient. A multichannel pump may have an advantage over a multiline device in cost savings, because it uses only one tubing cassette for delivery of all fluids.

4. What are the advantages of constant infusion with a peristaltic mechanism vs. linear/piston action?

Syringe pumps (linear/piston) deliver a smooth, nonpulsatile flow of drugs, ensuring a more stable pharmacokinetic response in the patient. Infusion pumps, such as the Imed, pull from a container or syringe in a pulsatile manner. Variations in flow rates may induce significant variations in blood pressure in vivo with infusion at slow rates. Therefore, the linear/piston devices offer the least variation in flow and possibly the most reliable mechanism of delivery. Linear/piston syringe pumps are an ideal choice for conscious sedation in the critical care setting.

5. Are pumps necessary for the delivery of intravenous solutions?

From a practical standpoint, the use of an infusion controller makes sense whenever close monitoring of fluid delivery is required. In the case of hypovolemia, delivery rates may be safely increased to the uppermost limit of the individual pump; an alarm signal will sound before the fluid container becomes empty.

6. Are specific infusion devices available for epidural pain control?

Several devices specifically address the needs of controlled analgesia. Two significant concerns are programmability and security. The delivery rate and pressure setting for infusions on epidural pumps are somewhat different. Although some all-purpose pumps allow pressure setting changes, it is best to select a pump that is specifically designed for epidural pain management. Thus delivery of narcotic into the epidural space will be consistent. An epidural pump must have the capability of microgram dosing; the risk of confusion is too great in a pump that allows only milligram dosing. Because an opioid infusion is most common, a method to lock in the solution should also be available to prevent siphoning of opioid or inadvertent overdosing by the patient. Dedication of pain control analgesia to a specific pump also prevents inadvertent infusion of intravenous medications into the epidural space. Two popular models are the Baxter PCA/Epidural Pump and the Abbott APM system. Both have dedicated tubing and the ability to program and lock.

7. What limiting factors should be considered in using an infusion pump?

Drug concentration often determines the type of infusion control that should be used. Some pumps accept only syringes, whereas others, like the Abbott ANNE, deliver from a bag, syringe, or bottle. Other primary considerations in selection of a delivery system should be expected length of use and patient location. Induction agents, muscle relaxants, and opioids are candidates for a simple system such as the Bard InfusOr or the Baxter AS40A. These systems require only the syringe, pump, and conventional microbore tubing. If the patient is transferred with an infusion pump in operation, the pharmacy can refill the syringes or provide the initial admixture solution used to prepare the syringes. This type of preparation and communication greatly reduces the cost to the patient, eliminating the need to discard or remix drugs for use with another system. Infusion rate ranges vary according to the size of the syringe. Many of the newer syringe pumps request confirmation of brand and size. The table below offers a guideline of typical rate ranges in most syringe pumps.

Syringe Specification from Different Manufacurers

SYRINGE MANUFACTURER	SYRINGE (SIZE (ml)	MINIMAL FLOW RATE (ml/hr)	MAXIMAL FLOW RATE (ml/hr)
B-D	1	0.01	10
	3	0.02	30
	5	0.03	50
	10	0.1	100
	20	0.1	150
	30	0.1	200
	60	0.1	360
Monoject	1	0.01	10
	3	0.02	30
	6	0.03	50
	12	0.1	100
	20	0.1	150
	35	0.1	200
	60	0.1	360
Terumo	1	0.01	10
	3	0.02	30
	5	0.03	50
	10	0.1	100
	20	0.1	150
	30	0.1	200
	60	0.2	360

8. Are any pumps preprogrammed?

At least three models are equipped with a drug library. Drug-specific information is programmed into the memory of the pump by the manufacturer. These libraries are meant to provide infusion parameters, common bolus amounts, and drip rates. Most pumps calculate delivery on the basis of the patient's weight and available drug concentration.

9. What are the most common problems with infusion devices?

One of the most common problems with infusion control is air in the patient's line. If the device is a controller, air in the cassette chamber will stop the pump. A change in the resistance of the tubing will signal both kinds of devices to alarm and halt infusion. The table below is a simple troubleshooting guide.

Syringe Pump Trouble Shooting

ALARM PROBLEM	SYRINGE PUMP	VOLUMETRIC/CONTROLLER
Pump will not turn on	Check power source Replace batteries, charger	Check power source
Occlusion	Check line for kinks Loosen barrel of syringe Check catheter site	Check line for kinks Check catheter site Reposition patient

Table continued on following page.

Syringe Pump Trouble Shooting (Continued)

ALARM PROBLEM	SYRINGE PUMP	VOLUMETRIC/CONTROLLER
Occlusion *(cont.)*	Reposition patient Clear tubing* Check slide clamps, stopcocks	Reinstall cassette Clear tubing Check slide clamps, stopcocks
Air in line	Clear tubing Refill drip chamber Remove air from all injection ports	Clear tubing Refill drip chamber Remove and flush cassette
Pump interruption	Replace faceplate Check volume limit settings Check lock button on key pad Check solution container Check power source Reposition patient	Check drip sensor, reposition Check volume limit settings Check solution container Check power source Check cassette Reposition patient
Low power	Replace batteries Switch to AC power	Plug device into AC Replace pump[†]

* Warning: Disconnect patient from administration line prior to purging.
[†] Some models do not maintain a charge when operation on AC.

10. What are the options for replacing high-volume loss?

Each manufacturer has setting limits for rate of infusion. One should refer to the operations manual for such information. Many pumps deliver at 999 ml/hr, such as the Lifecare series. However, for high-volume loss replacement, the Haemonetics Rapid Infusion System (RIS) is the proper choice. This system is capable of delivering $1\frac{1}{2}$ liters of fluid in one minute, and has the added advantage of warming the solution during delivery. Multiple peripheral lines can be replaced with two large-bore catheters connecting to the delivery tubing. The mechanism of delivery on the RIS is a high-speed roller pump head, which turns in synchronicity with the opening of control clamps. Air and pressure detectors are also incorporated in-line to prevent line block as well as air infusion. Because the system can deliver large volumes of blood, a 40-micron filter is placed distally in the tubing.

11. Is the use of the RIS confined to liver transplantation?

No. The benefits of the RIS include high flow rates for a prolonged period, flexibility in reinfusion, and temperature control of all solutions. Any major trauma or surgery involving massive blood loss, such as ruptured aortic aneurysm, may benefit from the use of the RIS. Cardiac stability and temperature maintenance are more easily controlled, preventing future complications in cardiac performance as well as defects in coagulation.

12. Is the Level 1 system considered an infusion device?

The Level 1 system is not an infusion pump, although some models come equipped with pressure infusion systems manufactured by Alton Dean. Level 1 systems are primarily blood warmers, capable of warming at high infusion rates.

13. Summarize the factors to be considered in selecting a pump.

Infusion devices are useful tools in managing the fluid replacement needs of almost every patient. Mechanism of delivery varies, as explained, and should play an important part in selection of a pump. Cost also factors into the decision-making process. If one needs both syringe and large container delivery, a pump such as the OmniFlow 4000 plus may offer the most affordable savings to the patient, because both needs are served with one pump and delivery cassette. For simple fluid maintenance and replacement therapy, a gravity-based controller is sufficient, and its cost is relatively low. Over 40% of all drugs and fluids in the hospital setting are administered intravenously, and most of these infusions are run by an electronic pump of some form. Proper selection is quite important in influencing cost as well as outcome.

BIBLIOGRAPHY

1. AS40A Infusion Pump Operation Manual. Baxter HealthCare Corporation, IV Systems Division, 1993.
2. Klem SA, Farrington DM, Leff RD: Influence of infusion pump operation and flow rate on hemodynamic stability during epinephrine infusion. J Crit Care Med 21:1216, 1993.
3. Kwan JW: High-technology I.V. infusion devices. Am J Hosp Pharm 48:S36–S51, 1991.
4. Kwan JW: Use of infusion devices for epidural or intrathecal administration of spinal opioids. Am J Hosp Pharm 47:S18–S22, 1990.
5. Pelletier SD: Patients' experience of technology at the bedside: Intravenous infusion control devices. J Adv Nurs 17:1274–1282, 1992.

IV. *Patient Monitoring and Procedures*

23. ELECTROCARDIOGRAPHY

James W. Rosher, M.D.

1. What is an electrocardiogram (ECG or EKG)?

An ECG is a surface recording of the electrical activity of the myocardium. The ECG displays cardiac electrical activity only; it says nothing about the adequacy of the myocardial pump function. The ECG is created by connecting various electrodes through which electrical potentials are measured. By using different lead configurations, various areas of the myocardium can be monitored. Myocardial activity may be displayed on the monitor (oscilloscope) or permanently recorded on paper (rhythm strips or 12-lead ECG).

Einthoven in 1906 invented the first ECG using a string galvanometer to measure the current generated during a cardiac impulse. It was not until the 1950s that the ECG was introduced commercially in the operating room (OR) setting. In the late 1960s, the ECG came into general use in the OR. Today the continuous ECG is a routine monitor for all anesthetic or surgical procedures.

American Society of Anesthesiologists (ASA) Standards for Basic Intraoperative Monitoring requires that any patient receiving an anesthetic have the ECG continuously displayed from the beginning of anesthesia until preparing to leave the OR.

2. Describe the anatomy and physiology of the cardiac conduction system.

The cardiac impulse originates in the sinoatrial (SA node), which rapidly conducts across the atria to the atrioventricular (AV node). There is a normal delay across the AV node of approximately 0.04 to 0.11 second. The impulse is then directed to the common bundle of His and the Purkinje fibers, resulting in ventricular depolarization. The normal cardiac impulse originating in the SA node requires less than 0.2 second to depolarize the entire myocardium.

Action potentials from different areas of the heart have characteristic shapes. The particular phases of the various action potentials correlate to the activation and inactivation of ion specific channels, especially sodium and calcium.

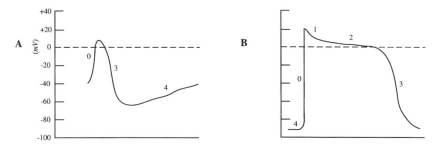

Action potentials demonstrating the action of the ion specific channels. **A.** SA node. **B.** Ventricular muscle.

- **Phase 0** correlates with the activation of the "fast" sodium channels with net movement of sodium into the myocardial cell producing depolarization.

139

- **Phase 1** represents the early repolarization phase and is the result of inactivation of the sodium channels and transient increases in potassium permeability.
- **Phase 2** represents the plateau phase resulting from activation of the "slow" calcium channels and influx of calcium ions into the cells.
- **Phase 3** represents the final repolarization phase resulting in inactivation of the calcium channels and efflux of potassium ions out of the cell.
- **Phase 4** is the resting potential phase during which normal ion permeability is restored.

Phase 4 of the SA node demonstrates an increase in voltage secondary to the spontaneous influx of sodium and calcium into the SA node, which results in spontaneous diastolic depolarization. This repetitive diastolic depolarization enables the pacing function of the SA node. Note that normal ventricular muscle does not have this capability.

3. What are the components of an ECG complex?

The ECG tracing is a recording of the summed electrical vectors produced during depolarization and repolarization of the heart. Electrical forces directed toward an electrode are represented as positive forces (upward deflections), whereas forces directed away from an electrode are represented as negative forces (downward deflections).

The standard representation of the cardiac cycle is seen in the ECG as the P wave, the QRS complex, and the T wave. These waves and complexes are separated by regularly occurring intervals.

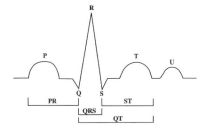

A single normal ECG cycle.

The **P wave** represents the atrial depolarization. The QRS complex represents the ventricular depolarization. The atrial repolarization is usually not seen because it occurs during the QRS complex. The **T wave** represents the repolarization of the ventricles. The **PR interval** represents the time required for an impulse to depolarize the atria, traverse the AV node, and enter the ventricular conduction system. The **QT interval** represents the duration of electrical systole and varies with heart rate. The **ST segment** represents the segment following ventricular depolarization and the preceding ventricular repolarization.

4. Who should have a preoperative 12-lead ECG?

- Any patient over 40 years of age without a recent ECG (within 1 year)
- Any other patient who has signs or symptoms of cardiac disease
- Patients with prior history of cardiac ischemia, dysrhythmias, or pacemaker placement

5. What disorders can be diagnosed perioperatively by the ECG?

- Dysrhythmias
- Conduction abnormalities (AV blocks, PACs, PVCs)
- Myocardial ischemia
- Myocardial infarctions
- Ventricular and atrial hypertrophy
- Pacemaker function
- Preexcitation (e.g., Wolff-Parkinson-White)

• Drug toxicity (digitalis, antiarrhythmics, tricyclic antidepressants)
• Electrolyte abnormalities (e.g., disturbances in calcium, potassium)
• Various medical conditions (e.g., pericarditis, hypothermia, pulmonary emboli, cor pulmonale, cerebrovascular accidents, or increased intracranial pressure)

6. What potential risks may be associated with intraoperative ECG monitoring?

If the patient is improperly grounded, shocks or burns could occur if the electrodes complete a short circuit. New ECG monitors have minimal risk secondary to patient isolation devices. Older ECG monitors lack these safety devices and may be hazardous.

7. What artifacts can alter the ECG monitor intraoperatively?

Artifacts on the ECG monitor may lead to inaccurate diagnosis. The following conditions may produce artifacts on the ECG:

1. Loose or misplaced ECG wires or electrodes
2. Improper electrode placement or adhesion (e.g., hair, burned tissue, inadequate skin preparation, surgical scrub, loose electrodes, or dry electrode gel)
3. Motion (e.g., shivering, tremor, hiccuping, surgical preparation, or diaphragmatic movement)
4. OR equipment (e.g., electrocautery, cardiopulmonary bypass pump, OR lasers, irrigation/suction devices, evoked potential monitoring, and surgical drills and saws)
5. Patient contact by surgeons, nurses, or anesthesia personnel

8. How do you adequately prepare the skin for ECG electrode placement?

Proper skin preparation helps decrease ECG artifact and improve the signal quality for monitoring and diagnostic electrocardiography.

1. Gentle abrasion of the superficial epithelial layer with alcohol and cotton swabs over the intended area of electrode placement helps to decrease the skin resistance and improve adhesion of the electrodes.
2. Hairy skin should be shaved before placement of the skin electrodes to allow optimal adhesion and to decrease discomfort with electrode removal.
3. Wet and oily skin should be cleansed and allowed to dry before electrode placement.
4. Skin electrodes should be completely covered with water-resistant drapes if they are likely to be loosened by preparation solutions.

9. Where do you place the skin electrodes for a unipolar system (5-lead configuration)?

One electrode is placed on the **right shoulder**, one on the **left shoulder**, one on the **left hip area**, one on the **right hip area**, and the V5 electrode in the **5th intercostal space in the left anterior axillary line**.

This 5-lead configuration allows the clinician to monitor 7 different ECG leads (I, II, III, AvR, AvL, AvF, and V5). Although many operating room ECG monitors have only 3-lead systems, the 5-lead system is preferred because it enhances the extent of ECG monitoring possible. If only 3 leads are available, one can create modified bipolar limb leads to help diagnose specific abnormalities in question.

10. What two leads would you select as primary ECG monitors?

The usefulness of ECG leads in the operative setting was studied by London et al. More than 100 patients with known coronary artery disease were monitored for ischemia during anesthesia and surgery. They found that 75% of the ischemic events occurred in lead V5. Combining leads V4 and V5 resulted in detection of approximately 85% of all the detected events. Lead II is usually best for monitoring P waves, enhancing diagnosis of dysrhythmias, and detecting inferior wall ischemia. Lead V5 is most sensitive for detection of anterior and lateral ischemia. By monitoring leads II and V5 simultaneously, the most information can be obtained.

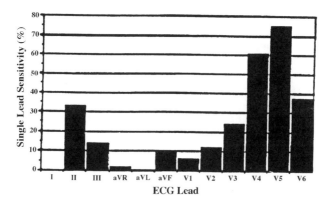

Sensitivity of ECG leads for detection of ischemic events. (From London MJ, Hollenberg M, Wong MG, et al: Intraoperative myocardial ischemia: Localization by continuous 12-lead electrocardiography. Anesthesiology 69:232–241, 1988, with permission.)

11. Which ECG leads monitor specific areas of myocardium?

Ischemia is usually detected as ST segment elevation or depression, T wave inversion, or development of Q waves in leads corresponding to the specific areas of myocardium.

Leads	Ischemia/Infarction
II, III, AvF	Inferior wall
I, AvL, V4–V6	Lateral wall
V1–V3	Anteroseptal
V1–V6	Anterolateral wall

12. What is the difference between diagnostic and monitoring modes for intraoperative electrocardiography?

The diagnostic mode uses ST segment and T wave analysis to diagnose ischemia accurately. The diagnostic mode filters out frequencies below 0.14 Hz but often results in excessive baseline drift and artifact.

The monitoring mode is used to filter out the baseline drift and artifact introduced in ECG signals. This mode filters out all frequencies below 4.0 Hz, which helps remove most of the OR interference. The monitoring mode can introduce artificial elevation and depression of the ST and T wave segments.

13. What invasive ECG electrodes are available? How are they used?

Epicardial	Bronchial
Esophageal	Pulmonary artery catheter

Endocardial or epicardial electrodes are sometimes used during open chest procedures for pacing, diagnosis of dysrhythmias, and ischemia detection.

Esophageal electrodes have been used for differentiation of various dysrhythmias (e.g., atrial fibrillation vs. atrial flutter) because P waves are usually prominent. Esophageal electrodes may be used for detection of posterior myocardial ischemia. The electrode is contained within an esophageal stethoscope, the electrodes being positioned for maximal P wave amplitude.

Pulmonary artery catheters with five ECG electrodes are available for invasive ECG. These intra-atrial and intraventricular electrodes allow for pacing (atrial, AV sequential, or ventricular pacing), stable ECG monitoring, and reliable QRS triggering mechanisms for intra-aortic pump devices.

14. What are new advances in computerized ECG analysis?

Computerized ECG analysis is being developed to detect dysrhythmias and ischemia. The ST segment monitoring mode is a computerized automated monitoring device used to analyze the continuous ECG for ischemia by comparing the ST segment in several leads to the baseline ST segment values.

The leads monitored can be selected (I, II, III, V), the isoelectric and J point locations can be adjusted, and the degree of ST segment deviation can be calibrated to meet specified sensitivity. The recognition of dysrhythmias is becoming precise and sophisticated with the computer programs available today.

15. After orthotopic heart transplantation, what changes can be seen on the ECG tracing?

During orthotopic heart transplantation, the patient's original heart is removed except for the posterior walls of the atria for anastomosis to the donor heart. The patient's original SA node often remains with the original atria, and two P waves can be seen on ECG tracing.

BIBLIOGRAPHY

1. Dubin D: Rapid Interpretation of the EKG's, 4th ed. Tampa, FL, Cover Pub. Co., 1989.
2. Kaplan JA: Cardiac Anesthesia, 2nd ed. Orlando, Grune & Stratton, 1987, pp 55–84.
3. Kotrly KJ, Kotter GS, Montana D, et al: Intraoperative detection of myocardial ischemia with an ST segment trend monitoring system. Anesth Analg 63:343–345, 1984.
4. London MJ, Hollenberg M, Wong MG, et al: Intraoperative myocardial ischemia: Localization by continuous 12-lead electrocardiography. Anesthesiology 69:232–241, 1988.
5. Marriot HJL: Practical Electrocardiography, 7th ed. Baltimore, Williams & Wilkins, 1983.
6. Rao TLK, Jacobs KH, El-Etr AA: Reinfarction following anesthesia in patients with myocardial infarction. Anesthesiology 59:499–505, 1983.
7. Slogoff S, Keats AS: Does perioperative myocardial ischemia lead to postoperative myocardial infarction? Anesthesiology 62:107–114, 1985.
8. Steen PA, Timber JH, Tarhan S: Myocardial reinfarction after anesthesia and surgery. JAMA 239:2566, 1978.
9. Thys D, Hillel Z: Electrocardiography. In Miller RD (ed): Anesthesia, 4th ed. New York, Churchill Livingstone, 1994, pp 1229–1252.

24. PULSE OXIMETRY

Julian M. Goldman, M.D.

1. What is pulse oximetry?

Pulse oximetry is the noninvasive measurement of the ratio of oxyhemoglobin to deoxyhemoglobin (expressed as a percent) measured by optical plethysmography and spectroscopy by transilluminating pulsatile capillary beds.

In English: Two light-emitting diodes (LEDs) emit red and infrared wavelengths of light that is detected by a tiny sensor on the other side of the finger (or earlobe or whatever). Because blood changes color in accordance with its degree of oxygenation, the proportion of transmission of red and infrared light may be analyzed to calculate the color of the intervening tissue as percent oxygen saturation. Saturation measured by pulse oximetry is denoted by SpO_2 ("p" is for pulse oximetry).

2. How does one know that the color measured by the two lights is due to the color of the blood and not to the color of skin or other tissue?

Simple. With each systolic ejection of blood from the heart, the capillaries and adjacent vessels increase in volume so that less LED light passes through the finger tip. Therefore, the pulsatile component of the light transmission signal is detected by the pulse oximeter; the non-pulsatile components (including venous blood) are ignored. It is an elegant concept.

3. How does the pulse oximeter differentiate between arterial or capillary blood and some other pulsatile entity?

The pulse oximeter cannot differentiate pulsatile venous blood from capillary blood. In fact, if one places a pulse oximeter probe on the earlobe of a patient with severe tricuspid valvular regurgitation, the right ventricular pressure pulsations are detected and the pulse oximeter reads venous pulsations. Similarly, one can measure the SpO_2 of a hot dog by wiggling it in the probe.

4. What is the normal SpO_2?

Partial pressure of oxygen in arterial blood (PaO_2) and hence SpO_2 vary with age, altitude, and health. Identifying abnormal values is helpful for screening people for cardiopulmonary disease, but perioperative assessment of SpO_2 has a different motive. In general, the SpO_2 should be above the "cliff" of the oxyhemoglobin dissociation curve (see figure, next page). At and below the cliff, which appears at a saturation of approximately 90%, a small decrease of PaO_2 results in swift desaturation. For example, on the steep part of curve, as PO_2 changes by 1 mmHg, SaO_2 changes by 3%. In the effort to keep the SpO_2 in the safe zone, supplemental oxygen is usually administered to patients who are receiving or recovering from general anesthesia.

5. Why is SpO_2 such a big deal?

One reason, of course, is that SpO_2 can be measured inexpensively and noninvasively. The second reason requires an understanding of oxygen carriage in the blood. The amount of oxygen carried by a sample of blood depends on the SaO_2 and hemoglobin concentration. If hemoglobin concentration remains constant, blood that is 50% saturated with oxygen binds one-half as much oxygen as a sample that is 100% saturated. Examination of the oxyhemoglobin dissociation curve tells the rest of the story, because it illustrates the nonlinear relationship between SaO_2 and PaO_2. For example, as PaO_2 increases from 60 mmHg to 100 mmHg, SaO_2 increases only about 6%. In contrast, as PaO_2 increases 33 mmHg, from 27 mmHg to 60 mmHg, SaO_2 increases by 25%.

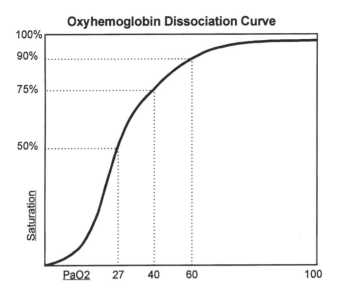

Oxyhemoglobin Dissociation Curve

The oxyhemyglobin dissociation curve describes the nonlinear relationship between PaO_2 and percentage saturation of hemoglobin with oxygen (SaO_2). Note that in the steep part of the curve (50% region), small changes in PaO_2 result in large changes in SaO_2. The converse is true when PaO_2 rises above 60 mmHg. Three regions of the curve have been marked (see question 6).

6. Memorizing the entire oxyhemoglobin dissociation curve is difficult. Are there any tricks to remembering it?

Remember the following key values:

- The PaO_2 at which hemoglobin is 50% saturated, called the P50, is approximately 27 mmHg.
- The saturation of mixed venous blood (in the pulmonary artery) is about 75%, which occurs at a PO_2 of 40 mmHg.
- A PaO_2 of 30 mm Hg produces 60% SaO_2, and a PaO_2 of 60 mm Hg produces 90% SaO_2.
- Little is gained by increasing PaO_2 above approximately 85 mmHg (SaO_2 96.5%).

7. What is the goal of preoxygenation (or denitrogenation) before induction of general anesthesia? How can one determine that it has occurred?

The goal of preoxygenation is to denitrogenate the functional residual capacity (FRC) of the lungs and thus to increase substantially the reservoir of O_2 available to an apneic patient. For example, an average adult breathing room air has about 1.5 L of available O_2 (0.45 L in the lung, with the remainder dissolved or bound in blood and other tissues). In contrast, complete denitrogenation provides about 4.25 L of O_2 storage, 3 L of which occupies the FRC. This 6-fold increase of O_2 storage in the FRC may provide sufficient O_2 to prevent hypoxemia after 5 minutes of apnea.

In practice, it is difficult to increase alveolar O_2 concentration above 85–90% by briefly breathing pure O_2 by mask. The 85–90% target end-tidal O_2 is verified by measuring expired gas concentration with a rapidly responding (or "fast") oxygen sensor. Alternatively, one can measure end-tidal N_2 and verify that it dropped below 10% (4–7%). (The third gas is CO_2—about 5%.) If 5–10 minutes of quiet (tidal volume) breathing or 4–5 deep (vital capacity) breaths do not give the desired effect, further efforts at preoxygenation may be a waste of time in view of the patient's pulmonary disease.

8. Many anesthesiologists use the SpO_2 as an indicator of adequate preoxygenation. If the SpO_2 reaches 100% during preoxygenation, does this indicate complete denitrogenation?

No. Typically, the average sedated patient has an SpO_2 of 92–98% while breathing room air. Administration of pure O_2 should rapidly bring the SpO_2 to 100%. However, the pulse oximeter typically has an error of about 1.5% (in the 90–100% range); thus a reading of 100% may represent an SpO_2 of only 98.5%. Patients with a normal oxyhemoglobin dissociation curve reach 98.5% saturation at a PaO_2 of about 160 mmHg, which can be achieved with approximately 30% alveolar O_2. In such patients only one-third of the potential FRC O_2 reservoir has been attained.

9. The SpO_2 has not risen to 100% despite preoxygenation. What does this mean?
If the SpO_2 has not reached 100% after 2–5 minutes of breathing pure O_2, the patient probably has serious ventilation-perfusion abnormalities (venous admixture or pulmonary shunt), and the SpO_2 will not improve in the next few minutes. Conversely, even complete preoxygenation may not increase SpO_2 to 100% in the presence of pulmonary shunt, because blood that bypasses the alveoli cannot be oxygenated. Before invoking such esoteric explanations, make sure that the patient has a good mask fit and sufficient fresh gas flow to prevent a reduction of inspired O_2 concentration.

10. Do carboxyhemoglobin and methemoglobin interfere with obtaining accurate pulse oximetry measurements?
Yes. Just as the patient with carboxyhemoglobin toxicity exhibits the classic cherry red appearance, the pulse oximeter sees carboxyhemoglobin as oxyhemoglobin. Thus oxygenation is overestimated. Therefore, in a victim of smoke inhalation oxygenation should be assessed by arterial blood gas analysis—not pulse oximetry.

The influence of methemoglobinemia on SpO_2 readings is a bit more complicated. If methemoglobin levels are less than about 20%, the pulse oximeter reads that amount as one-half oxyhemoglobin and one-half reduced hemoglobin. Higher levels of methemoglobin drive the displayed SpO_2 toward 85%.

11. The saturation plummets after injection of methylene blue. Is the monitor or the patient desaturating?
Methylene blue fools the pulse oximeter into thinking that more reduced hemoglobin is present. The apparent SpO_2 returns to normal within a few minutes.

12. Is it necessary to aggravate patients by removing their beautifully applied and buffed nail polish?
No. Simply apply the finger probe sideways so that it transilluminates the finger from one side to the other and avoids the nail polish. This technique usually works but should not be used if the probe does not fit well in the lateral position.

13. After a struggle to secure the patient's airway, the lungs are ventilated, but the saturation still decreases! What should be done next?
Patience, grasshopper. It takes time for O_2 delivered to the lung to influence oxygenation at the fingertip. If the lungs are in fact ventilated (a capnograph can be used for verification), the SpO_2 should rise within approximately 20 seconds.

14. What is the appropriate technique to obtain pulse oximetry readings in a cold, shivering patient?
Cold implies vasoconstriction. It is difficult to get an acceptable SpO_2 reading with a small plethysmographic pulsation (i.e., small signal) and lots of movement (i.e., noise). Try warming the patient or applying the probe to a site with better perfusion (earlobe). A digital nerve block improves finger perfusion and facilitates obtaining a reading, but it is a bit extreme. The next generation of pulse oximeters will perform much better under such conditions. Of course, if one cannot get a reliable reading, one cannot chart SpO_2 values.

BIBLIOGRAPHY
1. Goldman JM, Souders J: Respiratory monitoring. In Kirby R, Gravenstein N (eds): Clinical Anesthesia Practice. Philadelphia, W. B. Saunders, 1994.
2. Nunn JF: Nunn's Applied Respiratory Physiology, 4th Ed. Oxford, Butterworth-Heinemann, 1993.

25. CAPNOGRAPHY

Julian M. Goldman, M.D.

1. What is capnography?

The term **capnography** derives from kapnos, which means smoke in Greek. Capnography is the commonly used, catchall term for measuring and displaying the carbon dioxide concentration of expired and inspired gases. The gas is usually sampled at the connector-end of the tracheal tube, the y-piece, the mask, or from nasal cannulas. The tracheal tube or y-piece provides a more reliable sample than the mask or nasal cannula for measuring exhaled CO_2 concentration and evaluating the waveform.

2. Capnogram, capnograph, capnometer — what is the difference?

The **capnogram** is a continuous graphic recording or display of the respiratory CO_2 time-concentration curve. The **capnograph** is the instrument that displays the capnogram. The **capnometer** is an instrument which displays CO_2 concentration in a nongraphic format (such as a digital display). Capnometers are almost extinct. Confused? Let Dr. Manners provide a few examples: "Hey, Chuck, take a look at this bizarre **capnogram**." "Mr. Tightwad, can our unit purchase this new **capnograph**?" "Sally, I see that you picked up another old **capnometer** at a yard sale!"

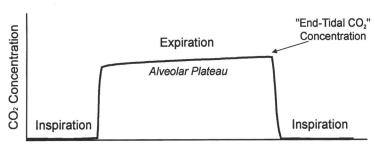

A normal capnograph has the following characteristics: the CO_2 concentration is zero during inspiration, it rises abruptly during expiration, and the alveolar plateau is flat or slightly upsloping. The highest CO_2 concentration is achieved at the end of exhalation and is called the end-tidal CO_2.

3. Why all the fuss about CO_2? What exactly can it tell us?

To get the most out of capnography, we must think about the chain of events required to generate a normal capnogram:

1. The body tissues must generate CO_2.
2. Blood must carry the CO_2 to the lungs.
3. CO_2-containing gas must be exhaled from the lungs and sampled at the mouth or tracheal tube.
4. The capnograph and its sampling line or detector must be in working order.
5. Another CO_2-free inhalation must come along to clear the previously exhaled CO_2 from the sample site.

When CO_2 is exhaled for several breaths in a row (about 5–7), we can be fairly certain that the heart is pumping blood, that ventilating gas is reaching the alveoli and being exhaled, and that the capnograph is functional. An abnormal capnogram may indicate a problem at any point in the chain.

4. Is it possible to see exhaled CO_2 after accidental intubation of the esophagus?

Yes—if the patient drank a can of Coca-Cola before induction of anesthesia and the Coke still has some fizz left. However, because CO_2 is not continuously generated in the stomach, the expired CO_2 concentration will quickly fall to zero after a few breaths. Suspect an inadvertent esophageal intubation if the capnogram does not last for more than 5 breaths. Coke is not the only way for CO_2 to get into the stomach. Sometimes during positive pressure mask ventilation, previously exhaled gas is forced from the mouth and pharynx into the stomach.

5. Can interpreting the shape of the capnogram be as informative as interpreting the ECG?

For some people, the capnograph is much more informative. In general, ECG reading is like bird watching—pure pattern recognition. In contrast, the phenomena that contribute to generating the capnogram are easy to understand, and their effects can be identified as changes in the capnogram.

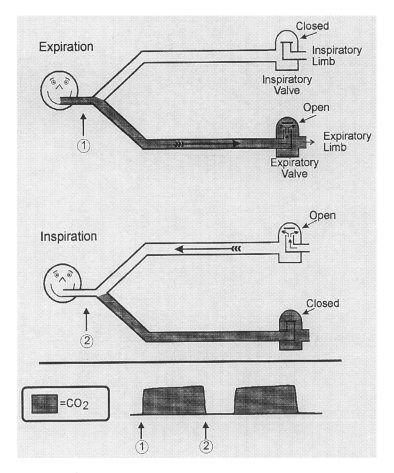

Generation of the capnogram. The capnogram represents the CO_2 concentration at the y-piece. 1. **Expiration.** CO_2 is present at the y-piece. Although expiratory gas flow stops at the end of expiration once the lungs have emptied, the capnogram remains elevated because CO_2-containing gas sits in the y-piece until the next inspiration. 2. **Inspiration.** No CO_2 is present at the y-piece.

6. Immediately after intubation of the trachea, the capnograph displays a CO_2 concentration of zero. What is the next step?

1. Consider the possibilities:
   - There is no pulmonary blood flow (e.g., cardiac arrest or huge pulmonary embolus)
   - There is no tidal ventilation (e.g., faulty circuit, severe asthma)
   - There is a problem with the capnograph or sampling line.
   - The tracheal tube is not actually in the trachea.
2. Tips for developing the diagnostic and therapeutic plan:
   - Did the tracheal tube pass through the vocal cords? An experienced laryngoscopist usually knows from observation of the initial insertion. Another quick look may be wise.
   - Rule out cardiac arrest by placing a finger on the carotid artery to check for a pulse or by glancing at the pulse oximeter waveform.
   - Assessing the performance of the capnograph is simple: disconnect the sampling line and exhale on it. If it does not register CO_2, the problem is in the instrument.
   - If (1) the patient has a pulse, (2) the capnograph works, (3) the clinical likelihood of severe acute pulmonary embolism is remote, (4) physical exam rules out airway obstruction, (5) the patient is cyanotic, and (6) the saturation continues to plummet, the tracheal tube probably did not go through the vocal cords. Consider performing another direct laryngoscopy or removing the tracheal tube and ventilating the patient's lungs via a mask.

7. The baseline of the capnogram is elevated. What are the possible causes?

The baseline of the capnogram may not return to zero at high respiratory rates with some capnographs. However, if the baseline is significantly elevated (above approximately 2 mmHg CO_2), the patient is receiving CO_2 during inspiration. Possible sources for the inspired CO_2 include:

1. An exhausted CO_2 absorber
2. An incompetent unidirectional inspiratory or expiratory valve
3. Deliberate or inadvertent administration of CO_2 from a CO_2-equipped anesthesia machine

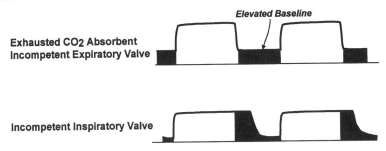

The above capnograms illustrate rebreathing of previously exhaled CO_2, which results in elevation of arterial CO_2 and exhaled CO_2 concentrations. Shaded areas represent CO_2 present during inspiration. Note that the CO_2 contributed by the exhausted CO_2 absorbent or incompetent expiratory valve mixes with CO_2-free inspiratory gas at the y-piece and elevates the inspiratory CO_2 concentration by a relatively constant amount. In contrast, when the inspiratory valve is incompetent, exhaled CO_2-containing gas flows (backward) into the inspiratory limb. During inspiration this previously exhaled CO_2 must flow back into the patient. As the CO_2-laden gas passes the y-piece during inspiration, it registers on the capnograph. The capnogram finally drops to zero after all previously exhaled gas is rebreathed, and fresh gas appears at the y-piece.

8. What other equipment problems can be detected by examining the capnogram?

A gas leak around a partially deflated tracheal tube cuff produces an abnormal capnogram. A kinked or partially obstructed tracheal tube delays expiration and produces a delayed rise of the capnogram.

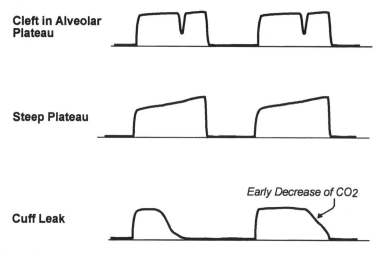

Cleft in Alveolar Plateau

Steep Plateau

Cuff Leak

Early Decrease of CO2

Several abnormal capnograms. The early decrease of CO_2 concentration due to a leak past the tracheal tube cuff is variable. In general, the larger the leak, the earlier the capnogram begins to taper off. This pattern is also evident during mask ventilation with a loose-fitting mask.

9. What other patient problems can be identified by the capnogram?

Many respiratory diseases affect ventilation–perfusion matching and expiratory gas flow. Consequently, such diseases may produce abnormal capnograms. For example, asthma and chronic obstructive pulmonary diseases cause a delayed upslope and steep alveolar plateau (see figure above). Pulmonary hypoperfusion, as in systemic hypotension or pulmonary embolism, decreases CO_2 excretion and reduces the end-tidal CO_2. However, the capnogram should still have a normal shape.

A commonly seen abnormal capnogram results when the patient makes spontaneous respiratory efforts and inhales before the next mechanical inspiration. This characteristic "cleft" in the alveolar plateau is a useful clinical sign that the patient has started to breathe.

BIBLIOGRAPHY

1. Goldman JM, Souders J: Respiratory monitoring. In Kirby R, Gravenstein N (eds): Clinical Anesthesia Practice. Philadelphia, W.B. Saunders, 1994.
2. Gravenstein JS, Paulus DA, Hayes TJ: Capnography in Clinical Practice. Butterworths, Stoneham, MA, 1989.
3. Nunn JF: Nunn's Applied Respiratory Physiology, 4th ed. Oxford, Butterworth-Heinemann, 1993.

26. MONITORING NEUROMUSCULAR FUNCTION

Theresa L. Kinnard, M.D.

1. Describe the anatomy of the neuromuscular junction (NMJ).

The NMJ is composed of a motor nerve ending separated from a highly folded membrane of skeletal muscle (populated with acetylcholine (ACh) receptors) by a synaptic cleft. The synaptic cleft is filled with extracellular fluid and the enzyme acetylcholinesterase. The NMJ transmits the action potential from the nerve to depolarize the muscle and produce muscle contraction.

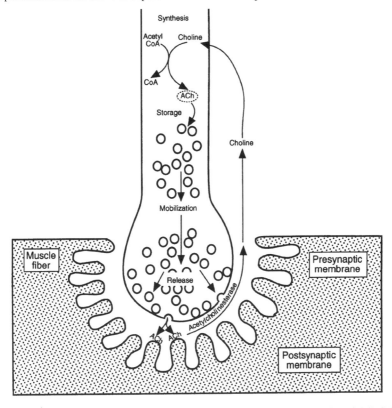

The neuromuscular junction. (From Lebowitz PW, Ramsey FM: Muscle relaxants. In Barash PG, Cullen BF, Stoelting RK (eds): Clinical Anesthesia. Philadelphia, J.B. Lippincott, 1989, pp 339–370, with permission.)

2. Name the steps involved in normal neuromuscular transmission.

1. Transmission of a nerve action potential and depolarization of the nerve terminal
2. Release of ACh from storage vesicles at the terminal
3. Binding of two ACh molecules to the ACh receptor, generating a conformational change
4. Flow of sodium, potassium, and calcium ions down their concentration gradients and through the receptor channel generating an endplate potential
5. When between 5 and 20% of the receptor channels are open and a threshold potential is reached, a muscle action potential (MAP) is generated.
6. Propagation of the MAP along the muscle membrane leads to muscle contraction

3. What is the structure of the ACh receptor?

The ACh receptor consists of 5 glycoprotein subunits: 2 alpha and 1 each of beta, delta, and epsilon. The receptor is contained within the membrane.

4. Where are the ACh receptors located?

The ACh receptors, also referred to as nicotinic cholinergic receptors, can be found in several areas:

    1. Postjunctional receptors are located on the postjunctional muscle membrane in large numbers, approximately 5 million ACh receptors per NMJ.

    2. Prejunctional receptors are present on the motor nerve endings and influence the release of ACh. The prejunctional and postjunctional receptors have different binding characteristics (affinity for ACh).

    3. Extrajunctional receptors are located throughout the skeletal muscle in relatively low numbers owing to suppression of their synthesis by normal neural activity. In cases of traumatized skeletal muscle or denervation injuries, these receptors proliferate.

5. What is the mode of action of muscle relaxants?

Muscle relaxants block transmission of nerve impulses at the NMJ. **Nondepolarizing muscle relaxants** (NDMR) bind competitively to the ACh receptor, preventing released ACh from binding to the receptor. They may also work by binding to the prejunctional receptors, modulating ACh release.

Depolarizing muscle relaxants (DMR) behave similarly to ACH in that they bind to the ACh receptor and depolarize the postsynaptic membrane at the NMJ. This action produces the characteristic muscle fasciculations of a depolarizing block. The DMR are not hydrolyzed by the acetylcholinesterase present at the junction; thus, they hold the channel open for an extended period of time, rendering the muscle flaccid.

6. Why monitor neuromuscular function?

Monitoring neuromuscular function can aid in the delivery of a correct dose of muscle relaxant, help detect patients who are sensitive to muscle relaxants, and help assess adequate neuromuscular recovery. Relying on standard pharmacokinetic data in dosing muscle relaxants is unreliable owing to great patient-to-patient variability.

7. How is neuromuscular function monitored?

Assessments of strength, including hand grip, head lift, tidal volume, vital capacity, and inspiratory pressure have all been used in predicting adequate neuromuscular function. In patients under general anesthesia, the measurement of these variables is often not possible, or their values may be affected by other centrally acting anesthetic agents. The most reliable method of monitoring neuromuscular function uses a portable nerve stimulator to stimulate a peripheral motor nerve and measures the response of the skeletal muscle innervated by that nerve. The stimulus is usually delivered to the nerve via surface electrodes, although needle electrodes have been used in obese patients or experimental situations.

8. What are the common methods of measuring the response of the muscle to stimulation?

The two most common methods of measuring response are via mechanomyography and electromyography. **Mechanomyography** measures the contractile responses of the whole muscle to stimulation. Force transducers have been used to make quantitative measurements. In clinical practice, visual or tactile assessment of motor activity is the most commonly used method. **Electromyography** measures the electrical activity associated with the propagation of an action potential in muscle cells. Measurement of the amplified electromyographic signal is related to the number of contracting muscle fibers. This method is not widely used clinically.

9. Which nerves can be chosen for stimulation?

The most common nerve stimulated is the ulnar nerve. The ulnar nerve supplies several hand muscles, including the adductor pollicis muscle. This muscle adducts the thumb at the metacarpophalangeal joint. The contraction of this muscle is most commonly monitored when evaluating the effects of muscle relaxants. It is crucial to monitor the response of the thumb because response of the other fingers may be due to direct stimulation of muscle groups of the hand. The ophthalmic branch of the facial nerve may also be stimulated, monitoring the contraction of the orbicularis oculi muscle. When access to the head and arms is difficult, the peroneal nerve or posterior tibial nerve of the leg can be stimulated. The degree of dorsiflexion of the foot and plantar flexion of the big toe are monitored.

10. Where should the stimulating electrodes be placed on the skin?

There is both a positive and a negative electrode to the nerve stimulator. A negative (black) electrode generates its action potential by depolarizing the membrane. Depolarization, versus hyperpolarization (produced by the positive electrode), makes it easier to stimulate the nerve. Therefore, maximal twitch height occurs when the negative electrode is placed in closest proximity to the nerve. Stimulation is also possible, however, if the positive electrode is placed close to the nerve.

11. Does it make a difference which nerve-muscle is monitored?

Different muscles have different sensitivities to muscle relaxants.

MUSCLE	SENSITIVITY
Vocal cord	Most resistant
Diaphragm	↑
Orbicularis oculi	
Abdominal rectus	
Adductor pollicis	
Masseter	
Pharyngeal	↓
Extraocular	Most sensitive

From Rupp SM: Monitoring neuromuscular blockade—twitch monitoring. Anesthesiol Clin North Am 11:361, 1993, with permission.

The fact that a patient is no longer breathing does not mean that he or she is ready to intubate (control of breathing is a complex process). If we attempt intubation based on when a patient becomes apneic, the patient may cough or move owing to the relative resistance of the vocal cords and diaphragm to muscle relaxants.

12. Discuss important characteristics of a nerve stimulator.

The stimulator chosen should be able to deliver impulses of 0.1–0.3 ms duration to prevent repetitive firing of the nerve. A supramaximal current output of 50–60 mA at all frequencies should be able to be delivered; this would guarantee that all nerve fibers depolarize with stimulation. The pulse waveform generated should be a monophasic square wave, delivering constant current for a specified interval. It should be capable of delivering single-twitch stimulation at 0.1 Hz (1 stimulus every 10 seconds), train of four (TOF) at 2 Hz (2 per second), and tetanic stimulation at 50 Hz (50 per second).

13. What are the different patterns of stimulation and their clinical applicability?

Single stimulus. The simplest mode of stimulation consists of the delivery of single impulses separated by at least 10 seconds (0.1 Hz). Clinically the use of this stimulus is limited owing to the necessity of establishing a baseline response. The single stimulus response is used when comparing effective doses of muscle relaxants, for instance, the ED 95 of a muscle relaxant is the effective dose for 95% single-twitch suppression of thumb adduction.

Train of four. A stimulus delivered at a frequency fo 2 Hz (2 per second) for a total of four stimuli is known as TOF. Each train is repeated every 10 seconds. The ratio of the amplitude of the fourth to the first response in a train permits the estimation of the degree of block without the need for a control stimulus (T4/T1 ratio). TOF stimulation is the most common modality used to assess degree of blockade. It causes significantly less discomfort in the awake patient than tetanic stimulation and does not affect the subsequent responses to a stimulus. During the onset of nueromuscular blockade, the fourth twitch in the TOF is eliminated at approximately 75% depression of the first twitch. The third twitch is abolished at 80% suppression of the first twitch, and the second twitch is abolished at about 90% block fo the first twitch.

Tetanus. Tetanic stimulation consists of repetitive, high-frequency stimulation at frequencies of 50 Hz or greater. Higher frequency stimulation (100 Hz) has been shown to produce fade in the absence of neuromuscular blocking agents owing to depletion of ACh at the NMJ. The response to tetanus is a more sensitive indicator of residual neuromuscular blockade than single twitch. An important consideration in applying a tetanic stimulus is that it changes the response of the NMJ to further stimulation for upward of 30 minutes, thus leading to overestimation of neuromuscular function on further testing. Clincally a tetanic stimulus is painful to apply in an awake patient, and it is best used in the context of posttetanic count.

Posttetanic facilitation and posttetanic count. This mode of stimulation is useful during periods of intense neuromuscular blockade (when there is no response to TOF stimulation) and extends our range of monitoring. It provides an indication as to when recovery of a single twitch is anticipated and, hence, when reversal of neuromuscular blockade is possible. An application of a 50-Hz stimulus for 5 seconds is followed in 3 seconds by single twitches at 1 Hz. The number of twitches observed is inversely related to the degree of blockade. The number of twitches also may be related to the time until the return of the first response in the TOF.

Double burst. The most recently introduced mode of stimulation that appears to be more sensitive than TOF stimulation for detecting small degrees of residual neuromuscular blockade is double burst. This type of stimulation involves the application of an initial burst of three 0.2-ms impulses at 50 Hz followed by an identical stimulation in 750 ms.[7] The magnitude of the responses to double burst is approximately 3 times greater than that of TOF stimulation, thus making it easier to assess degree of fade present. This method has not gained wide usage.

14. What are the characteristic responses to the various patterns of stimulation produced by nondepolarizing agents and depolarizing agents?
In the presence of a NDMR, repetitive stimulation (TOF or tetanus) is associated with fade of the muscle response. The other distinguishing feature of an NDMR blockade is the presence of posttetanic faciliation. Following a tetanic stimulus, the response to subsequent stimulations is increased. This is thought to be due to increased ACh release or increased sensitivity at the end plate.

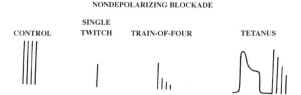

Response to NDMR blockade. (From Bevan DR, Bevan JC, Donati F: Muscle Relaxants in Clinical Anesthesia. Chicago, Year Book Medical Publishers, 1988, pp 49–70, with permission.)

DMR blockade does not exhibit fade in response to repetitive stimuli (TOF and tetanus). It also does not exhibit posttetanic facilitation. The single-twitch, TOF, and tetanus amplitudes are uniformly decreased in relation to the degree of blockade present. A phase II depolarizing or desensitization block (present with large doses of succinylcholine, over 2 mg/kg) exhibits the same characteristics as a NDMR blockade.

DEPOLARIZING BLOCKADE

Response to DMR blockade. (From Bevan DR, Bevan JC, Donati F: Muscle Relaxants in Clinical Anesthesia. Chicago, Year Book Medical Publishers, 1988, pp 49–70, with permission.)

15. Which responses to stimulation indicate adequate relaxation (blockade)?

The degree of neuromuscular blockade required for a surgical procedure varies greatly, depending on the type of surgery, amount of inhalational agent administered, coexisting disease, medications, and musculature of the patient. Adequate relaxation is generally present when one to two twitches of the TOF response are present, correlating with 80% depression of single-twitch height. To ensure paralysis of the more resistant muscle groups, there should be no response to posttetanic stimulation.

16. How does the response obtained to various patterns of stimulation correlate with the actual percentage of receptors occupied?

The response to single twitch is not reduced until approximately 75% of receptors are occupied, and the response disappears at 90–95% occupancy. The fourth twitch of the TOF disappears when there are 75–80% of the receptors occupied, the third twitch disappears at 85% occupancy, the second twitch disappears at 85–90% occupancy, and the first twitch disappears at 90–95% occupancy.[13] Sustained tetanus at 50 Hz can be present when up to 75% of receptors are occupied.

17. What results of neuromuscular stimulation indicate adequate muscle relaxant reversal?

Neuromuscular blockade can be reversed when the response to TOF stimulation is at least one twitch and preferably more. No tetanic stimulus should have been applied in the previous 10 minutes. TOF ratio of greater than 0.7 and sustained tetanus at 50 Hz correlate with restoration of neuromuscular function (ability to protect the airway and maintain respiratory function). Unfortunately the tactile evaluation of fade in TOF and tetanus can be unreliable even in experienced hands. This has led to the development of double-burst stimulation. With the strength of the contractions greater than in TOF, tactile evaluation of the response to double burst appears to be more reliable.

18. What clinical and respiratory parameters correlate with the restoration of neuromuscular function?

An adequate tidal volume is the most insensitive indicator of adequate strength (80% of receptors may still be occupied). The most sensitive respiratory parameter is inspiratory force (50% receptor occupancy) and of intermediate sensitivity is the vital capacity. A negative inspiratory force of -50 cm H_2O is thought to correlate with airway protection and adequate reversal of neuromuscular blockade.[2] The ability to sustain a headlift for 5 seconds and hand grasp are the most sensitive tests of adequate strength (33% receptor occupancy).

19. Which drugs or clinical conditions can prolong neuromuscular blockade?

- Respiratory acidosis
- Metabolic alkalosis
- Hypothermia
- Hypokalemia
- Hypercalcemia

- Hypermagnesemia
- Administration of certain antibiotics such as streptomycin, polymyxin, or neomycin

Cocaine, procaine, lidocaine, and etiodocaine have also been shown to have neuromuscular blocking properties. Prolonged blockade has also been shown following lithium therapy owing to its hypokalemic effect. Corticosteroids have been found to have a potentiating effect on neuromuscular blockade. Patients with impaired hepatic or renal function may exhibit increased sensitivity to muscle relaxants depending on their mode of elimination. An important interaction to remember is the potentiation of neuromuscular blockade in the presence of inhaled anesthetics.

20. Which drugs or clinical conditions are associated with resistance to neuromuscular blockade?

1. Antiepileptic drugs tend to shorten the duration of action of neuromuscular blockade drugs.
2. Long-term phenytoin therapy has been shown to shorten the duration of long-acting muscle relaxant blockade by 50%.
3. Patients with burns exhibit resistance to NDMR and sensitivity to succinylcholine with a hyperkalemic response.

21. What is the response to neuromuscular blockade drugs in patients with neuromuscular disease?

Patients with myotonic syndromes exhibit delayed muscle relaxation following contraction. Succinylcholine can induce severe contractions and should be avoided. The response to NDMR blockade in these patients is normal. The patient with myasthenia gravis tends to be extremely sensitive to NDMR blockade and resistant to DMR blockade. Patients with lower motor neuron disorders are sensitive to NDMR blockade and may show marked hyperkalemia in response to succinylcholine. Hemiplegia has been associated with resistance to NDMR, when neuromuscular transmission is monitored on the affected side, and hyperkalemia in response to succinylcholine. According to a theory by Brown and Charlton, the level of neurologic lesion determines the response of the NMJ to stimulation.[6] Intracranial lesions cause resistance to muscle relaxants, and spinal cord lesions tend to cause increased sensitivity.

BIBLIOGRAPHY

1. Ali HH: Monitoring of neuromuscular function. In Katz L (ed): Muscle Relaxants: Basic and Clinical Aspects. Orlando, Grune & Stratton, 1985, pp 53–68.
2. Ali HH, Wilson RS, Savarese JJ, et al: The effect of tubocurarine on indirectly elicited train-of-four muscle response and respiratory measurements in humans. Br J Anaesth 47:570–573, 1975.
3. Azar I: Complications of neuromuscular blockers. Anesthesiol Clin North Am 11:379–389, 1993.
4. Berger JJ, Gravenstein JS, Munson ES: Electrode polarity and peripheral nerve stimulation. Anesthesiology 56:402–404, 1982.
5. Bevan DR, Bevan JC, Donati F: Muscle Relaxants in Clinical Anesthesia. Chicago, Year Book, 1988, pp 49–70.
6. Brown JC, Charlton JE: A sensitivity to curare in certain neurological disorders using a regional technique. J Neurol Neurosurg Psychiatry 38:34–39, 1975.
7. Engbaek J, Ostergaard D, Viby-Mogensen J: Double burst stimulation (DBS). A new pattern of nerve stimulation to identify residual neuromuscular block. Br J Anaesth 62:274–278, 1989.
8. Lebowitz PW, Ramsey FM: Muscle relaxants. In Barash PG, Cullen BF, Stoelting RK (eds): Clinical Anesthesia. Philadelphia, J.B. Lippincott, 1989, pp 339–370.
9. Patane PS, Condon BF: Neuromuscular blocking agents and trauma patients. Am J Anesthiol 22:13–22, 1995.
10. Pavlin EG: Clinical tests of recovery from neuromuscular blocking agents. Anesthesiol Clin North Am 11:379–389, 1993.
11. Rupp SM: Monitoring neuromuscular blockade—twitch monitoring. Anesthesiol Clin North Am 11:361–378, 1993.
12. Siverman DG, Brull SJ: Monitoring neuromuscular block. Anesthesiol Clin North Am 12:237–260, 1994.
13. Waud BE, Waud DR: The relation between the response to "train-of-four" stimulation and receptor occlusion during competitive neuromuscular block. Anesthesiology 37:413–416, 1972.

27. CENTRAL VENOUS CATHETERIZATION AND PRESSURE MONITORING

Lyle E. Kirson, D.D.S.

1. What is central venous catheterization?

Central venous catheterization involves inserting a catheter into the venous circulation and advancing it so that its distal orifice is positioned immediately adjacent to, or within, the right atrium of the heart (see figure below). The catheter is introduced into the venous circulation from one of several venous access points.

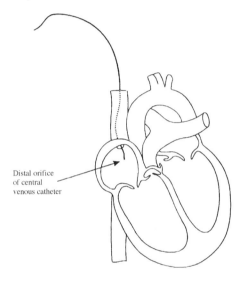

Distal orifice of central venous catheter

2. What is central venous pressure?

Central venous pressure refers to the hydrostatic pressure generated by the blood within either the right atrium of the heart or the great veins of the thorax at a point immediately adjacent to the right atrium of the heart.

3. How is central venous pressure measured?

The proximal orifice of the central venous catheter is attached to a fluid-filled manometer. The pressure at the distal orifice is transmitted through the fluid path within the catheter and supports the fluid column within the manometer. If the base of the fluid column is placed at the level of the heart, then the height of the fluid column represents the pressure at the distal orifice of the catheter, the central venous pressure.

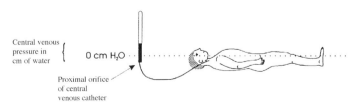

Central venous pressure in cm of water

0 cm H$_2$O

Proximal orifice of central venous catheter

In the past, central venous pressure was measured by connecting the catheter to a water manometer and reading the pressure in centimeters (cm) of water. Today, it is more common to attach the catheter to a pressure transducer. The transducer converts the pressure generated at the distal orifice of the catheter into an electrical signal that is then displayed in torr or millimeters of mercury (mm Hg) on a real-time display screen. The use of a transducer is more convenient than the manometer and has the added capability of displaying the central venous pressure waveform on the display screen. The waveform provides additional information to the clinician regarding the patient's cardiac function (see #19). As with a water manometer, the pressure transducer must be positioned at the level of the heart in order to obtain consistently accurate pressure measurements.

4. How is central venous pressure regulated?

Central venous pressure is regulated by a balance between two factors: the volume of blood returning to the heart from the systemic circulation, and the ability of the right ventricle to pump the returning blood through the pulmonary circulation.[7] Any physiologic process or event that affects either of these two factors will alter the balance between the two factors and may vary the central venous pressure.[8] Vasodilatation, hemorrhage, fluid infusion, alterations in local tissue metabolism, myocardial ischemia, or changes in sympathetic stimulation of the heart can all alter this balance.

5. At what point on the body should central venous pressure be measured?

The ideal point at which to measure central venous pressure is at the level of the tricuspid valve. It is at this point that, in the healthy heart, hydrostatic pressures caused by changes in body position are almost zero. This phenomenon exists because as the pressure at the tricuspid valve increases from the position change, the right ventricle will fill to a greater degree, right ventricular cardiac output will transiently increase, and the change in pressure at the tricuspid valve will be brought back toward zero. The opposite will occur if pressure at the tricuspid valve decreases.[7]

It is of course difficult to consistently find the precise level of the tricuspid valve in a clinical setting. Therefore, ongoing adjustment is necessary to assure that the transducer or manometer is at a constant reference point whenever the patient's position or bed height is altered.

6. How does central venous pressure relate to right ventricular preload?

Central venous pressure reflects the preload for the right ventricle. While preload is more accurately defined as the right ventricular end-diastolic volume (RVEDV), RVEDV cannot be easily monitored clinically. Therefore, central venous pressure is the best indicator of right atrial preload currently available to the clinician. Preload is often used to guide the clinician in intravenous fluid replacement. A low or decreasing preload may indicate a need for intravenous fluid administration. An increasing or elevated preload (above 15 mm Hg) may indicate over-resuscitation or impaired cardiac performance.

7. Does central venous pressure relate to left ventricular preload?

Central venous pressure is representative of **right** ventricular preload only. It is possible that, in patients whose left and right ventricles are functioning identically, central venous pressure equals or parallels the preload for the **left** ventricle. However, in patients with pulmonary hypertension, pulmonary disease, or right or left ventricular damage, a pulmonary artery catheter provides better information with regard to left ventricular preload than does a central venous catheter.

8. Is there a single normal central venous pressure reading?

There is no single central venous pressure that is normal for all patients, or for that matter, for any individual patient. Measurements may range from 1–15 torr and depend on the patient's stage of hydration, presence or absence of positive pressure ventilation, position, cardiac function, and chamber compliance. Use several clinical signs (signs of hydration, urine output, blood pressure, etc.) to determine the appropriate range of central venous pressure for any one individual patient.

9. What are the indications for placement of a central venous catheter?
There are perioperative and nonoperative indications for central venous catheterization.

Perioperative indications include:
1. Guiding fluid replacement;
2. Evaluating cardiac function;
3. Providing access for:
    a. aspiration of air emboli that can occur during neurosurgical procedures;
    b. drug infusion;
    c. blood and fluid infusion;
    d. introduction of a pulmonary artery catheter or transvenous pacer;
    e. blood sampling.

Nonoperative indications include providing access for:
1. Hyperalimentation;
2. Temporary hemodialysis;
3. Long-term chemotherapy;
4. Frequent therapeutic plasmapheresis.[1]

10. Describe several approaches to introduction of the central venous catheter into the venous circulation.
Numerous access points are available for introduction of a catheter into the venous circulation. All approaches carry risks, and none will work successfully for every single patient. Therefore, it is recommended that the clinician become familiar with several different approaches.

The following approaches require that the patient be placed in Trendelenburg position prior to venous puncture. Placing the access point below the level of the heart distends the target vessel and promotes positive venous pressure within the vessel.

As the needle is advanced toward a vessel, slight and constant aspiration is required. However, it is possible that during needle penetration, the vessel walls will collapse upon themselves, allowing the needle to pass through the vessel without demonstrating blood aspiration. Therefore, if blood is not aspirated as the needle is advanced, aspiration should be maintained as the needle is slowly withdrawn.

Finally, be familiar with the anatomy surrounding the vessel and needle puncture site. Advancing the introducer needle too far or in the wrong direction can injure adjacent structures.

The most common approaches to the central venous circulation are:

1. **Subclavian vein**. The subclavian approach is commonly used in the operating room and for quick access in emergency room settings because of the ease of access to the vessel. The subclavian vein is best cannulated from the subclavicular approach. The skin puncture is made just lateral to the costoclavicular ligament, one fingerwidth below the clavicle. The needle is directed along the posterior border of the clavicle in the direction of the sternal notch until the subclavian vein is entered and blood is aspirated.

2. **Internal jugular vein.** There are several approaches to the internal jugular vein, three of which are briefly described here.

• *Low anterior.* Locate the point at which the sternal and clavicular heads of the sternocleidomastoid muscle join. Introduce the needle at this point and direct it at an angle of 30 degrees to the skin. Advance the needle toward the ipsilateral nipple until the internal jugular vein is entered and blood is aspirated.

• *High anterior.* Palpate the carotid artery at the level of the cricothyroid membrane. Introduce the needle just lateral to the carotid pulsation and advance it toward the ipsilateral nipple at a 30-degree angle to the skin until the internal jugular vein is entered and blood is aspirated. This approach frequently requires penetration of the body of the sternocleidomastoid muscle by the introducer needle.

- **Posterior.** Locate the junction of the posterior border of the sternocleidomastoid muscle and the external jugular vein. Introduce the needle just posterior to this point and advance it along the deep surface of the muscle toward the ipsilateral corner of the sternal notch until the internal jugular vein is entered and blood is aspirated.

3. **External jugular vein.** When the patient is in Trendelenburg position, the external jugular vein frequently can be visualized where it crosses the sternocleidomastoid muscle. The needle is advanced in a direction paralleling the vessel and introduced into the vein approximately two fingerwidths below the inferior border of the mandible. **Warning:** difficulty may arise in advancing the catheter or guide wire into the central circulation from the external jugular vein approach because the patient's anatomy frequently directs the catheter into the subclavian vein.

11. Describe the different techniques for introducing the central venous catheter into the venous circulation.

The two most common techniques for introducing a central venous catheter into the venous circulation are passing the catheter through a needle or passing the catheter over a guide wire. In the former, a 14-gauge needle is introduced into the vessel and the catheter then threaded through the needle and into the vein. The needle is then removed. In the latter, commonly referred to as the Seldinger technique (named after the individual who first described this technique for arterial catheterization in 1953),[15] an 18- or 20-gauge needle is introduced into the vessel. A guide wire is threaded through the needle and into the vein. The needle is removed, leaving the guide wire in place. The catheter is then passed over the guide wire and into the vessel. Finally, the guide wire is removed. The obvious benefit of the Seldinger technique rests in the use of a smaller gauge introducer needle.

12. Are there different types of central venous catheters?

Several different styles of catheters are available for central venous catheterization. Single-lumen catheters are most commonly used and are available with single port and multiport tips. Triple-lumen catheters are basically three single-lumen, single-port catheters joined together. Each of the three lumens is of slightly different length. The purpose of the triple-lumen catheter is to provide ports for simultaneous drug infusion, blood drawing, and central venous pressure monitoring.

A percutaneous introducer sheath is designed to introduce a pulmonary artery catheter into the central circulation. The introducer sheath is a large-bore catheter (8.5 Fr) with a side-port extension attached at its superior aspect. The side port of the introducer sheath can be used as a central venous catheter, whether or not the pulmonary artery catheter is in place.

13. Where should the distal orifice of the catheter be positioned?

The indication for catheter insertion dictates where the catheter tip should be located. When pressure measurements are to be followed for guidance in fluid management, the tip of the catheter can be positioned within either the atrium or the vena cava near the cava–atrial junction. When monitoring pressures, do not change the position of the catheter tip by advancing or withdrawing the catheter or change the external landmark (approximate level of the tricuspid valve) to which you are referencing your measurements.

For monitoring the waveform of the central venous pressure tracing, position the catheter within the atrium. By so positioning, the waveform will not be damped and will accurately reflect the pressure changes within the right atrium.

Placement of the catheter for aspiration of air emboli during neurosurgical cases requires positioning of the catheter tip (preferably multiport) in the right atrium near the superior vena cava–atrial junction. Embolized air flows past this point and accumulates in the superior aspect of the atrium. Positioning the catheter tip at the superior vena cava–atrial junction allows for optimal aspiration. Locating the tip of the catheter further toward the tricuspid valve reduces its effectiveness for aspirating air emboli.[3]

14. How can you judge the correct positioning of the distal orifice of the catheter?

Judging the appropriate distance for catheter advancement can be accomplished in several ways. Prior to insertion, measurement of the distance from the point of insertion to the right atrium (external projection—immediately right of the third costal cartilage) helps initially define the correct distance for intravascular advancement of the catheter.

When position of the catheter tip is critical, techniques for judging exact catheter location should be employed. Advancement of the catheter under fluoroscopy represents the most accurate method for positioning the catheter tip, but it may be time-consuming and cumbersome in the crowded confines of an operating room or intensive care suite.

An alternative method is to use an electrocardiogram (ECG) to guide placement of the catheter. This technique was first described in 1959[9] and relies upon transforming the catheter into an extension of an ECG lead. After insertion of the central venous catheter at the site of choice, the catheter is filled with electrolyte solution—normal saline or 8.4% $NaHCO_3$—and the "V" lead of the ECG attached to the proximal port.[4] The catheter is then advanced toward the right atrium. The axis and voltage of the P wave on the "V" lead tracing are indicative of the catheter tip position. As the catheter tip passes the area of the sinoatrial node, the P wave becomes equal in height to the R wave of the ECG. The catheter tip passing the mid-atrial position is demonstrated by a decreasing or biphasic P wave. Low atrial positioning is indicated by an inverted P wave or absence of the P wave.

15. Are complications associated with placement of the central venous catheter?

Yes. Considering the proximity of the carotid artery to the internal jugular vein, it is not surprising that carotid artery puncture is one of the more common complications associated with all the internal jugular vein approaches. Pneumothorax may occur[5] and is more commonly associated with a subclavian, low anterior (internal jugular), or junctional approach (junction of the internal jugular vein and subclavian vein). Hemothorax is associated primarily with the subclavian vein approach and occurs secondary to subclavian artery laceration.

The thoracic duct, as it wraps around the internal jugular vein, can reach as high as 3 or 4 cm above the sternal end of the clavicle. This places the duct in a vulnerable position for puncture or laceration when a left internal jugular vena puncture is attempted.[10]

A serious complication can occur when a catheter cannot be advanced through an introducer needle and the catheter is then withdrawn from that needle. This maneuver can result in shearing and embolization of the catheter tip. Therefore, if a catheter cannot be advanced through an introducer needle, remove the needle and catheter in unison. A similar event can occur with the Seldinger technique when the tip of the guide wire is sheared and embolized. If a wire cannot be advanced through an introducer needle, remove the needle and wire in unison.

An uncommon but potentially devastating complication is air embolism during central venous catheterization. In order to avoid this problem, the patient should be positioned head down (if entry is at a point superior to the heart) until the catheter is inserted and the hub of the catheter is occluded.

16. What are the *late* complications associated with central venous catheterization?

Late complications include infection, vascular damage, hematoma formation, dysrhythmia, and extravascular catheter migration.[2,6,12,13]

17. Can you use the central venous catheter for blood transfusions?

Certain clinical implications should be understood before using the central venous catheter for blood transfusions. Most central venous catheters have narrow lumens and long lengths. This configuration creates high resistance, which restricts the flow of blood and creates increased shear force on blood cells. An alternative to the long, narrow catheter is the percutaneous introduce sheath (8.5 Fr) used for pulmonary artery catheter introduction. Caution must be exercised when using this sheath for transfusion. Because the sheath has a large lumen, a great volume of blood can be transfused into the central circulation in a short period of time. The high infusion rate can result in transient right heart volume overload.

18. Are any special precautions needed when removing a central venous catheter?

Before a central venous catheter is removed, the insertion site should be positioned lower than the level of the right atrium. This puts the patient in the head-down position for removal of an internal jugular vein or subclavian vein catheter. The purpose of this positioning is to increase venous pressure at the point of removal and thereby prevent air aspiration into the vein through the evacuated catheter tract. Following removal of the catheter, external pressure should be maintained on the area from which the catheter is withdrawn until clot formation has sealed the vessel.

19. Describe the normal central venous pressure waveform and relate its pattern to the cardiac cycle.

The normal central venous pressure waveform shows a pattern of three upstrokes and two descents that correspond to certain events in the cardiac cycle (see figure below).

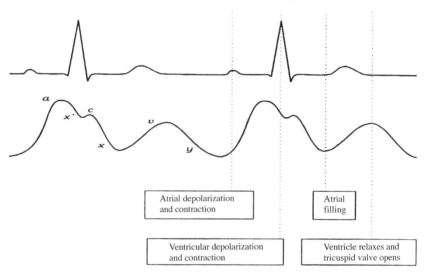

| Atrial depolarization and contraction | Atrial filling |
| Ventricular depolarization and contraction | Ventricle relaxes and tricuspid valve opens |

1. The "a" wave represents the increase in atrial pressure which occurs during atrial contraction.

2. The "x′" descent is the decrease in atrial pressure as the atrium begins to relax.

3. Before total relaxation is completed, the "c" wave occurs, which is caused by the bulging of the tricuspid valve into the atrium during the early phases of right ventricular contraction.

4. The "x" descent follows the "c" wave and is a continuation of the "x′" descent. The "x" descent is caused by a drop in pressure brought about by a downward movement of the ventricle and tricuspid valve during the later stages of ventricular contraction.

5. The "v" wave represents the increase in atrial pressure that occurs while the atrium fills against a closed tricuspid valve.

6. Finally, the "y" descent represents a drop in pressure as the ventricle relaxes, the tricuspid valve opens (because atrial pressure is higher than ventricular pressure), and blood passively enters the ventricle.

20. What is the significance of the central venous pressure waveform?

The significance of the central venous pressure waveform is that it may be used to assist in diagnosis of pathophysiologic events affecting right heart function that may not be detected easily by other monitors. For example, atrial fibrillation is characterized by absence of the normal "a" wave component. Tricuspid regurgitation results in a "giant V wave" that replaces the normal "c," "x," and "v" waves. Other events that can change the normal shape of the central venous pressure waveform include, but are not limited to, atrioventricular dissociation, asynchronous atrial contraction during ventricular pacing, tricuspid stenosis, tamponade, pericardial effusion, increased ventricular afterload, pulmonary hypertension, and right ventricular ischemia and failure.[11,14] Any occurrence, or variation in rhythm, that alters the normal relationship between the events described in #19 above will alter the normal central venous pressure wave morphology.

BIBLIOGRAPHY

1. Blitt CD: Monitoring the anesthetized patient. In Barash PG, Cullen BF, Stoelting RK (eds): Clinical Anesthesia. Philadelphia, J.B. Lippincott, 1989, pp 567–573.
2. Brown CS, Wallace CT: Chronic hematoma—a complication of percutaneous catheterization of the internal jugular vein. Anesthesiology 45:368–369, 1976.
3. Bunegin L, Albin MS, Helsel PE, Hoffman A, Hung T: Positioning the right atrial catheter: A model for reappraisal. Anesthesiology 55:343–348, 1981.
4. Colley PS, Artru AA: ECG-guided placement of Sorenson CVP catheters via arm veins. Anesth Analg 63:953–956, 1984.
5. Cook TL, Dueker CW: Tension pneumothorax following internal jugular cannulation and general anesthesia. Anesthesiology 45:554–555, 1976.
6. Dodson T, Quindlen E, Crowell R, McEnany MT: Vertebral arteriovenous fistulas following insertion of central monitoring catheters. Surgery 87:343–346, 1980.
7. Guyton AC: The systemic circulation. In Textbook of Medical Physiology, 7th ed. Philadelphia, W.B. Saunders, 1986, pp 218–210.
8. Guyton AC: Cardiac output, venous return, and their regulation. In Textbook of Medical Physiology, 7th ed. Philadelphia, W.B. Saunders, 1986, pp 272–286.
9. Hughes RE, McGovern GJ: The relationship between right atrial pressure and blood volume. Arch Surg 79:238–243, 1959.
10. Khalil KG, Parker FB Jr, Mukherjee N, Webb WR: Thoracic duct injury—a complication of jugular vein catheterization. JAMA 221:908–909, 1972.
11. Mark JB: Central venous pressure monitoring: Clinical insights beyond the numbers. J Cardiothorac Vasc Anesth 5:163–173, 1991.
12. Nakayama M, Fujita S, Kawamata M, et al: Traumatic aneurysm of the internal jugular vein causing vagal nerve palsy: A rare complication of percutaneous catheterization. Anesth Analg 78:598–600, 1994.
13. Otto CW: Central venous pressure monitoring. In Blitt CD (ed): Monitoring and Anesthesia Critical Care, 2nd ed. New York, Churchill Livingstone, 1989, pp 169–210.
14. Reich DL, Kaplan JA: Hemodynamic monitoring. In Kaplan JA (ed): Cardiac Anesthesia, 3rd ed. Philadelphia, W.B. Saunders, 1993, pp 269–276.
15. Seldinger SI: Catheter replacement of the needle in percutaneous arteriography. Acta Radiol 39:369–376, 1953.

28. PULMONARY ARTERY CATHETERIZATION

Michael B. Ochs, D.O.

1. When and by whom was the pulmonary artery catheter developed?

Catheterization of the pulmonary artery (PA) with a balloon-tipped catheter was first described by Lategalo and Rahn in 1953. The first report of clinical usefulness of a balloon-tipped PA catheter was in 1970 by Swan and Ganz. Their original PA catheter was a double-lumen catheter designed for measuring PA and pulmonary capillary wedge pressures. Catheters currently used are based on the original design by Swan and Ganz and are frequently called Swan-Ganz catheters.

2. What are the different types of PA catheters?

The basic PA catheter in current use is a balloon-tipped, flow-directed, multilumen catheter inserted percutaneously into the central venous system. These catheters are capable of measuring central venous pressure (CVP), pulmonary artery pressure (PAP), and pulmonary capillary wedge pressure (PCWP). They are also capable of measuring cardiac output using the thermodilution method. A fiberoptic channel capable of continuously measuring mixed venous oxygen saturation is incorporated into some catheters. Other catheters allow pacing of the heart, and some can measure right ventricular ejection fraction. Many catheters contain a lumen known as the VIP lumen, which is usually used for the infusion of vasoactive drugs. New technology allows development of catheters that measure cardiac output continuously instead of intermittently.

3. During which surgical procedures are PA catheters most likely to be placed?

PA catheters are useful in patients undergoing cardiac surgery, cardiac transplantation, lung transplantation, and liver transplantation. PA catheters also may be used to guide the resuscitation of trauma victims who have sustained major blood loss or multiple organ system injury. PA catheters also may be of benefit in patients with poor left ventricular function, left ventricular ejection fraction < 40%, cardiac index < 2 L/min/m^2, recent complicated myocardial infarction, severe ischemic heart disease, pulmonary hypertension, shock states, sepsis, or toxemia of pregnancy, as well as any patient undergoing surgery with anticipated large volume shifts. Many centers also place PA catheters in patients undergoing vascular surgery that involves cross-clamping of the abdominal or thoracic aorta.

4. Are PA catheters useful outside the operating room?

Yes. Swan and Forester stratified patients by data obtained from PA catheters after acute myocardial infarction into one of four groups based on PCWP and cardiac index (CI). Group 1 patients have a CI > 2.2 L/min/m^2 and PCWP < 18 mmHg with an estimated mortality of 3%; group 2 patients have a CI > 2.2 L/min/m^2 and PCWP > 18 mmHg with an estimated mortality of 9%; group 3 patients have a CI < 2.2 L/min/m^2 and PCWP < 18 mmHg with an estimated mortality of 23%; group 4 patients have a CI < 2.2 L/min/m^2 and a PCWP >18 mmHg with an estimated mortality of 51%. Shoemaker has shown that the use of a PA catheter to guide oxygen delivery in high-risk surgical patients and shock victims may improve survival. PA catheters also are useful for diagnoses and treatment of intracardiac shunts, sepsis, pulmonary hypertension, adult respiratory distress syndrome, and cardiac tamponade. PA catheters may be used to perform pulmonary angiograms, although typically this procedure is not done with the Swan-Ganz catheters.

5. What equipment is required for a pulmonary artery catheter insertion?

The specific equipment required depends largely on the type of catheter that is inserted. The basic equipment must include a percutaneous sheath introducer, a PA catheter, pressure transducers, and a monitor capable of displaying pressure waveforms. More specialized equipment is necessary for determination of thermodilution cardiac output, mixed venous oxygen saturation, and right ventricular ejection fraction. Pacemaker generators and wires may be needed if the PA catheter is used for cardiac pacing. Fluoroscopy is usually not necessary for placement of a PA catheter but may be useful in patients in whom the anatomy of the great veins, right atrium, tricuspid valve, right ventricle, or pulmonary artery may be abnormal.

6. Which medical specialists commonly use PA catheters?

Any physician who cares for critically ill patients should be skilled in the placement and interpretation of data from PA catheters, including surgeons, anesthesiologists, intensivists, cardiologists, pulmonologists and anyone else who cares for critically ill patients in intensive care settings.

7. What are the contraindications to placement of a PA catheter?

There are no absolute contraindications for PA catheterization. Suggested relative contraindications include severe coagulopathies, significant thrombocytopenia, prosthetic right-heart valve, endocardial pacemaker leads, and infection or tissue breakdown at the proposed cannulation site. Some clinicians believe that complete left bundle-branch block is a contraindication to PA catheterization because of the risk that the catheter may cause a right bundle-branch block as it passes through the right ventricle and thus lead to complete heart block.

8. What common complications are seen with PA catheters?

Complications may occur during venous access or catheter insertion, while the PA catheter is in place, and during removal of the PA catheter and/or introducer sheath. Shah et al. prospectively studied 6,245 patients who were to have PA catheters inserted in the perioperative period. The great majority of catheters were placed in the right internal jugular vein. In 1.9% of patients the carotid artery was inadvertently cannulated, and in 4 patients a 7.5 French introducer sheath was actually placed in the carotid artery. In 31 patients (0.5%) pneumothorax resulted from attempts at central vein cannulation. Cardiac rhythm disturbances occurred in over 70% of the patients, whereas only 3.1% required a bolus of lidocaine to suppress ventricular dysrhythmias. One patient with preexisting left bundle-branch block developed complete heart block and required pacemaker insertion. Four patients (0.064%) suffered an intrapulmonary hemorrhage secondary to pulmonary artery rupture; three occurred during cardiopulmonary bypass. Pulmonary infarction occurred in 4 patients, perforation of the right ventricle in 1 patient, and pulmonary embolus was suspected in 4 patients. The incidence of a positive PA catheter tip culture varies from 5–45% depending on the method used. The risk of developing catheter-related sepsis ranges from 0.3–0.5% per day.

9. Are any of the complications life-threatening?

Although rare, rupture of the pulmonary artery is the most serious complication associated with PA catheterization. Major risk factors for pulmonary artery rupture include cardiopulmonary bypass, hypothermia, and excessively prolonged balloon inflation and catheter manipulation. Pulmonary artery rupture usually manifests as rapid hypotension with hemoptysis. Management includes reversal of anticoagulation, leaving the PA catheter in place, placement of a double-lumen endotracheal tube to isolate the lung with the bleeding problem, and preparation of the patient for a possible emergent lobectomy or pneumonectomy. Positive end-expiratory pressure (PEEP) also may be useful in cases of hemorrhage.

10. What are the best sites for insertion of a pulmonary artery catheter?

Most anesthesiologists prefer the right internal jugular vein because of its relatively low incidence of complications and its anatomic alignment with the superior vena cava and right atrium. The second best site is the left subclavian vein, which allows continuous smooth catheter curvature from the insertion site downward into the right side of the heart and outward into the pulmonary artery. Less desirable sites are the left internal jugular vein (because of the risk of injury to the thoracic duct) and the right subclavian vein (because the catheter must make a series of turns to gain access to the pulmonary artery). Large veins in the upper arms as well as the femoral vein also may be used for PA catheter placement. Most anesthesiologists do not prefer arm veins because they are generally smaller than central veins and catheter passage into the right heart may be difficult. Arm veins are useful in the presence of severe coagulopathies. The femoral vein is not usually chosen by anesthesiologists because it does not allow catheter manipulation during most surgical procedures.

11. How does one know where the tip of the catheter is?
During placement or flotation of the PA catheter, a pressure transducer is connected through extension tubing to the distal or pulmonary artery port of the catheter. This lumen of the catheter is filled with fluid, the pressure is monitored, and the pressure waveform is continuously displayed on the monitor screen. As the catheter enters the central vein, a central venous pressure waveform is apparent. As the catheter passes the tricuspid valve, a right ventricular wave form is present. When the catheter goes through the pulmonic valve into the main pulmonary artery, the pulmonary arterial waveform is seen; with continued catheter advancement the balloon wedges into a small branch of a pulmonary artery and the waveform reflects PCWP.

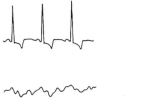

This shows the tip of the catheter in the central venous system.

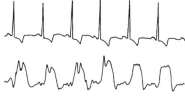

Now in the right ventricle.

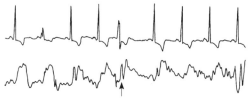

Moving from the right ventricle to the pulmonary artery (at the arrow). Note the presence of a premature ventricular contraction as the catheter passes through the pulmonary outflow tract. This is very common.

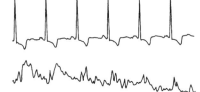

Continued advancement of the catheter causes it to wedge in a branch of the pulmonary artery.

12. Does it matter in which pulmonary artery or which branch of the pulmonary artery the catheter finally comes to rest?
In some cases, yes, and in some cases, no. Balloon-tipped catheters typically go into the pulmonary artery, which receives the majority of blood flow. Once it enters the main pulmonary artery, it then usually enters the branch that receives the most flow, which most often is the dependent portion of the lung. It is best to have the tip of the catheter in a branch of the pulmonary artery in which both pulmonary arterial and pulmonary venous pressures are greater than alveolar pressure. This positioning minimizes the effects of positive pressure ventilation on hemodynamic measurements. If the pulmonary artery is to be ligated (i.e. pneumonectomy, transplant), it is usually desirable to have the catheter in the opposite pulmonary artery. Unless fluoroscopy is used or a chest radiograph obtained after catheter placement, it is generally not known in which pulmonary artery (left or right) the catheter lies. If the surgeon plans to manipulate one of the pulmonary arteries, it is wise to remind the surgeon to palpate the pulmonary artery and check for the presence of the catheter before manipulation is begun. If the catheter is found to be in the pulmonary artery undergoing surgery, it should be withdrawn either into the main pulmonary artery or the right ventricle and refloated to the opposite pulmonary artery, with the surgeon assisting its placement.

13. What hemodynamic parameters are measured by the pulmonary artery catheter?

The most frequently measured hemodynamic parameters are right atrial or central venous pressure, pulmonary arterial pressure, and intermittent measurement of PCWP. All other hemodynamic data are calculated rather than measured.

Calculation of Hemodynamic Variables

VARIABLES	FORMULA	NORMAL VALUES
CI	$\dfrac{CO\ (L/minute)}{body\ surface\ area\ (m^2)}$	2.8–4.2 L/minute/m^2
SV	$\dfrac{CO\ (L/minute) \times 1000}{heart\ rate\ (beats/minute)}$	60–90 ml/minute
SI	$\dfrac{SV\ (ml/beat)}{body\ surface\ area\ (m^2)}$	30–65 ml/beat/m2
RVSWI	0.0136 (MPAP – CVP) × SI	5–10 gm-m/beat/m^2
LVSWI	0.0136 (MAP – PCWP) × SI	45–60 gm-m/beat/m^2
SVR	$\dfrac{MAP - CVP}{CO\ (L/minute)} \times 80$	1200–1500 dynes-second/cm^{-5}
PVR	$\dfrac{MPAP - PCWP}{CO\ (L/minute)} \times 80$	100–300 dynes-second/cm^{-5}

CI = cardiac index, SV = stroke volume, SI = stroke index, RVSWI = right ventricular stroke work index, LVSWI = left ventricular stroke work index, SVR = systemic vascular resistance, PVR = pulmonary vascular resistance, CO = cardiac output, MPAP = mean pulmonary artery pressure, MAP = mean arterial pressure, PCWP = pulmonary capillary wedge pressure.

14. What is the thermodilution method of measuring cardiac output?

The thermodilution method involves injecting a known volume of fluid with a known temperature (colder than blood) into the proximal or right atrial port of the PA catheter and monitoring the temperature change produced by the cold fluid at the distal end of the PA catheter. The change in temperature of the blood over time is inversely proportional to blood flow. Usually a computer is used to assist with the determination of cardiac output. Typically 10 ml of iced or room-temperature crystalloid solution is injected, and the change in temperature over time is measured by the thermistor at the distal end of the PA catheter. A computation constant based on the type of PA catheter and the volume and temperature of the injected solution should be entered into the cardiac output computer to ensure accurate results. Usually at least three consecutive measurements are obtained a little more than 1 minute apart and then averaged. If the results vary significantly, more determinations should be made to increase the accuracy of the result. The injection for cardiac output should be made at the same point in the respiratory cycle for each determination. Meticulous attention to sterile technique as well as to absence of air in the injectate are absolutely necessary. If room-temperature injectate is used, there must be at least a 10° C difference between the patient's blood temperature and the injectate temperature to ensure accurate results.

15. Are there any ways to verify that the cardiac output obtained by thermodilution is accurate?

If thermodilution cardiac outputs are performed correctly, the data are generally accurate and reproducible. If one wants to verify the validity of the results, the Fick equation can be used:

$$CO = \frac{\dot{V}O_2}{CaO_2 - C\bar{v}O_2}$$

where CO = cardiac output, VO_2 = oxygen consumption, CaO_2 = oxygen content of arterial blood, and $C\bar{v}O_2$ = oxygen content of mixed venous blood.

To obtain accurate calculations using the Fick principle, oxygen consumption must be known. Oxygen consumption is relatively easy to calculate in ventilated patients if one knows the alveolar minute ventilation as well as inspired and expired oxygen concentrations. In spontaneously breathing patients it is much more difficult to obtain accurate numbers for oxygen consumption. The cardiac output determined either by thermodilution or the Fick method should always be viewed in light of the patient's clinical condition. If discrepancies exist between the numerical data and the patient's clinical condition, a reason for the discrepancy must be sought.

16. What is the wedge pressure? How do we measure it?
If the balloon at the tip of the catheter is inflated and the catheter is advanced, eventually the catheter will wedge itself into a small branch of the pulmonary artery. If the balloon is left inflated, the pressure monitored distal to the balloon reflects the pulmonary capillary pressure, pulmonary venous pressure, and left atrial pressure. The characteristic venous pressure waveform should be observed on the monitor with its usual A-wave, C-waves and V-waves.

The A-wave represents an increase in left atrial pressure during atrial contraction and usually correlates with the PR interval on the ECG. The C-wave, which may not always be readily apparent, represents closure of the mitral valve and a small increase in atrial pressure at closure. The next large pressure increase, the V-wave, represents filling of the left atrial chamber concomitantly with left ventricular contraction. An adequate wedge position of the PA catheter may be confirmed using three criteria: (1) the contour of the waveform changes from an arterial to a venous pressure waveform; (2) mean pulmonary artery pressure should drop as the catheter is wedged; and (3) the partial pressure of oxygen of a blood sample taken from the tip of wedge catheter should be at least 19 mmHg higher than a sample taken from a systemic artery, and/or oxyhemoglobin saturation should be approximately 20% higher than that recorded from a freely floating catheter in the pulmonary artery. Just as CVP is proportional to the preload of the right heart, PCWP is proportional to the preload of the left side of the heart. In many patients with cardiac disease, CVP may or may not correlate with PCWP.

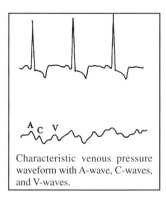

Characteristic venous pressure waveform with A-wave, C-waves, and V-waves.

17. At what point during the cardiac cycle should wedge pressure be determined?
Wedge pressure is often measured to evaluate the preloading conditions of the left ventricle and correlates with left ventricular end-diastolic pressure (LVEDP). Therefore, to make this correlation accurate, the wedge pressure tracing should be analyzed for the point that correlates with the end of the left ventricular diastolic period. This point correlates with the point on the pressure tracing after the A-wave but before the C-wave. The C-wave represents mitral valve closure, which occurs at the beginning of left ventricular systole. A strip chart recorder that simultaneously records the ECG as well as the wedge pressure tracing is useful for determining pulmonary capillary wedge pressure. Wedge pressure measurements also should be taken at the end of exhalation to eliminate any variation caused by the respiratory cycle.

18. What is the importance of a wedge pressure measurement?
Usually it is desirable to optimize the cardiac output of critically ill patients. Increasing left ventricular end-diastolic volume usually results in an increased cardiac output, but only to a certain point. Further increases in left ventricular end-diastolic volume provide too much stretch of myocardial muscle fibers, and left ventricular performance declines. If wedge pressure can be measured at the end of left ventricular diastole, the result is thought to correlate with left ventricular end-diastolic pressure. Because increases in volume should result in an increase in pressure, there should be some correlation between left ventricular end-diastolic pressure and left ventricular end-diastolic volume. In the normal heart, increases in left ventricular end-diastolic volume result in increases in left ventricular end-diastolic pressure. This correlation is not necessarily found in the failing heart. Obviously any factor that decreases left ventricular compliance (e.g., myocardial

ischemia, myocardial contusions, constrictive pericarditis) will result in much larger changes in left ventricular pressures with small changes in left ventricular volumes.

CONTROVERSY

19. Do PA catheters improve outcome in critically ill patients?

This controversy centers on the complications that may occur with catheterization and the ability of clinicians to understand and use the data obtained in a cardiovascular profile. Tuman et al. failed to demonstrate any difference in outcome of patients undergoing coronary artery surgery with or without the use of a PA catheter. Rao et al. showed a decrease in perioperative myocardial infarction in high-risk surgical patients undergoing noncardiac surgery. The investigators used invasive hemodynamic monitoring, including PA catheters in the perioperative period. Shoemaker argues that use of PA catheters to guide therapy that increases cardiac output and oxygen delivery to supranormal values in high-risk surgical patients increases survival rates.

The controversy surrounding the use of PA catheters is likely to continue. Large-scale outcome studies are difficult to control. With appropriate training and vigilance, however, the complication rate associated with PA catheterization is acceptable. Some patients clearly benefit from the data obtained from PA catheters, but only if the clinician interpreting the data has a thorough understanding of the patient's pathophysiology and makes appropriate therapeutic decisions. The following are just three examples of how data from a PA catheter may affect patient care:

Example 1: A 65-year-old man with coronary artery disease undergoing a bowel resection begins to have a progressive decrease in cardiac output, with a concomitant increase in PCWP.

Interpretation. This finding may well represent acute left ventricular dysfunction secondary to myocardial ischemia. If such is the case, the patient probably will benefit from therapy with nitroglycerin.

Example 2: Four hours after surgical repair of fractures of both lower extremities and a ruptured spleen, the urine output of a 35-year-old victim of a motorcycle accident has decreased to 10 ml (over the last hour); cardiac output is low normal, as are CVP and PCWP.

Interpretation. The clinical situation and the data suggest inadequate intravascular volume. Other causes of low urine output (renal dysfunction, urinary obstruction) also should be considered.

Example 3: A 40-year-old woman who underwent laparoscopic cholecystectomy 7 days ago is discovered to be lethargic with low blood pressure at home. She is brought to the hospital and a PA catheter is placed. Blood pressure = 80/40, cardiac index = 6 L/min/m², CVP = 3 mmHg, PCWP = 6 mmHg.

Interpretation. Such data are consistent with septic shock.

BIBLIOGRAPHY

1. Ermakov S, Hoyt JW: Pulmonary artery catheterization. Crit Care Clin 8:773–806, 1992.
2. Fiddian-Green RG, Haglund U, Gutierrez G, Shoemaker WC: Goals for the resuscitation of shock. Crit Care Med 21:S25–S31, 1993.
3. Finegan BA: The pulmonary artery catheter: When and why it should be used. Can J Anaesth 39:R71–R75, 1992.
4. Rao TL, Jacobs KH, El-Etr AA: Reinfarction following anesthesia in patients with myocardial infarction. Anesthesiology 59:499–505, 1983.
5. Shah KB, Rao TLK, Laughlin S, El-Etr AA: A Review of pulmonary artery catheterization in 6,245 patients. Anesthesiology 61:271–275, 1984.
6. Shoemaker WC, Appel PL, Kram HB: Measurement of tissue perfusion by oxygen transport patterns in experimental shock and in high-risk surgical patients. Intens Care Med 16(Suppl 2):S135–S144, 1990.
7. Shoemaker WC: Use and abuse of the balloon tip pulmonary artery (Swan-Ganz) catheter: Are patients getting their money's worth? Crit Care Med 18:1294–1296, 1990.
8. Shoemaker WC, Patil R, Appel PL, Kram HB: Hemodynamic and oxygen transport patterns for outcome prediction, therapeutic goals, and clinical algorithms to improve outcome. Feasibility of artificial intelligence to customize algorithms. Chest 102:617S–625S, 1992.
9. Shoemaker WC, Appel PL, Kram HB: Hemodynamic and oxygen transport responses in survivors and nonsurvivors of high-risk surgery. Crit Care Med 21:977–990, 1993.
10. Spodick DH: Analysis of flow-directed pulmonary artery catheterization. JAMA 261:1946–1947, 1989.

29. ARTERIAL CATHETERIZATION AND PRESSURE MONITORING

Paige Latham, M.D., and Charles W. Whitten, M.D.

1. Why is arterial blood pressure monitored?

Blood pressure monitoring is fundamental in determining the effects of anesthesia on the cardiovascular system. Because decisions about patient care may be based on blood pressure data, it is important to understand how the data are obtained. Arterial pressure is monitored either noninvasively with a blood pressure cuff or invasively with arterial cannulation and pressure transduction.

2. How do noninvasive blood pressure devices work?

Blood pressure is usually measured either manually (ausculatory method) or with an automated device (oscillometric method).

With the **ausculatory method,** a pneumatic cuff is inflated to occlude arterial blood flow. As the cuff is deflated, audible frequencies called Korotkoff sounds are created by turbulent blood flow in the artery. The pressure at which the sounds are first audible is taken as the systolic pressure and the pressure at which the sounds become muffled or disappear is taken as the diastolic pressure. Errors in measurement may be due to (1) long stethoscope tubing, (2) poor hearing in the observer, (3) calibration errors in the sphygmanometer, (4) decreased blood flow in the extremities due to either hypovolemia or to the use of vasopressors, (5) severe atherosclerosis that prevents occlusion of the artery at suprasystolic pressures, (6) inappropriate cuff size, or (7) too rapid of a deflation rate.

With the **oscillometric method,** a pneumatic cuff is also inflated to occlude the arterial blood flow. As the cuff is deflated, the arterial pulsations cause pressure changes in the cuff that are analyzed by a computer. The systolic pressure is taken as the point of rapidly increasing oscillations, the mean arterial pressure as the point of maximal oscillation, and the diastolic pressure as the point of rapidly decreasing oscillations. Errors in measurement may occur from inappropriate cuff size or factors that prevent detection of cuff pressure variations, such as patient shivering. Prolonged use of the stat mode, in which the cuff reinflates immediately after each measurement is obtained, may lead to complications such as ulnar nerve paresthesia, thrombophlebitis, and/or compartment syndrome.

3. What are the indications for intraarterial blood pressure monitoring?

Intraarterial blood pressure monitoring is indicated when (1) blood pressure changes may be rapid, (2) moderate blood pressure changes may cause end-organ damage, (3) frequent arterial blood gases may be needed, or (4) noninvasive blood pressure monitoring is inaccurate. Clinical examples include anticipated cardiovascular instability (e.g., massive fluid shifts, intracranial surgery, significant cardiovascular disease, valvular heart disease, diabetes), direct manipulation of the cardiovascular system (cardiac surgery, major vascular surgery, deliberate hypotension), frequent sampling of blood gases for pulmonary disease or single lung ventilation, or morbid obesity, which prevents accurate noninvasive measurements.

4. What are the complications of invasive arterial monitoring?

Complications include distal ischemia, arterial thrombosis, hematoma formation, catheter site infection, systemic infection, necrosis of the overlying skin, and potential blood loss due to disconnection. The incidence of infection increases with duration of catheterization. The incidence of arterial thrombosis increases with (1) duration of catheterization, (2) increased catheter size, (3) catheter type (Teflon catheters cause more thrombosis than catheters made of polypropylene), (4) proximal emboli, (5) prolonged shock, and (6) preexisting peripheral vascular disease.

5. How is radial artery catheterization performed?

The wrist is dorsiflexed and immobilized, the skin is cleaned with an antiseptic solution, the course of the radial artery is determined by palpation, and local anesthetic is infiltrated into the skin overlying the artery. A 20-gauge over-the-needle catheter apparatus is inserted at a 30–45° angle to the skin along the course of the radial artery. After arterial blood return, the angle is decreased, and the catheter is advanced slightly to ensure that both the catheter tip and the needle have advanced into the arterial lumen. The catheter is then threaded into the artery. Alternatively, the radial artery may be transfixed. After arterial blood return, the apparatus is advanced until both the catheter and the needle pass completely through the front and back walls of the artery. The needle is withdrawn into the catheter, and the catheter is pulled back slowly. When pulsatile blood flow is seen in the catheter, the catheter is advanced into the lumen. If the catheter will not advance into the arterial lumen and blood return is good, a sterile guidewire may be placed into the lumen through the catheter and the catheter advanced over the wire. After the catheter is fully advanced into the lumen, low-compliance pressure tubing is fastened to the catheter, a sterile dressing is applied, and the catheter is securely fastened in place. Care must be taken to ensure that the pressure tubing is free from bubbles before connection.

6. Describe Allen's test. Explain its purpose.

Allen's test is performed before radial artery cannulation to determine whether ulnar collateral circulation to the hand is adequate in case of radial artery thrombosis. The hand is exsanguinated by having the patient make a tight fist. The radial and ulnar arteries are occluded by manual compression, the patient relaxes the hand, and the pressure over the ulnar artery is released. Collateral flow is assessed by measuring the time required for return of normal coloration. Return of color in less than 5 seconds indicates adequate collateral flow; whereas 5–10 seconds suggests an equivocal test and more than 10 seconds indicates inadequate collateral circulation.

7. Is Allen's test an adequate predictor of ischemic sequelae?

Although some clinicians advocate use of Allen's test, others have demonstrated that Allen's tests of radial artery patency have no relationship to distal blood flow as assessed by fluoroscein dye injection. There are many reports of ischemic sequelae in patients with normal Allen's tests; conversely patients with abnormal Allen's tests may have no ischemic sequelae. Apparently Allen's test alone does not reliably predict adverse outcome.

8. What alternative cannulation sites are available?

When the radial arteries are unavailable for cannulation, the ulnar, brachial, axillary, femoral, dorsalis pedis, and posterior tibial arteries have been cannulated for arterial pressure monitoring. The ulnar artery is a good choice, especially when collateral flow via the radial artery is adequate. The brachial artery does not have the benefit of collateral circulation, but many studies have demonstrated the relative safety of this technique. Complications with cannulation of the axillary artery are infrequent; however, the left side is preferred because of a lower incidence of carotid artery obstruction and embolization. Vertebral artery impingement may occur with equal frequency on either side. Cannulation of the femoral artery is thought to be as safe as it is for other sites, but it may be associated with a slightly higher incidence of infection. The small size of the dorsalis pedis and posterior tibial arteries may make cannulation difficult. Because of the increased risk for ischemic sequelae, cannulation of the dorsalis pedis and posterior tibial arteries is relatively contraindicated in patients with peripheral vascular disease or diabetes mellitus.

9. How does a central waveform differ from a peripheral waveform?

As the arterial pressure is transmitted from the central aorta to the peripheral arteries, the waveform is distorted. Transmission is delayed, high frequency components such as the dicrotic notch are lost, the systolic peak increases, and the diastolic trough is decreased. The changes in systolic and diastolic pressures result from a decrease in the arterial wall compliance and from resonance (the addition of reflected waves to the arterial waveform as it travels distally in the arterial tree).

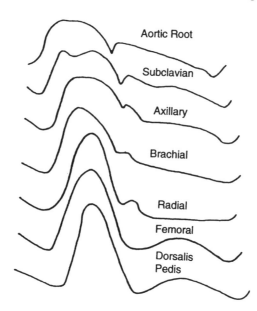

Configuration of the arterial waveform at various sites in the arterial tree. (From Blitt CD, Hines RL: Monitoring in Anesthesia and Critical Care Medicine, 3rd ed. Churchill Livingstone, 1995, with permission).

10. What information can be obtained from an arterial waveform?

The arterial waveform provides valuable information about the patient's hemodynamic status: (1) the waveform determines the heart rate during ECG electrocautery interference and whether the electrical spikes from a pacemaker result in ventricular contractions; (2) the slope of the upstroke may be used to evaluate myocardial contractility; (3) large respiratory variations suggest hypovolemia; and (4) the waveform provides a visual estimate of the hemodynamic consequences of various arrhythmias.

11. How is the arterial waveform reproduced?

Reproduction of the arterial waveform requires the following equipment: (1) an intravascular catheter, (2) fluid-filled pressure tubing and a stopcock, (3) electromechanical transducer, and (4) electronic analyzer and display system. The mechanical energy at the catheter tip is transmitted to the transducer by the fluid-filled tubing and then converted to an electrical signal. The electrical signal is then converted to a waveform by the analyzer and displayed.

12. Describe the conversion of the mechanical energy of a pressure wave to an electrical signal.

Transducers convert the mechanical energy of a pressure wave into electrical current or voltage. The design of most transducers is based on the strain-gauge principle, which states that stretching a wire or silicone crystal changes its electrical resistance. Consequently, distortion in the shape of the diaphragm in the transducer (due to changes in mechanical pressure) results in a small electrical current. The sensing elements are arranged as a Wheatstone-Bridge circuit so that the voltage output is proportionate to the mechanical pressure applied to the diaphragm.

13. How is the waveform reproduced from an electrical signal?

The waveform is reproduced by the summation of a series of sinusoidal waves. Waveforms consist of the fundamental waveform and ten harmonics. The frequency of the fundamental waveform depends on the patient's heart rate. If the heart rate is 60 bpm, the fundamental frequency is 1 Hz (cycles/second), and frequencies up to 10 Hz contribute to the waveform.

14. Define damping coefficient and natural frequency.

Natural frequency, a property of the catheter-stopcock-transducer apparatus, is the frequency at which the monitoring system resonates and amplifies the signals it receives. The natural frequency is directly proportional to the diameter of the catheter lumen and inversely proportional to (1) the square root of the length of the tubing connection, (2) the square root of the system compliance, and (3) the density of the fluid contained in the system. Because the natural frequency of most monitoring systems is in the same range as the frequencies used to recreate the arterial waveform, significant amplification and distortion of the waveform may occur.

The **damping coefficient** reflects the rate of dissipation of the energy of a pressure wave. This property may be adjusted to counterbalance the erroneous amplification that results when the natural frequency of the monitoring system overlaps with the frequencies used to recreate the waveform.

15. What are the characteristics of overdamped and underdamped monitoring systems?

The damping coefficient is estimated by evaluating the time for the system to settle to zero after a high-pressure flush. An underdamped system continues to oscillate for 3–4 cycles; it overestimates the systolic and underestimates the diastolic blood pressure. An overdamped system settles to baseline slowly without oscillating; it underestimates the systolic and overestimates the diastolic blood blood pressure. In both cases, however, the mean blood pressure is relatively accurate.

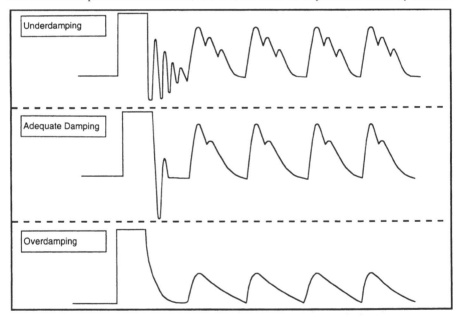

Underdamped, adequately damped, and overdamped arterial pressure tracings after a high pressured flush.

16. How can the incidence of artifacts in arterial monitoring systems by reduced?

The incidence of artifacts can be reduced by meticulous care of the monitoring system:

1. The connecting tubing should be rigid with an internal diameter of 1.5–3 mm and a maximal length of 120 cm.

2. The lines should be kept free of kinks, clots, and bubbles, which cause overdamping of the system.

3. Only one stopcock per line should be used to minimize possible air introduction.

4. The mechanical coupling system should be flushed with heparinized saline to maintain patency of the arterial line and to minimize the risk of distal embolization and nosocomial infection.

5. The transducer should be placed at the level of the right atrium, the midaxillary line in the supine position.

6. The transducer should be electrically balanced or rezeroed periodically because the zero point may drift if the room temperature changes.

BIBLIOGRAPHY

1. Bedford RF, Shah NK: Blood pressure monitoring: Invasive and non-invasive. In Blitt CD, Hines RL (eds): Monitoring in Anesthesia and Critical Medicine. New York, Churchill Livingstone, 1995, p 100.
2. Gilbert HC, Vender JS: Monitoring the anesthetized patient. In Barash PG, Cullen BF, Stoelting RK (eds): Clinical Anesthesia. Philadelphia, J.B. Lippincott, 1992, pp 747–749.
3. McGregor AD: The Allen test—An investigation of its accuracy by fluorescein angiography. J Hand Surg 12:82–85, 1987.
4. Meyer RM, Katele GV: The case for a complete Allen's test. Anesth Analg 62:947, 1983.
5. Reich DL, Kaplan JA: Hemodynamic monitoring. In Kaplan JA (ed): Cardiac Anesthesia. Philadelphia, W.B. Saunders, 1993, pp 263–266.
6. Skeehan TM, Thys DM: Monitoring the cardiac surgical patient. In Hensley FA, Martin DE (eds): The Practice of Cardiac Anesthesia. Boston, Little, Brown, 1990, pp 131–144.
7. Slogoff S, Keats AS, Arlund C: On the safety of radial artery cannulation. Anesthesiology 59:42, 1983.
8. Stanley TE, Reves JG: Cardiovascular monitoring. In Miller RD (ed): Anesthesia. New York, Churchill Livingstone, 1990, pp 1034–1043.

30. INTRAOPERATIVE TRANSESOPHAGEAL ECHOCARDIOGRAPHY

Olivia V. Adair, M.D., and Douglas Paul Voorhees, R.R.T.

1. In what situations has transesophageal echocardiography (TEE) become a valuable tool in the intraoperative evaluation of surgical patients?

Over the past decade TEE has expanded to include multiple intraoperative uses. The most notable use has been in cardiac surgical procedures, including primary and prosthetic valvular disease, congenital heart disease, thoracic aorta disease, hypertrophic obstructive cardiomyopathy, sequelae of myocardial infarction (e.g., aneurysm, ventricular septal rupture, papillary muscle rupture), and neoplastic and traumatic cardiac disease. In addition, TEE has become more common in noncardiac operations, especially in peripheral vascular, orthopedic, and neurologic procedures, and is expected to continue to be used in high-risk patients for detecting cardiac ischemia. This use would be especially important, for example, in diabetic patients who have a history of coronary artery disease and must undergo a procedure characterized by significant fluid shifts or hemodynamic fluctuations.

2. How is TEE performed in the operating room without interfering with access to the patient?

The TEE probe is usually introduced after induction of general anesthesia and endotracheal intubation but before sterile draping. After placement of the TEE probe, continuous monitoring is possible without interfering with the sterile field or surgical personnel. The TEE system is placed to one side of the anesthesia screen, and the operator stands about 60 cm from the patient's head, with controls located on the distal end of the probe. This positioning does not impede the anesthesiologist's access to the patient or monitors.

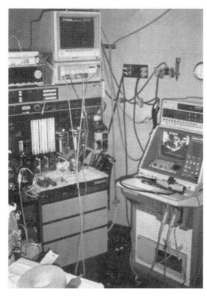

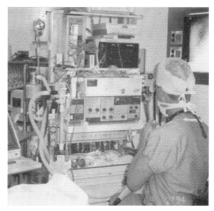

Equipment is easily placed in OR without interference with sterile field.

Personnel can operate the probe and monitor the images about 60 cm from the patient

3. How should echocardiography be included in the planning and management of the surgical patient?

TEE should be considered at three specific stages during surgical management: baseline, intraoperative, and postoperative. The initial examination should include a transthoracic echocardiogram to evaluate chambers, valves, cardiac function, and pericardium, with color Doppler evaluation of flow characteristics. If further evaluation or clarification of images is needed, a TEE should be performed. Possible findings include thrombus (alerting the surgeon to a possible embolic source), aortic disease (e.g., plaque or thrombus, which, if identified, would be instructive for choice of site for aortic cross-clamping or anastomosis of coronary bypass grafting), or even unsuspected left ventricular dysfunction. Specific intraoperative objectives should be discussed with input from surgeons, anesthesiologist, and echocardiologist. In patients with valvular disease it is essential to evaluate all valves and their function before repair or prosthetic placement is undertaken as well as after the procedure. The effect of the procedure on other valvular function can be evaluated intraoperatively; for example, after aortic valve replacement tricuspid or mitral valves can be evaluated for either severe stenosis or regurgitation. In addition, before closure a complete evaluation of the repair should be included.

Postoperatively, all patients with valve repair and valve replacement should have a TEE with color flow Doppler before discharge or shortly thereafter to evaluate baseline gradients, flow patterns, and valve images. Thus follow-up evaluations can be done when clinically indicated, with patients acting as their own control. In addition, if a patient does not improve or fares poorly postoperatively, TEE should be used to evaluate chamber functions, complications (e.g., ischemia, shunts, perivascular leaks, or endocarditis), and valve repair.

4. What are the indications for intraoperative TEE?

When intraoperative echocardiography is needed, TEE is almost exclusively the technique of choice because of (1) ease of use in the operating room, (2) lack of interference with staff or sterile field, and (3) clarity of images. Although TEE was used initially in mitral and prosthetic valve surgery, the scope of its use has markedly increased with the prevalence of congenital heart disease in adults as well as the development of smaller probes for adolescents and children. Other uses include the identification of intracardiac shunts in valvular procedures or septal defect repair, hypertrophic obstructive cardiomyopathy, intracardiac masses, and thoracic aortic disease. In noncardiac surgery intraoperative TEE is often used in selected patients undergoing vascular or orthopedic surgery; it also is used in surgery on patients at high risk for cardiac complications to evaluate left ventricular segmental function. During neurosurgery, intraoperative TEE is often used to monitor potential for air embolism.

5. What are the contraindications for intraoperative TEE?

The contraindications for intraoperative TEE are the same as for nonoperative patients. Absolute contraindications include (1) esophageal disease (strictures, fistula, laceration, perforation, diverticula, or carcinoma); (2) active upper gastrointestinal bleeding; and (3) severe cervical spine instability. Relative contraindications requiring special consideration include (1) recent gastroesophageal operation; (2) esophageal varices; (3) severe cervical arthritis; and (4) unexplained symptoms of dysphagia or odynophagia. In addition, patients with a history of extensive mediastinal radiation have increased risk of abnormal esophageal anatomy, which may cause problems with introduction and manipulation.

6. What are the complications and risks of intraoperative TEE?

TEE can be performed intraoperatively with the same minimal risk of complications as in the nonoperative patient. TEE is considered semiinvasive but is generally quite safe. Two large studies showed major complications were unusual (0.18%–0.5%). Complications should be considered as related to three aspects of the procedure: (1) probe introduction, (2) procedure, and (3) medications.

Probe injuries are rarely related to pressure contact; however, in prolonged procedures in patients who have gastroesophagitis or are fully anticoagulated (e.g. cardiopulmonary bypass), there are rare case reports of hemorrhage or Mallory-Weiss tears. Of note are the few reported cases of buckling of the tip of the probe in the esophagus, making it difficult to advance and unfold the tip into the stomach. This complication may be associated with flaccidity of the probe tip due to loose rotary controls. It is best to check rotary controls and the tip of the probe after each procedure and to submit for repair if flaccid or loose. Transient vocal cord paralysis also has been reported, especially with large probes and lengthy monitoring (e.g., neurosurgical procedures with patients in an upright position); sore throat with pharyngeal irritation has also been described. Of note, the administration of drying agents may increase the irritating effect of the probe. Procedure-related complications include development of occasional benign, self limiting ventricular and supraventricular arrhythmias. There are rare reports of hemodynamically significant arrhythmias, which usually are terminated by repositioning or removing the probe. There are reports of significant bradyarrhythmias, with one death due to bradycardia secondary to vagal stimulation. Atropine should be available on the procedure table; although rarely needed, it quickly reverses bradycardia.

Transient episodes of hypotension or hypertension and hypoxia have occurred in less than 1% of patients, but in most intubated patients one needs only to adjust oxygen flow. In a large European study of 10,419 patients, the incidence of unsuccessful TEE probe induction was 1.9%. Only 0.88% of the procedures were interrupted before completion; causes included patient intolerance (72%), significant arrhythmias (0.07%), and respiratory compromise (0.07%).

7. Does prolonged TEE intubation for a surgical procedure provide additional risk?

A double-blind study of 48 patients undergoing cardiac surgery evaluated postoperative side effects of intraoperative TEE. The mean duration of intraoperative TEE was 5.4 ± 2.3 hours. On the second postoperative day, there were no significant differences in local discomfort, swallowing, nausea, minor oropharyngeal trauma, or time to first oral intake.

8. Is there ever a problem with TEE probe introduction?

The TEE probe is usually introduced after the patient has undergone endotracheal intubation and is therefore already under general anesthesia in a supine position. Usually the index finger can be used successfully to guide the probe around the endotracheal tube. At our institute we have rarely needed to use a laryngoscope to aid in introduction of the TEE probe.

9. Of what value is left ventricular function and wall motion intraoperatively?

Left ventricular (LV) function can be assessed continuously with the transgastric short-axis view of the LV at the midcavity (papillary muscle). The use of omniplane also provides an additional long-axis (parasternal view) and a deep gastric 5-chamber view for wall motion evaluation. This technique enables evaluation of LV function with assessment of LV wall thickness, endocardium contraction, and relaxation, and LV chamber changes. The left ventricular function is calculated by the change in chamber size or volume from diastole to systole. Clinical signs such as tachycardias can be evaluated; for example, a small and hyperdynamic LV chamber suggests hypovolemia and the need for volume resuscitation. Likewise, an enlarged LV chamber with diminished function indicates depressed LV function and the need for an inotropic agent.

10. How sensitive is TEE in detecting myocardial ischemia during a surgical procedure?

A new regional wall motion abnormality (RWMA) is probably the most sensitive indicator of ischemia and predicts an increased risk of adverse outcome. RWMA occurs early, preceding ECG evidence of ischemia, and is 4 times more sensitive than ECG. However, TEE may be oversensitive and therefore less specific. A transient new RWMA is consistent with myocardial ischemia, whereas a persistent change is consistent with acute infarction. The echocardiologist must consider three potential situations of decreased specificity: (1) large changes in LV loading conditions may alter LV systolic function without indicating ischemia; (2) the area of dysfunction is larger than the ischemic area; and (3) areas of stunned or hibernating myocardium may represent diminished perfusion or persistent RWMA after relief of ischemia without loss of myocardial viability.

11. For what specific patients or specific procedures is intraoperative TEE considered especially appropriate?

High-risk patients are most likely to benefit from intraoperative TEE, including elderly patients, diabetics, patients with known coronary artery disease or a history of congestive heart failure, and all emergency or trauma cases. Specific procedures in which TEE may improve outcome include orthopedic surgery, especially long-bone and hip replacement with cement; major vascular surgery, including abdomen and thoracic aorta; valve repair and replacement; congenital heart surgery; and surgery for intracardiac masses.

12. How has TEE affected operative outcome?

Clinical observations suggest that intraoperative TEE is a good predictor of ischemic events and adverse outcome in coronary bypass surgery, but TEE is less predictive of ischemic events in noncardiac procedures. Smith et al. observed that in patients undergoing coronary artery bypass surgery or vascular surgery a new RWMA correlated strongly with perioperative myocardial infarction. In another study London et al. observed 156 high-risk patients undergoing noncardiac surgery and demonstrated poor correlation between intraoperative RWMA and postoperative cardiac complications.

13. How is intraoperative TEE used in assessment of mitral valve repair?

Mitral valve repair has become the procedure of choice for mitral regurgitation (MR). Initially, intraoperative TEE with color-flow Doppler helps to establish the primary mechanism of MR to aid in decisions for repair. For example, in posterior leaflet prolapse or failed leaflet an eccentric regurgitant jet is directed anteromedially. A central jet is seen with annular dilatation or rheumatic disease that causes restriction of leaflets; alternatively, an asymmetric central jet with unequal restriction may be observed. In addition, mitral leaflet perforation can be localized.

Of the utmost importance is intraoperative evaluation to assess mitral competence after repair, which may include contrast as well as Doppler color-flow echocardiography. The leaflets, annulus, and whole support apparatus are well visualized with real-time high resolution. In addition, the LV can be evaluated for the effect of the repair on function and coronary perfusion. Residual mitral regurgitation is evaluated before closure in multiple planes and views with color-flow Doppler mapping.

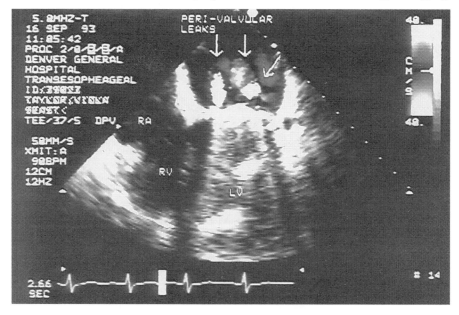

Intraoperative TEE detects significant mitral regurgitation of the prostatic valve that requires correction before chest wall closure. Without correction, mortality is markedly increased.

14. What is the impact on outcome of TEE for mitral valve repair?

Studies have shown that intraoperative TEE identifies significant residual MR (grade ≥ III/IV) in about 8% of cases, especially those involving anterior leaflet or bilateral disease, and thus leads to successful revision. In patients undergoing coronary artery bypass surgery (CABG) TEE aided in decisions to include a mitral valve repair during the procedure. Survival after CABG is 50% lower in patients with grade II–III MR without an MV procedure vs. patients with grade I or less MR (45% vs. 90% at 1 year). This difference emphasizes the importance of intraoperative diagnosis and treatment of MR. Another study showed that in 17% of patients undergoing MV repair, TEE identified significant MR, allowing immediate revision or replacement before closure. Intraoperative TEE for MV repair has also been shown to identify unsuspected findings that influence the surgical plan in 3–8% of patients. Such findings include previously unknown intracardiac shunts, other valve disease, and intracardiac masses.

15. How can intraoperative TEE be an aid during repair of congenital heart defects?

Several studies have shown that intraoperative TEE has a significant positive influence on the management of congenital heart disease. The focus is on both accurate diagnoses (with sensitivity in detecting residual lesions) and postoperative management. The results of TEE have altered preoperative diagnosis in 9–31% of cases, and operation in 4–13%; postoperative TEE also has helped in medical management of 6–10% of reported cases. Furthermore, clear evidence indicates that intraoperative TEE becomes increasingly valuable with more complex cases. In one study of 42 adults undergoing operations for congenital heart disease, TEE clarified or detected unsuspected lesions in 36% of those studied and altered the planned surgical procedure in 12%. One limitation of TEE is failure to detect clinically insignificant residual ventricular septal defects < 3 mm in diameter.

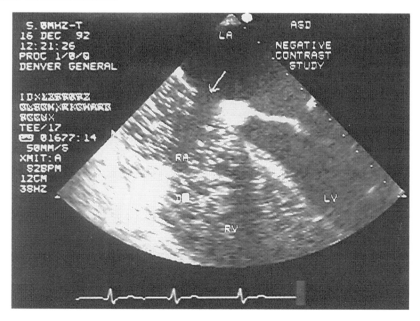

Positive contrast study for atrial septal defect (RA = right atrium, RV = right ventricle, LV = left ventricle).

16. Does intraoperative TEE have a role in aortic valve (AV) surgery?

Intraoperative TEE used for sizing of AV allografts correlates well with direct surgeon measurement of the AV annulus and thus helps to minimize the delay between thawing and implantation. In addition, evaluation of the calcific extension into the annulus is important. An additional measurement after debridement is recommended, because enlargement of the annulus may be significant. Intraoperative TEE for evaluating the cause of aortic regurgitation and color-flow Doppler mapping of the regurgitant jet in a short-axis view also help to guide the repair. One study emphasized the importance of postprocedure evaluation before closure; 7% of cases required successful revision of the repair secondary to significant residual aortic regurgitant flow.

17. Does preoperative TEE have a role in aortic dissection repair?
Yes. TEE can characterize the extent of the intimal flap, the location of intimal tears, and involvement of the aortic root and valve as well as provide important information about potential complications, such as aortic rupture, cardiac tamponade, and saccular aneurysm formation.

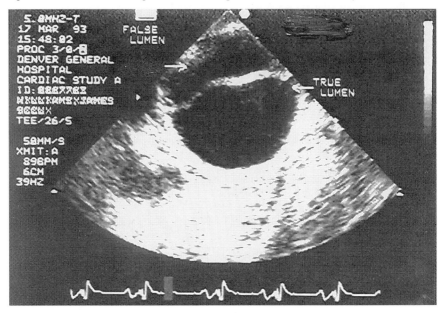

Aortic dissection showing false and true lumen.

18. For what other thoracic aortic diseases is TEE useful in making technical surgical decisions?
During repair of coarctation TEE may identify an intraluminal thoracic aortic thrombus that requires surgical removal. In addition, patients undergoing coronary bypass surgery may have extensive as well as mobile atheromatous disease of the thoracic aortic arch, which presents a significant risk factor for perioperative cerebrovascular accidents. Thoracic arch atheromatous disease has been observed in about 20% of patients undergoing coronary bypass surgery or vascular surgery: TEE evaluation may be useful in diagnosis and management.

19. What are the limitations of intraoperative TEE?
TEE images are sometimes limited by electrocautery artifacts, but this problem is easily avoided by currently available systems that shield the emission. In addition, after the patient is removed from cardiopulmonary bypass, the imaging system may turn off and interrupt TEE images because of intravascular rewarming to 39° C. This may activate the automatic cooling circuit of the probe. Although some systems allow override of the automatic cooling function or reprogramming of the temperature, most systems require cooling before imaging can resume.

20. What are potential pitfalls of intraoperative TEE?

Potential pitfalls include hemodynamic changes, especially when procedures involve cardiopulmonary bypass. General anesthesia has many effects on peripheral vascular tone, especially development of vasodilation and, in many patients, myocardial depression. Global and segmental evaluation of myocardial function also may be influenced by the recovery of myocardial function, hypothermia, cardioplegia, coronary artery bypass, and arrhythmias. Paced rhythms may mimic myocardial dysfunction, as does dyssynergy between valve closure and myocardial contraction. Both markedly increase the degree of regurgitant flow on color flow Doppler. Reduction in afterload also significantly underestimates valvular regurgitant flow as well as the significance of intracardiac shunts.

21. A 36-year-old woman presented with marked shortness of breath and exercise intolerance. She had progressed in approximately 2 months to the point of not being able to lie flat. The chest radiograph revealed a large mass in close proximity to or involving the heart. CT was inconclusive for cardiac involvement. The surgical plan was to perform a transbronchial biopsy under general anesthesia. Does intraoperative TEE have a role in this setting?

Biopsy of a mass that may involve the pericardium or even erode into the myocardium may lead to tamponade or death. Therefore, if there is any question whether a lung mass involves the heart, transthoracic echocardiography (TTE) and, most likely, TEE, which is more sensitive, should be performed. Because of marked respiratory problems, it was decided that the patient would undergo bronchoscopy with nasal intubation and general anesthesia. Because the exact border of the mass could not be ascertained from TTE or CT, TEE was done intraoperatively before bronchoscopy. On TEE examination the mass was identified as impinging on but not involving the pericardium. The mass appeared by TEE to have a consistency consistent with a bronchogenic cyst rather than a solid tumor. This finding changed the surgical plan from biopsy to excision, which proved to be wise. The tumor lifted out nicely and was indeed a bronchogenic cyst filled with thick mucus material, not amendable to biopsy. This case illustrates the importance of TEE and of using all available information to help in planning management strategies.

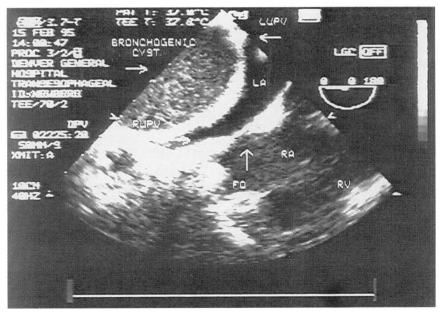

Bronchogenic cyst collapsing the right and left upper pulmonary vein (RUPV, LUPV) and the left atrium (LA). (RA = right atrium, FP = foramen ovale, RV = right ventricle).

22. What other intraoperative uses of TEE have been found to improve patient outcome?
Liver transplant surgery
   To evaluate myocardial dysfunction
   To evaluate right ventricular failure
   To recognize air embolism
Neurosurgery
   To monitor for air embolism
   To aid in verification of correct placement of ventriculoatrial shunts
   To identify a patent foramen ovale
Orthopedic surgery
   To detect causes of hypotension, hemodynamic deterioration, and embolization of air, fat,
   or cement.

BIBLIOGRAPHY

1. Daniel WG, Erbel R, Kasper W, et al: Safety of transesophageal echocardiography: A multicenter survey of 10,419 examinations. Circulation 83:817–821, 1991.
2. Eisenberg MJ, London MJ, Leung JM, et al: Monitoring for myocardial ischemia during non-cardiac surgery. A technology assessment of transesophageal echocardiography and 12-lead electrocardiography. The Study of Peri-operative Ischemia Research Group. JAMA 268:210–216, 1992.
3. Grigg LE, Wigle ED, Williams WG, et al: Transesophageal Doppler echocardiography in obstructive hypertrophic cardiomyopathy: Clarification of pathophysiology and importance in intraoperative decision making. J Am Coll Cardiol 20:42–52, 1992.
4. Johnston SR, Freeman WK, Schaff HV, Tajik AJ: Severe tricuspid regurgitation after mitral valve repair: Diagnosis by intraoperative transesophageal echocardiography. J Am Soc Echocardiogr 72:1083–1085, 1990.
5. Klein AL, Stewart WJ, Salcedo EE, et al: The role of intraoperative echocardiography in tricuspid valve repair [abstract]. J Am Coll Cardiol 15:61A, 1990.
6. London MJ, Tubau JF, Wong MG, et al: The "natural history" of segmental wall motion abnormalities in patients undergoing noncardiac surgery. Anesthesiology 73:644–655, 1990.
7. O'Kelly BF, Tubau JF, Knitht AA, et al: Measurement of left ventricular contractility using transesophageal echocardiography in patients undergoing coronary artery bypass grafting. Am Heart J 122: 1041–1049, 1991.
8. Pell ACH, Keating JF, Christie J, Sutherland GR. Use of transesophageal echocardiography to predict patients at risk of the fat embolism syndrome following traumatic injuries [abstract]. J Am Coll Cardiol 21:264A, 1993.
9. Rafferty T, Durkin MA, Sittig D, et al: Transesophageal color flow Doppler imaging for aortic insufficiency in patients having cardiac operations. J Thorac Cardiovasc Surg 104:521–525, 1992.
10. Ribakove GH, Katz ES, Galloway AC, et al: Surgical implications of transesophageal echocardiography to grade the atheromatous aortic arch. Ann Thorac Surg 53:758–761, 1992.
11. Savage RM, Duffy CI, Thomas JD, et al: Transesophageal echocardiography (TEE) is indicated in the placement of the implantable left ventricular assist device [abstract]. J Am Coll Cardiol 21:321A, 1993.
12. Shintani H, Nakano S, Matsuda H, et al: Efficacy of transesophageal echocardiography as a peri-operative monitor in patients undergoing cardiovascular surgery: Analysis of 149 consecutive studies. J Cardiovasc Surg 31: 564–570, 1990.
13. Smith JS, Cahalan MK, Benefiel DJ, et al: Intraoperative detection of myocardial ischemia in high-risk patients: Electrocardiography versus two-dimensional transesophageal echocardiography. Circulation 72:1015–1021, 1985.
14. Thwaites BK, Stamatos JM, Crowl FD, et al: Transesophageal echocardiographic diagnosis of intra-aortic thrombus during coarctation repair. Anesthesiology 76:638–639, 1992.

V. Perioperative Problems

31. HYPOXEMIA AND PULMONARY PHYSIOLOGY

Jeff Nabonsal, M.D., and Michael Owens, R.R.T.

1. In the operating room the patient's oxygen saturation begins to decrease. What is the appropriate response?

When a true hypoxic event is identified, apply 100% oxygen immediately; then adequacy of ventilation must be assessed by whatever means is available. The problem usually represents an intrapulmonary process, but one must rule out mechanical causes first. If the patient is not intubated, attempt mask ventilation; if the patient is intubated, hand ventilation by bag is appropriate. At this point check the inspired oxygen concentration, capnograph, and peak pressures required to move the chest. Oxygen concentration should be increased to 100%. A calibrated oxygen analyzer is the only way to ensure that a hypoxic mixture is not delivered to the patient. In the intubated patient a ruptured endotracheal tube cuff is recognized by an audible leak with bagging, whereas poor compliance should make one consider obstruction, bronchospasm, or tension pneumothorax. Listen to the chest for bilateral breath sounds, decreased breath sounds, wheezing, or rales. Inspect the endotracheal tube for kinks, plugging (if one can pass a suction catheter, the tube is most likely patent), and position. If necessary, perform laryngoscopy to check for endotracheal tube placement. Check the circuit for mechanical problems and for possible failure of the oxygen supply. If there is any question about the machine, do not hesitate to switch to an Ambu bag and an alternate oxygen tank. As a last resort, reintubate; do not allow the patient to deteriorate before intervening. If pneumothorax is high on the differential diagnosis, consider decompressing the chest, first with a needle, then with a chest tube if appropriate. Obtain arterial blood gases, chest radiograph, and ECG and review recent events.

Other causes to consider after ruling out mechanical problems and endotracheal tube problems include surgical causes (anemia, hypotension, compression of vital structures) and other patient-related causes (ventilation/perfusion mismatch, pulmonary embolism, pulmonary edema, fat embolism, anemia, decreased cardiac output). Lastly, consider positive end-expiratory pressure (PEEP) and a pulmonary artery catheter to aid in diagnosing and treating a hypoxic event.

2. Discuss the determinants of pulmonary blood flow and include the effects of hypotension and PEEP.

The major determinants of pulmonary blood flow are gravity and hypoxic pulmonary vasoconstriction (HPV). The actual perfusion to an alveolus depends on multiple factors. West describes four zones of perfusion in an upright lung, starting at the apices and moving downward to the bases:

In **zone 1** alveolar pressure (P_{Alv}) exceeds pulmonary artery pressure (P_{pa}), leading to ventilation without perfusion (alveolar deadspace). Zone 1 is essentially nonexistent in healthy patients.

In **zone 2** arterial pressure exceeds alveolar pressure, but alveolar pressure still exceeds venous pressure (P_{pv}). Blood flow in zone 2 is determined by arterial-alveolar pressure differences, which steadily increase down the zone.

In **zone 3** pulmonary venous pressure now exceeds alveolar pressure, and flow is determined by the arterial-venous pressure difference.

In **zone 4** interstitial pressure ($P_{interstitium}$) is greater than venous and alveolar pressures; thus flow is determined by the arterial-interstitial pressure difference.

To simplify: Zone 1 $P_{Alv} > P_{pa} > P_{pv}$
                     Zone 2 $P_{pa} > P_{Alv} > P_{pv}$
                     Zone 3 $P_{pa} > P_{pv} > P_{Alv}$
                     Zone 4 $P_{pa} > P_{interstitium} > P_{pv} > P_{Alv}$

Decreased pulmonary artery pressure increases the size of zones 1 and 2 at the expense of zones 2 and 3; this may occur with hypotension or extreme blood loss. Increased pulmonary artery pressure has the opposite effect. PEEP increases P_{Alv} and the size of zones 1 and 2 at the expense of zones 2 and 3.

3. What is meant by the term ventilation/perfusion (V/Q) mismatch? Describe how HPV aids in avoiding this problem.

Both ventilation and perfusion increase toward the gravity-dependent portion of the lungs but at different rates. Thus, V/Q is >1 at the top of the lungs, 1 at the third rib in the upright lung, and <1 below the third rib. HPV is a local response of pulmonary artery smooth muscle that decreases blood flow when a low alveolar oxygen pressure is sensed. This response aids in keeping normal V/Q relationships by diversion of blood from underventilated areas but is effective only when normoxic areas of the lungs are available to receive the diverted blood flow. HPV is inhibited to a degree by the volatile anesthetics and some vasodialators but is not affected by intravenous anesthesia.

V/Q = infinity = deadspace
V/Q = 0 = absolute shunt
V/Q inequalities or mismatch implies relative shunt, which is amenable to oxygen therapy.

4. Why does general anesthesia worsen V/Q mismatch?

Under general anesthesia functional residual capacity (FRC) is reduced by approximately 400 ml in an adult. The supine position decreases FRC another 800 ml. Obesity, pregnancy, ascites, abdominal surgery, and multiple other causes may further decrease FRC. A large enough decrease in FRC may bring end-expiratory volumes or even the entire tidal volume to levels below the closing volumes. Closing volumes are the volumes at which small airways begin to close. When small airways begin to close, low V/Q areas develop. Closing capacity is equal to the sum of the closing volume and the residual volume. Surgical compression or clamping of the pulmonary vasculature creates high V/Q areas or increased pulmonary deadspace, which is also a source of V/Q mismatch.

5. Define the terms anatomic, alveolar, and physiologic deadspace.

Deadspace (V_D) is the portion of the tidal volume that does not participate in gas exchange. **Anatomic deadspace** is the volume of gas that ventilates the conducting airways. **Alveolar deadspace** is the volume of gas that reaches the alveoli but does not take part in gas exchange because the alveoli are not perfused (West zone 1). In awake, healthy, supine patients alveolar deadspace is negligible. **Physiologic deadspace is the sum of anatomic and alveolar deadspace.**

V_D/V_T is the ratio of the physiologic deadspace to the tidal volume and is usually approximately 33%.

Clinically, V_D/V_T is determined by the Bohr method, which assumes that all expired CO_2 comes from perfused alveoli and not deadspace.

$$V_D/V_T = \frac{(\text{alveolar } P_{CO_2} - \text{expired } P_{CO_2})}{\text{alveolar } P_{CO_2}}$$

where we assume alveolar P_{CO_2} = arterial P_{CO_2}, and expired P_{CO_2} = the average P_{CO_2} in an expired gas sample (not the same as end-tidal P_{CO_2}).

6. What is meant by a diffusion defect? Name some causes and a clinical test used to assess it.

A diffusion defect occurs when pulmonary capillary blood oxygen tension does not equilibrate with alveolar oxygen tension. Under normal conditions the capillary PO_2 equals alveolar oxygen tension after about 0.25 seconds of exposure. The normal transcapillary exposure time is 0.75 seconds, leaving 0.5 seconds of buffer or reserve time in normal lung.

Diseases that contribute to diffusion defects include diffuse pulmonary granulomatosis, fibrosis, sarcoidosis, healed destructive tuberculosis, and collagen vascular disease of the lungs. Hypoxemia caused by diffusion defects can be corrected by increasing FiO_2 to 100%.

DL_{CO}, the diffusing capacity of carbon monoxide, measures the diffusion of carbon monoxide across the alveolar-capillary membrane. A diffusion defect is demonstrated when this value decreases below 20–30 ml/mm·mmHg. Clinically patients with a known diffusion defect tolerate poorly tachycardia and high-flow states (e.g., exercise), both of which decrease total trancapillary red blood cell transit time in an already diseased lung.

7. What is the significance of the alveolar-arterial oxygen gradient? What is the most common reason for an increase in this value?

The alveolar-arterial oxygen gradient (A-a gradient or $A-aDO_2$) is a gradient that normally exists in humans and occurs for three reasons:
1. Absolute shunting
2. V/Q mismatch
3. Diffusion impairment

$$A-aDO_2 = \text{alveolar oxygen pressure} - \text{arterial oxygen pressure.}$$

$$\text{Alveolar oxygen pressure} = P_AO_2 = FiO_2\,(P_B - P_{H_2O}) - P_aCO_2/RQ,$$

where P_B = barometric pressure, P_{H_2O} = vapor pressure of water = 47 mmHg, RQ = respiratory quotient (approximately 0.8; this value changes with diet), and arterial oxygen pressure (P_aO_2) is determined by blood gas analysis.

The most common cause of a widened $A-aDO_2$ is shunt.

8. Define absolute shunt. How does one calculate the shunt fraction (Q_S/Q_T)?

Absolute shunt is defined as blood that reaches the arterial system without passing through ventilated regions of the lung. The fraction of cardiac output that passes through a shunt is determined by the following equation:

$$Q_S/Q_T = C_c - C_a/C_c - C_v$$

where C_c = oxygen content of end pulmonary capillary blood, C_v = mixed venous oxygen content, and C_a = arterial oxygen content.

The formula for calculating blood oxygen content is discussed in question 11.

9. What are the five causes of hypoxemia and how can they be differentiated?

Differential Diagnosis of Hypoxemia

CAUSES	$PaCO_2$	$A-aDO_2$	RESPONSE TO 100% OXYGEN*
Hypoventilation	↑	Normal	Often improves
Absolute shunt (V/Q = 0)	Normal	↑	None
V/Q mismatch	Normal	↑	Improves
Diffusion abnormality	Normal	↑	Improves
Decreases FiO_2	Normal	Normal	Improves

* All causes are improved by 100% oxygen therapy except absolute shunt.

10. What is responsible for normal physiologic shunt?
It is estimated that 2–5% of cardiac output is normally shunted through pulmonary shunts, thus accounting for the normal A-aDO$_2$. There are thought to be three different types of shunt.
1. Physiologic—atelectasis and consolidated alveoli
2. Postpulmonary—thebesian, bronchial, mediastinal, and pleural veins
3. Pathologic—congenital or traumatic anomalies as well as intrapulmonary tumors

11. Calculate normal arterial and venous oxygen content.
Oxygen content is calculated by summing the oxygen bound to hemoglobin and the dissolved oxygen of blood:

$$\text{Oxygen content (ml O}_2\text{/dl)} = 1.34 \text{ ml O}_2\text{/gm Hgb} \times [\text{Hgb}] \times S_aO_2 + (P_aO_2 \times 0.003)$$
$$\underbrace{\hspace{3.5cm}}_{\text{Bound}} \qquad \underbrace{\hspace{2.5cm}}_{\text{Dissolved}}$$

where S_aO_2 is the percent of saturated hemoglobin. If [Hgb] = 15 gm/dl, arterial saturation = 96% and P_aO_2 = 90 mmHg, mixed venous saturation = 75%, and P_vO_2 = 40 mmHg, then

$$C_aO_2 = (1.34 \text{ ml O}_2\text{/gm Hgb} \times 15 \text{ gm Hgb/dl} \times .96) + (90 \times 0.003) = 19.6 \text{ ml O}_2\text{/dl}$$
$$C_vO_2 = (1.34 \text{ ml O}_2\text{/gm Hgb} \times 15 \text{ gm Hgb/dl} \times .75) + (40 \times 0.003) = 15.2 \text{ ml O}_2\text{/dl}$$

12. How is oxygen consumption determined?
According to the Fick equation, oxygen consumption is determined when the difference between the C_aO_2 and the C_vO_2 is multiplied by cardiac output.

$$VO_2 = \text{Cardiac output (L/min)} \times (C_aO_2 - C_vO_2) \text{ in ml O}_2\text{/dl}$$

Thus, if cardiac output is 5 L/min or 50 dl/min:

$$50 \text{ dl/min} \times 4.4 \text{ ml O}_2\text{/dl} = 220 \text{ ml O}_2\text{/min}.$$

13. What are the normal P_AO_2, P_aO_2, and Aa gradient at sea level on room air?
The P_AO_2 can be calculated using the alveolar gas equation (see question 7):

$$P_AO_2 = FiO_2 (P_B - PH_2O) - P_aCO_2/RQ$$
$$P_AO_2 = .21 (760 - 47) - 40/0.8 = 99.7$$

The P_aO_2 of normal room air is about 90–100 at sea level (P_B = 760) and can be estimated by the equation:

$$P_aO_2 = 102 - (\text{age in years})/3$$
$$\text{A/a gradient} = P_AO_2 - P_aO_2 = 100 - 90 = 10$$

A normal Aa gradient on room air is about 10–15 mmHg and increases with age. If the A/a gradient is negative, consider the possibility of a bubble in the sample.

14. Estimate normal P_aO_2 for Denver (P_B = 630), where normal P_aCO_2 = 32. Guess where this chapter was written.

$$P_AO_2 = .21 (630 - 47) - 32/0.8 = 82$$

Assuming an Aa gradient of 10, then 82 – P_aO_2 =10 and P_aO_2 = 72. Yes, this chapter was written in Denver.

15. Define compliance. Give the normal value as well as the value considered to be abnormal.
Compliance is defined as the change in volume per unit change in pressure. Normal compliance is 100 ml/cm H$_2$O; compliance is considered abnormal when it decreases to less than 50 ml/cm H$_2$O.

16. Describe the nature of the elastic forces taking place between the chest wall and the lungs.
The lungs have elastic recoil forces that attempt to collapse the lung. The chest wall has elastic recoil forces that try to expand the chest. Under normal circumstances the chest wall and lung

pleura are attached, and the two opposite forces balance one another. However, when two entities separate, as in pneumothorax, the lung collapses and the chest wall expands because of elastic recoil properties.

17. A fetus is born at 32 weeks' gestation, appears dusky after delivery, and is difficult to ventilate. What is the likely cause?

Infant respiratory distress syndrome (IRDS), which is found in premature infants with an immature surfactant system, is characterized by respiratory failure secondary to poor lung compliance. Surfactant is a substance that decreases the alveolar surface tension and thus the pressure required to distend the alveolus. The alveoli are made up of two different types of cells. Type II cells manufacture surfactant, otherwise known as dipalmityl phosphatidylcholine (DPPC). DPPC, a phospholipid, is synthesized from fatty acids. Surfactant molecules appear hydrophobic on one end and hydrophilic on the other. The hydrophobic portion projects into the alveolar cavity, whereas the hydrophilic end lies within the alveolar fluid. The molecule is confined to the alveolar surface, where, during expiration, the area of the alveolus diminishes, leaving the surfactant molecules more densely packed. Just as soap reduces the surface tension of water, surfactant reduces the normal forces between surface molecules, thus lowering surface tension and increasing lung compliance.

18. Discuss the law of Laplace with respect to the alveolus.

The Laplace equation states:

$$P = 2 \times T/R$$

where P = distending pressures within the alveolus (dynes/cm^2), T = surface tension of the alveolar fluid (dynes/cm), and R = radius of the alveolus (cm). The relationship shows that the pressure necessary to expand the alveolus is (1) directly proportional to the surface tension and (2) inversely proportional to the radius. Thus, the combination of lowering surface tension and increasing alveolar diameter lowers the pressure required to expand alveoli.

19. Internists are having difficulty with weaning a 100-kg man from mechanical ventilation. The patient has a 7.0-mm endotracheal tube that is 29 cm long. The internists want to know whether cutting off 4 cm of endotracheal tube length will be as helpful as changing to a tube of larger diameter. What is the correct answer?

Because pressure = flow $\times$ resistance (Ohm's law), resistance = pressure/flow. For laminar gas flow, according to Poiseuille's law,

$$resistance = 8NL/\pi R^4$$

where R = radius, N = viscosity (poises), and L = length.

The single most important factor in determining airway resistance is the radius of the tube. If the radius is halved, the resistance within the tube increases to 16-fold; if the length of the tube is doubled, however, the resistance is also doubled. The clinical significance is that cutting the length of the tube minimally affects resistance; however, increasing the tube diameter makes a dramatic difference in resistance. Therefore, to reduce the work of breathing and the driving pressure necessary for the patient, the endotracheal tube should be changed to a larger size.

20. What determines the velocity profile of a gas?

Laminar flow, which has stream lines that are parallel with the tube, occurs at low flows. Turbulent flow has an uneven flow characteristic. As flow rates increase, laminar stream lines break away from parallel and become turbulent. Laminar flow is more dependent on viscosity, whereas turbulent flow is more dependent on density.

21. A 5-year-old child with multiple large laryngeal papillomas is stridorous before arrival at the OR for laser removal of the lesions. The surgeon requests helium to help ventilate the child. Discuss the physical explanation behind the use of helium. Is it acceptable to use helium with a laser?

Helium's utility as a therapeutic gas is based on its low density. As stated in question 20, when flow is turbulent, driving pressure is mostly related to gas density. Because flow in large airways is mainly turbulent, use of low-density gas mixtures in place of air or oxygen lowers the driving pressure needed to move gas in and out of the area. With less pressure required to move the gas through the large airways, the patient or ventilator's work of breathing decreases. Helium also can be used in the treatment of bronchospastic disease, but this effect is limited strictly to large airway obstruction.

Because helium is inert (one of the noble gases), it can be used safely with laser without the worry of combustion. But some oxygen must be delivered with the helium; therefore, all patients are at risk of airway fires with laser.

22. What is Reynolds' number?

In 1883 Osborne Reynolds showed that the transition from laminar to turbulent flow in a tube is determined by the value of a dimensionless parameter known as the Reynolds' number.

$$\text{Reynolds' number} = \frac{2rvd}{N}$$

where d = density, v = average velocity, r = radius, and N = viscosity. Reynolds showed that for any sized tube, transition from laminar to turbulent flow occurs when the Reynolds' number reaches a value of approximately 2100.

BIBLIOGRAPHY

1. Barash PG, Cullen BF, Stoelting RK (eds) : Clinical Anesthesia. Philadelphia, J.B. Lippincott, 1989.
2. Harrison RA: Physiologic basis for evaluation and treatment of hypoxemia. In ASA Regional Refresher Course Lectures. Park Ridge, IL, American Society of Anesthesiologists, 1985.
3. Miller RD (ed): Anesthesia, 3rd ed. New York, Churchill Livingstone, 1990.
4. Scanlan CL, Spearman CB, Sheldon RL (eds): Egan's Fundamentals of Respiratory Care. St. Louis, Mosby, 1995.
5. West JB: Respiratory Physiology: The Essentials, 3rd ed. Baltimore, Williams & Wilkins, 1989.

32. HYPERCARBIA

Teresa J. Youtz, M.D.

1. What is the normal range for arterial partial pressure of carbon dioxide ($PaCO_2$)?
At sea level, the normal range of $PaCO_2$ is 36–44 mmHg. Hypercarbia is defined as $PaCO_2$ > 44 mmHg and hypocarbia as $PaCO_2$ < 36 mmHg. $PaCO_2$ of 90–120 mmHg produces carbon dioxide (CO_2) narcosis, an inert gas narcotic effect that may produce unconsciousness. At inhaled CO_2 concentrations of 30%, anesthesia is induced.

2. How is CO_2 transported in the blood?
CO_2 is transported to the lungs as dissolved CO_2, bicarbonate ions (HCO_3^-) and carbaminohemoglobin, which transport an average of 4 ml CO_2 per 100 dl of blood. Of the 4 ml of CO_2, 7% is dissolved CO_2, 23% carbaminohemoglobin, and 70% HCO_3^-.

3. What are the clinical signs of hypercarbia?
The initial response to hypercarbia is sympathetic in origin. Signs of hypercarbia are hyperventilation, hypertension, tachycardia, elevated pulse pressure, warm flushed skin, and hiccups. Symptoms of hypercarbia may include headache, restlessness, excitement, and hallucinations. Under general anesthetic, many or all of these may be attenuated or abolished.

4. Discuss the mechanisms of hypercarbia.
 1. **Hypoventilation**
    - Increased difficulty in breathing may be due to surgical position, increased airway resistance, or decreased compliance.
    - Decreased respiratory drive secondary to anesthetic drugs' effect on central respiratory drive.
 2. **Increased dead space ventilation** (the portion of minute ventilation or tidal volume that does not participate in gas exchange)
    - Decreased pulmonary artery pressure (e.g., during deliberate hypotention) may increase zone I (alveolar pressure > arterial pressure > venous pressure) and alveolar dead-space ventilation (the volume of gas that enters nonperfused lung).
    - Increased airway pressure (i.e., positive end-expiratory pressure) may increase zone I and dead-space ventilation.
    - Pulmonary embolus, thrombosis, and vascular obliteration may result from kinking, clamping, or blocking of the pulmonary artery during surgery.
    - Short, rapid inspirations may be distributed preferentially to noncompliant and poorly perfused alveoli. Slow inspiratory time allows more compliant distribution and better perfused alveoli.
    - Anesthetic apparatus increases total dead space. Normal apparatus increases total dead space by 33–46% in intubated patients and by 64% in patients breathing by mask. Anesthetic circuits may cause rebreathing of expired gases if fresh gas flow is insufficient or if valves are defective.
 3. **Increase in CO_2 production**. All causes of increased oxygen (O_2) consumption increase CO_2 production:
    - Hyperthermia (temperature of 40° C may increase CO_2 production by 25%)
    - Shivering
    - Catecholamine release
    - Hypertension
    - Hyperthyroidism

   • Malignant hyperthermia
   • Hyperalimentation.
4. **Inspired CO$_2$**
   • CO$_2$ absorber channeling or exhaustion
   • CO$_2$ directly into circuit

5. What should be done when a patient has an elevated PaCO$_2$?

The first step is to determine the cause of the elevation of PaCO$_2$ (see question 4). In mechanically ventilated patients, most increases in PaCO$_2$ can be treated with an increase in minute ventilation until the cause is found. In spontaneously ventilating patients, the usual cause of hypocarbia is hypoventilation from a relative overdose of sedatives, which results in central nervous system depression. The spectrum of interventions includes verbal and physical stimuli, decreasing the dose of anesthetic, pharmacologic reversal of anesthetic agent, assisted ventilation by mask, endotracheal intubation, and mechanical ventilation.

During controlled ventilation, if the increased PaCO$_2$ is due to inadequate ventilation, an increase in tidal volume and/or respiratory rate will lower the PaCO$_2$. Increased airway resistance as the cause of increased CO$_2$ may be due to kinking or blockage of the endotracheal tube (ETT), which responds to suctioning, or bronchospasm, which may be treated with inhaled symphathomimetics.

Rebreathing of CO$_2$ may be a cause of increased PaCO$_2$. Increasing the gas flow to the patient will temporize the situation until the cause is found, e.g., replacing leaking valves or replacing exhausted CO$_2$ absorbent.

Increased CO$_2$ production may be the cause of hypercarbia. Malignant hyperthermia has a standard treatment; sepsis should be treated with antibiotics; and increased minute ventilation and shivering may be treated by warming the patient or with intravenous meperidine.

Hypercarbia is often seen during certain procedures such as laparoscopy, aortic repurfusion after the cross-clamp is relieved, or limb reperfusion after use of a tourniquet. These problems are easily corrected with a brief period of increased minute ventilation.

6. What is normal CO$_2$ production? How does it change during general anesthesia?

A 70-kg man at rest produces approximately 200 ml/min. of CO$_2$. General anesthesia produces a 10–40% decrease in CO$_2$ production secondary to decreased oxygen demand. Decreased oxygen demand is secondary to hypothermia, no work of breathing with controlled ventilation, and decreased myocardial work secondary to decreased blood pressure and cardiac output. Postoperatively the patient's CO$_2$ production and oxygen consumption return to normal and may result in a transient hypercarbia if ventilation is depressed by residual anesthetics or relaxants.

7. Define adequate ventilation.

Adequate ventilation is the minute volume that ensures normal or satisfactory levels of PaCO$_2$. If the CO$_2$ production remains constant, a rise in PaCO$_2$ during anesthesia must result from either a decrease in alveolar ventilation or an increase in inspired CO$_2$. For example, it is possible to have normal minute ventilation and greatly inadequate alveolar ventilation.

$$PaCO_2 = \frac{VCO_2 \text{ (ml/min) STPD} \times 0.863}{VA \text{ (L/min) BTPS}} = \frac{200 \times 0.863}{4} = 43 \text{ mmHg}$$

Note: 0.863 is a correction factor for different units of measure; VCO$_2$ is CO$_2$ production per minute; STPD is standard temperature pressure dry; BTPS is body temperature ambient pressure saturated with water vapor; and VA is alveolar minute ventilation.

With an increase of dead-space ventilation (mechanical or physiologic) by 50% of each tidal volume and with an adequate minute ventilation of 6 L/min, by the above equation the PaCO$_2$ will be 56 mmHg.

$$PaCO_2 = \frac{200 \times 0.863}{6 \times 50\%} = 56 \text{ mmHg}$$

8. What is the rate of increase of $PaCO_2$ during apnea?

During steady-state where CO_2 production equals CO_2 elimination, there is about a 6 mmHg gradient between alveolar partial pressure of CO_2 (P_ACO_2) and mixed venous CO_2 ($PvCO_2$). If CO_2 elimination is stopped, P_ACO_2 and $PvCO_2$ equilibrate rapidly during the first minute of apnea, as is reflected by a 5–10 mmHg increase in the $PaCO_2$. Subsequently, there is a 2–4 mmHg increase in $PaCO_2$ per minute, up to 80 mmHg.

9. Define apneic threshold. At what level of $PaCO_2$ does it occur?

Apneic threshold is the maximal $PaCO_2$ that does not initiate spontaneous ventilation, which is about 5 mmHg below resting $PaCO_2$ regardless of its baseline level.

10. What is the ventilatory response to an increase in inspired CO_2?

In awake patients, in the range of 20–80 mmHg, for each mmHg increase in $PaCO_2$ minute ventilation increases by 2 L/min.

CO_2 RESPONSE CURVE

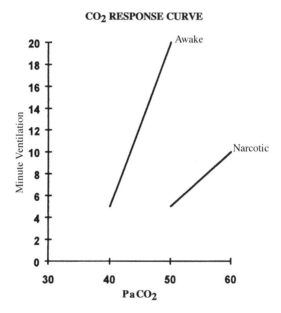

Ventilating response to increase in inspired CO_2.

11. What can change the slope of the CO_2 response curve?

A depressed CO_2 response curve equates to less increase in minute ventilation with increasing $PaCO_2$. When the CO_2 response curve is shifted to the right, higher $PaCO_2$ is required to get the same response in minute ventilation. When normal physiologic sleep shifts the CO_2 response curve to the right and depresses the slope, the $PaCO_2$ may increase to 50–52 mmHg. Under spontaneous ventilation, inhaled anesthetics show a dose-dependent increase in $PaCO_2$; enflurane produces the greatest increase in $PaCO_2$, whereas halothane produces the least decrease. The CO_2 response curve is shifted to the right and the slope depressed. Opioids, barbiturates, and other intravenous anesthetics shift the CO_2 response curve to the right and depress the slope. The magnitude of $PaCO_2$ elevation is less after 5–6 hours of volatile anesthetic compared with 1–3 hours of the same dose. The CO_2 response curve returns toward normal after 5–6 hours of volatile anesthetic. The reason for less depression is unknown.

12. What are the effects of hypercarbia on the circulatory system? How are these effects modified by inhaled anesthetics ?

Moderate hypercarbia directly stimulates the sympathoadrenal system with an increase in catecholamines, which compensates for the direct cardiac and vascular depression. Increases in $PaCO_2$ between 20–80 mmHg are associated with a linear increase in heart rate and cardiac output. Direct sympathetic stimulation of the cerebral nervous system is mediated at the vasomotor level and indirect stimulation by afferent impulses from peripheral chemoreceptors. CO_2 acts as a direct vasodilator except in pulmonary vasculature, in which it is a direct vasoconstrictor. The overall effects in awake patients are increases in systolic blood pressure, pulse pressure, stroke volume, myocardial contractility, and heart rate and a decrease in systemic vascular resistance.

Halothane and enflurane, which reduce preganglionic sympathetic activity, partially suppress the circulatory response to CO_2. Cyclopropane, ether, and fluroxene, which augments sympathetic activity, are associated with marked elevations of circulating catecholamines in response to increased $PaCO_2$.

13. Discuss mechanisms by which oxygenation can be affected by CO_2.

1. An increase in P_ACO_2 must displace oxygen from the alveoli. At sea level, a P_ACO_2 of 80 mmHg decreases the alveolar partial pressure of oxygen (P_AO_2) from 100 to 60 mmHg, with a resulting decrease in arterial partial pressure of oxygen (PaO_2).

2. Increased $PaCO_2$ produces a decrease in pH, with a resulting shift to the right of the oxyhemoglobin dissociation curve. The result is a decreased affinity of hemoglobin for oxygen.

14. What are the advantages and disadvantages of using an opioid antagonist to treat hypercarbia due to an opioid-induced decrease in ventilatory drive?

The advantage is rapid reversal of narcosis. The disadvantages are nausea, vomiting, pulmonary edema, hypertension, tachycardia, and reversal of analgesia.

15. When is mechanical ventilation needed for ventilatory failure?

Many signs and symptoms need to be considered: whether the patient shows changes in mental status; whether the $PaCO_2 > 80$; whether the rate of $PaCO_2$ increase is progressive or stable; whether the patient is in distress, tachypneic or dyspneic; whether the work of breathing increases with intercostal retractions and tracheal tug, and whether the patient is hypoxic.

16. What is the effect of $PaCO_2$ on cerebral blood flow (CBF)?

Cerebral blood flow increases or decreases 1 ml/100 g/min for every mmHg increase or decrease in $PaCO_2$ from baseline. The cerebral vasculature maximally dilates at a $PaCO_2$ of 80 mmHg.

17. How does $PaCO_2$ affect the convulsive threshold of local anesthetics? What are the mechanisms for this change?

The $PaCO_2$ is inversely related to the convulsive threshold. The mechanisms for the decrease are as follows:

1. Increased $PaCO_2$ increases CBF,; thus more anesthetic is delivered to the brain.

2. Diffusion of CO_2 into neural cells decreases intracellular pH. This decrease facilitates the conversion of the unionized form of local anesthetic to the ionized form, which does not diffuse across the nerve membrane. The resultant increase in ion trapping increases CNS toxicity;

3. Hypercarbia and/or acidosis decreases plasma protein binding of local anesthetics, with a resulting increase in the proportion of free drug available for diffusion into the brain.

18. How does end-tidal CO_2 ($ETCO_2$) monitoring correlate with $PaCO_2$?

$ETCO_2$ monitors gas from end exhalation of the lungs, which is measured by spectrophotometry or mass spectrometry. The exhaled CO_2 from the alveoli mixes with the gas from the conducting airways and the breathing circuit that was not involved in gas exchange. The exhaled CO_2 is diluted so that the $ETCO_2$ is usually lower than the $PaCO_2$. In healthy lungs the $ETCO_2$ is usually

5 cm less than the $PaCO_2$. With increasing dead-space ventilation, the difference between the $ETCO_2$ and $PaCO_2$ becomes greater.

19. What is the preterm infant's response to hypercarbia?
The preterm infant has smaller increases in minute ventilation than full-term infants and adults.

20. How does hypercarbia affect uteroplacental blood flow?
Moderate hypercarbia has no effect on uteroplacental blood flow. Uterine blood flow increases with $PaCO_2 > 60$, secondary to increase in mean arterial pressure (MAP). Uterine vascular resistance is unchanged.

21. Discuss some electrolyte changes associated with hypercarbia.
Increased $PaCO_2$ creates respiratory acidosis. The CO_2 combines with water to form carbonic acid, and the carbonic acid then breaks down to a hydrogen ion and a bicarbonate ion. Chronic hypercarbia (e.g., chronic lung disease) increases the reabsorption of bicarbonate by the kidneys, causing a compensatory metabolic alkalosis.

Hypercarbia also produces a leakage of potassium ions from cells into the plasma. This increase is associated with an increase in glucose, which is a response to the increased catecholamines that mobilize glucose from cells, especially in the liver. Because it takes time for potassium ions to reenter the cells, repeated episodes of hypercarbia at brief intervals may result in an increase of plasma potassium.

BIBLIOGRAPHY

 1. Benumof JL: Respiratory physiology and respiratory function during anesthesia. In Miller RD (ed): Anesthesia, 4th ed. New York, Churchill Livingstone, 1994, pp 611–615.
 2. Don H: Hypoxemia and hypercarbia during and after anesthesia. In Orkin FK, Cooperman LH (eds): Complications in Anesthesiology. Philadelphia, J.B. Lippincott, 1983, pp 196–204.
 3. Gal TJ: Causes and consequences of impaired gas exchange. In Benumof JL, Saidman LJ (eds): Anesthesia and Perioperative Complications. St. Louis, Mosby, 1992, pp 205–208.
 4. Kopman AF: Differential diagnosis of hypercarbia. In Ravin MB (ed): Problems in Anesthesia: A Case Study Approach. Boston, Little, Brown, 1981, pp 29–36.
 5. Jerome EH: Recovery of pediatric patient from anesthesia. In Gregory GA (ed): Pediatric Anesthesia. New York, Churchill Livingstone, 1989, p 638.
 6. Mecca RS: Postoperative recovery. In Barash PG, Cullen BF, Stoelting RK (eds): Clinical Anesthesia 2nd ed. Philadelphia, J.B .Lippincott, 1992, pp1524–1528.
 7. Nunn JF: The effects of changes in the carbon dioxide tension. In Nunn's Applied Respiratory Physiology 4th ed. Oxford, Butterworth-Heinemann, 1993, pp 526–527.
 8. Sakabe T, Nakakimu K: Cerebral and spinal cord blood flow. In Cottrell JE, Smith DS (eds): Anesthesia and Neurosurgery. St. Louis, Mosby, 1989, pp 27–28.
 9. Shnider SM, Levinson G, Cosmi EV: Obstetric anesthesia and uterine blood flow. In Shnider SM, Levinson G (eds): Anesthesia for Obstetrics. Williams & Wilkins, 1993, pp 45–46.
10. Stoelting RK, Miller RD: Effects of inhaled anesthesia on ventilation and circulation. In Basics of Anesthesia, 3rd ed. New York, Churchill Livingstone, 1994, pp 47–51.

33. HYPOTENSION

Cindy Griffiths, M.D., and Rita Agarwal, M.D.

1. Define hypotension.
Hypotension occurs when the mean arterial pressure falls below 20–30% of "normal" values for that person. Hypertensive patients with less vascular compliance may have decreased organ perfusion at pressures that are ordinarily considered normotensive.

2. Broadly categorize the causes of hypotension.
The mnemonic "DDD VITAMINS" is useful for differential diagnoses.

		EXAMPLE
D	**Developmental**	Valvular heart lesions
D	Drugs	Anesthetics and other drugs
D	Degenerative	Neurologic
V	Vascular	Cardiovascular instability
I	Infectious/Iatrogenic	Adverse reactions, surgical
T	Toxic/Traumatic	Hemorrhage, sepsis
A	Autoimmune/Anoxic	Anoxic brain injury
M	Metabolic/Medical	Medical causes
I	Endocrine	Pregnancy
N	**Neoplastic**	(Self-explanatory)
S	Special	Postoperative, deliberate

3. What is orthostatic hypotension?
Orthostatic hypotension is commonly defined as a decrease in systolic blood pressure of greater than 20% accompanied by an increase in heart rate of 20 beats per minute or more when the patient goes from the supine to upright position. It is variable with age and vascular compliance. Young people may maintain normal blood pressure despite a 20% reduction in circulating volume, whereas elderly patients may become orthostatic with a normal blood volume.

4. How do valvular heart lesions produce hypotension?
1. **Mitral stenosis.** Tachycardia can decrease blood pressure by limiting diastolic time, impairing left ventricular filling. Also, left ventricular pressures increase, producing pulmonary hypertension and right ventricular dysfunction, all contributing to decreased cardiac output. Hypotension can be treated by augmenting preload and judicious use of vasoconstricting agents (ephedrine) or inotropes (dobutamine, epinephrine).
2. **Aortic stenosis.** The heart relies on volume to overcome increased afterload and a noncompliant ventricle. Decreased perfusion to a greatly distended ventricle produces ischemia, decreasing cardiac output and producing hypotension. Extremes of heart rate may likewise decrease cardiac output.
3. **Mitral regurgitation.** Left ventricular ejection fraction is reduced from regurgitation of some of each stroke volume to the left atrium through an incompetent mitral valve. Hypotension occurs if the heart rate decreases or systemic vascular resistance (SVR) increases. Maintain intravascular volume to ensure adequate filling and ejection fraction. Use agents that mildly increase heart rate and decrease SVR. Keep the heart "full and fast."
4. **Aortic regurgitation.** "Forward" stroke volume is decreased by regurgitation through an incompetent aortic valve. Decreased diastolic blood pressure produces coronary hypoperfusion. Treatment is directed toward avoiding extremes of heart rate or increased afterload, while maintaining contractility and intravascular volume.

5. Which drugs common to the operating room have hypotension as a side effect?

1. **Antihypertensive agents** may inadvertently cause hypotension, especially in hypovolemic patients.

2. **Intravenous contrast agents** may cause hypotension in 5–8% of patients by anaphylaxis, release of vasoactive substances, or activating the complement system.

3. **Methylmethacrylate,** a cement used in joint replacement, undergoes an exothermic reaction that causes it to adhere to imperfections in the bony surface. Hypotension usually occurs 30–60 seconds after placement of the cement but can occur up to 10 minutes later. Postulated mechanisms include tissue damage from the reaction, release of vasoactive substances when it is hydrolyzed to methacrylate acid, embolization as the bone is reamed, and vasodilation caused by absorption of the volatile monomer.

4. **Epinephrine** is used in local anesthetic preparations. At low doses, epinephrine may cause hypotension early after injection by stimulating peripheral beta$_2$-adrenergic receptors, causing vasodilation. Subsequent beta$_1$-adrenergic stimulation produces a compensatory increase in heart rate and cardiac output.

5. **Drug allergy to anesthetic agents.** Usually an anaphylactoid reaction mediated by histamine release occurs; neuromuscular blocking agents are the most common anesthetic drugs that cause this reaction. **Latex** products can cause delayed-onset anaphylaxis. Hypotension and cardiovascular collapse occur approximately 40 minutes after exposure. Presumably, time is needed for allergenic proteins to be extruded from gloves. Predisposed individuals include 40% of patients with spina bifida, patients requiring repeated urinary catheterization, and up to 7% of operating room personnel. Prevention is all important. A good history is invaluable.

6. **Narcotics** may cause hypotension by decreasing sympathetic tone. More commonly, they cause bradycardia. Histamine release from rapidly injected morphine can also decrease blood pressure.

7. **Antibiotics** are the most common drug class to cause allergic reactions. Vancomycin, if rapidly infused, can cause "red man syndrome," an anaphylactoid reaction due to histamine release and characterized by flushing and hypotension.

6. By what mechanism(s) do commonly used anesthetic agents cause hypotension?

1. **Inhalational agents:** Halothane lowers cardiac output by directly depressing myocardial contractility. Isoflurane, by contrast, reduces preload and afterload through vasodilation.

2. **Hypnotics:** Both propofol and sodium pentothal cause hypotension through vasodilation.

3. **Neuromuscular blocking agents:** A side effect of rapidly injected atracurium and mivacurium is histamine release with resultant hypotension.

7. How do local anesthetics cause hypotension?

Systemic absorption or inadvertent intravascular injection of local anesthetics causes a central toxic reaction. Severity varies with the type of anesthetic, serum levels, metabolism, uptake, distribution, and excretion. Signs and symptoms of local anesthetic toxicity include tinnitus, metallic taste, dysphoria, dizziness, and central nervous system (CNS) excitability (including seizures) followed by CNS depression. Epinephrine added to local anesthetics decreases systemic absorption by vasoconstriction and by limiting uptake of the drug. Local anesthetics used in regional anesthesia produce a sympathectomy, leading to hypotension. (See question 8.)

8. In what ways can regional anesthetics lead to hypotension?

1. **Epidural anesthesia.** Conduction blockade of sympathetic fibers causes vasodilation below the level of the block. There is less chance of hypotension with blocks lower than the fifth thoracic level (T-5) because of compensatory vasoconstriction of the upper extremities. Blocks higher than T-2 may affect cardioaccelerator nerves, reducing cardiac output and heart rate. The vagus nerve may remain unaffected, causing further vasovagal reductions in heart rate and blood pressure. Rapid-acting agents such as chloroprocaine and etidocaine produce a faster sympathectomy and more abrupt hypotension.

2. Spinal (subarachnoid) anesthesia. Because the local anesthetic is injected directly into the cerebrospinal fluid, spinal blockade generally has a faster onset than epidural blockade and may decrease blood pressure faster and more dramatically. Hypovolemic patients are especially susceptible to hypotension after regional blockade. They have compensated by vasoconstriction, and when sympathetic tone is abolished, they vasodilate and become profoundly hypotensive.

9. Which neurologic conditions cause hypotension?

1. **Head injury.** A transient decrease in blood pressure is common. Suspect occult bleeding, as prolonged hypotension is likely due to hemorrhage. The injured brain is more vulnerable to the ischemic effects of hypotension. Scalp and facial lesions are deceptive and may be a source of significant blood loss.

2. **Brain death.** There is loss of descending vascular control, exacerbated by hypovolemia from hemorrhage or the diuresis used to reduce cerebral edema.

3. **Spinal shock.** For 24–72 hours after a spinal cord injury, neurologic assessment may be unreliable. Spinal shock causes disruption of motor, sensory, and reflex impulses. Loss of sympathetic tone leads to bradycardia, vasodilation, and hypotension. Keep patients well hydrated. Pressors may be required if hypotension persists despite normovolemia. Bradycardia can be treated with atropine.

10. Describe some iatrogenic causes of hypotension.

The most common **iatrogenic** causes of hypotension are side effects from drugs and regional anesthetic techniques.

Aortic cross-clamping and unclamping can lead to hypotension. Clamping the abdominal aorta, to repair an aneurysm for example, leads to hypertension in the segment proximal to the clamp with hypoperfusion distally. **Infrarenal clamping** leads to a mild increase in afterload and usually preserves myocardial contractility. **Suprarenal clamping** elevates mean arterial pressure (MAP), central venous pressure, pulmonary artery pressure, and pulmonary capillary wedge pressure, and decreases cardiac index. The increase in afterload may lead to overdistention of an impaired left ventricle, impairing performance and producing hypotension.

"Unclamping shock" is a short-lived, moderately hypotensive episode (approximately 40% reduction in MAP) associated with increased oxygen requirements and metabolic acidosis, usually for approximately 30 minutes after unclamping. Two theories as to the cause of unclamping shock have been developed. The first theory, which is not as strongly supported, proposes that hypotension is due to washout of vasoactive mediators and acids from ischemic limbs. The second theory is that there is a reactive hyperemia at the newly revascularized area, causing a relative hypovolemia when fluid is redistributed after unclamping. Vascular resistance diminishes, producing hypotension.

11. Review some miscellaneous medical conditions associated with hypotension.

1. **Guillain-Barré syndrome.** This syndrome is associated with wide fluctuations in heart rate and blood pressure secondary to autonomic dysfunction. Cardiac output may be sensitive to positive pressure ventilation, position change, hypovolemia, and effects of anesthetic agents.

2. **Dialysis.** Approximately one-fourth of dialysis patients, especially those who are critically ill or septic, become hypotensive owing to impaired carotid and aortic body reflexes. Acetate used in dialysis solutions may produce vasodilation in these hypovolemic patients. Overdiuresis while on dialysis may also contribute to hypotension.

3. **Biliary obstruction.** Bile acids may contribute to vasodilation. These patients are intolerant to moderate blood loss because they have decreased sensitivity to vasoactive drugs.

4. **Carcinoid syndrome.** Hormone-releasing tumors may affect blood pressure by releasing kinins, serotonin, or histamine.

12. What causes of hypotension are associated with pregnancy and childbirth?

1. **Supine hypotension syndrome.** Beyond the first trimester, weight of the gravid uterus produces aortocaval compression, decreasing venous return as well as compromising uteroplacental perfusion. Only 10% of women at term are symptomatic (dizziness, nausea, hypotension),

although 90% have complete caval obstruction when supine. All pregnant patients should have a wedge under the right hip when supine, displacing the uterus to the left.

2. Hypotension after **regional block.** Prehydration is important. If the patient remains hypotensive, ensure that the uterus is displaced, increase fluids, place the patient in slight head-down position, and administer ephedrine, which is conventionally thought to preserve uterine blood flow better than phenylephrine.

3. **Postpartum hemorrhage.** Normal blood loss is approximately 500 ml from a vaginal delivery and 1000 ml from a cesarean section. Further losses, from uterine atony, an unidentified bleeding source, or severe lacerations, may significantly diminish the parturient's blood volume.

4. Rapid infusion of **intravenous oxytocin (Pitocin).** Bolus administration of intravenous oxytocin produces systemic vasodilation, tachycardia, hypotension, and antidiuresis.

5. **Amniotic fluid embolism.** Absorption of amniotic fluid and particulate fetal matter through large uterine blood vessels occurs in approximately 3/100,000 births. The biphasic response consists initially of pulmonary vasospasm in response to vasoactive substances, followed by right-sided heart failure, decreased cardiac output, pulmonary edema, hypoxia, hypotension, and death.

13. How is hypotension treated intraoperatively?

First, determine the cause. Estimate blood loss and prior fluid resuscitation, check hematocrit, urine output, and electrocardiogram (ECG). Invasive monitoring may be indicated.

CAUSES	TREATMENT
Decreased preload	Fluids then pressors
Decreased cardiac output	
ST segment depression	Treat ischemia with nitroglycerin
Decreased contractility	Chronotropes
Increased afterload	Decrease afterload (sodium nitroprusside [Nipride])
Decreased afterload	Volume, inotropes

14. Describe the major causes of postoperative hypotension.

- **Spurious:** Incorrect readings may be obtained using a blood pressure cuff that is too large, or an arterial line that is improperly zeroed, malpositioned, or damped.
- **Decreased SVR** caused by a sympathectomy from regional anesthesia.
- **Hypovolemia** caused by unreplaced fluid deficit, unrecognized blood loss, third spacing, or ongoing fluid loss. The patient may require reoperation to investigate persistent occult bleeding.
- **Ventricular dysfunction** can be produced by ischemia, impaired contractility, fluid overload, or mobilization of fluid after regional anesthesia.
- **Mechanical problems** such as a tension pneumothorax or tamponade may impair venous return.
- **Arrhythmias** are more common in patients with preexisting heart disease. They can be triggered by ischemia; decreasing cardiac output; or medications including alpha blockers, venodilators, and histamine-releasing drugs.

15. How is postoperative hypotension treated?

When to treat

When MAP is 20–30% below baseline, the patient displays signs of decreased organ perfusion (pale, cool, moist skin, oliguria, confusion, angina, diaphoresis). Supplement oxygen and increase IV fluid rate. Trendelenburg position may be helpful. **Hypovolemia** is by far the most common cause. Examine the patient for pulses and blood pressure, and check the surgical site. Review medications the patient has received both preoperatively and postoperatively. Immediately discontinue any hypotensive agents. If hypovolemia does not seem to be the cause, decrease the fluid rate and obtain a 12-lead ECG, arterial blood gases, and chest x-ray. Does the patient need to be intubated? Hypercapnea produces sympathetic stimulation resulting in hypertension, increased cardiac output, and tachycardia. After compensatory mechanisms are exhausted, direct myocardial depression develops, manifested by decreased cardiac output as well as decreased SVR. If crystalloid infusion is ineffective, consider myocardial dysfunction and give blood or colloid and sympthomimetic drugs.

16. Discuss concerns about hypotension in pediatrics.

Mask induction with halothane causes hypotension by directly depressing the myocardium. Children have an increased incidence of bradycardia, hypotension, and cardiac arrest compared with adults because they have rapid anesthetic uptake, immature baroreflexes that are blunted by anesthesia, and less vasoconstrictive responses to hemorrhage than adults.

17. What techniques are used to cause deliberate hypotension?

Sodium nitroprusside, an afterload reducer, is commonly used because it has a rapid onset and short half-life and is easy to titrate. Perfusion is preserved at pressures greater than 50 mmHg in normal patients. Disadvantages of sodium nitroprusside include rebound hypertension, tachyphylaxis, increased intracranial pressure, and cyanide toxicity.

Nitroglycerin has a short half life and no toxic metabolites. It causes increased cerebral blood flow by venodilation.

Esmolol is a cardioselective beta$_1$-adrenergic blocking agent with a half-life of 9 minutes and is easily titratable. Advantages in neurosurgery include a lack of cerebral vasodilation, tachycardia, rebound hypertension, or toxic metabolites.

Less commonly used agents include ganglionic blockers (trimethaphan), alpha antagonists (phentolomine), and inhalational agents. Modest hypotension can also be a benefit of a regional technique that causes a sympathectomy.

CONTROVERSY

18. Describe surgical conditions in which deliberate hypotension would be either desirable or not recommended.

Desirable

Hypotensive techniques have been used, with some controversy, in cerebral aneurysm repair and in arteriovenous malformation surgeries. The goals of deliberate hypotension are to decrease systemic pressure to prevent rupture of vascular lesions and to decrease blood loss. Opponents of this technique suggest that hypotension may contribute to vasospasm of the cerebral arteries and thrombosis of arteriovenous malformations.

Not recommended

Cerebral blood flow autoregulation occurs at MAPs between 50 and 150 mmHg in normotensive individuals: that is, the brain is protected from hypoperfusion by automatic regulation of flow at MAPs in this range. In chronically hypertensive patients, autoregulation is "shifted to the right," meaning that decreased cerebral blood flow may occur at pressures considered normotensive. Deliberate hypotension is contraindicated in patients with fever, ischemic heart disease, renal insufficiency, anemia, occlusive cerebral vascular disease, and intracerebral hematomas.

BIBLIOGRAPHY

1. Chestnut DH: Obstetrical Anesthesia: Principles and Practice. St. Louis, Mosby, 1994.
2. Cotrell JE, Hartung J: Induced hypotension. In Cotrell JE, Smith DS (eds): Anesthesiology and Neurosurgery. St. Louis, Mosby, 1994, pp 425–434.
3. Covino BG, Lambert DH: Epidural and spinal anesthesia. In Barash PG, Cullen BF, Stoelting RK (eds): Clinical Anesthesia, 2nd ed. Philadelphia, J.B. Lippincott, 1992, pp 831–860.
4. Friesen RH, Henry DH: Cardiovascular changes in preterm neonates receiving isoflurane, halothane, fentanyl, and ketamine. Anesthesiology 64:238–242, 1986.

5. Malhotra V: Abdominal aortic aneurysm. In Yao FS, Artusio JF (eds): Anesthesiology: Problem-Oriented Patient Management, 2nd ed. Philadelphia, J.B. Lippincott, 1994, pp 148–160.
6. Mecca RS: Postoperative recovery. In Barash PG, Cullen BF, Stoelting RK (eds): Clinical Anesthesia, 2nd ed. Philadelphia, J.B. Lippincott, 1992, pp 1517–1521.
7. Nunn JF: Causes of hypercapnea. In Nunn JF: Nunn's Applied Respiratory Physiology. Oxford, UK, Butterworth-Heinemann, 1993, pp 237–238.
8. Nunn JF: Effects of changes in CO_2 tension. In Nunn JF: Nunn's Applied Respiratory Physiology. Oxford, UK, Butterworth-Heinemann, 1993, pp 518–528.
9. Roizen MF, Ellis J: Anesthesia for vascular surgery. In Barash PG, Cullen BF, Stoelting RK (eds): Clinical Anesthesia, 2nd ed. Philadelphia, J.B. Lippincott, 1992, pp 1075–1080.
10. Stoelting RK, Dierdorf SF: Anesthesia and Co-Existing Disease, 3rd ed. New York, Churchill Livingstone, 1993, pp 30–35.
11. Weis FR: Cardiovascular effects of Pitocin. Obstet Gynecol 46:211–214, 1975.

34. HYPERTENSION

Tanya Argo, M.D., and Terri Kinnard, M.D.

1. What is hypertension?

Hypertension (HTN) is a disease process in which the patient has higher than normal blood pressure (BP) on more than one occasion. As a rule, the upper limit of normal BP is considered around 140/90. Over time, elevated BP leads to end-organ damage.

2. Contrast systolic and diastolic hypertension.

Systolic HTN is associated with advancing age and is related to a decreased compliance of the aorta and arterioles. In adults with a diastolic BP (DBP) < 90 mmHg, a systolic BP (SBP) of 140–159 mmHg is borderline isolated systolic HTN, whereas SBP > 160 mmHg is isolated systolic HTN.

Diastolic HTN is associated with an increase in systemic vascular resistance and believed to be the major contributor to hypertensive morbidity. In adults, a diastolic BP of 90–104 mmHg is mild HTN; 105–114 mmHg is moderate HTN; and > 115 mmHg is severe HTN.

3. What are the causes of hypertension?

1. Essential hypertension—unknown cause; > 90% of all cases fall into this category.
2. Endocrine—adrenocortical dysfunction, pheochromocytoma, myxedema, acromegaly, birth control pills, thyrotoxicosis.
3. Renal—chronic pyelonephritis, renovascular stenosis, acute and chronic glomerulonephritis, polycystic kidney disease.
4. Neurogenic—psychogenic, familial dysautonomia, increased intracranial pressure, spinal cord transection, polyneuritis.
5. Systolic hypertension with wide pulse pressure—arteriosclerosis, aortic valvular insufficiency, patent ductus arteriosus, AV fistula.
6. Miscellaneous—increased intravascular volume, polyarteritis nodosa, hypercalcemia, toxemia of pregnancy, coarctation of the aorta, acute intermittent porphyria.

4. Why should hypertension be treated?

Many hypertensive patients develop smooth muscle hypertrophy in the precapillary resistance arterioles. Hypertrophied arterioles develop increased resting resistance and an exaggerated response to vasomotor stimuli. Uncontrolled HTN is also associated with early arteriosclerosis, which leads to coronary artery disease; intracerebral occlusions or hemorrhage; and renal failure. Men with isolated systolic HTN have a 2–3-fold increase in cardiovascular disease. Recently, however, the results of the Systolic Hypertension in the Elderly Program (SHEP) suggested that treatment with a thiazide diuretic decreases the risk of cerebrovascular accident by 36%. Decreasing DBP to a normal range also has been associated with a decrease in morbidity and mortality of HTN-related diseases.

5. Identify current drug therapies for hypertensive patients.

Five classes of drugs are used in the medical treatment of hypertension:

1. Diuretics
2. Antiadrenergics—alpha and beta blockers
3. Calcium channel blockers
4. Vasodilators
5. Angiotensin-converting enzyme (ACE) inhibitors

6. What are the doses, mechanism of action, and complications associated with antihypertensive drugs?

Doses, Mechanism of Action, and Complications of Antihypertensive Drugs

DRUG AND DOSE	MECHANISM OF ACTION	COMPLICATIONS
Diuretics		
Thiazide 25–50 mg/day	Increases urinary excretion of sodium (Na) and water by inhibiting Na reabsorption in cortical diluting tubule in nephron; exact mechanism of antihypertension is unknown—may be partially from direct arteriolar vasodilation.	Hypokalemia, dehydration, hyperglycemia, hyperuricemia, decreased lithium clearance.
Loop diuretics 40–240 mg/day	Inhibits Na and chloride reabsorption in proximal ascending loop of Henle; also has renal and peripheral vasodilatory effects.	Hypokalemia, dehydration, hypochloremic alkalosis.
Spironolactone 50–100 mg/day	Potassium-sparing—competitively inhibits aldosterone effects on distal renal tubules (increases Na and water excretion); may also block aldosterone effect on vascular smooth muscle.	Hyperkalemia, gynecomastia, dehydration.
Central antiadrenergics		
Alpha-methyldopa PO 500–2000 mg/day IV 250–500 mg over 30–60 min every 6 hr	Metabolite (alpha methylnorepinephrine) stimulates inhibitory alpha$_2$ adrenergic receptors and inhibits sympathetic nervous system outflow, thus decreasing total peripheral resistance.	Sedation, hepatic dysfunction, lupuslike symptoms, rebound hypertension, positive Coomb's test.
Clonidine PO 0.1–2.4 mg/day Topical transdermal patch every 7 days	Stimulates inhibitory alpha$_2$ receptors and inhibits sympathetic outflow.	Sedation, xerostomia, rebound HTN, 50% decrease in minimal alveolar concentrations of volatile anesthetic.
Peripheral antiadrenergics		
Prazosin (Minipres) 2–20 mg/day	Selective and competitive postsynaptic alpha$_1$ receptor blockade leading to arteriolar and vasodilation.	Alters test result for pheochromocytoma, false-positive test for ANA, increase liver function tests.
Terazosin (Hytrin) 1–5 mg PO/day	Selectively inhibits alpha$_1$ receptors in vascular smooth muscles. Dilates both arterioles and venules.	Decreases hematocrit, hemoglobin, albumin, leukocytes, and total protein.
Guanethidine (Ismelin) 100–300 mg/day	Peripherally inhibits alpha1 receptors and release of norepinephrine (NE); depletes stores of NE in adrenergic nerve endings.	Use with direct-acting sympathomimetics may precipitate a hypertensive crisis.
Labetalol 100–400 mg PO twice daily, 10–80 IV every 10 min	Competitive antagonist at beta and alpha$_1$ adrenergic receptors	Contraindicated in asthmatic, 2nd- or 3rd-degree AV block, congestive heart failure, or "brittle" diabetic.
Vasodilators		
Hydralazine 10–50 mg PO 4 times/day 5–10 mg IV every 20 min	Direct relaxing effect on vascular smooth muscle (arterioles > veins).	Lupuslike syndrome in 1—20% of patients on chronic therapy, decreases DBP > SBP, increases heart rate.
Minoxidil 5–100 mg/day PO	Direct relaxation of arteriolar smooth muscle.	Fluid retention, pericardial effusion, hypertrichosis.

Table continued on following page.

Doses, Mechanism of Action, and Complications of Antihypertensive Drugs (Continued)

DRUG AND DOSE	MECHANISM OF ACTION	COMPLICATIONS
Antiotensin-converting enzyme (ACE) inhibitors Benazepril (Lotensin) (10–40 mg/day PO) Captopril (Capoten) 6.25–150 mg PO 3 times/day Enalapril (Vasotec) 5–40 mg/day PO 1.25 mg/IV every 6 hr Lisinopril (Zestril) 10–40 mg/day PO	Competes with ACE, preventing pulmo-nary conversion of angiotensin I to angiotensin II (a potent vasoconstrictor). Decreases peripheral arterial resistance; leads to decreased aldosterone secretion, thereby reducing Na and water retention.	10% get rash with fever and joint pain, pro-teinuria neutropenia, cough.
Calcium channel blockers Diltiazem (Cardizem) 30–90 mg PO 4 times/day 0.25 mg/kg IV over 2 min 5–15 mg/hr IV drip Isradipine (DynaCirc) 2.5–5 mg PO twice daily Nifedipine (Procardia) 10–30 mg PO 3 times/day Verapamil (Calan, Isoptin) 0.075–0.3 mg/kg IV over 2 min 80–120 PO 3 times/day	Blocks calcium movement across cell membranes, causing arterial vaso-dilation. Nifedipine is the most potent peripheral and coronary artery vasocilator of calcium channel blockers. Diltiazem has less negative inotropic effects than verapamil and has some selective coronary vasodilatory effects.	Congestive heart failure, nodal changes, edema, headaches, hyper-kalemia, flushing. Tachycardia (with nifedipine only).

PO = orally, IV = intravenously, HTN = hypertension, ANA = antinuclear antibody, DBP = diastolic blood pressure, SDP = systolic blood pressure, AV = atrioventricular.

7. Describe common preanesthetic considerations in hypertensive patients.

1. What is the cause of the hypertension? Surgical mortality is fairly high in patients with renovascular hypertension. Undiagnosed pheochromocytoma may have devastating operative consequences, such as catecholamine-induced coronary artery spasm or sustained malignant hypertension.

2. When did the patient become hypertensive? If HTN was of sudden onset, it probably has an identifiable cause.

3. How long has the patient had hypertension? A longer duration of disease may mean more severe end-organ damage.

4. What medications is the patient taking now?

5. What medications has the patient taken in the past?

6. Has the patient been compliant with medication?

7. Have medications adequately controlled the HTN? Poorly controlled HTN leads to an in-creased incidence of end-organ damage.

8. Is there any evidence of end-organ damage? More than 50% of untreated hypertensives develop end-organ disease, including left ventricular hypertrophy, congestive heart failure, car-diomyopathy, renal insufficiency, strokes, and retinopathy.

9. Are the electrolytes within normal limits, especially in patients taking diuretics?

8. What findings from physical and laboratory exams may indicate end-organ damage from hypertension?

1. Left ventricular lift with cardiac palpation
2. Loud A2 and S4 upon cardiac auscultation
3. Left ventricular hypertrophy on an ECG suggests long-term HTN
4. Arteriovenous nicking on retinal exam
5. Orthostatic hypotension
6. Elevated serum creatinine
7. Abdominal bruits
8. Congestive heart failure

9. What antihypertensive medications should be taken until the time of surgery?

A well-controlled hypertensive patient has less intraoperative lability in blood pressure. Acute withdrawal of antihypertensives may precipitate rebound hypertension and/or myocardial ischemia. In general, antihypertensive therapy should be maintained until the time of surgery and restarted as soon as possible after surgery. However, Coriate et al. found that discontinuation of ACE inhibitors 24 hours before the scheduled surgery decreased the incidence of severe hypotension on induction. Diuretics may be withheld when depletion of intravascular volume is a concern.

10. What preoperative premedication is appropriate for hypertensive patients?

Hypertensive patients, like all patients, have increased anxiety before surgery and may benefit from anxiolytics such as the benzodiazepines. Clonidine, an alpha$_2$-adrenergic agonist, also has been shown to decrease preoperative anxiety and to reduce lability of intraoperative blood pressure and anesthetic requirements. If an anticholinergic is required, glycopyrrolate is a better choice that atropine, because it is associated with a lower incidence of tachycardia.

11. Discuss alternative induction agents for general anesthesia in hypertensive patients.

Any induction agent can be successfully used with careful titration and monitoring.

- Barbiturates, benzodiazepines, and propofol are likely to lead to an exaggerated decrease in BP if not titrated slowly to effect. Untreated or poorly controlled hypertensive patients are often volume-depleted and especially prone to significant falls in BP.
- Propofol, a diisopropylphenol, exhibits dose-dependent cardiovascular depression.
- Ketamine is rarely recommended, because its sympathomimetic effects may exaggerate HTN.
- Etomidate is a nonbarbiturate hypnotic with a lower incidence of cardiovascular effects. It is probably the most cardiovascularly stable drug available for induction of hypertensive patients.
- Opioids also may be used with minimal cardiovascular effects but may require doses not conducive to immediate extubation at the end of surgery.
- Intravenous or topical laryngotracheal lidocaine (1.5 mg/kg) before intubation may help to minimize the sympathetic response to the stimulation of intubation.
- Sodium nitroprusside (1–2 μg/kg), nitroglycerin (1–2 μg/kg), or esmolol also help to blunt rise in BP and heart rate with laryngoscopy and intubation.
- The most important factor for limiting the exaggerated BP response to intubation is to limit the duration of laryngoscopy to 15 seconds or less.

12. Is regional anesthesia a viable option for hypertensive patients?

Yes, but a high level of sympathetic blockade in hypertensive patients may produce excessive reductions in BP, because decreased intravascular fluid volume exacerbates vasodilatation. Regional blocks should be administered to an adequately medicated and sedated patient to prevent stress-related release of catecholamines. Epinephrine should not be added to local anesthetics because of its association with tachycardia and exacerbation of HTN.

13. Discuss common intraoperative considerations for hypertensive patients.

Long-term hypertension often leads to **left ventricular functional abnormalities**. Left ventricular hypertrophy (LVH) results from the increased pressure against which the left ventricle is required to eject. The hypertrophied left ventricle requires a greater filling pressure to produce adequate end-diastolic stretching of heart muscle to maintain stroke volume, as illustrated by the Frank-Starling curve (see p. 239). The left ventricle also may exhibit diastolic dysfunction, in which the ventricle does not relax enough to allow adequate filling for maintenance of stroke volume (unless end-diastolic pressures increase). Subsequently, hypertensive patients with LVH depend on preload to maintain cardiac output and arterial blood pressure.

The autoregulation curve of cerebral blood flow (CBF) also shifts to the right. Autoregulation is the ability of the brain to maintain a constant cerebral blood flow over a range of BPs. In hypertensive patients the higher pressure required for normal blood flow is reflected in the shifting

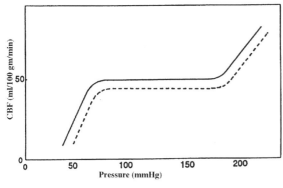

Autoregulation of cerebral blood flow.

of the curve. Symptoms of cerebral ischemia are more likely to occur at higher pressures in hypertensive patients than in normotensive controls.

Other considerations include constant monitoring of the electrocardiogram (ECG) for evidence of myocardial ischemia, keeping in mind that an increase in heart rate and BP may lead to increased myocardial oxygen consumption. Intraoperative hypertension also promotes increased bleeding in the operative site. Renal dysfunction may influence choice of agents and/or dosage requirement. Centrally acting antihypertensives (e.g., clonidine, methyldopa) promote sedation and therefore may decrease anesthetic needs.

14. Provide a differential diagnosis for intraoperative HTN.

Related to preexisting disease

Preexisting hypertension	Elevated intracranial pressure
Early acute myocardial infarction	Autonomic hyperreflexia
Aortic dissection	

Related to surgery

Prolonged tourniquet time	Postmyocardial revascularization
Aortic cross-clamping	Postcarotid endarterectomy

Related to anesthetic

Pain/catecholamine release	Malignant hyperthermia
Inadequate depth of anesthesia	Shivering
Hypoxia	Improperly sized (too small) BP cuff
Hypervolemia	Transducer artifact-increased resonance
Hypercarbia	(improperly low position of transducer)

Related to medication

Rebound hypertension (from discontinuation of clonidine, beta blockers, or methyldopa
Systemic absorption of vasoconstrictors
Intravenous indigo carmine dye

Others

Bladder distention, hypothermia and vasoconstriction, hypoglycemia

15. Is acute postoperative HTN significant?

It is fairly common for postoperative patients to exhibit hypertension. Prompt diagnosis of cause and appropriate treatment are needed to prevent associated complications. Acute hypertension increases afterload and therefore myocardial work and thus may precipitate myocardial ischemia. Increased systemic vascular resistance also may impair left ventricular ejection of blood, decreasing cardiac output and leading to pulmonary edema. Other complications include wound hematomas, intracerebral hemorrhage, arrhythmias, acute renal failure, headache, and changes in mental status.

16. How is postoperative hypertension managed?

Pain is the most common cause of postoperative hypertension, but the first step is thorough assessment for other causes. The best approach is to diagnose the problem and to individualize treatment. Normally careful titration of labetalol or esmolol is sufficient to gain quick control of postoperative HTN. Occasionally, one may need to consider a nitroprusside drip, especially if tight control is required (i.e., postoperative craniotomy patients, patients prone to myocardial ischemia).

CONTROVERSIES

17. Are hypertensive patients undergoing general anesthesia at increased risk for perioperative cardiac morbidity?
The hypertensive patient's risk for perioperative cardiac complications is difficult to assess because of differences in study design and patient selection. A study by Pry-Roberts noted that poorly controlled hypertensive patients with an average mean blood pressure of 129.5 mmHg demonstrated an increased incidence of hypotension and ECG changes, suggesting myocardial ischemia during maintenance of general anesthesia. Other studies also suggest that a DBP > 110 mmHg is a risk factor for cardiac morbidity.

18. Is there a BP above which elective surgery should be cancelled?
The answer to this question is highly individualized and depends on the anesthesiologist, surgeon, surgical procedure, and patient. Elevated BP in a patient who is normally well controlled but very nervous preoperatively should be treated with an anxiolytic and reevaluated. The available data suggest that the patient with a diastolic BP $\geq$ 110 mmHg should not undergo elective anesthesia because of an increased incidence of cardiac complications (myocardial ischemia, congestive heart failure, or cardiac death).

19. Was HTN included among Goldman's criteria as a predictor of poor operative outcome?
In 1979 Goldman et al. conducted a prospective study to derive the cardiac risk index. They studied 1001 consecutive patients undergoing a wide variety of surgical procedures and demonstrated that nine factors increase cardiac risk:
1. Myocardial infarction within the past 6 months
2. Preoperative S_3 heart sound or jugular venous distention
3. History of 6 or more premature ventricular contractions per minute
4. Nonsinus rhythm
5. Age > 70 years
6. Significant aortic valvular stenosis
7. Emergency operation
8. Intraperitoneal, intrathoracic, or aortic operation
9. Poor medical condition

Although Goldman found an increased cardiac risk in hypertensive patients, the number of patients in the study with a DBP > 110 mmHg was too small for a definitive conclusion.

BIBLIOGRAPHY

1. Coriate P, Richer C, Douraki T, et al: Influence of chronic angiotensin converting enzyme inhibition on anesthetic induction. Anesthesiology 81:299–307, 1994.
2. Goldman L, Caldera DL: Risks of general anesthesia and elective operation in the hypertensive patient. Anesthesiology 50:285–292, 1979.
3. Miller ED: New developments in the management of perioperative hypertension. In American Society of Anesthesiology Annual Refresher Course Lectures. San Francisco, 1994, pp 522–527.
4. Murad F: Drugs used for the treatment of angina. In Gilman AG, Rall TW, Nies AS, Taylor P (eds): Pharmacological Basis of Therapeutics, 7th ed. New York, Pergamon Press, 1990, pp 774–783.
5. Prys-Roberts C: Anesthesia and hypertension. Br J Anaesth 56:711–724, 1984.
6. SHEP Cooperative Research Group: Prevention of stroke by antihypertensive drug treatment in the older persons with isolated systolic hypertension. JAMA 265:3255–3264, 1991.
7. Steen PA, Tinker JH, Tarhan S: Myocardial reinfarction after anesthesia and surgery. JAMA 239:2566, 1978.
8. Stoelting RK, Dierdorf SF: Anesthesia and Co-existing Disease, 3rd ed. New York, Churchill Livingstone, 1993, pp 79–86.
9. Williams GH: Hypertensive vascular disease. In Wilson JD, Braunwald E, Isselbacher KJ, Petersdorf RG, et al (eds): Harrison's Principles of Internal Medicine, 12th ed. New York, McGraw-Hill, 1991, pp 1001–1015.

35. AWARENESS DURING ANESTHESIA

James A. Ottevaere, M.D.

1. What is awareness under anesthesia?

Patient perception under general anesthesia takes the form of either explicit or implicit memory. Anesthetic awareness refers to explicit memory of intraoperative events, which involves spontaneous or conscious recall. In contrast, implicit memory is subconscious processing of information by the brain. Explicit recall of intraoperative events may occur with or without the sensation of pain, and recollections may be vivid, such as operating room conversation, or vague, such as dreams or unpleasant sensations associated with the operation. Implicit memory during anesthesia has been tested by hypnosis and behavioral suggestion. A commonly used behavioral suggestion is intraoperative instructions to touch a designated body part during the postoperative interview. The results of such investigations are variable but indicate that implicit memory during anesthesia exists in some form.

2. What is the significance of implicit memory during general anesthesia?

Implicit memory in anesthetized patients has prompted investigation into improving postoperative outcomes by using intraoperative suggestion. Patients listen to audiotapes containing positive messages while undergoing general anesthesia. Studies using this technique have demonstrated a decrease in both hospital stay and use of postoperative analgesia. Patients also report an improved sense of well-being. The subject, however, remains controversial because some studies found no difference in outcomes after positive suggestion.

3. Discuss the incidence of awareness during anesthesia.

The incidence of awareness during anesthesia varies greatly, depending on clinical situation and anesthetic technique. Awareness under anesthesia is divided into two categories, consciousness with pain and consciousness without pain. Awareness with painful sensation has the greatest effect on postoperative sequelae. The incidence of awareness with pain is approximately 1 in 3000 general anesthetics. Consciousness without pain has a higher incidence—approximately 3 in 1000 general anesthetics. Absence of pain may result from the concomitant use of local anesthetics or opioids or the analgesic properties of volatile anesthetics at low doses. Evidence suggests that the incidence of awareness under anesthesia has decreased over the last two decades.

4. Describe common clinical situations associated with awareness.

Anesthesiologists often intentionally use light general anesthesia when it is indicated by the clinical situation. Common surgeries associated with an increased incidence of awareness are cesarean section, major trauma, and cardiac procedures. General anesthesia in obstetric patients may produce neonatal suppression; therefore, doses and concentrations of anesthetics have traditionally been minimized. As a result, the incidence of awareness in obstetric patients is approximately 1%. The hemodynamic instability associated with major trauma often requires reduced dosages of anesthetics. The incidence of postoperative awareness in trauma patients may be as high as 48%, depending on the severity of trauma. Patients undergoing cardiac surgery with cardiopulmonary bypass also have a higher incidence of postoperative recall because of the reliance on narcotic-based anesthesia, which minimizes myocardial depression but produces unreliable amnesia. Recent data suggests an incidence of 1%.

5. Describe the clinical signs and symptoms of light anesthesia.

Signs of light anesthesia reflect both motor and autonomic response to stimulation. Motor signs in response to light anesthesia frequently precede hemodynamic changes or sympathetic activation.

Specific motor signs include eyelid or eye motion, swallowing, coughing, grimacing, and movement of the extremities or head. Increased respiratory effort is due to activity of intercostal and abdominal muscles, which are suppressed at deeper levels of anesthesia. With the use of neuromuscular blockade, motor signs do not provide information about anesthetic depth. Consequently, sympathetic activation represents an additional method for assessing light anesthesia. Sympathetic effects associated with light anesthesia include hypertension, tachycardia, mydriasis, tearing, sweating, and salivation. Such findings are nonspecific and modified by anesthetic agents; thus their presence or absence is an unreliable indicator of awareness.

6. What is the last sensory modality suppressed by anesthesia?

The auditory pathway is the most metabolically active part of the conscious brain. Thus, hearing is the last sense suppressed by anesthesia. This fact has significant implications. Because hearing plays an important role in implicit memory, intraoperative events or conversation may affect postoperative well-being both positively and negatively. In addition, monitoring of auditory-evoked potentials (AEPs) provides a window into anesthetic depth and may be used to evaluate the effects of anesthetic drugs.

7. Are there adequate monitors for detecting awareness during anesthesia?

Various techniques have been evaluated as indicators of awareness during anesthesia. However, no monitoring technique has proved reliable in predicting recall, although some demonstrate good correlation with anesthetic depth. Clinical signs of light anesthesia led to the development of Pressure, Rate, Sweating, and Tears (PRST) scale. As described above, however, these signs are unreliable indicators of awareness. The isolated forearm technique, which uses a tourniquet to isolate the forearm from the effects of muscle relaxants, demonstrated patient movement in response to verbal commands but correlated poorly with postoperative recall. Monitoring of lower esophageal contractility, frontalis muscle activity, and EEG during anesthesia have proved unreliable at predicting anesthetic awareness. AEPs undergo characteristic changes with increasing concentrations of anesthetics, suggesting that they reflect anesthetic depth. Although this approach is promising, the complexity and size of equipment for monitoring AEP limit its clinical use. Measurement of respiratory sinus arrhythmia (RSA), which is the degree of variation of heart rate with respiration, reflects parasympathetic tone from the brainstem. Early data suggest that decreases in RSA correlate with anesthetic depth but reliability has not been proved. This method is easy to apply with standard monitors.

8. Which anesthetic techniques are associated with increased risk of intraoperative awareness?

Several anesthetic techniques increase the risk of awareness. Use of muscle relaxants, particularly in combination with nitrous oxide and opioids alone, may mask signs of light anesthesia and contribute to increased incidence of intraoperative awareness. Incidence of recall is also increased in opioid-based anesthetics used in cardiac and other selected surgeries. Total intravenous anesthesia (TIVA) may predispose patients to awareness under anesthesia because of the variability in dosage requirements and elimination rates, which is not seen with volatile agents. Outpatient anesthesia, which emphasizes rapid patient recovery, relies on short-acting agents and an intentionally light plane of anesthesia; thus the risk of awareness is increased.

9. What are the common preventable causes of intraoperative awareness?

Aside from intentionally light planes of anesthesia, awareness may result from equipment malfunction or clinical misjudgment by the anesthesiologist. Empty or malfunctioning vaporizers and leaks or partial disconnection of the breathing circuit are examples of equipment problems that may lead to decreased anesthetic delivery and subsequent intraoperative awareness. Equipment malfunction is largely preventable by adequate preoperative check-out procedures, familiarity with apparatus, and intraoperative vigilance. Clinical errors also may lead to intraoperative awareness. An unanticipated difficult intubation with inadequate anesthesia may lead to recall. Failure to recognize increased anesthetic requirements, excessive reliance on muscle re-laxants, and unfamiliarity with the chosen technique are additional examples of clinical misjudg-ments that result in intraoperative awareness. The anesthesiologist may prevent such errors with adequate preoperative evaluation and preparation.

10. What dose of volatile agent is sufficient to prevent awareness?
Volatile agents have amnestic properties. However, the concentration of volatile anesthetics nec-essary to eliminate intraoperative awareness is not clearly established. Variability among patients and clinical situations contributes to altered alveolar concentrations necessary to suppress recall. Evidence indicates that 0.4 to 0.6 minimum alveolar concentration (MAC) of isoflurane prevents response to commands and eliminates awareness in volunteers. The fact that these volunteers did not receive surgical stimulation has led to recommendations of at least 0.8 MAC to guarantee un-consciousness during surgery when volatile agents are used as the primary anesthetic. Addition of amnestic agents such as benzodiazepines, scopolamine, and intravenous anesthetics lower the concentration of volatile agent necessary to prevent recall.

11. Identify common clinical situations that increase anesthetic requirements.
Unrecognized increases in anesthetic requirements may contribute to intraoperative awareness. Certain clinical situations are associated with increased minimum alveolar concentration (MAC) of volatile anesthetics. Multiple general anesthetics may produce long-term tolerance to subse-quent anesthetics. Chronic alcoholism, hypernatremia, and hyperthermia increase MAC. Drugs that increase central nervous system catecholamines, such as monoamine oxidase inhibitors, tri-cyclic antidepressants, cocaine, and amphetamines, also increase the MAC of inhaled anesthetics.

12. Describe postoperative signs and symptoms of anesthetic awareness.
The postoperative interview allows the anesthesiologist to elicit information about anesthetic recall. Because few patients spontaneously complain of intraoperative awareness, underreporting is common. Direct inquiry about the patient's subjective feelings about the anesthetic may elicit complaints of fear, anger, sadness, or simply a feeling that something is "not quite right." Complaints involving recall of intraoperative conversation, pain, weakness or paralysis, or intu-bation should be pursued to determine their validity. Some cases of awareness may manifest months to years postoperatively as posttraumatic stress disorder (PTSD). PTSD results from dis-tressing events outside normal human experience; in anesthesia, it is usually associated with in-traoperative awareness involving pain. PTSD symptoms include flashbacks or nightmares, avoidance behaviors, emotional numbing, preoccupation with death, and hyperarousal.

13. How should patients who have experienced intraoperative awareness be managed?
When a case of awareness is identified either by staff or during the postoperative interview, sev-eral steps should be taken immediately. The anesthesiologist should determine the validity of the claim by eliciting details from the patient and comparing them with intraoperative events. The timing of any recollection of pain should be assessed, because patients may confuse postopera-tive and intraoperative pain. The anesthesiologist should question patients compassionately and acknowledge belief in their accounts. Detailed documentation of the interview and findings should be recorded in the hospital chart. Prompt referral to a psychologist or psychiatrist trained in treatment of PTSD is warranted, particularly in patients who exhibit psychological symptoms or experience pain as part of their intraoperative recall.

14. How can the anesthesiologist help to prevent intraoperative awareness?
Prevention of awareness is an important consideration in the proper administration of anesthesia. Research and experience have led to the development of specific recommendations for preven-tion. Preoperatively the anesthesiologist should perform a thorough machine check. Amnestic agents such as benzodiazepines or scopolamine are helpful when used as premedicants or adju-vants to anesthesia. Additional doses of induction agents during prolonged or difficult intubations

helps to ensure adequate levels of anesthesia. Intraoperatively, muscle relaxants should be avoided unless necessary for surgical conditions. Nitrous oxide and opioids alone or in combination are unreliable in the prevention of awareness and should be supplemented with volatile or intravenous agents. Volatile agents should be administered in at least 0.8 MAC when used as the sole anesthetic. Finally, given the potential effect of auditory input on postoperative outcomes, discouraging negative comments or using headphones or earplugs during anesthesia may have some value in the prevention of explicit and implicit recall.

BIBLIOGRAPHY

1. Aitkenhead AR: Awareness during anaesthesia: What should the patient be told? [editorial]. Anaesthesia 45;351–352, 1990.
2. Bailey PL, Stanley TH: Intravenous opioid anesthetics. In Miller RD (ed): Anesthesia, 4th ed. New York, Churchill Livingstone, 1994, pp 300–303.
3. Bennett HL: Treating psychological sequelae of awareness. ASA Newlett 58(10):12–15, 1994.
4. Eldor J, Frankel DZN: Intra-anesthetic awareness. Resuscitation 21:113–119, 1991.
5. Ghoneim MM, Block RI: Learning and consciousness during general anesthesia. Anesthesiology 76:279–305, 1992.
6. Heneghan C: Clinical and medicolegal aspects of conscious awareness during anesthesia. Int Anesthesiol Clin 3194):1–11, 1993.
7. Jones JG: Perception and memory during general anesthesia. Br J Anaesth 73:31–37, 1994.
8. Liu WHD, Thorp TAS, Graham SG, Aitkenhead AR: Incidence of awareness with recall during general anesthesia. Anaesthesia 46:435–437, 1991.
9. Lyons G, Macdonald R: Awareness during caesarean section. Anaesthesia 46:62–64, 1991.
10. McLeskey CH, Aitkenhead AR: Prevention of awareness. ASA Newslett 58(1):16–21, 1994.
11. Newton DEF, Thornton C, Konieczko K, et al: Levels of consciousness in volunteers breathing sub-MAC concentrations of isoflurane. Br J Anaesth 65:609–615, 1990.
12. Phillips AA, McLean RF, Devitt JH, Harrington EM: Recall of intraoperative events after general anaesthesia and cardiopulmonary bypass. Can J Anaesth 40:922–926, 1993.
13. Pomfrett CJD, Barrie JR, Healy TEJ: Respiratory sinus arrhythmia: An index of light anaesthesia. Br J Anaesth 71:212–217, 1993.

36. CARDIAC DYSRHYTHMIAS

Kelli Lambert Weiner, M.D.

1. Describe the relationship between the electrocardiogram (ECG) tracing and the intracellular action potential.

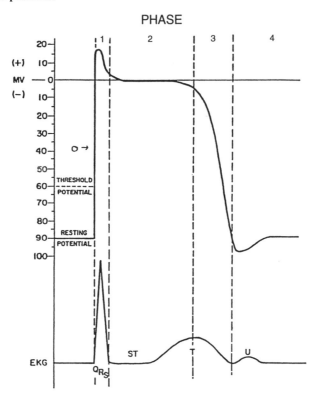

Action potential and surface ECG.

There are five phases to the action potential. The **resting membrane potential** is predominantly determined by the concentration gradient between intracellular and extracellular potassium and, to a lesser extent, the sodium gradient. As demonstrated in the figure above, phase 0 is the rapid depolarization of the action potential and corresponds to the initiation of the QRS complex of the ECG. This occurs when an electrical stimulus causes an increase in sodium permeability and allows an influx of sodium into the cell.

There are four phases to repolarization. The earliest phase of recovery—**phase 1**—proceeds quickly to the plateau portion of the action potential—**phase 2**—corresponding to the QT interval. **Phase 3** is related to the T wave of the ECG. Repolarization is due to the efflux of potassium from the cell and the inactivation of the sodium and calcium channels. **Phase 4** is the time when the cell is at its resting membrane potential, between the end of the T wave and the beginning of the QRS complex.

Each portion of the conduction system has a specific type of action potential, designated either as fast or slow action potentials. The primary current for the fast action potentials is sodium movement, and for the slow channels, calcium. The sinus node and the arterioventricular node have slow action potentials. The atrium, His-Purkinje network, and the ventricle have fast action potentials.

2. Interpret the following 12-lead ECG.

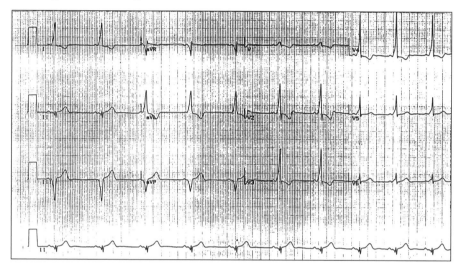

This tracing is a classic example of the **Wolff-Parkinson-White** (WPW) phenomenon. The ECG findings are a short P-R interval of ≤ 0.12 seconds, initial slurring of the QRS, and prolongation of the QRS. The slurring of the QRS—the delta wave—is caused by early depolarization of the portion of the ventricle due to an accessory pathway.

In the past, two patterns of WPW have been described: type A and type B. When aberrant conduction occurs down a left-sided accessory pathway, a pattern resembling right bundle branch block exists, and this is known as type A. With a right-sided accessory pathway, a pattern resembling left bundle branch block is seen and is known as type B. In patients with WPW, the atrial stimulus may conduct only through the normal pathway, down both pathways, or down the accessory pathway. Accessory atrioventricular (AV) connections may be capable of conduction in the retrograde direction only, and these are termed "concealed pathways," as there are no delta waves present on the ECG.

3. What are the mechanisms of reentry and of AV reentrant tachycardia?

Reentrant tachycardia can occur when there are two conduction pathways available which form a potentially circular path. If an unidirectional block is present in one pathway, and conduction time is slow enough over the nonblocked pathway to allow recovery time in the blocked pathway, this allows retrograde conduction over the previously blocked pathway.

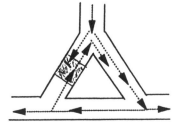

Requirements for a Reentry Circuit.
1. A potentially circular pathway
2. A zone of depressed conduction
3. An area of unidirectional block

Orthodromic AV reentrant tachycardia is the most frequent form of tachycardia that utilizes an accessory pathway (see figure below).

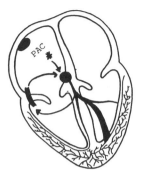

Orthodromic AV reentry.

This term refers to the propagation of an impulse down the normal AV conduction system and retrograde conduction over the accessory pathway back to the atrium. The QRS morphology is narrow, unless an underlying bundle branch block is present. This type of tachycardia can be initiated by either a premature atrial contraction (PAC) or premature ventricular contraction (PVC). **Antidromic tachycardia** uses the accessory pathway for anterograde conduction, with retrograde conduction through the normal ventricular to atrial (VA) conduction system. This pattern also can be started by either a PAC or PVC, and during the tachycardia, the QRS will be broad and often bizarre.

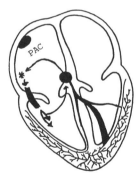
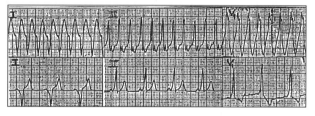

Antidromic AV reentry. Note the rhythm strip with the broad QRS, and after conversion, delta waves are present in the second strip.

4. What is the treatment of AV reentry tachycardia?

The first step in treatment is to determine if the patient is hemodynamically stable. If the patient is not stable, the first choice is synchronized cardioversion. If the patient is stable, the first choice is to increase vagal tone by carotid massage or Valsalva maneuver. The next step is to administer verapamil, 5–10 mg intravenously, or adenosine, 6 mg intravenously, followed by 12 mg if necessary. These measures can be repeated, if necessary, and followed by synchronized cardioversion if the rhythm persists or the patient becomes unstable.

5. Identify this patient's rhythm.

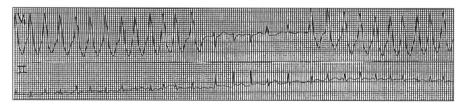

In this ECG, the rhythm is **atrial fibrillation** in a patient with an **AV accessory pathway**. The normal and abnormal QRS complexes indicate two possible pathways for conduction. This combination of an irregular rhythm with narrow and wide QRS complexes is virtually diagnostic of atrial fibrillation with preexcitation. It is important to recognize this pattern, as the treatment differs from that for a patient with atrial fibrillation without preexcitation. Lead II is uninformative in this ECG and demonstrates the importance of multiple ECG lead analysis.

6. What is the treatment of atrial fibrillation with preexcitation?

In the usual patient with atrial fibrillation, digitalis is often used to decrease the number of stimuli that are conducted through the AV node. However, in Wolff-Parkinson-White, digitalis may increase the conductivity of the accessory pathway and lead to ventricular fibrillation. Beta-adrenergic blockers prolong conduction time and increase the refractoriness in the AV node; however, they do not terminate AV reentry tachycardia and can cause profound hypotension. Although calcium channel blockers can terminate orthodromic AV reentry, they are dangerous during atrial fibrillation because they can increase the ventricular rate by increasing the number of preexcited ventricular complexes. The use of adenosine in these patients is controversial, because adenosine can terminate reentrant supraventricular arrhythmias involving the AV node. However, the drug can also cause increased conduction through the accessory pathway, possibly leading to ventricular fibrillation. The recommended treatment for atrial fibrillation with an accessory pathway in a hemodynamically stable patient is **procainamide**, 50 mg/min intravenously, to a total dose of 10 mg/kg. If the patient is hemodynamically unstable, the treatment is **synchronized cardioversion**.

7. Discuss the anesthetic considerations for patients with preexcitation syndromes.

Adequate suppression of the sympathetic response is the key to avoiding these potentially serious arrhythmias. **Halothane** is a poor choice for a volatile anesthetic because it sensitizes the myocardium to catecholamines. It also has the least effect on refractoriness. **Droperidol** depresses accessory pathway conduction and may prevent the rapid ventricular response during AV reentrant tachycardia. **Opiates** and **barbiturates** have no proven electrophysiologic effect on accessory pathways. **Pancuronium** enhances AV conduction and is contraindicated.

8. What is the differential diagnosis for the following 12-lead ECG?

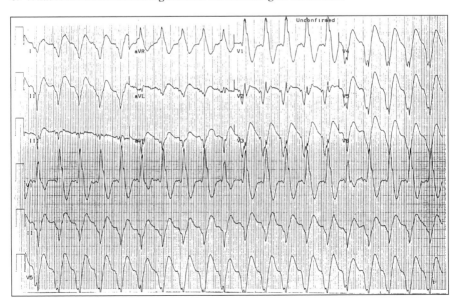

The differential diagnosis of a **wide complex tachycardia** includes ventricular tachycardia, supraventricular tachycardia with aberrant conduction, supraventricular tachycardia with a preexisting bundle branch block, or antidromic AV reentrant tachycardia.

9. What is the interpretation of the preceding ECG?

Determining the etiology of a wide complex tachycardia is often difficult. The following criteria can be seen in the ECG in question 8, supporting the diagnosis of **ventricular tachycardia**:

1. QRS duration > 0.14 seconds
2. Axis: quadrant III (negative in lead I, negative in lead aVF)
3. AV dissociation
4. VA association (ventricular to atrial conduction)
5. Morphology is unlike the pattern of right or left bundle branch block
6. Concordance: QRS complexes in all precordial leads are positive or negative

10. What is Brugada's rule?

Brugada et al. addressed the difficulty of interpreting wide complex tachycardias. They measured the interval from the onset of the R wave to the deepest part of the S wave in all tachycardias showing an RS complex in at least one precordial lead. An RS interval of > 100 msec was consistent with ventricular tachycardia. **The absence of an RS complex in all precordial leads or an RS interval > 100 msec was 100% specific for ventricular tachycardia** in their study. The ECG in question 8 illustrates the absence of RS complexes in all precordial leads.

11. What is a fusion beat?

A fusion beat occurs when there is activation of the ventricle from an atrial stimulus and from a ventricular focus simultaneously. This beat has a morphology intermediate between the normal beat and ventricular complex and identifies **AV dissociation**.

12. What is a Dressler beat?

A Dressler beat also indicates AV dissociation—a "capture beat." It occurs when there is a normal QRS due to ventricular activation from an atrial stimulus. If these beats are present during a wide complex tachycardia, the diagnosis is ventricular tachycardia. Fusion (F) and capture (C) beats are demonstrated in this ECG strip.

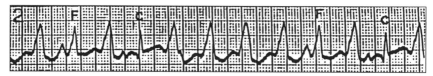

ECG courtesy of Dr. Henry J.L. Marriott.

13. Interpret the following ECG.

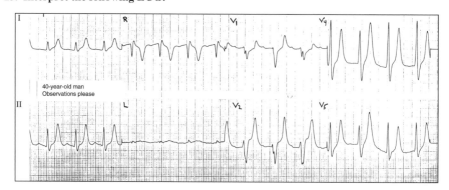

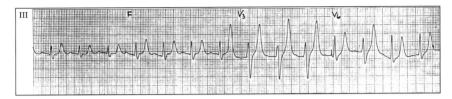

This ECG reveals the characteristic findings of **hyperkalemia**. Hyperkalemia causes a decrease in the resting membrane potential, therefore making the potential less negative. There is a decrease in the velocity of phase 0, leading to slowing of intraventricular conduction and a variable widening of the QRS on ECG. Hyperkalemia also causes acceleration of repolarization by increasing the steepness of the slope of phase 3. This is caused by increased membrane permeability to potassium and accounts for the tall and peaked T waves that are characteristic of hyperkalemia. This ECG was obtained in a 40-year-old man with diabetic ketoacidosis with a potassium concentration of 7.8 mmol/L. Note the prolonged PR interval, moderate increase in QRS duration, and marked increase in T-wave amplitude.

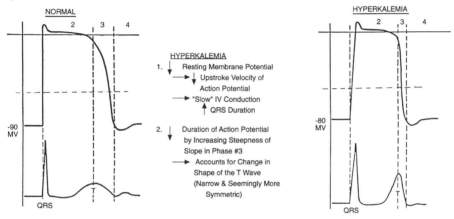

Effects of hyperkalemia on the action potential.

14. Describe the electrophysiologic changes that occur with hypokalemia.

Hypokalemia causes an increase in the resting membrane potential and an increase in the duration of the action potential (see figure on following page). Phase 3 increases in duration, prolonging repolarization. A decrease in phase 2 and the increase in phase 3 cause shortening of the ST segment, flattened T waves, and the appearance of a U wave. The QRS may widen if hypokalemia is severe. The height of the P wave may be increased and the PR segment prolonged. ECG below reveals a U wave in a patient with an aldosterone-secreting tumor and a potassium level of 1.8 mmol/L.

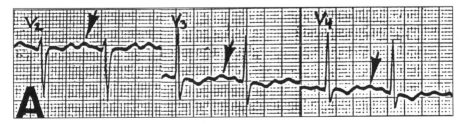

HYPOKALEMIA

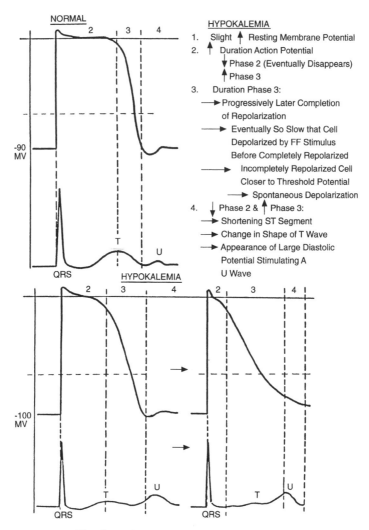

The effects of hypokalemia on the action potential.

15. What electrolyte abnormality is detected on this ECG strip?

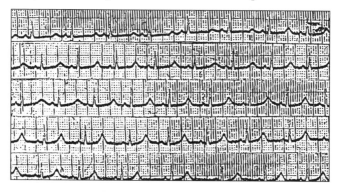

This ECG reveals a prolonged QT interval, primarily affecting the interval between the beginning of the QRS and the onset of the T wave. **Hypocalcemia** results in such prolongation. During the preceding rhythm strip, the QT normalizes as calcium is being administered.

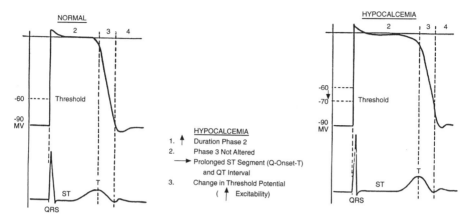

16. Describe the causes of QT prolongation.
The causes of a prolonged QT can be grouped as either congenital or acquired. The acquired causes can be due to **antiarrhythmic drugs** that prolong repolarization, such as quinidine, procainamide, sotolol, and amiodarone. Other offending drugs include phenothiazines, tricyclic antidepressants, and lithium. **Electrolyte imbalances** can result in QT prolongation, particularly hypokalemia, hypomagnesemia, and hypocalcemia. **Central nervous system disturbances**, such as subarachnoid or intracerebral hemorrhage, head trauma, and cerebral tumors, may cause marked repolarization abnormalities. **Myocarditis** and **myocardial ischemia** are additional causes.

17. What arrhythmia can occur with prolonged QT syndrome?
The arrhythmia associated with this syndrome is torsade de pointes. It is initiated by a ventricular beat in the setting of prolonged ventricular repolarization. This arrhythmia frequently spontaneously resolves, but it can lead to ventricular fibrillation.

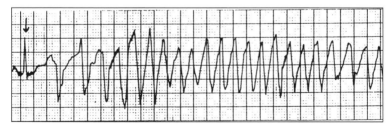

An example of torsade de pointes. A single sinus beat (arrow) is followed by ventricular tachycardia with an oscillating or swinging pattern of the QRS complexes.

ACKNOWLEDGMENT

The author thanks Dr. William P. Nelson, Saint Joseph's Hospital, Denver, Colorado, for his assistance with this chapter and the use of his illustrations.

BIBLIOGRAPHY

1. Brugada P, Brugada J, Mont L, et al: A new approach to the differential diagnosis of a regular tachycardia with a wide QRS complex. Circulation 83:1649–1659, 1991.
2. Durakovie Z, Durakovie A, Kastelan A: The preexcitation syndrome: Epidemiological and genetic study. Int J Cardiol 35:181–186, 1992.
3. Exner DV, Muzyka T, Gillis AM: Proarrhythmia in patients with the Wolff-Parkinson-White syndrome after standard doses of intravenous adenosine. Ann Intern Med 122:351–352, 1995.
4. Gursoy S, Brugada R, Brugada J: Which ventricular tachycardia is dangerous? Clin Cardiol 15:43–44, 1992.
5. Kaplan JA: Cardiac Anesthesia, 3rd ed. Philadelphia, W.B. Saunders, 1993, pp 781–818.
6. Lowenstein SR, Harken AH: A wide, complex look at cardiac dysrhythmias. J Emerg Med 5:519–531, 1987.
7. Lubarsky D, Kaufman B, Turndorf H: Anesthesia unmasking benign Wolff-Parkinson-White syndrome. Anesth Analg 68:172–174, 1989.
8. Podrid PJ, Kowey PR: Cardiac Arrhythmia: Mechanisms, Diagnosis, and Management. Baltimore, Williams & Wilkins, 1995.
9. Prystowky EN: Diagnosis and management of the preexcitation syndromes. Curr Probl Cardiol 13:225–310, 1988.
10. Sager PT, Khandari AK: Wide complex tachycardias: Differential diagnosis and management. Cardiol Clin 9:595–640, 1991.
11. Sharpe MD, Dobkowski WB, Murken JM, et al: The electrophysiologic effects of volatile anesthetics and sufentanil on the normal atrioventricular conduction system and accessory pathways in Wolff-Parkinson-White syndrome. Anesthesiology 80:63–70, 1994.
12. Steurer G, Gursoy S, Frey B, et al: The differential diagnosis of the electrocardiogram between ventricular tachycardia and preexcited tachycardia. Clin Cardiol 17:306–308, 1994.
13. Surawicz B: Electrophysiologic Basis of ECG and Cardiac Arrhythmias. Baltimore, Williams & Wilkins, 1995.
14. Wolff L, Parkinson J, White PD: Bundle-branch block with short P-R interval in healthy young people prone to paroxysmal tachycardia. Am Heart J 5:685–704, 1930.
15. Wrenn K: Management strategies in wide QRS complex tachycardia. Am J Emerg Med 9:592–597, 1991.

37. TEMPERATURE MONITORING AND DISTURBANCES

John H. Yang, M.D.

1. What are acceptable sites for temperature monitoring?

Monitoring temperature is a standard of care in anesthesia. The site for monitoring temperature during anesthesia depends on the surgical procedure, type of anesthesia, and reason for temperature monitoring:

1. **Skin**—may not reflect core temperature (as much as 3–4°C lower).

2. **Axilla**—temperature monitored over the brachial artery with the arm adducted to the side is approximately 1°C below core.

3. **Rectum**—does not reflect rapid changes; rectal perforation is a rare complication.

4. **Esophagus**—a probe in the lower one-third of the esophagus accurately reflects core and blood temperature; combined with an esophageal stethoscope, the temperature probe is also useful for auscultation.

5. **Nasopharynx**—reflects brain temperature because of its proximity to the internal carotid artery; complications include nosebleed, especially if the patient is pregnant or has a coagulopathy; contraindicated in head trauma or with evidence of cerebrospinal fluid rhinorrhea.

6. **External auditory meatus**—because the tympanic membrane is in close proximity to the internal carotid artery, it reflects core temperature well; eardrum perforation is a possible complication.

7. **Bladder catheter**—approximates core temperature when urine flow is high.

8. **Pulmonary artery catheter**—an accurate measure of core temperature but expensive and invasive.

2. Define hypothermia.

Hypothermia is a clinical state of subnormal body temperature in which the body is unable to generate enough heat for bodily functions. A core temperature of 35°C (95°F) is the upper limit of hypothermia. Cold signals travel to the hypothalamus primarily via delta fibers traversing the spinothalamic tracts in the anterior spinal cord. Below this temperature shivering and autonomic and endocrinologic responses are unable to compensate completely without assisted warming.

3. How does anesthesia predispose to hypothermia?

Heat loss is common in all patients during general anesthesia, because anesthetics alter thermoregulation, prevent shivering, and produce peripheral vasodilation. Volatile anesthetics impair the thermoregulatory center in the hypothalamus and also have direct vasodilatory properties. Opioids reduce the vasoconstrictive mechanisms of heat conservation by their sympatholytic properties. Barbiturates cause peripheral vasodilation. Muscle relaxants reduce muscle tone and prevent shivering thermogenesis. Regional anesthesia also may produce sympathetic blockade, muscle relaxation, and sensory blockade of thermal receptors, thus inhibiting compensatory responses.

4. What are the clinical signs of hypothermia?

Shivering, decreased sweating, and vasoconstriction are early signs of hypothermia. If hypothermia is prolonged, patients may present with altered mental status and muscle weakness. Anesthetized patients behave as poikilotherms, reflecting the temperature of the external environment. Decreased motor activity is also an early manifestation of hypothermia.

The physiologic effects of hypothermia depend on the degree of temperature depression. With mild hypothermia (32–35°C, 90–95°F), one sees central nervous system (CNS) depression, decreased basal metabolic rate, tachycardia, and shivering. The patient also may have dysarthria, amnesia, ataxia, and apathy. Moderate hypothermia (27–32°C, 80–90°F) involves further depression in level of consciousness, mild depression of vital signs, arrhythmias, and cold diuresis. In severe hypothermia (< 27°C, 80°F), the patient may be comatose and areflexic and have significantly depressed vital signs.

5. Which patients are at risk for hypothermia?

Patients at risk include the elderly, who have reduced autonomic vascular control, and infants, who have a large surface area-to-mass ratio. Patients with burns, spinal cord injuries that involve autonomic dysfunction, and endocrine abnormalities are also at risk.

6. What is the function of shivering?

Shivering is the spontaneous, asynchronous, random contraction of skeletal muscles in an effort to increase the basal metabolic rate. Shivering is modulated through the hypothalamus and can increase the body's heat production by up to 300%. Shivering increases oxygen consumption and carbon dioxide production. This effect may be undesirable in the patient with coronary artery disease or pulmonary insufficiency.

Nonshivering thermogenesis increases metabolic heat production without producing mechanical work. Infants less than 3 months of age cannot shiver and mount a caloric response by nonshivering thermogenesis. Skeletal muscle and brown fat tissue are the major energy sources for this process, which does not occur in anesthetized adults.

7. What are the pathophysiologic effects of hypothermia?

1. **Vascular**—vasoconstriction leads to hypoperfusion of peripheral tissues and promotes tissue hypoxia. Systemic vascular resistance and central venous pressure are increased; the reliability of pulse oximetry and intrarterial pressure monitoring is decreased

2. **Cardiac**—shivering increases oxygen consumption by up to 300% and thus increases myocardial oxygen demand. As hypothermia worsens, heart rate, cardiac output, and oxygen consumption decrease. Later symptoms include ventricular arrhythmias and further myocardial depression.

3. **Pulmonary**—pulmonary vascular resistance increases and hypoxic pulmonary vasoconstriction decreases, resulting in increased ventilation/perfusion mismatch and hypoxemia. Ventilatory drive is depressed. Bronchomotor tone is diminished, thus increasing anatomic deadspace. The carbon dioxide content of blood (PCO_2) drops 50% per 8°C-decrease in temperature; thus there is little respiratory stimulus to breathe. In blood the carbon dioxide and oxygen solubility increase with cooling. The pH of arterial blood gases rises 0.015 units per centigrade decrease in temperature. The rule of thumb is that the body temperature in centigrade should approximate arterial carbon dioxide partial pressures ($PaCO_2$).

4. **Renal**—renal blood flow is decreased, glomerular filtration is reduced, and protein catabolism and diuresis are increased, with spilling of urinary nitrogen. Cold diuresis due to impaired sodium reabsorption may lead to hypovolemia. The ability to concentrate or dilute urine is decreased.

5. **Hepatic**—hepatic blood flow is decreased and the metabolic and excretory functions of the liver are diminished.

6. **Central nervous system**—cerebral blood flow is decreased, and cerebral vascular resistance is increased. Cerebral metabolic oxygen consumption decreases by 7% per centigrade decrease in temperature. Both motor and somatosensory evoked potential latencies are increased by hypothermia. At about 33°C sedation occurs, and at 30°C cold narcosis results. The minimal alveolar concentration (MAC) of volatile agents is decreased, resulting in delayed emergence, drowsiness, and confusion.

7. **Hematologic**—decreased platelet function, visceral sequestration, and platelet aggregation result in thrombocytopenia. Activity of clotting factors is reduced, resulting in impaired coagulation, whereas fibrinolysis is increased. Leukocytes are also sequestered. Blood viscosity increases about 3% with each centigrade decrease in temperature. Increases in hematocrit (2–3% per centigrade decrease in temperature) are associated with rouleaux formation. The oxygen-hemoglobin dissociation curve shifts to the left, and hemoglobin affinity for oxygen increases 6% per centigrade decrease in temperature. Plasma volume decreases 25% for each 11°C decrease because of cold diuresis and impaired sodium resorption.

8. **Metabolic**—the basal metabolic rate and tissue perfusion decrease, leading to metabolic acidosis. Acute hyperkalemia is a risk with rewarming. Moderate hyperglycemia may result from the catecholamine response, decreased insulin levels, and decreased insulin responsiveness. Oxygen consumption and carbon dioxide production decrease by 8% per centigrade decrease in temperature.

9. **Intraocular pressure**—decreases because of a decrease in aqueous humor production and vasoconstriction.

10. **Healing**—hypothermia may contribute to wound infection by directly impairing the immune system and by triggering thermoregulatory vasoconstriction that reduces oxygen delivery to the wound.

8. Describe the electrocardiographic (ECG) manifestations of hypothermia.

Mild hypothermia may be associated only with sinus bradycardia. Moderate hypothermia may result in prolonged PR intervals, widened QRS complexes, and a prolonged QT interval. Below 32°C an elevation of the junction of the QRS and ST segments known as the hypothermic hump or Osborne or J wave may be seen. Its size increases with decreasing body temperature; it usually is seen in leads II and V6 and may spread to leads V3 and V4. The J wave is not specific for hypothermia; it also may be seen in hypothalamic lesions and cardiac ischemia. Nodal rhythms are common below 30°C. Below 28°C, premature ventricular contractions, atrioventricular blocks, and spontaneous atrial or ventricular fibrillation also occur. Ventricular fibrillation or asystole below 28°C is relatively unresponsive to atropine, countershock, or pacing. Resuscitative efforts should persist until the patient is rewarmed.

9. What are the pharmacologic effects of hypothermia?

Drug effects are prolonged by decreased hepatic blood flow and metabolism and decreased renal blood flow and clearance. Protein binding increases as body temperature decreases. The MAC of inhalational agents is decreased about 5–7% per centigrade decrease in core temperature, but decreased cardiac output and increased blood solubility result in no change in speed of inhalational induction. Hypothermia may prolong the duration of neuromuscular blocking agents because of decreased metabolism. Monitoring of neuromuscular function may also be impaired. Hypothermia delays discharge from the postanesthetic care unit and may prolong the need for mechanical ventilation.

10. Describe the major mechanisms of heat loss.

1. **Radiation** (i.e., dissipation of heat to cooler surroundings) accounts for about 60% of heat loss, depending on cutaneous blood flow and exposed body surface area.

2. **Evaporation** accounts for 20% of heat loss due to the latent heat of vaporization, which is the energy required to vaporize liquid from serosal and mucosal surfaces. Evaporation depends on exposed surface area and the relative humidity of ambient air.

3. **Convection** is responsible for about 15% of heat loss and depends on the air flow over exposed surfaces.

4. **Conduction** depends upon the transfer of heat between adjacent surfaces and accounts for about 5% of the total heat loss. The degree of loss is a function of the temperature gradient and thermal conductivity.

11. What are the major causes of heat loss in the operating room?

Cool rooms, cold intravenous and prepping solutions, and exposure of the patient contribute significantly to hypothermia. One unit of refrigerated blood or 1 liter of room-temperature crystalloid decreases the body temperature about 0.25°C. Cutaneous heat loss is proportional to exposed surface area and accounts for 90% of heat loss. General anesthetics cause vasodilation and decrease heat production. In addition, loss of hypothalamic responsiveness due to volatile anesthetics results in the inability to mount a caloric response to decreasing body temperature. Neuromuscular blocking agents prevent muscle heat production by shivering. Less than 10% of heat loss is through the respiratory tract.

12. What disease processes are associated with hypothermia?

Hypothyroidism and hypothalamic lesions may predispose a patient to intraoperative hypothermia. Difficulty in maintaining normothermia during general anesthesia is age-related. The elderly and the very young are at increased risk of hypothermia because of poor temperature regulation. The basal metabolic rate declines by approximately 1% per year after age 30. Infants also may become hypothermic more easily because of their decreased ability to shiver.

13. Discuss methods of rewarming.

Passive rewarming uses the body's ability to provide necessary heat if continued heat loss is minimized by covering exposed areas. Because passive rewarming relies on shivering thermogenesis, hypothalamic mechanisms must be intact and sufficient glycogen stores must be available.

Active rewarming involves methods readily available in the operating room, including the administration of warmed intravenous fluids and use of radiant heat lamps and warming blankets, especially those that blow warm air over body surfaces. Airway rewarming is less effective, because the heat content of gases is poor. Heated irrigation fluids administered by peritoneal lavage or bladder instillation and extracorporal rewarming with cardiopulmonary bypass may be required. A core temperature afterdrop (a secondary decline in core temperature with rewarming) may result from the return of cold blood from the periphery.

14. Describe ways to prevent hypothermia in the surgical patient.

Operating rooms are commonly cool. Use of a passive heat and moisture exchanger (artificial nose) is beneficial. Humidification of respiratory gases is important to prevent airway drying and to maintain normal ciliary function, but it is not a major method of rewarming. Other steps include the following:

1. Raise the ambient temperature in the operating room; all patients become hypothermic at common operating room temperatures.

2. Cover exposed areas to minimize conductive and convective losses.

3. Use intravenous fluid warmers when administering intravenous fluids and transfusing blood. Depending on the rate of infusion, fluids may be warmed up to 40–42°C.

4. Use heated humidifiers to the anesthetic circuit to minimize evaporative losses and to warm compressed gases.

5. Maintain closed or low-flow semiclosed circuits to decrease evaporative losses and conserve anesthetic vapors.

6. Use warming blankets for conductive transfer of heat.

7. Use radiant warmers and heat lamps, especially in pediatric patients, who have a high surface area-to-weight ratio and cannot mount a caloric response.

8. Irrigate with warm solutions if possible.

15. Define hyperthermia.

Hyperthermia is a rise in body temperature of 2°C per hour. Because it is uncommon in the operating room, its cause must be investigated. The usual cause is sepsis or fever secondary to the stress of surgery. Hypothalamic lesions and hyperthyroidism are less common. Malignant hyperthermia, catecholamine surges, and production of bacteremia in the course of surgery may elevate body temperature. Occasionally overly vigorous warming techniques, usually in peripheral surgical procedures, may be responsible.

16. Describe the manifestations of hyperthermia.

The awake patient may manifest general malaise, nausea, lightheadedness, and tachycardia, accompanied by sweating, vasodilation, and increased basal metabolic rate. With prolonged hyperthermia the patient may exhibit symptoms of heat exhaustion or even heat stroke. In the anesthetized patient signs and symptoms include tachycardia, hypertension, increased end-tidal carbon dioxide, increased drug metabolism, and possibly dehydration, as suggested by a decline in urine output and decreased skin turgor. Hyperthermia is a hypermetabolic state with increased oxygen consumption, increased minute ventilation, sweating, and vasodilation. Intravascular volume and venous return are decreased. Heart rate increases by 10 bpm per centigrade increase in temperature.

17. What is heat exhaustion?

Heat exhaustion is a syndrome of volume depletion and heat stress that results in mild hyperpyrexia, somatic complaints (nausea, vomiting, and lightheadedness), and signs of dehydration, but mental status is unaltered. Active cooling of the patient is therapeutic, and the prognosis is good because major organ systems are minimally affected.

18. Define heat stroke.

Heat stroke is defined as body temperature above 40°C or 106°F with associated changes in mental status. The body's mechanisms for heat dissipation are overwhelmed at this point. Thermoregulatory mechanisms cannot overcome the exogenous heat stress, and the patient is at risk for multisystem organ failure.

19. What conditions are associated with hyperthermia?

1. Malignant hyperthermia is a possible cause in patients with a genetic predisposition. However, it may manifest initially as tachycardia, hypercapnia, muscle rigidity, tachyarrhythmias, ventilatory difficulties, and metabolic acidosis. Treatment consists of discontinuing triggering agents, administering dantrolene, cooling the patient, and ensuring adequate renal output. Blood gases should be checked and metabolic acidosis corrected.
2. Hypermetabolic states, including sepsis, infection (endogenous pyrogens), thyrotoxicosis (thyroid storm), and pheochromocytoma
3. Hypothalamic lesions secondary to trauma, anoxia, or tumor
4. Neuroleptic malignant syndrome
5. Transfusion reaction
6. Medications

20. Do any drugs increase the risk of hyperthermia?

Sympathomimetic drugs, monoamine oxidase inhibitors, cocaine, amphetamines, and tricyclic antidepressants increase the basal metabolic rate and heat production. Anticholinergics may elevate temperature by unopposed vasodilation and suppression of sweating. Antihistamines likewise decrease sweating.

21. What are the pharmacologic effects of hyperthermia?

Increases in basal metabolic rate and hepatic metabolism decrease the half-life of anesthetic drugs. Anesthetic requirements may be increased.

22. What is the treatment for the hyperthermic patient in the operating room?

Exposure of skin surfaces is helpful, as are cooling blankets and cool intravenous fluids. Administration of antipyretics is prudent. Vasodilators may increase conductive heat loss. Correctible causes of hyperpyrexia should be ruled out.

23. Discuss ways to prevent hyperthermia in the surgical patient.
Rarely a problem in the operating room, any patient who comes to surgery with an elevated body temperature should be monitored closely and the cause of the hyperthermia determined. Surgery should be postponed if the fever cannot be controlled and the temperature is a threat to organ system functions, unless the procedure is directed at the cause of the temperature elevation.

BIBLIOGRAPHY

1. Danzl DF: Hypothermia outcome score: Development and implications. Crit Care Med 17:227-231, 1989.
2. Davison JK: Clinical Anesthesia Procedures of the Massachusetts General Hospital, 4th ed. Boston, Little, Brown, 1993, pp 130–131, 256–259, 539–540.
3. Frank SM: Epidural vs. general anesthesia: Ambient operating room temperature and patient age as predictors of inadvertant hypothermia. Anesthesiology 77:252–257, 1992.
4. Kramer MR: Mortality in elderly patients with thermoregulatory failure. Arch Intern Med 149:1521–1523, 1989.
5. Lockwood SA: Physiologic and metabolic effects of hypothermia. In Faust RJ (ed): Anesthesiology Review, 2nd ed. New York, Churchill Livingstone, 1994, pp 82–83.
6. Mecca RS: Postoperative recovery. In Barash PG, Cullen BF, Stoelting RK (eds): Clinical Anesthesia, 2nd ed. Philadelphia, J.P. Lippincott, 1992, pp 1538–1539.
7. McMahon JC: Hypothermia and perioperative temperature control. In Faust RJ (ed): Anesthesiology Review, 2nd ed. New York, Churchill Livingstone, 1994, pp 84–85.
8. Sessler DI: Physiologic responses to mild perianesthetic hypothermia in humans. Anesthesiology 75:594–610, 1991.
9. Sessler DI: Skin surface warming: Heat flux and central temperature. Anesthesiology 73:218–224, 1990.
10. Sessler DI: Temperature monitoring. In Miller RD (ed): Anesthesia, 4th ed. New York, Churchill Livingstone, 1994, pp 1363–1382.
11. Solomon A: The electrocardiographic features of hypothermia. J Emerg Med 7:169–173, 1989.
12. Slotman GJ: Adverse effects of hypothermia in postoperative patients. Am J Surg 149:495–501, 1985.
13. Stoelting RK, Miller RD: Basics of Anesthesia, 3rd ed. New York, Churchill Livingstone, 1994, pp 207–208, 434, 496.
14. Zoll RH: Temperature monitoring. In Ehrenwerth J, Eisenkraft JB (eds): Anesthesia Equipment: Principles and Applications. St. Louis, Mosby, 1993, pp 264–273.

38. POSTANESTHETIC CARE AND COMPLICATIONS

Roger A. Mattison, M.D.

1. Which patients should be cared for in the postanesthetic care unit (PACU)?
Following anesthesia and surgery, perioperative care should be continued in the PACU for all patients who are likely to require a period of physiologic stabilization. However, a mandatory period of high-intensity care for every postoperative patient is an obsolete requirement. PACU care is generally divided into phase 1, during which monitoring and staffing ratios are equivalent to an intensive care unit (ICU), and phase 2, during which a transition is made from intensive observation to stabilization for care on a surgical ward or at home. Most patients who receive general anesthesia recover initially in phase 1, whereas after regional anesthesia or monitored anesthesia care only phase 2 may be required. However, preexisting disease, surgical procedure, and pharmacologic implications of the perioperative anesthetic agents ultimately determine the most appropriate sequence of postoperative care for each patient. Alterations in preoperative status during postoperative recovery are often more intense but usually shorter in duration than alterations caused by systemic illness.

2. How long should a patient stay in the PACU?
No specific period is required for PACU care. On admission to the PACU a report is given by the anesthesiologist or anesthetist to the PACU nurse about the patient's prior health status, surgical procedure, intraoperative events, and anesthetic course. This report guides the planning of the type and duration of observations in the PACU. Anesthetic technique, choice of agents, administration of intraoperative opioids and sedatives, and type and reversal of neuromuscular blocking agents should be included in the report. Initial assessment of the patient by the PACU nurse includes baseline determinations of responsiveness, ventilation, pain, and hemodynamic stability as well as vital signs. Initial PACU vital signs become the final entry on the intraoperative anesthetic record. Subsequent PACU nursing observations are recorded on a flow sheet. Various scoring systems have been used to allow numeric scoring of subjective observations as an indicator of progress toward discharge. The Aldrete scoring system tracks five observations: activity, respiratory effort, circulation, consciousness, and oxygenation. Scales for each are 0–2, and a total score of 8–10 indicates readiness to move to the next phase of care. Other important indicators of readiness for discharge from the PACU include regression of motor block in the case of regional anesthesia and absence of signs or symptoms that may indicate a change in previous health status.

The Aldrete Score

Activity	• Able to move four extremities	2
	• Able to move two extremities	1
	• Not able to move extremities voluntarily or on command	0
Respiration	• Able to breathe and cough	2
	• Dyspnea or limited breathing	1
	• Apneic	0
Circulation	• BP ± 20% of preanesthetic level	2
	• BP ± 21–49% of preanesthetic level	1
	• BP ± 50% of preanesthetic level	0

Table continued on following page.

The Aldrete Score (Cont.)

Consciousness	• Fully awake	2
	• Arousable on calling	1
	• Not responding	0
O_2 Saturation	• Maintain O_2 sat > 92% in room air	2
	• Needs O_2 to maintain O_2 sat > 90%	1
	• O_2 saturation < 90% with O_2 supplement	0

Modified from Aldrete AJ, Krovlik D: The postanesthetic recovery score. Anesth Analg 49:924–933, 1970, with permission.

3. What problems should be resolved during postanesthetic care?

1. Poor respiratory effort: the patient should be breathing easily and able to cough on command and oxygenate to preanesthesia levels.

2. Hemodynamic instability: blood pressure should be within 20% of preanesthetic measurements with stable heart rate and rhythm.

3. Attenuated sensorium: the patient should be fully awake and able to move all extremities voluntarily.

4. Postoperative pain: pain management should no longer require continuous nursing intervention.

4. How does use of muscle relaxants during surgery relate to poor respiratory effort?

Residual muscle weakness is immediately apparent in the PACU because of the effect on respiratory effort. An unresponsive patient appears "floppy" with poorly coordinated and ineffective abdominal and intercostal muscle activity. A patient who can verbalize complains that breathing is restricted and that efforts to deliver supplemental oxygen are suffocating. Although apparently willing to respond to commands, the patient is not able to sustain a head lift or hand grasp. In the worst case weakness of the pharyngeal muscles results in upper airway collapse and respiratory obstruction after extubation. Nether a good response to train-of-four testing in the operating room nor a report of spontaneous rhythmic ventilation before extubation rules out the presence of residual neuromuscular blockade. The clinical mismatch of the pharmacology of relaxant and reversal agents is termed "recurarization."

5. How do opioids and residual volatile anesthetics affect breathing?

Slow rhythmic breathing or apneic pauses in a patient who is hard to arouse indicate residual narcosis. In contrast to the patient with residual muscle relaxation, the narcotized patient often is unconcerned about ventilation despite obvious hypoxia. Because adequate degrees of analgesia and narcotic depression of ventilation are both dose-dependent, the patient may appear quite comfortable. Because narcosis slows ventilation, the route of elimination of inhalation agents is suppressed. The volatile anesthetic effect at clinical levels well below minimal alveolar concentration (MAC) reduces tidal volume and depresses respiratory effort. This synergism may cause significant postoperative hypoventilation.

6. How should these causes of hypoventilation be treated?

Hypoventilation due to residual neuromuscular blockade should be treated urgently and aggressively. Additional reversal agents may be given in divided doses up to the usual dose limitations. Cholinergic effects of reversal agents at the sinoatrial node may result in significant bradycardia and dictate incremental, titrating administration until reversal is satisfactory. Usually after failure of reversal in the operating room, a longer-duration reversal agent is chosen.

Treatment decisions for residual narcosis are not as readily apparent. Opioid antagonism for the sake of ventilatory support reverses adequate analgesia. The agonist/antagonist class of analgesic drugs seldom yields a net improvement in ventilation when used for reversal and may excessively obtund the patient without adding to analgesia. Usually, the best alternatives are ventilatory support with nasal or oral airway and continuous tactile and verbal stimulation until the shorter-duration opioid used in the operating room is sufficiently eliminated. Other supportive measures include increasing inspired oxygen concentrations (FiO_2) by switching from nasal cannula to mask.

Volatile anesthetic agents are eliminated through the lungs after transport from the central nervous system site of action. All of the agents in current use have low blood-gas partition coefficients and thus should be eliminated effectively in the PACU if minute ventilation is sufficient. In severe respiratory depression of any cause, reintubation and mechanical ventilation are reasonable interventions.

Ventilation Problems in the PACU

PROBLEM	SIGNS/SYMPTOMS	TREATMENT
Inadequate reversal of neuro-muscular block	Uncoordinated, ineffectual respiration effort	Neostigmine, 0.05 mg/kg intravenously
Narcosis	Slow ventilation, sedated or asleep	Respiratory support. Naloxone 0.04–0.40 mg intravenously
Residual inhalation anesthesia	Sleepy, shallow breathing	Encourage deep breathing, tactile stimulation

7. What other problems with ventilation should be considered in the PACU?

Whereas residual effects of the anesthetic drugs reduce respiratory effort, other intraoperative events interfere with ventilation in various ways. Aspiration of gastric contents or reactive airway disease leads to segmental bronchiolar obstruction resulting in wheezing, prolonged expiratory phase, and hypoxia. Bronchial foreign body and pneumothorax present with asymmetric breaths sounds and hypoxia but can be differentiated readily by postoperative chest radiography. Supraglottic obstruction may result in stridor and hypercarbia in excess of hypoxia. Rarely, in susceptible patients (poor cardiac output, compromised renal function, hypoproteinemia), fluid overload results in pulmonary edema with hypoxia. The common physiologic pathway for any of these difficulties is extreme ventilation-perfusion mismatch. The secondary physiologic effect is a hypertensive response to hypercarbia or hypoxia. Review of the operative procedure and the intraoperative anesthetic record will suggest possible etiologies. Past medical history of smoking, asthma, or chronic obstructive pulmonary disease are also important for the recognition of patients at higher risk for reactive small airway obstruction.

8. What is negative pressure pulmonary edema?

A phenomenon unique to the postextubation period and thus pertinent to the PACU is negative pressure pulmonary edema. Findings include coarse breath sounds and production of pink frothy sputum, as with other causes of pulmonary edema, but often hypoxia and hypertension precede the telltale physical signs. The cause of this phenomenon is the patient's vigorous ventilatory effort against a partially closed glottis or occasionally a small endotracheal tube. The clinical presentation follows a rapid emergence, often when the patient has been intoxicated at the time of induction. This phenomenon should be anticipated in young muscular individuals but may occur in any patient with some degree of laryngospasm after extubation. Often reversal of opioids has been required to achieve sufficient responsiveness for extubation. Chest radiographs confirm the presence of a normal-sized heart and rarely show any lung parenchymal changes corresponding to the degree of respiratory signs but may reveal alveolar infiltrates. The edema usually responds to supportive measures and minimal diuretic treatment.

9. Describe an orderly approach to treatment of respiratory emergencies in the PACU.

1. Supplemental oxygen plus measures to support airway patency:
   - Chin lift, neck extension, steady positive pressure ventilation by mask to overcome supraglottic obstruction.
   - Occasionally inhalation of nebulized epinephrine or intravenous steroid for mucosal swelling.

2. Subcutaneous or inhaled beta-adrenergic agonists (e.g., albuterol) are appropriate if respiratory difficulties are related to distal bronchoconstriction:
   • Inhaled route is less likely to exacerbate hypertension from other causes.
   • If bronchoconstriction is part of a full-blown anaphylactic episode, a more aggressive approach (beyond the scope of this chapter) is required.
3. Mechanical causes of lower airways obstruction should be vigorously sought out and treated. (Simple atelectasis, which is most common, is treated with supplemental oxygen; instructions to breathe deeply and cough are more appropriate than incentive spirometry in the PACU.)
4. Maximize treatment of postoperative pain.
5. Avoid treatment of hypertension and tachycardia with drugs until hypercarbia and hypoventilation are ruled out.

Predicted FiO_2 with Supplemental Oxygen Delivery

SYSTEM	DELIVERY FLOW	FiO_2 PREDICTED
Nasal cannula	2 L/min	0.28
Nasal cannula	4 L/min	0.36
Face mask	6 L/min	0.50
Partial rebreathing mask	6 L/min	0.6
Partial rebreathing mask	8 L/min	0.8

10. What other causes of hemodynamic alterations should be treated?

Several causes of tachycardia and hypertension require intervention but not drug treatment. Bladder distention, mild hypothermia, shivering, excitement, and errors of measurement are common and easily treated causes of postoperative hypertension. In many cases, blood pressure elevations up to 20% above baseline in the absence of symptoms will resolve without further treatment. Postoperative pain is a potent stimulus of heart rate and blood pressure which requires analgesic therapy. Tachyarrhythmias may reemerge in the presence of other postoperative events. In addition, preexisting hypertensive disease, clonidine withdrawal, or compromised myocardial or renal function that may be adversely affected by elevated blood pressure demand primary treatment by heart rate and blood pressure reduction.

Treatment options include beta-adrenergic blockade, calcium channel blockade, angiotensin-converting enzyme inhibitors, and direct vasodilator therapy. Direct vasodilator therapy is often chosen after craniotomy or coronary artery bypass grafting because of the concern for leakage or loss of hemostasis at the operative sites.

Treatment of Hypertension (Intravenous Preparations)

	BENEFIT	HAZARD	PREPARATION
Beta-adrenergic antagonist (cardioselective)	Short-acting preparation available; slows heart rate	Bradycardia, decreased contractility	Esmolol,* 0.3 mg/kg intravenous
			Labetalol, 5–50 mg/kg intravenous
Calcium channel blocker	Less effect on contractility	Not given as bolus	Nicardipine infusion, 0.1 mg/ml; up to 5 mg over 1 hour
Angiotensin-converting enzyme inhibitors	Least effect on contractility	Long-acting effects	Enalapril, 1.25–2.5 mg intravenous
Direct vasodilator	Infusion administration	Potent; requires continuous monitor	Sodium nitroprusside, 0.2–8 μg/kg/min

* Bolus may be followed by infusion.

11. What is the relationship between postanesthetic events and hypotension?

Emergence from inhalation anesthesia is characterized by decreasing vasodilation, increasing muscle tone, and increasing sympathetic tone, which usually results in an expansion of central blood volume and at least a temporary increase in blood pressure at the end of the operative procedure. As the patient is warmed and pain control is begun in the PACU, sympathetic tone is reduced and blood volume is redistributed to the periphery. In addition to these physiologic changes, the effects of surgical blood loss, third-space sequestration of fluid, ongoing hemorrhage and inadequate volume replacement in the operating room are manifested as hypotension. Less commonly, failure of the myocardial pump may present as hypotension. Dysrhythmia and preexisting ischemic heart disease may lead to pump failure. Sepsis or anaphylactic release of vasoactive mediators may result in expansion of peripheral capillary beds that exceeds cardiac output capacity and results in severe hypotension. Although such cases are rare, intervention must be swift and aggressive. Volume expansion is generally the first step in the resolution of hypotension in the PACU because rapid fluid administration treats most causes and provides the necessary first step before pressor therapy. Pressors may be given by bolus (ephedrine, phenylephrine, epinephrine) or by infusion (dopamine or epinephrine).

12. When should hypotension be treated?

Treatment of presumed hypovolemia should be initiated while other causes are evaluated. An indwelling urinary catheter is particularly useful in such circumstances to monitor urinary output. Reduced urine output may suggest poor renal perfusion even without hypovolemia. Electrocardiographic (ECG) monitoring may reveal irregularities of rhythm or ischemia, which can be confirmed with a diagnostic 12-lead ECG and compared with preoperative tracings. Signs and symptoms reveal early sepsis or anaphylaxis, both of which cause a relative hypotension by vasodilation. Such observations may help to direct continuing therapy but should not delay resuscitation. Elevation of lower extremities and Trendelenburg position transiently augment return of intravascular volume to the central compartment. Colloid or crystalloid can be given in 10–20 ml/kg doses initially while hematocrit is assessed to guide further volume replacement. In planning for volume repletion, the ultimate goal is delivery to tissues of sufficient oxygen to meet metabolic demands. In each patient, a target hematocrit should be determined with consideration of coexisting disease and coronary perfusion needs. Indications for administration of packed red blood cells are then readily apparent. Oxygen supplementation is always indicated.

13. Under what circumstances is a patient slow to awaken?

Most patients do not achieve a state of complete conscious awareness during the PACU stay because short-term memory function remains unreliable. However, they are said to be "awake" if they are capable of recalling preoperative details, stating orientation to time, place, and person, and responding to normal conversation. Minimal lapses are not generally considered deficits in awakening. Usually the diagnosis that a patient is slow to awaken in the PACU indicates failure to progress beyond demonstration of adequate airway protective reflexes and minimal conscious awareness. Some patients may make transient progress only to lapse to a lower level of consciousness.

The initial consideration in patients who are slow to awaken is that residual drug effects are depressing the sensorium. In patients who make no progress in level of consciousness, this is rarely the cause; other metabolic or catastrophic events altering cortical or subcortical brain function must be considered. Medical problems include intraoperative hypoxia or poor oxygen delivery due to anemia, central nervous system ischemia due to hypotension or coronary insufficiency, and embolic cerebrovascular occlusion. Hyponatremia, withdrawal from intoxication, hypoglycemia, and hyperglycemia with hyperosmolarity are readily predicted from clinical history and easily excluded. Postseizure stupor is harder to anticipate if the seizure occurs while the patient is anesthetized but may be anticipated from preoperative history. Hypoxic central nervous system injury is a significant concern in patients with a history of previous ischemic stroke or cerebrovascular insufficiency or after intraoperative hypotension or hypoxia. Review of the details of the conduct of the operative procedure is equally important to understand why a patient remains obtunded. Difficult clip placement on an intracerebral aneurysm with regional hypoperfusion; partial resection of cerebral arteriovenous malformation or supratentorial tumor causing subsequent brain swelling; and cardiopulmonary bypass with the possibility of embolism of particulate matter or air should be considered among the more likely causes of slow awakening.

14. When are aggressive evaluation and management of slow awakening necessary?

Patients who have had carotid endarterectomy or craniotomy require prompt radiographic (computerized tomography or angiography) evaluation if slow to awaken. Early in the postoperative course, surgically correctable causes of continuing coma such as increased intracranial pressure, intracranial hemorrhage, or major cerebral vascular occlusion cannot be distinguished by clinical examination in the PACU. Radiologic evaluation is necessary. Patients who awaken slowly over several hours to days but have no surgically correctable lesion usually have sustained some insult to the microcirculation to the brainstem and may make substantial recovery with time.

15. What is postoperative delirium?

Between the state of postanesthetic awakening and depressed consciousness, most patients pass briefly through a state of delirium in which responsiveness to commands is obtunded and primitive responses to pain, hypoxia, and disorientation predominate. If this state lasts more than a few minutes, the patient is said to suffer "emergence delirium." Adolescents and young adults seem to be more susceptible. Often the anesthetic course of such patients is no different from that in patients whose emergence is uneventful, but if specific drugs are implicated, they are usually atropine and opioids. Among the anticholinergics, atropine crosses the blood-brain barrier and may cause central nervous system stimulation. Similarly, the individual reaction to opioids may include a predominance of dysphoria. Abnormal neurologic signs are present in such patients, including Babinski reflex and abnormal pupillary responses. Usually the patient does not recall this phase of recovery accurately. If simply waiting for a better level of conscious awareness to emerge (and protecting the patient from self-injury) is not acceptable, physostigmine (0.5–2.0 mg by intravenous infusion) sometimes provides dramatic resolution of symptoms.

16. Why is pain management important in the PACU?

Problems with achieving adequate pain management are second only to problems of managing nausea and vomiting as causes of prolonged stay in the PACU. During the process of care nonspecific measures are directed to modulating the pain stimulus, including oxygen administration, rewarming, and verbal support and reassurance. Pain management with analgesic agents is a continuum of incremental analgesic administration weighed against individual respiratory and sedation responses to the analgesic agent. Nausea caused by analgesics is a limiting factor in pain treatment, but inadequately treated pain also may cause nausea. Initial pain management also may have implications in the longer-term recovery of postsurgical patients. Patients with inadequately managed pain are less able to participate in postoperative mobilization and physical therapy. Hospital stays in patients with inadequate analgesia may be longer. Ongoing pain interferes with the balance of autonomic influences on heart rate, leading to less heart rate variability and potential myocardial ischemia. An aggressive and carefully planned pain control regimen is critical to successful postoperative management plans.

17. How should analgesic drugs be selected for PACU use?

    1. Choose an analgesic agent that avoids previous allergies and adverse reactions.
       • Nausea with one opioid may predict similar reaction to others.
       • Documented allergic reaction may be avoided by choosing a structurally different drug.
    2. Avoid dose-dependent adverse reactions to opioids by adding nonsteroidal antiinflammatory drugs (NSAIDs) for nonnarcotic analgesia; consider epidural analgesia in the anesthetic plan.
    3. Substitute ketorolac for minimal-to-moderate pain if NSAID contraindications (compromised renal function, history of easy bleeding, previous peptic ulcer disease) are absent.

4. Coordinate initial analgesic with longer-range pain management modalities, such as patient controlled analgesia (PCA) or epidural infusion.

5. Consider whether the patient will be discharged to home postoperatively or remain an inpatient who can be given supplemental oxygen and more intense observation.

6. Review the patient's history for preoperative opioid use, which would predict greater tolerance and higher dosage limits for postoperative opioid analgesia.

18. Should ambulatory patients be treated differently in the PACU?

Postanesthetic care of the ambulatory patient is driven by the goal that the patient must be ready to be "on the street" after a period of recovery. Nausea and vomiting are treated aggressively, while avoiding drugs of the butyrophenone class (e.g., droperidol), which may be excessively sedating. Insofar as possible, pain should be treated with short-acting agents such as fentanyl. Nonnarcotic agents should be used whenever possible. Oral analgesics should be used in phase 2 recovery as prescribed for postoperative care. After regional anesthesia extremities should be protected while the patient is mobilized and ambulation should be assisted if transient segmental paresthesia makes movement unsteady. No ambulatory surgery patient should be discharged after any anesthetic, analgesic or sedative administration without a companion to ensure safe transportation to a place of residence.

19. What are safe guidelines for discharging a patient to home after ambulatory surgery?

By the time the patient arrives in phase 2, issues of cardiovascular stability, orientation and conscious awareness, and ventilation should be resolved. Resolution of postoperative nausea or pain may extend into phase 2, but the continued use of intravenous agents should rarely be required. Patients should be able to stand and to take a few steps (or to sit upright if the surgical procedure will not permit standing). They should sip fluids and urinate. They should be able to repeat postoperative management and follow-up instructions and to identify their escort home (allowing for baseline cognitive function). Prescriptions for postoperative care at home should be provided to patients in phase 2 recovery so that a separate pharmacy stop is not required. Conditions that require further intervention after discharge should be manageable with oral therapy. Finally, the patient and any companions should be provided with telephone number(s) for contacting health care providers at the facility if any untoward postoperative events occur. It is good practice to plan on a follow-up telephone call from the ambulatory PACU to the patient 24 hours after discharge to review postoperative progress and satisfaction.

BIBLIOGRAPHY

1. Aldrete AJ, Krovlik D: The postanesthetic recovery score. Anesth Analg 49:924–933, 1970.
2. Bellati RG Jr: Common post anesthesia problems. In Vendor JS, Speiss BD (eds): Post Anesthesia Care. Philadelphia, W.B. Saunders, 1992, pp 9–20.
3. Don H: Hypoxemia and hypercapnia during and after anesthesia. In Orkin EK, Cooperman LH (eds): Complications in Anesthesiology. Philadelphia, J.B. Lippincott, 1983, pp 191–194, 200–202.
4. Malley RA: Delayed return to consciousness. In Frust EAM, Galdiner PL (eds): Postanesthetic Care. Norwalk, CT, Appleton & Lange, 1990, pp 9–16.
5. Marymount JH, O'Connor BS: Postoperative cardiovascular complications. In Vendor JS, Spiess BD (eds): Post Anesthesia Care. Philadelphia, W.B. Saunders, 1992, pp 25–33.
6. Rosenberg H: Postoperative emotional responses. In Orkin EK, Cooperman LH (eds): Complications in Anesthesiology. Philadelphia, J.B. Lippincott, 1983, pp 355–361.
7. Wetchler BV: Problem solving in the postanesthesia care unit. In Wetchler BV (ed): Anesthesia for Ambulatory Surgery, 2nd ed. Philadelphia, J.B. Lippincott, 1990, pp 400–410.

VI. Anesthesia and Systemic Disease

39. ISCHEMIC HEART DISEASE AND MYOCARDIAL INFARCTION

Richard B. Allen, M.D.

1. How common is ischemic heart disease in the United States?
Ten million Americans currently have ischemic heart disease (IHD), which causes approximately 500,000 deaths annually. Of the 25 million patients undergoing surgical procedures each year, 7 million are at high risk for the presence of IHD. Over 50,000 patients suffer a perioperative myocardial infarction annually with a mortality rate approaching 50%. Efforts to identify patients with IHD and optimize their perioperative care are vital.

2. Name the known risk factors for the development of IHD.
Age, male gender, positive family history, hypertension, smoking, hypercholesterolemia and diabetes mellitus. Sedentary lifestyle and obesity are often associated factors.

3. Explain the determinants of myocardial oxygen supply and demand.
   Oxygen (O_2) supply to the myocardium is determined by oxygen content and coronary blood flow. Oxygen content can be calculated by the following equation:

$$O_2 \text{ content} = [1.39 \text{ ml } O_2/\text{gm of hemoglobin} \times \text{hemoglobin (gm/dl)} \times \% \text{ saturation}] + [0.003 \times PaO_2]$$

Coronary blood flow occurs mainly during diastole, especially in the ventricular endocardium. Coronary perfusion pressure is determined by the difference between diastolic blood pressure and left ventricular end-diastolic pressure (LVEDP). Anemia, hypoxemia, tachycardia, diastolic hypotension, hypocapnia (coronary vasoconstriction), coronary occlusion (IHD), vasospasm, increased LVEDP, and hypertrophied myocardium all may adversely affect myocardial O_2 supply.
   Myocardial O_2 demand is determined by heart rate, contractility, and wall tension. Increases in heart rate increase myocardial work as well as decrease the relative time spent in diastole (decreased supply). Contractility increases in response to sympathetic stimulation which increases O_2 demand. Wall tension is the product of intraventricular pressure and radius. Increased ventricular volume (preload) and increased blood pressure (afterload) both increase wall tension and O_2 demand.

4. What is the pathophysiology of ischemia?
Normal coronary vasculature vasodilates to increase blood flow in the setting of increased myocardial O_2 demand. Ischemia occurs when coronary blood flow is inadequate to meet the needs of the myocardium, usually due to atherosclerotic stenosis of one or more coronary arteries which decreases oxygen delivery distal to the occlusion. Lesions that occlude 50–75% of the vessel lumen are considered hemodynamically significant. Nonstenotic causes of ischemia include aortic valve disease, left ventricular hypertrophy, ostial occlusion, coronary embolism, coronary arteritis, and vasospasm.
   The right coronary artery system is dominant in 80–90% of people and supplies the sinoatrial node, atrioventricular node, and right ventricle. Right-sided coronary artery disease often

manifests as heart block and dysrhythmias. The left main coronary artery gives rise to the circumflex artery and left anterior descending artery, which supply the majority of the interventricular septum and left ventricular wall. Significant stenosis of the left main coronary artery (left main disease) or the proximal circumflex and left anterior descending arteries (left main equivalent) may cause severely depressed myocardial function during ischemia.

5. Describe the pathogenesis of a perioperative myocardial infarction.
A myocardial infarction (MI) is usually caused by platelet aggregation, vasoconstriction, and thrombus formation at the site of an atheromatous plaque in a coronary artery. Sudden increases in myocardial O_2 demand (tachycardia, hypertension) or decreases in O_2 supply (hypotension, hypoxemia, anemia), as can occur in the perioperative period, can precipitate MI in patients with IHD. Necrosis of the myocardium occurs quickly in the absence of blood flow. Complications of MI include dysrhythmias, hypotension, shock, congestive heart failure, acute mitral regurgitation, pericarditis, ventricular thrombus formation, ventricular rupture, and death.

6. What clinical factors increase the risk of a perioperative MI following noncardiac surgery?
Ischemic heart disease (prior MI or angina) and congestive heart failure are historically the strongest predictors of an increased risk for perioperative MI. Other risk factors include valvular heart disease (particularly aortic stenosis), arrhythmias due to underlying heart disease, advanced age, type of surgical procedure, and poor general medical status. Hypertension alone does not place a patient at increased risk for perioperative MI, but these patients are at increased risk for IHD, congestive heart failure, and stroke.

7. How can cardiac function be evaluated on history and physical examination?
If a patient's exercise capacity is excellent, even in the presence of IHD, then chances are good that the patient will be able to tolerate the stresses of surgery. Poor exercise tolerance in the absence of pulmonary or other systemic disease indicates an inadequate cardiac reserve. All patients should be questioned about their ability to perform daily activities, such as cleaning, yard work, shopping, and golfing, for example. The ability to climb two to three flights of stairs without significant symptoms (angina, dyspnea, syncope) is usually an indication of adequate cardiac reserve. Signs and symptoms of congestive heart failure including dyspnea, orthopnea, paroxysmal nocturnal dyspnea, peripheral edema, jugular venous distension, a third heart sound, rales, and hepatomegaly must be recognized preoperatively.

8. What is the significance of a history of angina pectoris?
Angina is the symptom of myocardial ischemia, and nearly all patients with angina have coronary artery disease. Stable angina is defined as no change in the onset, severity, and duration of chest pain for at least 60 days. Syncope, shortness of breath, or dizziness that accompanies angina may indicate severe myocardial dysfunction due to ischemia. Patients with unstable angina are at high risk for developing a MI and should be referred for medical evaluation immediately. Patients with diabetes mellitus and hypertension have a much higher incidence of ischemia without angina (silent ischemia or silent MI) and should be evaluated with a high index of suspicion. Perioperatively, most ischemic episodes are silent (as determined by ambulatory and postoperative ECG) but probably significant in the final outcome of surgery.

9. Should all cardiac medications be continued throughout the perioperative period?
Patients with a history of IHD are usually taking medications intended to decrease myocardial oxygen demand by decreasing the heart rate, preload, or contractile state (beta-blockers, calcium channel antagonists, nitrates) and to increase the oxygen supply by causing coronary vasodilation (nitrates). These drugs are generally continued throughout the perioperative period. Abrupt withdrawal of beta-blockers can cause rebound increases in heart rate and blood pressure. Calcium channel blockers can exaggerate the myocardial depressant effects of inhaled anesthetics but

should be continued perioperatively. Digoxin has a relatively long half-life and may need to be discontinued 24 hours preoperatively if there is a risk that hypokalemia could occur causing digitalis toxicity (cardiopulmonary bypass, diuretics).

10. What ECG findings support the diagnosis of IHD?
The resting 12-lead ECG remains a low cost, effective screening tool in the detection of IHD. It should be evaluated for the presence of ST-segment depression or elevation, T wave inversion, old MI as demonstrated by Q waves, disturbances in conduction and rhythm, and left ventricular hypertrophy. Ischemic changes in leads II, III, and aVF suggest right coronary artery disease, leads I and aVL monitor the circumflex artery distribution, and leads V3 to V5 look at the distribution of the left anterior desending artery. Poor progression of anterior forces suggests significant left ventricular dysfunction, possibly related to IHD.

11. What tests performed by medical consultants can help further evaluate patients with known or suspected IHD?
Exercise ECG is a noninvasive test, tthat attempts to produce ischemic changes on ECG (ST depression ≥ 1 mm from baseline) or symptoms suggestive of IHD by having the patient exercise to maximum capacity. Information obtained relates to the thresholds of heart rate and blood pressure that can be tolerated. A decrease in blood pressure or syncope during testing are ominous signs of poor dynamic myocardial function.

Exercise thallium scintigraphy increases the sensitivity and specificity of the exercise ECG. The isotope thallium is almost completely taken up from the coronary circulation by the myocardium and can then be visualized radiographically. Poorly perfused areas that later refill with contrast delineate areas of myocardium at risk for ischemia. Fixed perfusion defects indicate infarcted myocardium.

Dipyridamole thallium imaging is useful in patients who are unable to exercise. This testing is frequently required in patients with peripheral vascular disease who are at high risk for IHD and limited by claudication. Dipyridamole is a potent coronary vasodilator that causes differential flow between normal and diseased coronary arteries detectable by thallium imaging.

Echocardiography can be used to evaluate left ventricular and valvular function and to measure ejection fraction. Stress echocardiography (dobutamine echo) can be used to evaluate new or worsened regional wall motion abnormalities in the pharmacologically stressed heart. Areas of wall motion abnormality are considered at risk for ischemia.

Coronary angiography is the gold standard for defining the coronary anatomy. Valvular and ventricular function can be evaluated and measurements of hemodynamic indices taken. Because angiography is invasive, it is reserved for patients who require further evaluation based on previous tests or who have a high probability of severe coronary disease and are considered candidates for coronary artery revascularization.

12. Based on the initial evaluation, which patients should be referred for further testing?
Patients at risk for IHD but with good exercise tolerance may not require further workup, especially if they are undergoing procedures with a low to moderate risk of perioperative MI. Patients with decreased exercise tolerance for unclear reasons or with unreliable histories should be evaluated with dipyridamole thallium testing.

Patients with documented IHD (prior MI or chronic stable angina) with good exercise tolerance can sometimes proceed with low-risk surgery without further evaluation. Exercise thallium imaging may provide useful information for higher risk procedures in these patients. Patients with known IHD and poor exercise tolerance should be referred for dipyridamole thallium testing or coronary angiography prior to all but the most minor surgical procedures.

13. Which surgical procedures carry the highest risk of perioperative MI?
In general, major abdominal, thoracic, and emergency surgery carry the highest risk of perioperative MI. The highest-risk noncardiac procedure is aortic aneurysm repair. These patients have a

high incidence of IHD, and cross-clamping of the aorta during surgery and postoperative complications can place great stress on the heart.

14. How long should a patient with a recent MI wait before undergoing elective noncardiac surgery?
The risk of reinfarction during surgery after a prior MI has traditionally depended on the time interval between the MI and the procedure. The highest risk of reinfarction is between 0 and 3 months post-MI, lower risk is from 3 to 6 months, and a baseline risk level is reached after 6 months (approximately 5% in most studies).

15. What if surgery cannot safely be delayed for 6 months?
The patient's functional status following rehabilitation from a MI is probably more important than the absolute time interval. Patients with ongoing symptoms may be candidates for coronary revascularization prior to their noncardiac procedure. Patients who quickly return to good functional status following a MI can be considered for necessary noncardiac surgery between 6 weeks and 3 months without undue added risk.

16. How is premedication useful in the setting of IHD and surgery?
Patient anxiety can lead to catecholamine secretion and increased oxygen demand. In this regard, the goal of premedication is to produce sedation and amnesia without causing deleterious myocardial depression, hypotension, or hypoxemia. Morphine, scopolamine, and benzodiazepines, alone or in combination, are popular choices to achieve these goals. All premedicated patients should receive supplemental oxygen. Patients who use sublingual nitroglycerin should have access to their medication. Transdermal nitroglycerin can be applied in the perioperative period as well.

17. Outline the hemodynamic goals of induction and maintenance of general anesthesia in patients with IHD.
The anesthesiologist's goal must be to maintain the balance between myocardial O_2 supply and demand throughout the perioperative period. Induction should be smooth without hypotension. A variety of induction agents can produce this result if used judiciously. Ketamine should be avoided due to its potential for central nervous system stimulation with resultant tachycardia and hypertension. Prolonged laryngoscopy should be avoided, and the anesthesiologist may wish to blunt the stimulation of laryngoscopy and intubation by the addition of opiates, beta-blockers, or laryngotracheal or intravenous lidocaine.

Maintenance drugs are chosen with knowledge of the patient's ventricular function. In patients with good left ventricular function, the cardiac depressant and vasodilatory effects of inhaled anesthetics may reduce myocardial O_2 demand. A narcotic-based technique may be chosen to avoid undue myocardial depression in patients with poor left ventricular function. Muscle relaxants with minimal cardiovascular effects are usually preferred.

Blood pressure and heart rate should be maintained near baseline values. This can be accomplished by blunting sympathetic stimulation with adequate analgesia and aggressively treating hypertension (anesthetics, nitroglycerin, nitroprusside, beta-blockers), hypotension (fluids, sympathomimetics, inotropic drugs), and tachycardia (fluids, anesthetics, beta-blockers).

18. What monitors are useful for detecting ischemia intraoperatively?
The V5 precordial lead is the most sensitive single ECG lead for detecting ischemia and should be monitored routinely in patients at risk for IHD. Lead II can detect ischemia of the right coronary artery distribution and is the most useful lead for monitoring P waves and cardiac rhythm.

Transesophageal echocardiography can provide continuous intraoperative monitoring of left ventricular function. Detection of regional wall motion abnormalities with this technique is the most sensitive monitor for myocardial ischemia.

The pulmonary artery occlusion (wedge) pressure gives an indirect measurement of left ventricular end-diastolic pressure and volume and is a useful guide to optimizing intravascular fluid therapy. Sudden increases in the wedge pressure may indicate acute left ventricular dysfunction due to ischemia. The routine use of pulmonary artery catheters in patients with IHD has not been shown to improve outcome. However, close hemodynamic monitoring (including pulmonary artery catheter data) may be beneficial depending on the patient's condition and the nature of the surgical procedure.

19. Discuss postoperative physiologic considerations in the patient with IHD.

A smooth emergence from anesthesia and adequate ventilation and oxygenation are of obvious importance. Pain, shivering, hypovolemia, anemia, and tachycardia all frequently occur in the postoperative period and can adversely affect myocardial oxygen supply and demand. Close supervision of patients in the recovery room and a rapid response to emerging problems are essential.

BIBLIOGRAPHY

1. Eagle KA, Coley CM, Newell JB, et al: Combining clinical and thallium data optimizes preoperative assessment of cardiac risk before major vascular surgery. Ann Intern Med 110:859–866, 1989.
2. Fleisher LA, Barash PG: Preoperative cardiac evaluation for noncardiac surgery: A functional approach. Anesth Analg 74:586–598, 1992.
3. Goldman L: Cardiac risk in noncardiac surgery: An update. Anesth Analg 80:810–820, 1995.
4. Mangano DT: Perioperative cardiac morbidity, Anesthesiology 72:153–184, 1990.
5. Stoelting RK, Dierdorf SF: Ischemic heart disease. In Stoelting RK, Dierdorf SF (eds): Anesthesia and Coexisting Disease, 3rd ed. New York, Churchill Livingstone, 1993, pp 1–20.

40. CONGESTIVE HEART FAILURE

Richard D. Abbott, M.D.

1. Define congestive heart failure.

Heart failure is defined as the inability of the heart to maintain a circulation sufficient to meet the body's metabolic needs. It is commonly termed congestive heart failure (CHF) because symptoms of circulatory congestion (pulmonary edema and/or peripheral edema) accompany heart failure.

2. Name the classifications and causes of heart failure.

Heart failure may be classified as left-sided vs. right-sided, high output vs. low output, backward vs. forward, acute vs. chronic, and compensated vs. decompensated. One needs to be cautious in recognizing the difference between underlying causes and precipitating factors. The causes may be classified as cardiac or noncardiac. The cardiac causes may be divided further into conditions that directly alter myocardial or ventricular function and conditions that do not.

Causes of Heart Failure Conditions

CARDIAC	NONCARDIAC
Ischemia	Hypertension
Cardiomyopathy	Pulmonary embolus
Toxic	High output states
Metabolic	Thyrotoxicosis
Infectious inflammatory	
Infiltrative	
Genetic	
Idiopathic	
Vavlular heart diseases	
Aortic stenosis, regurgitation	
Mitral stenosis, regurgitation	
Restrictive disease	
Pericardial	
Myocardial	
Congenital disease	
Electrical abnormalities	
Tachydysrhythmias	
Ventricular dyssynergy	

3. What major alterations in physiology occur in patients with heart failure?

Perfusion is altered by the interaction of impedance, preload, and contractility. The heart adapts in a number of ways. Myocardial hypertrophy allows the heart to overcome pressure overload, whereas dilation occurs with volume overload. Ventricular dilation allows the chamber to eject an adequate stroke volume with less muscle shortening, but wall stress is increased, as described by the Laplace relationship.

The peripheral vasculature undergoes functional and structural alterations that result in arteriolar narrowing and decreased compliance of conduit arteries. This process includes vascular smooth muscle hypertrophy and/or remodeling and activation of vasoconstrictor mechanisms. Vasoconstrictor mechanisms include elevated sympathetic nervous system (SNS) activity, activation of the renin-angiotensin system, increased levels of circulating arginine vasopressin and endothelin, and possibly decreased local release of endothelium-derived relaxing factor (nitric oxide).

Further evidence of elevated SNS activity includes the presence of increased inotrophy, tachycardia, and diaphoresis. Plasma levels of norepinephrine are often elevated, whereas cardiac catecholamine stores may eventually become depleted as CHF progresses. Downregulation of systemic sympathetic receptors occurs. The renin-angiotensin-aldosterone system is activated by decreased renal perfusion and sympathetic stimulation, leading to sodium and water retention and vasoconstriction. Such alterations in physiology result in a vicious cycle of worsening ventricular performance and increased compensatory responses.

4. What are the presenting symptoms of heart failure?
Exertional dyspnea and fatigue are most often the primary complaint. However, ankle swelling may be the first symptom recognized by the patient. Dyspnea that is more prominent in the supine position, particularly if proxysmal nocturnal dyspnea (PND) occurs during the early hours of sleep, is strongly suggestive of heart failure. Nocturia, coughing, wheezing, right upper quadrant pain, anorexia, nausea and vomiting, and palpitations also may be prominent complaints.

5. What physical signs suggest heart failure?
Much of the physical examination can be directed toward the heart, lungs, and jugular veins. Cardiac palpation may reveal an expanded impulse area with ventricular dilatation or a forceful sustained impulse with left ventricular hypertrophy (LVH). Auscultation frequently reveals a protodiastolic gallop rhythm (S_3) or an S_4 secondary to forceful atrial contraction. Murmurs of valvular diseases should be looked for. Severe failure may result in cyanosis, both peripheral and central.

Pulmonary examination often reveals rales located most prominently over the lung bases. Decreased breath sounds secondary to pleural effusions occur more often in patients with chronic heart failure.

Jugular venous distention (JVD) > 10 cm H_2O above the right atrium is considered abnormal. Close examination may reveal a large A-wave with a noncompliant right ventricle, a large v-wave with tricuspid regurgitation or a rapid y-descent secondary to restrictive disease.

Further signs of vascular congestion may be prominent, including hepatomegaly, splenomegaly, and peripheral edema that may extend to chest level in severe cases.

6. What laboratory studies are useful in evaluating the patient with heart failure?
The posteroanterior and lateral chest radiograph may detect cardiomegaly or evidence of pulmonary vascular congestion, including perihilar engorgement of the pulmonary veins, cephalization of the pulmonary vascular markings, and/or pleural effusions. The ECG is often nonspecific, although 70–90% of patients may demonstrate ventricular or supraventricular dysrhythmias. Left ventricular imaging is considered mandatory by some clinicians in the evaluation of the patient with a failing heart. Echocardiography evaluates chamber size, wall motion, valvular function, and left ventricular wall thickness. Radionuclide angiography provides a fairly reproducible and accurate assessment of left ventricular ejection fraction.

Blood work, including serum electrolytes, arterial blood gases (ABG), liver function tests (LFTs), and blood counts (CBC), is frequently evaluated. Many patients with heart failure are hyponatremic from activation of the vasopressin system. Treatment with diuretics and aldosterone activation may lead to hypokalemia and hypomagnesemia. Some degree of prerenal azotemia is often present; renal injury may occur secondary to hypoperfusion or other underlying diseases, such as hypertension or diabetes mellitus. Hypocalcemia and hypophosphatemia also are often present. Hepatic congestion may result in elevated bilirubin levels and elevated LFTs. Patients may be hypoxic secondary to pulmonary congestion and acidotic from poor organ perfusion; lactate levels may be elevated.

7. Why is it important to differentiate between compensated and decompensated heart failure preoperatively?
Patients with a history of heart failure who are found to have JVD, pulmonary edema, and/or an S_3 gallop rhythm during the preoperative assessment are considered to be in a decompensated state. Cardiac output (CO) and oxygen transport are usually markedly reduced in such patients.

Severe ventilation perfusion mismatching and hypoxemia may be present secondary to pulmonary edema and pleural effusions. The combined cardiopulmonary dysfunction of heart failure predisposes to intraoperative hypoxemia, hypotension, metabolic acidosis, overt pulmonary edema, and malignant arrhythmias. Patients with stable, hemodynamically compensated heart failure may have diminished signs of reserve such as orthopnea, cardiomegaly, basilar rales, and decreased exercise tolerance, but JVD, pulmonary edema, and an S_3 gallop are not present.

An important study by Goldman et al. prospectively evaluated cardiac risk factors and complications in > 1,000 patients undergoing noncardiac surgery. Their study indicated that patients who demonstrated an S_3 or JVD preoperatively had approximately a 20-fold increased risk for postoperative cardiac death compared with patients without such risk factors. Patients presenting with pulmonary edema had a 14-fold risk, whereas patients with pulmonary rales or cardiomegaly, as evidenced by chest radiograph, had a 5-fold risk. They also found that patients with a history of heart failure who were not in failure preoperatively were significantly less likely to develop pulmonary edema than patients in whom CHF was still evident preoperatively.

8. Differentiate between systolic and diastolic dysfunction.

Systolic dysfunction occurs when myocardial sarcomere shortening is reduced and may result from global or regional reduction in contractility or high impedance to ventricular ejection. Elevated preload, as evidenced by elevated left ventricular end-diastolic volume, provides at least short-term compensation (see question 9). Myocardial hypertrophy and new sarcomere generation provide longer-term compensation. With diastolic dysfunction the principal abnormality involves impaired relaxation of the ventricle. Ventricular relaxation is energy-dependent and relies on reuptake of calcium into the sarcoplasmic reticulum of the myocyte. It is also related to myocardial mass, collagen content, and extrinsic forces such as pericardial disease. It is often difficult to assess in a clinical setting, but for practical purposes demonstration of an elevated left ventricular end-diastolic or left atrial pressure when the ventricle is not grossly dilated can be accepted as indicative of diastolic dysfunction. Most patients with heart failure have some degree of systolic dysfunction coexisting with some degree of diastolic dysfunction.

9. What is the Frank-Starling law?

The Frank-Starling law basically states that the force or tension developed in a muscle fiber depends on the extent to which the fiber is stretched. There is an optimal sarcomere length and thus an optimal fiber length from which the most forceful contraction occurs. The left ventricle normally operates at a left ventricular end-diastolic volume (LVEDV) that results in less than optimal fiber lengths. Stroke volume increases with increasing preload to an extent. A heart with elevated contractility, as occurs with sympathetic stimulation, and a failing heart respond differently to changes in preload (below).

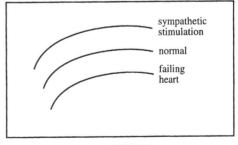

Effects of changes in preload on normal, failing, and sympathetically stimulated hearts.

10. How is the severity of heart failure classified?

Typically, the status of patients with CHF can be classified on the basis of either symptoms and impairment of lifestyle or severity of cardiac dysfunction. The New York Heart Association classification is used to assess symptomatic limitations of heart failure and response to therapy:

Class I—ordinary physical activity does not cause symptoms.
Class II—ordinary physical activity will result in symptoms.
Class III—less than ordinary activity results in symptoms.
Class IV—symptoms occur at rest.

Evaluation of left ventricular (LV) chamber size and left ventricular ejection fraction (LVEF) is used to estimate the degree of cardiac dysfunction. Exercise testing with measurement of gas exchange also has been used to assess severity of the syndrome on the basis of peak exercise capacity.

Prognosis of the patient with CHF does not necessarily relate to classifications used to assess the severity of the syndrome. LVEF has been linked to mortality rates in some studies. An EF < 25% has been associated with an annual mortality rate as high as 40%, whereas an EF > 35–40% has been associated with mortality rates below 10%. Decreased exercise capacity based on gas exchange measurements, episodes of nonsustained ventricular tachycardia, elevated plasma norepinephrine levels, hyponatremia, and azotemia also have been identified as markers of a poorer prognosis.

11. What treatment strategies are used in heart failure?

Treatment may be divided into pharmacologic and nonpharmacologic approaches. Nonpharmacologic treatment includes diet, exercise, and appropriate rest.

Diuretics are used when patients with heart failure exhibit signs or symptoms of circulatory congestion. Thiazide diuretics are often used for mild fluid retention. Loop diuretics such as furosemide may be substituted with evidence of more severe congestion or when thiazides fail to result in an adequate response. Addition of a second diuretic, such as metolazone, may induce an effective diuresis in patients resistant to loop diuretics alone.

Angiotensin-converting enzyme (ACE) inhibitors are effective therapy for patients who can tolerate them. Data demonstrates that therapy with ACE inhibitors improves LV function and exercise tolerance and may prolong life. Hypotension and azotemia are the major side effects. A dry cough is fairly common but rarely necessitates discontinuation of therapy. A combination of the vasodilators hydralazine and isosorbide dinitrate also has been shown to be effective in improving exercise tolerance and life span and may be substituted for or even combined with ACE inhibitors.

Currently used **calcium channel blockers** may produce favorable hemodynamic responses but negative inotropic effects. These agents are used in patients with concurrent myocardial ischemia.

Digitalis is effective in patients with underlying atrial fibrillation or a dilated LV with poor systolic function. **Beta blockers** may produce favorable long-term effects on symptoms and LV function when gradually titrated to effective dose ranges.

Patients who present with acutely decompensated heart failure are treated with the goal of restoring hemodynamics to baseline if possible. Resolution of pulmonary edema, decreased or eliminated oxygen requirements, improved tolerance for physical activity, and improvement of metabolic and electrolyte disturbances are the goals of therapy. Such patients are usually treated in hospital, often in an intensive care unit. Precipitating factors, such as recent ischemic events, are evaluated and treated appropriately. High-dose diuretics are used to treat volume overload. Afterload reduction is effective when pulmonary capillary wedge pressures (PCWP) are elevated in the face of a low cardiac output and adequate arterial pressures. **Sodium nitroprusside** is often used in this setting. When response is inadequate to afterload reduction alone or when arterial pressures are low, **dopamine and/or dobutamine** are often effective. **Phosphodiesterase inhibitors**, such as amrinone or milrinone, have been used to improve inotropy and perfusion in patients failing to respond to catecholamines. Some patients who respond inadequately to continuation of oral therapy have been treated successfully with outpatient dobutamine therapy or recurrent hospital admissions for dobutamine therapy (dobutamine holidays).

12. What clinical findings would you expect in a patient with digitalis toxicity?

Patients may present with complaints of anorexia, nausea, and vomiting. Other symptoms include abdominal pain, confusion, paresthesias, amblyopia, and scotomata.

ECG manifestations are nonspecific. Increased automaticity, as evidenced by atrial or ventricular dysrrhythmias such as premature ventricular contractions, bigeminy, trigeminy, or ventricular tachycardia, may be present. Delayed atrioventricular node conduction is common, with complete heart block sometimes occurring. Advanced age, hypothyroidism, decreased renal function, hypokalemia, hypercalcemia and hypomagnesemia predispose to digitalis toxicity.

13. Should digitalis be administered prophylactically before anesthetic procedures?

Prophylactic administration of digitalis to patients scheduled for elective operations, without evidence of CHF, is controversial. Preoperative administration to geriatric patients undergoing thoracic or abdominal procedures may reduce the incidence of atrial fibrillation. Patients with coronary artery disease who are recovering from anesthesia and have received prophylactic digitalis have reduced evidence of impaired cardiac function. However, digitalis has a narrow toxic/therapeutic ratio, and it may be difficult to differentiated anesthetic-induced cardiac dysrrhythmias from those occurring secondary to digitalis toxicity. Impaired renal function, altered acid-base status, hypokalemia, increased sympathetic activity, and calcium administration may predispose the patient to digitalis toxicity.

14. What should be considered in preparing to conduct an anesthetic on the patient with heart failure?

The initial preoperative assessment should include determination of the cause of heart failure and evaluation of current and baseline signs and symptoms and current medication regimen, including recent medication changes. The initial evaluation should reveal whether the patient is in a decompensated state. In patients with decompensated failure planned procedures should be postponed, if possible, until physiologic status is optimized. This may require admission preoperatively if the patient is not already inhouse. Treatment needs to be vigorous, and adequate treatment is rarely accomplished in a few hours. Attempts to treat the patient overnight so that he or she is ready for surgery the next day are discouraged.

Choice of anesthetic approach is based on the patient's status, planned surgical procedure, and the anesthesiologist's experience and preferences (see questions 16 and 17). The goal of the anesthetic should be to maintain cardiac output and organ perfusion. This goal may require pharmacologic support, as described in question 11. Intraoperative monitoring also depends on the patient's status, planned procedure, and individual preferences of the anesthesiologist. Arterial catheterization is useful when infusions of vasopressors or vasodialators are planned. Pulmonary artery catheters provide useful data about response to therapeutic measures such as changes in CO, oxygen delivery, vascular resistance, and PCWP.

Finally, initial plans should be made for postoperative care. This may require intensive care admission, including cardiovascular and ventilatory support.

15. What are the goals of intraoperative fluid management in patients with heart failure?

Fluid management is directed to maintain optimal cardiac preload, to correct electrolyte disturbances, to diminish edema, and to avoid overadministration of sodium. Such goals may be difficult to achieve with the rapid fluid shifts that may occur perioperatively. Patient care is enhanced by direct or indirect measurements of preload, such as central venous pressure (CVP), PCWP, left atrial pressure (LAP), stroke volume, ejection fraction, or stroke work. In patients with a history of heart failure who are scheduled for major or prolonged surgery, monitoring should be begun preoperatively. Assessment of response to IV fluid challenges can then be made preoperatively. Early replacement of blood loss with colloids or blood products instead of crystalloid solutions may decrease perioperative tissue edema.

16. When conducting a general anesthetic in patients with a history of or active CHF, is there a perfect choice of anesthetic agents?

No. Patients with decreased myocardial reserve are more sensitive to the cardiovascular depressant effects caused by anesthetic agents, but careful administration with close monitoring of hemodynamic responses can be accomplished with most agents. This is true for both induction and maintenance of general anesthesia.

The barbiturates and propofol generally produce the most profound depression of cardiac function and blood pressure when used for induction of general anesthesia. Etomidate produces few aberrations in cardiovascular status, although hypotension may occur in the setting of hypovolemia. Ketamine administration may result in elevated cardiac output and blood pressure secondary to increased sympathetic activity, although this effect may be blunted in patients with CHF and when ketamine is coadministered with benzodiazepines, inhalational anesthetics, or thiopental. Cardiovascular side effects are mild when the benzodiazepines are given in sedative doses but become more pronounced when induction doses are given or when administered in combination with opioids. Induction doses of opioids are usually well tolerated by patients with decreased cardiac reserve but may not be well suited to short surgical procedures. Slower administration, smaller induction doses, and infusions of the IV anesthetics generally result in less dramatic alterations of blood pressure and myocardial function. Each of the inhaled anesthetics produces some degree of myocardial depression, which is more pronounced with halothane and enflurane than with isoflurane or desflurane.

17. Is regional anesthesia contraindicated in patients with heart failure?

No. Blockade of peripheral nerves of the upper extremity, including brachial plexus and bier blocks, or lower extremity generally produce few cardiovascular alterations, except in the setting of local anesthetic toxicity. Sympathetic nervous system blockade with concomitant decreases in systemic vascular resistance, as occurs with epidural or subarachnoid techniques, may be beneficial when gradual in onset. However, preload reduction also occurs. Because many patients depend on an elevated preload to maintain cardiac output, significant reductions in blood pressure and perfusion may result. Epidural or continuous spinal techniques or use of isobaric local anesthetics for spinal blockade generally result in more gradual reductions in blood pressure than administration of hyperbaric local anesthetics for spinal blockade. Treatment of excessive reductions in blood pressure with fluid administration may not be well tolerated in patients who are already fluid-overloaded. Response to vasopressors may be depressed secondary to adrenergic receptor downregulation and decreased myocardial catecholamine reserves, as occurs with heart failure.

Many patients with heart failure do not tolerate supine positioning because of symptoms of orthopnea and therefore may be poor candidates for awake regional anesthetic techniques.

BIBLIOGRAPHY

1. Chee TP, Prakash NS, Desser KB, Bechinol A: Postoperative supraventricular arrhythmias and the role of prophylactic digoxin in cardiac surgery. Am Heart J 104:974–977, 1982.
2. Chesler, Elliot: Clinical Cardiology. New York, Springer-Verlag, 1993, pp 166–188.
3. Clark NH, Stanley TH: Anesthesia for vascular surgery. In Miller RD (ed): Anesthesia, 4th ed. New York, Churchill Livingstone, 1994, pp 1857–1858.
4. Cohn JN: Heart failure. In Willerson JT, Cohn JN (eds): Cardiovascular Medicine. New York, Churchill Livingstone, 1995, pp 947–979.
5. Goldman L, Caldera DL, Nussbaum SR, et al: Cardiac risk factors and complications of non-cardiac surgery. Medicine 57:357–370, 1978.
6. Kemmotso O, Hashimoto Y, Shimosato S: The effects of fluroxene and enflurane on contractile performance of isolated papillary muscle from failing hearts. Anesthesiology 40:252–260, 1974.
7. Tonnessen AS: Crystaloids and colloids. In Miller RD (ed): Anesthesia, 4th ed. New York, Churchill Livingstone, 1994, pp 1595–1619.
8. Lake CL: Chronic treatment of congestive heart failure. In Kaplan JA (ed): Cardiac Anesthesia, 3rd ed. Philadelphia, W.B. Saunders, 1993, pp 125–149.
9. Pinaud MLJ, Blanoeil YAG, Souron RJ: Preoperative prophylactic digitalization of patients with coronary artery disease—a randomized echocardiographic and hemodynamic study. Anesth Analg 62:865–869, 1983.
10. Stoelting RK: Pharmacology and Physiology in Anesthetic Practice, 2nd ed. Philadelphia, J.B. Lippincott, 1991, pp 289–291.

41. VALVULAR HEART DISEASE

Richard B. Allen, M.D.

1. Discuss the basic pathophysiology of cardiac valvular disease.

Mitral and aortic stenosis cause pressure overload of the left ventricle, which produces hypertrophy with a cardiac chamber of normal size. Mitral and aortic regurgitation cause volume overload, either acute or chronic, which leads to hypertrophy with a dilated chamber. The net effect of left-sided valvular lesions is an impedance to forward flow of blood into the systemic circulation. Although right-sided valvular lesions occur, left-sided lesions are more common and usually more hemodynamically significant. This chapter deals only with left-sided lesions.

2. Describe common findings of the history and physical exam in patients with valvular disease.

A history of rheumatic fever, intravenous drug abuse, or heart murmur should alert the examiner to the possibility of valvular disease. Exercise tolerance is frequently decreased. Patients may exhibit signs and symptoms of congestive heart failure, including dyspnea, orthopnea, fatigue, pulmonary rales, jugular venous congestion, hepatic congestion, and dependent edema. Compensatory increases in sympathetic nervous system tone manifest as resting tachycardia, anxiety, and diaphoresis. Angina may occur in patients with a hypertrophied left ventricle even in the absence of coronary artery disease. Atrial fibrillation frequently accompanies diseases of the mitral valve.

3. Which tests are useful in the evaluation of valvular disease?

The electrocardiogram should be examined for evidence of ischemia, arrhythmias, atrial enlargement, and ventricular hypertrophy. The chest radiograph may show enlargement of cardiac chambers, suggest pulmonary hypertension, or reveal pulmonary edema and pleural effusions. Cardiac catheterization is the gold standard in the evaluation of such patients and determines pressures in various heart chambers as well as pressure gradients across valves. Cardiac angiography allows visualization of the coronary arteries and heart chambers.

4. How is echocardiography helpful?

Doppler echocardiography characterizes ventricular function and valve function. It can be used to measure the valve orifice area and transvalvular pressure gradients, which are measures of the severity of valvular dysfunction. The function of prosthetic valves is also measured echocardiographically.

5. Which invasive monitors aid the anesthesiologist in the perioperative period?

An arterial catheter provides beat-to-beat blood pressure measurement and continuous access to the bloodstream for sampling. Pulmonary artery catheters enable the anesthetist to measure cardiac output and provide central access for the infusion of vasoactive drugs. The pulmonary capillary wedge pressure is an index of left ventricular filling and is useful for guiding intravenous fluid therapy. Transesophageal echocardiography can be used intraoperatively to evaluate left ventricular volume and function, to detect ischemia (segmental wall motion abnormalities) and intracardiac air, and to examine valve function before and after repair.

6. What is a pressure-volume loop?

A pressure-volume loop plots left ventricular pressure against volume through one complete cardiac cycle. Each valvular lesion has a unique profile that suggests compensatory physiologic changes by the left ventricle.

7. How does a normal pressure-volume loop appear?

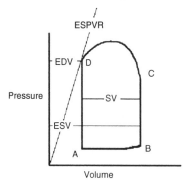

Basic Flow-Volume Loop

A = mitral opening, B = mitral closure, C = aortic opening, and D = aortic closure.

The segment DA is isovolumetric relaxation, AB is ventricular filling, BC is isovolumetric contraction, and CD is ejection. Stroke volume (SV), end-systolic volume (ESV), and end-diastolic volume (EDV) are labelled. The end-systolic pressure–volume relationship (ESPVR) slope is a measure of contractility. A horizontal/clockwise shift of the slope represents a decrease in contractility.

8. Discuss the pathophysiology of aortic stenosis.
Aortic stenosis is a fixed outlet obstruction to left ventricular ejection. Concentric hypertrophy (thickened ventricular wall with normal chamber size) develops in response to the increased intraventricular systolic pressure and increased wall tension necessary to maintain forward flow. Ventricular compliance decreases, and end-diastolic pressures increase. Contractility and ejection fraction are usually maintained until late in the disease process. Atrial contraction may account for up to 40% of ventricular filling (normally 20%). Aortic stenosis is usually secondary to calcification of a congenital bicuspid valve or rheumatic heart disease. Patients often present with angina, dyspnea, syncope, or sudden death. Angina occurs in the absence of coronary artery disease because the thickened myocardium is susceptible to ischemia (increased oxygen demand) and elevated end-diastolic pressure reduces coronary perfusion pressure (decreased oxygen supply).

9. How are the compensatory changes in the left ventricle represented by a pressure-volume loop?

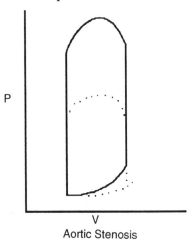

Aortic Stenosis

The dotted line represents a normal pressure-volume loop. Note the significant increase in left ventricular end-diastolic pressure and end-systolic pressure.

10. What are the hemodynamic goals in the anesthetic management of patients with aortic stenosis?

Patients must have adequate intravascular volume to fill the noncompliant ventricle. Reductions in afterload lead to reduced blood pressure and coronary perfusion because cardiac output is relatively fixed by the stenotic valve. Extremes of heart rate should be avoided. Bradycardias lead to a decrease in cardiac output, whereas tachycardias may produce ischemia as well as limit ejection time. A sinus rhythm is imperative, and emergent cardioversion is indicated if the patient suffers severe hemodynamic compromise due to supraventricular arrhythmia (remember the importance of the atrial "kick").

11. Discuss the pathophysiology of aortic insufficiency.

Chronic aortic insufficiency is usually rheumatic in origin. Acute aortic insufficiency may be secondary to trauma, endocarditis, or dissection of a thoracic aortic aneurysm. The left ventricle experiences volume overload, because part of the stroke volume regurgitates across the incompetent aortic valve in diastole. Eccentric hypertrophy (dilated and thickened chamber) develops. A dilated orifice, slower heart rate (relatively more time spent in diastole), and increased systemic vascular resistance increase the amount of regurgitant flow. Compliance and stroke volume may be markedly increased in chronic aortic insufficiency, whereas contractility gradually diminishes. Ideally, such patients should have valve replacement surgery before the onset of irreversible myocardial damage. In acute aortic insufficiency, the left ventricle is subjected to rapid, massive volume overload with elevated end-diastolic pressures and displays poor contractility. Hypotension and pulmonary edema may necessitate emergent valvular replacement.

12. What does the pressure-volume loop look like in acute and chronic aortic insufficiency?

The dotted line represents a normal flow-volume loop. Note the markedly increased ventricular volumes. In chronic aortic insufficiency the ventricle has time to dilate massively without a large increase in end-diastolic pressure. In acute aortic insufficiency the end-diastolic pressures increase significantly, and the compliance is diminished. Also note the increase in ventricular volume in diastole due to regurgitant flow.

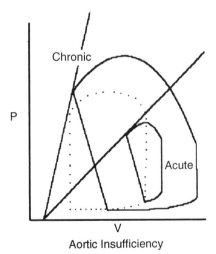

Aortic Insufficiency

13. What are the hemodynamic goals in the anesthetic management of patients with aortic insufficiency?

"Fast, full, and forward" is a phrase to remember in managing such patients. Afterload reduction augments forward flow, and additional intravascular volume may be necessary to maintain preload. Modest tachycardia reduces ventricular volumes and limits the time available for regurgitation. The natural heart rate should be maintained if the heart has had time to compensate for the disease state.

14. What is the pathophysiology of mitral stenosis?

Mitral stenosis is usually secondary to rheumatic disease. Critical stenosis of the valve occurs 10–20 years after the initial infection. As the orifice of the valve narrows, the left atrium experiences pressure overload. In contrast to other valvular lesions, the left ventricle shows relative volume underload due to the obstruction of forward blood flow from the atrium. The elevated atrial pressure may be transmitted to the pulmonary circuit and thus lead to pulmonary hypertension and right-heart failure. The overdistended atrium is susceptible to fibrillation with resultant loss of atrial systole, leading to reduced ventricular filling and cardiac output. Symptoms (fatigue, dyspnea on exertion, hemoptysis) may be worsened when increased cardiac output is needed, as with pregnancy, illness, anemia, and exercise. Blood stasis in the left atrium is a risk for thrombus formation and systemic embolization.

15. How is the pressure-volume loop changed from normal in mitral stenosis?

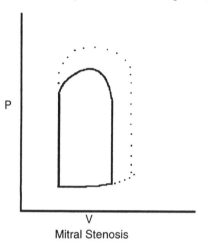

P

V

Mitral Stenosis

The dotted curve represents a normal flow-volume loop. Note that the peak systolic pressure and stroke volume are reduced in the volume-underloaded left ventricle.

16. What are the anesthetic considerations in mitral stenosis?

The intravascular volume must be adequate to maintain flow across the stenotic valve. Increases in pulmonary vascular resistance may exacerbate right ventricular failure, and treatment of hypotension with systemic vasoconstrictor drugs must be undertaken cautiously. Hypoxemia, hypercarbia, and acidosis increase pulmonary vascular resistance. For this reason, the respiratory depressant effects of preoperative medications may prove particularly deleterious. A slower heart rate is beneficial to allow more time for blood to flow across the valve and to increase ventricular filling.

17. Describe the pathophysiology of mitral regurgitation.

Chronic mitral regurgitation is usually due to rheumatic heart disease, ischemia, or mitral valve prolapse. Acute mitral regurgitation may occur in the setting of myocardial ischemia and infarction with papillary muscle dysfunction or chordae tendineae rupture. In chronic mitral regurgitation, the left ventricle and atrium show volume overload, which leads to eccentric hypertrophy. Left ventricular systolic pressures decrease as part of the stroke volume escapes through the incompetent valve into the left atrium, leading to elevated left atrial pressure, pulmonary hypertension, and eventually right-heart failure. As in aortic insufficiency, regurgitant flow depends on valve orifice size, time available for regurgitant flow, and transvalvular pressure gradient. The valve orifice increases in size as the left ventricle increases in size. In acute mitral regurgitation, the pulmonary circuit and right heart are subjected to sudden increases in pressure and volume in the absence of compensatory ventricular dilatation, which may precipitate acute pulmonary hypertension, pulmonary edema, and right-heart failure.

18. How is the pressure-volume loop in mitral regurgitation changed from normal?

The dotted curve represents a normal pressure-volume loop. The left ventricle shows volume overload but does not develop increased end-diastolic pressures. Systolic pressures are low. Note that intraventricular volume begins decreasing at the onset of systole rather than after a period of isovolumetric contraction as the blood flows across the incompetent valve into the left atrium.

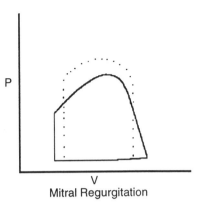

Mitral Regurgitation

19. What are the hemodynamic goals in anesthetic management of mitral regurgitation?
The intravascular volume should remain full, although slight decreases in volume may decrease the regurgitant fraction by shrinking the size of the ventricle. A slightly elevated heart rate also helps to decrease ventricular volume. Decreasing systemic vascular resistance augments forward flow. As in mitral stenosis, drugs and maneuvers that increase pulmonary vascular resistance must be avoided.

BIBLIOGRAPHY

1. Barash PG, Mathew JP: Mitral stenosis. In Bready LL, Smith RB (eds): Decision Making in Anesthesiology, 2nd ed. St. Louis, Mosby, 1992, pp 188–189.
2. Barash PG, Mathew JP: Mitral regurgitation. In Bready LL, Smith RB (eds): Decision Making in Anesthesiology, 2nd ed. St. Louis, Mosby, 1992, pp 190–191.
3. Deutsch N, Hantler CB: Aortic stenosis. In Bready LL, Smith RB (eds): Decision Making in Anesthesiology, 2nd ed. St. Louis, Mosby, 1992, pp 192–193.
4. Deutsch N, Hantler CB: Aortic regurgitation. In Bready LL, Smith RB (eds): Decision Making in Anesthesiology, 2nd ed. St. Louis, Mosby, 1992, pp 194–195.
5. Reich DL, Brooks JL III, Kaplan JA: Uncommon cardiac diseases. In Katz J, Benumof J, Kadis L (eds): Anesthesia and Uncommon Diseases, 3rd ed. Philadelphia, W.B.Saunders, 1990, pp 333–377.
6. Thomas SJ: The patient with valve disease for non-valve, non-cardiac surgery. American Society of Anesthesiologists 1994 Annual Refresher Course Lectures, 1994, no. 431.
7. Wray DL, Fine RH, Hughes CW, Thomas SJ: Anesthesia for cardiac surgery. In Barash PG, Cullen BF, Stoelting RK (eds): Clinical Anesthesia, 2nd ed. Philadelphia, J.B. Lippincott, 1992, pp 1021–1057.

42. AORTO-OCCLUSIVE DISEASE

Michael Leonard, M.D.

1. Define aorto-occlusive disease.

Aorto-occlusive disease is characterized by pathophysiologic, atherosclerotic changes within the aorta (almost always abdominal) that extend into the iliac or even femoral arteries and result in inadequate perfusion of vital organs and the lower extremities. Aneurysmal changes are common.

2. List pathophysiologic changes commonly present during anesthesia for vascular surgery on the aorta and its major branches.

- Acute hemodynamic changes
- Hypoperfusion of vital organs from underlying disease or vascular cross-clamping
- Potential for massive transfusion and attendant complications
- Severe increases in left ventricular afterload from aortic cross-clamping
- Acid-base disturbances

3. How significant is the incidence of coexisting disease in patients undergoing major vascular surgery?

Because peripheral vascular disease is clinically evident between the fifth and eighth decades of life, the majority of these patients have multiple medical problems.

Coronary artery disease 65%	Angina pectoris 15%
History of myocardial infarction 25%	Hypertension 35%
Congestive heart failure (CHF) 10% to 15%	Renal insufficiency 10%
Pulmonary disease 25%	Diabetes mellitus 8%
Cerebrovascular disease 13%	

4. What is the risk associated with major vascular surgery in patients with coexisting disease?

A mortality rate of roughly 5% is associated with elective abdominal aortic aneurysm (AAA) repair. The major cause of postoperative death is cardiac, primarily myocardial infarction. Some 30% of these patients have their postsurgical course complicated by CHF. Patients presenting for surgery with poorly controlled CHF, as evidenced by S3 gallop or distended neck veins, have a 20% mortality with AAA repair.

5. What are the perioperative concerns arising from concurrent disease?

Cardiac. Because cardiac problems are so prevalent in this population, careful evaluation and perioperative management are paramount. Optimal control of CHF, angina, and hypertension is critically important. Patients with a clinical history of ischemic heart disease may require extensive testing. Holter monitoring, exercise treadmill testing, dipyridamole-thallium scanning, and coronary arteriography are appropriate to assess these patients. Current practice is to continue all cardiac medications up to surgery with the possible exception of angiotensin-converting enzyme inhibitors in hypertensives because these patients may experience marked intraoperative hypotension.

Pulmonary. Many vascular patients are heavy smokers. Chronic obstructive pulmonary disease (COPD), chronic bronchitis, and bronchospasm are common problems. Preoperative intervention with antibiotics in chronic bronchitics, cessation of smoking, incentive spirometry, and appropriate use of bronchodilators minimizes the incidence of atelectasis, pneumonia, and respiratory failure after surgery.

Renal. The presence of renal insufficiency necessitates careful evaluation of renal function. These patients are more sensitive to the toxicity associated with arteriographic contrast agents and must be watched closely to ensure renal function is not diminished during the diagnostic evaluation. Postoperative renal failure in this population carries a 50% mortality.

Cerebrovascular disease. A decreased ability to autoregulate cerebral blood flow may be present in these individuals, and they require tighter control of blood pressure intraoperatively. The presence of ongoing symptoms of the cerebral circulation dictates further workup.

Diabetes. These patients have a high incidence of cardiac, vascular, and renal disease. They are also prone to silent myocardial ischemia. Autonomic neuropathy in diabetics frequently results in hemodynamic instability intraoperatively.

6. Describe the primary aspects of management when a patient presents with an acute abdominal aortic rupture.

If the rupture is retroperitoneal, enough blood may be contained for the patient to maintain hemodynamic stability. With free intraperitoneal rupture, survival is unusual. Patients should be stabilized in the operating room (not the emergency room) to a systolic blood pressure of 80 to 100 mmHg. At least 10 units of blood should be set up, multiple large-bore intravenous (IV) lines placed, and anesthesia induced gently. Invasive monitoring may be obtained either preinduction or postinduction, depending on the clinical situation. In cases of acute rupture, poor outcome is associated with advanced age, cardiac disease, free rupture, preoperative shock, acute coronary ischemia, and cardiac arrest.

7. Enumerate the appropriate intraoperative monitors for aortic surgery.
- ECG monitoring (preferably both lead II for rhythm assessment and V5 for detecting intraoperative ischemia)
- Arterial line for continuous pressure monitoring and blood gas analysis
- Pulmonary artery catheter
- Esophageal stethoscope and temperature probe

Critically important in patient management:
- Indwelling urinary catheter
- Estimation of intravascular volume
- Ability to detect myocardial ischemia
- Assessment of hematologic, acid-base, and electrolyte values

In high-risk patients, transesophageal echocardiography to assess the effect of aortic cross-clamping on left ventricular function can be helpful.

8. What are the factors to consider in choosing alternative anesthetic agents?
Hemodynamic stability and **cardiac function** are major determinants in the choice of anesthetic agents. Unstable patients are best induced with ketamine, etomidate, or small amounts of opioids and benzodiazepines. In stable patients, gradual and gentle inductions are preferred with the goals being avoidance of tachycardia and hypertension. Intratracheal lidocaine is useful in blunting the response to intubation. Patients with poor ventricular function are candidates for high-dose opioid anesthetics, which depress cardiac contractility less than inhalation agents. Combinations of regional epidural anesthetics and light general anesthetics offer the benefit of less intraoperative myocardial depression and airway control; local anesthetic and opioid infusions for postoperative pain control are an additional benefit. In the past, concerns have been raised about the risk of epidural hematomas resulting from regional anesthesia in patients receiving surgical anticoagulation, but studies have shown this to be a safe practice.

9. What percentage of AAAs involve the renal arteries?
Approximately 70% are infrarenal, whereas 30% include renal arteries.

10. Discuss the physiologic implications of cross-clamping the abdominal aorta.

Aortic cross-clamping produces an acute, tremendous increase in left ventricular afterload. Cardiac ischemia, acute left ventricular failure, and severe hypertension can all accompany cross-clamping. This abrupt increase in afterload can be treated through use of vasodilators such as nitroprusside and nitroglycerin and alpha-adrenergic blockers such as phentolamine. Renal ischemia and interruption of spinal cord perfusion are possible. Lack of perfusion below the cross- clamp produces metabolic acidosis in the lower extremities.

11. Does infrarenal clamping adversely affect renal function?

Infrarenal clamping causes increases in plasma renin activity, alterations in intrarenal blood flow, and decreases in glomerular filtration rate and renal perfusion. In addition, the surgery itself may result in arterial emboli to the kidney and hypoperfusion. These emboli are usually composed of atheromatous debris or thrombus from within the diseased vessel.

12. What physiologic changes can be expected with removal of the cross-clamp?

The decrease in peripheral vascular resistance from the maximally dilated vascular beds below the clamp results in an acute decrease in arterial blood pressure. Additionally, washout of the lactate and accumulated metabolites in the ischemic extremities produces an acute metabolic acidosis. Maneuvers to ameliorate the effects of cross-clamp removal include increasing arterial and central venous pressure by fluid loading the patient before the clamp comes off. Also, infusion of bicarbonate before clamp removal can buffer the acid load and minimize the acute acidosis.

13. What considerations for intraoperative fluid and blood replacement are warranted?

1. Adequate hydration must be maintained intraoperatively to maximize perfusion and urine output.
2. Volume loading before clamp removal.
3. The ability to replace blood loss quickly because rapid, severe hemorrhage is common.
4. Use of a cell saver may minimize or prevent use of products from the blood bank.
5. Massive transfusion may necessitate administration of clotting factors and platelets.
6. Use of IV fluid warmers helps maintain patient's body temperature.

14. Discuss important elements of postoperative care.

All patients should be admitted to the intensive care unit. The patient's cardiac status requires careful observation. The peak incidence of postoperative myocardial infarction is at about 72 hours postoperatively. This is probably related to the reabsorption of fluid "third spaced" during the operation, which can lead to CHF and myocardial ischemia. Pulmonary function can be enhanced with incentive spirometry, pulmonary toilet, and bronchodilators when appropriate. Close attention should be given to renal function and urine output, as postoperative renal failure has ominous implications. Pain must be well controlled to minimize physiologic stress. Other miscellaneous postoperative complications include gastrointestinal ischemia, bleeding, stroke, graft infection, distal arterial thrombosis, and pulmonary embolism.

BIBLIOGRAPHY

1. Clark NJ, Stanley TH: Anesthesia for vascular surgery. In Miller RD (ed): Anesthesia. New York, Churchill Livingstone, 1994.
2. Eagle KA, Coley CM, Nussbaum SR, et al: Combining clinical and thallium data optimizes preoperative assessment of cardiac risk before major vascular surgery. Ann Intern Med 110:859–866, 1989.
3. Goldman L, Caldera DL, Nussbaum SR, et al: Multifactorial index of cardiac risk in patients in noncardiac surgical procedures. N Engl J Med 297:845–850, 1977.
4. Lunn JK, Dannemiller FJ, Stanley TH: Cardiovascular responses to clamping of the aorta during epidural and general anesthesia. Anesth Analg 58:372, 1979.
5. Rao TKL, El-Etr A: Anticoagulation following placement of epidural and subarachnoid catheters: An evaluation of neurologic sequalae. Anesthesiology 55:618, 1981.

43. CEREBROVASCULAR INSUFFICIENCY

Cynthia K. Hampson, M.D.

1. What is cerebrovascular disease?
Cerebrovascular disease refers to abnormalities in both extracranial and intracranial blood vessels that may lead to an inadequate supply of blood and therefore oxygen to the brain. When the supply of oxygen is inadequate to meet the needs of the brain, cerebral ischemia results; this is termed cerebrovascular insufficiency.

2. What are the neurologic manifestations of cerbrovascular insufficiency?
The two major groups of symptoms include transient ischemia attack (TIA) and stroke. A TIA develops suddenly, involves neurologic dysfunction for minutes to hours (by definition, never lasting more than 24 hours), clears spontaneously, and is associated with a normal computed tomography (CT) scan. Strokes may develop rapidly or in a stepwise fashion over a period of hours, days, or weeks. Their major differentiating feature from TIAs is that the resultant neurologic dysfunction either requires a period of months to years to resolve or, more commonly, never resolves completely. Strokes can be classified as minor, with eventual full or nearly full recovery, or major, with severe and permanent disability or death. In addition to cerebrovascular abnormalities, strokes are associated with many other disease states, including but not limited to hypertension, diabetes, coagulopathies, atrial fibrillation, mitral valve disease, substance abuse, and endocarditis. A third group of patients experiences neurologic dysfunction for longer than 24 hours with spontaneous and complete recovery within 1–2 weeks. This phenomenon is termed reversible ischemic neurologic deficit (RIND) and should be pathophysiologically grouped with TIAs.

3. What is the major cause of TIAs?
TIAs have two presumed causes, depending on the area of brain affected. Ischemia of the frontal and parietal lobes or the retina of the eye are believed to be caused by embolism of platelet aggregates and debris from atheroscerotic plaques in the extracranial carotid arteries and vertebrobasilar arteries. The quick resolution of TIAs (within 24 hours) is the result of the body's inherent mechanisms for dissolving and breaking down such emboli. In contrast, ischemia of the brainstem or the temporal and occipital lobes is believed to be caused by a transient decrease in blood flow or blood pressure in the vertebrobasilar system.

4. Contrast the symptoms of vertebrobasilar and carotid TIAs.
Carotid artery emboli usually present as transient ipsilateral visual loss, contralateral motor or sensory disturbance, or both. The visual loss results from the passage of emboli into the first branch of the internal carotid, the ophthalmic artery. The visual loss is often described as a shade pulled down over one eye, a syndrome called amaurosis fugax. Motor or sensory loss, including tingling, numbness, clumsiness, altered mentation, and difficulty with speaking, is caused by the passage of emboli into a cerebral hemisphere; consciousness is rarely affected. In contrast, symptoms of vertebrobasilar artery disease result from ischemia to the occipital lobes and the brainstem. Visual disturbance is common, but it is bilateral and frequently described as dim or blurry. Diplopia, nausea, vomiting, vertigo, and unsteadiness are also common. A characteristic of vertebrobasilar disease is the "drop-attack," a sudden loss of postural tone in the legs. Transient episodes of global amnesia, probably resulting from ischemia to the temporal lobes of the thalamus, are most likely due to basilar insufficiency. Vertebrobasilar symptoms, in contrast to carotid symptoms, are often linked to patient position or movement. Abrupt changes in position resulting in orthostatic hypotension may precipitate symptoms, and turning the head or reaching above the head may cause compression of the involved arteries.

5. What is the incidence of stroke in the United States?

Stroke affects approximately 500,000 persons annually; it is the third most common cause of death in the United States.

6. List the risk factors for stroke.

Hypertension is the strongest risk factor. Both systolic and diastolic elevations in blood pressure are associated with increased risk, and the degree of elevation is directly proportional to the risk of stroke. Two other major risk factors are cardiac disease (left ventricular hypertrophy, atrial fibrillation, cardiovascular disease) and smoking. Other less significant factors include age, diabetes, and hyperlipidemia.

7. What is the significance of an asymptomatic carotid bruit?

Asymptomatic bruits are heard in 5–10% of the adult population. A 1989 prospective study of 566 patients with asymptomatic carotid bruits revealed a 1-year stroke or TIA rate of 2.5% compared with a rate of 0.7% in patients without carotid bruits. The rate of stroke or TIA increases dramatically with increasing stenosis, reaching a rate greater than 5% annually for stenoses greater than 75%. Progression to stenosis of greater than 80% was associated with a 1-year stroke or TIA rate of 46%.

8. What are the two most common means of evaluating carotid disease?

The most common noninvasive means of evaluating carotid stenosis is the duplex scan. A duplex scan involves B-mode ultrasonography of the carotid bifurcation, which provides a two-dimensional assesment of plaques, ulcerations, and patency; Doppler ultrasonography measures red blood cell velocity and further defines the degree of stenosis. Angiography, an invasive test that carries a low risk of stroke, is the most accurate means of assessing carotid stenosis and of measuring the size of plaques. The accuracy of the duplex scan in estimating the degree of stenosis is 95% compared with angiography.

9. List the most common coexisting medical problems of symptomatic patients presenting for carotid endarterectomy (CEA).

Analysis of patients enrolled in the North American Symptomatic Carotid Endarterectomy Trial (NASCET) made it possible to determine the prevalence of specific coexisting medical conditions.

Coexisting Medical Conditions

MEDICAL CONDITION	PREVALENCE (%)
Angina	24
Previous myocardial infarction	20
Hypertension	60
Claudication	15
Smoking, current	37
Smoking, previous	40
Diabetes	19

10. What is the major cause of morbidity and mortality in patients undergoing CEA?

Cardiac complications, mainly myocardial infarction, are the primary source of mortality associated with CEA. A study of 1,546 endarterectomies noted that patients with a preoperative history of angina had a mortality of 18% compared with less than 5% in patients free of cardiac symptoms. The overall incidence of fatal infarction in patients undergoing CEA is 0.5–4%, which represents approximately 40% of the total 30-day perioperative mortality. Other factors predictive of increased cardiac mortality with CEA are congestive heart failure, myocardial infarction within the previous 6 months, and severe hypertension.

11. Describe a risk stratification scheme that considers medical status, neurologic status, and extent of carotid disease.

Carotid Endarterectomy and Risk Stratification

RISK GROUP	CHARACTERISTICS	TOTAL MORBIDITY AND MORTALITY (%)
1	Neurologically stable, no major medical or angiographic risk	1
2	Neurologically stable, significant angiographic risk, no major medical risk	2
3	Neurologically stable, major medical risk, ± major angiographic risk	7
4	Neurologically unstable, ± major medical or angiographic risk	10

TYPE OF RISK	RISK FACTORS
Medical	Angina Myocardial infarction (< 6 months ago) Congestive heart failure Severe hypertension (>180/110 mmHg) Chronic obstructive pulmonary disease Age > 70 years Severe obesity
Neurologic	Progressing deficit New deficit (< 24 hours) Frequent daily TIAs Multiple cerebral infarcts
Angiographic	Contralateral internal carotid artery occlusion Internal carotid artery siphon stenosis Proximal or distal plaque extension High carotid bifurcation Presence of soft thrombus

From Herrick IA, Gelb AW: Occlusive cerebrovascular disease: Anesthetic considerations. In Cottrell JE, Smith DS (eds): Anesthesia and Neurosurgery. St. Louis, Mosby, 1994, p 484, with permission.

12. Define cerebral autoregulation. How is it affected in cerebrovascular disease? What are the anesthetic implications?
Cerebral autoregulation is the ability of the brain to maintain cerebral blood flow relatively constant (40–60 ml/100 gm/min) over a wide range (50–150 mmHg) of mean arterial pressure. Stenosis or obstruction in the internal carotid artery causes a pressure drop beyond the obstruction. In an effort to maintain cerebral blood flow and avoid ischemia, the cerebral vasculature dilates. As the degree of carotid obstruction progresses, the cerebral vasculature distal to the obstruction maximally dilates. At this point, the cerebral vasculature loses its autoregulatory ability. Cerebral blood flow becomes passive and depends on systemic blood pressure. It thus becomes critically important to maintain the blood pressure of the CEA patient within very narrow limits, because they have minimal or no autoregulatory reserve to counter anesthetic-induced reductions in blood pressure. The anesthesiologist must have multiple preoperative blood pressures and heart rates to define the range over which the patient's cerebral blood flow is currently maintained.

13. How are the cerebral responses to hyper- and hypocapnia altered in cerebrovascular disease? What are the anesthetic implications?
Normal cerebral vessels are highly sensitive to arterial carbon dioxide partial pressure ($PaCO_2$), dilating in response to hypercapnia and constricting in response to hypocapnia. Cerebral blood

flow normally increases approximately 4% (1–2 ml/100 gm/min) for each 1 mmHg increase in $PaCO_2$ between 20 and 100 mmHg. However, in ischemic, already maximally vasodilated areas of the brain, this relationship breaks down, and responses to hyper- and hypocapnia may be paradoxical. Because cerebral vessels in an area of ischemia are already maximally dilated, hypercapnia may result in dilation of only normally responsive vessels outside the area of ischemia. This phenomenon, termed "steal," may divert blood flow away from the ischemic area, further compromising perfusion. On the other hand, hypocapnia may cause vessels in the ischemic area and in marginally perfused areas to undergo constriction, converting marginally perfused areas to truly ischemic areas. This phenomenon is termed the "Robin Hood" or "inverse steal" effect. It is therefore recommended that normocapnia be maintained in patients undergoing endarterectomy.

14. What is normal cerebral blood flow? At what level is cerebral blood flow considered ischemic?

Normal cerebral blood flow in humans is 40–60 ml/100 gm/min (15% of cardiac output). The cerebral metabolic rate for oxygen in adults is 3–4 ml/100 gm/min (20% of whole-body oxygen consumption). The cerebral blood flow at which ischemia becomes apparent on EEG, termed the critical regional cerebral blood flow (rCBF), is 18–20 ml/100 gm/min. Metabolic failure occurs at approximately 10–12 ml/100 gm/min.

15. How do inhalational anesthetics affect cerebral perfusion and cerebral metabolic rate?

In the normal, unanesthetized brain, cerebral blood flow varies directly with the cerebral metabolic rate for oxygen. Inhalational agents are said to "uncouple" this relationship. They decrease the cerebral metabolic rate for oxygen but concurrently cause dilation of cerebral blood vessels, thus increasing cerebral blood flow. Isoflurane reduces rCBF to less than 10 ml/100 gm/min, thus providing relative brain protection. In comparison, enflurane reduces rCBF to about 15 and halothane to about 20 ml/100 gm/min. Although it has not been proved or disproved by formal studies, isoflurane is theoretically the inhaled anesthetic of choice for CEA.

16. How should patients scheduled for CEA be monitored?

All patients undergoing CEA should be monitored with leads II and V of the electrocardiogram, noninvasive arterial blood pressure, end-tidal capnometry, temperature and pulse oximetry. Because of the need to maintain the patient's blood pressure within a specified range and to perform repetitive blood gas and coagulation studies, intraarterial blood pressure monitoring is also indicated. As always, additional monitors should be guided by individual patient characteristics. Carotid surgery does not involve large fluid shifts and does not require a pulmonary artery catheter in the patient with normal ventricular function. A 16-gauge or larger intravenous line is the recommended peripheral venous access for the typical CEA. Additional intravenous lines are started to administer vasoactive or anesthetic infusions.

17. Is regional or general anesthesia preferred for the endarterectomy patient?

No studies demonstrate a long-term benefit of one technique over the other. Ultimately, the choice between regional and general anesthesia is based on patient suitability and preference, on surgeon and anesthesiologist experience and expertise, and on the availability of cerebral perfusion monitoring.

18. Describe a regional anesthetic technique suitable for CEA.

Suitable anesthesia requires sensory blockade of cervical nerves C2 through C4, which is provided by blockade of the deep cervical plexus. This block is performed with the patient in the supine position, with the head and neck slightly extended and turned away from the side which is to be blocked. The anesthesiologist should stand at the shoulder of the side to be blocked. A line is drawn from the tip of the mastoid process to Chassaignac's tubercle (the transverse process of the sixth cervical vertebra, the most easily palpable transverse process of the cervical vertebra). A second line 1 cm posterior and parallel to this line overlies the the tips of the transverse processes of C2 through C4. Each of these three processes should be located and marked before injection. The C2 process is located 1–2 cm below the mastoid process and is the most difficult to palpate. The C3 process is approximately 1.5 cm below the C2 process (along the second line), and the C4 process is approximately 1.5 cm more cauded than C3. A 2-inch 22-gauge needle is then inserted just superior and posterior to the marks and is angled slightly anterior and caudad. This angle decreases the chance of inadvertently advancing the needle between the transverse processes and into the vertebral artery. The needle should contact C2 process at a depth of 2.5–3 cm; the C3 and C4 processes are slightly more superficial. After aspiration, 6 ml of local anesthesia is injected at each of the three locations. An alternate technique (attributed to Winnie) involves location of all three processes but injection only at the C4 process of 10–12 ml of local anesthesia. A paresthesia should be obtained with this technique, which relies on spread within the neurovascular space to achieve adequate anesthesia. If a paresthesia is not obtained with initial needle placement, the needle should be walked in an anteroposterior plane in a stepwise manner. Sensory blockade is provided by lower concentrations of local anesthetics, such as 0.5–1% lidocaine or 0.25% bupivacaine. Contraindications to this block are relative, including coagulopathy, previous surgery in the area of blockade, and poor patient cooperation. Patients with significant chronic obstructive pulmonary disease or otherwise borderline respiratory status may not be good candidates, because phrenic nerve palsy is a frequent complicaton of deep cervical plexus blockade. Care should be taken not to palpate the neck excessively, because the carotid plaque may fragment and embolize.

19. What are the advantages and disadvantages of regional anesthesia for CEA?
The main advantage of regional anesthesia is the ability to perform continuous neurologic assessment of the awake, cooperative patient and to evaluate the adequacy of cerebral perfusion. This, however, can quickly become a disadvantage if the patient develops cerebral ischemia. Cerebral ischemia in this setting may lead to disorientation, inadequate ventilation and oxygenation, and a disrupted surgical field. Providing maximal cerebral protection often requires conversion to a general anesthetic, but endotracheal intubation in this setting may prove difficult. In addition, sedation may impair the value of the awake neurologic assessment and therefore must be titrated carefully. Proponents of regional anesthesia believe that greater inherent control of blood pressure is maintained, thus reducing the need for vasopressors and perioperative myocardial ischemia. However, studies supporting this claim are limited.

A recognized complication of deep cervical block is phrenic nerve block, which may cause ventilatory compromise in some patients and is the major contraindication for bilateral deep cervical blocks. Other disadvantages of the deep cervical block include seizures from intraarterial injection of local anesthetic, total spinal or epidural anesthesia, and recurrent laryngeal nerve block.

20. Describe a general anesthetic technique for a typical patient CEA.
Many general anesthetic techniques are acceptable for CEA. Any technique that provides prompt awakening of the patient at the end of surgery and affords myocardial and cerebral protection is acceptable. The following guidelines are designed to attain these goals.

Because of the desire to have the patient awake and responsive soon after the completion of CEA, heavy premedication with long-acting agents is to be avoided. Anxiety generally is alleviated by an effective preoperative interview. The intraarterial catheter is placed before induction, as induction often involves unacceptable hemodynamic changes. The patient is preoxygenated, and induction is begun with a short-acting opioid until the patient is comfortably sedated but able to maintain relative normocapnea. The patient is then induced with 2–3 mg/kg of thiopental; controlled ventilation is begun with 100% oxygen by mask with isoflurane added as tolerated. Paralysis is generally instituted with a muscle relaxant possessing hemodynamic stability, such as vecuronium or rocuronium. Succinylcholine may be used, but it is contraindicated in hemiparetic patients because of the risk of hyperkalemia. Additional opioid is also given to reach a preinduction dose of 3–5 μg/kg of fentanyl; this dose helps to blunt the sympathetic response to intubation but is not likely to prolong the patient's awakening. In addition, 1–1½ minutes before intubation, 100 mg of lidocaine is given intravenously to help to blunt the response to intubation. With complete paralysis verified by train-of-four monitoring, intubation is then performed.

A light general anesthetic is maintained with oxygen—up to 50% nitrous oxide and isoflurane. Additional opioids are administered judiciously as needed, with the goal of a smooth but prompt awakening. Light general anesthesia is associated with a decreased incidence of myocardial ischemia compared with deep anesthesia with phenylephrine to maintain blood pressure.

Blood pressure is usually maintained within a narrow predefined range based on multiple observations of the patient's baseline vital signs. This range is defined by the highest preoperative value that is not associated with myocardial ischemia and the lowest preoperative value that is not associated with cerebral ischemia. Vasoactive agents, such as phenylephrine, dopamine, nitroglycerin, and nitroprusside, are commonly used as necessary to maintain blood pressure within this range.

Before carotid occlusion, anesthetic depth is minimized and blood pressure is allowed to rise to the upper limit previously defined as acceptable. This goal may require the addition of vasopressors. To insure that the patient does not move during carotid clamping, muscle relaxants may be added. Stretching of the carotid baroreceptor and significant bradycardia and hypotension can be avoided by having the surgeon infiltrate the carotid bifurcation with 1% lidocaine.

21. Discuss the conflicting goals of myocardial protection and cerebral protection during CEA.

The main goals of CEA anesthesia are to protect the heart and the brain from ischemia. However, the means of achieving these goals are often in direct conflict. Decreasing myocardial oxygen requirements involves decreasing heart rate, blood pressure, and contractility, whereas increasing cerebral perfusion involves increasing blood pressure and contractility, and avoiding bradycardia. Suggested compromises, which have been incorporated into the general guidelines described in question 20, include injecting the carotid bifurcation to avoid sudden and severe bradycardia and hypotension, decreasing both cerebral and myocardial metabolic rate with anesthetics such as thiopental and isoflurane, and maximizing afterload reduction while monitoring the EEG for ischemia.

Conflicts in Myocardial and Cerebral Protection

HEMODYNAMIC VARIABLE	TO PROTECT THE HEART FROM ISCHEMIA	TO PROTECT THE BRAIN FROM ISCHEMIA
Heart rate	Slow	Do not slow
Blood pressure	Decrease	Increase cerebral perfusion pressure
Contractility	Decrease	Increase

Compromise solutions:
1. Inject area of carotid bifurcations with 1% lidocaine for 10–15 minutes.
2. Decrease cerebral and myocardial metabolic rate and contractility.
3. Use normal findings of EEG or processed EEG to guide afterload reduction.

From Roizen MF, Ellis JE: Anesthesia for vascular surgery. In Barash PG, Cullen BF, Stoelting RK (eds): Clinical Anesthesia. Philadelphia, J.B. Lippincott, 1992, pp 1059–1072, with permission.

22. What are the advantages and disadvantages of general anesthesia for patients undergoing CEA?

Advantages of general anesthesia include control of the airway, a quiet operative field, and the ability to maximize cerebral perfusion if ischemia develops. The main disadvantage of general anesthesia is loss of the continuous neurologic evaluation of the awake patient.

23. What methods of monitoring cerebral perfusion during general anesthesia are available?

Several methods currently in use provide adequate cerebral perfusion, including stump pressure monitoring, intraoperative EEG, monitoring of somatosensory-evoked potentials, monitoring of jugular venous or transconjunctival oxygen saturation, transcranial Doppler, and tracer wash-out techniques. None is as reliable as an awake cooperative patient. None of the methods has been demonstrated to improve outcome, and none has gained widespread acceptance as the monitor of choice. In addition, the availablity of proper equipment and personnel to perform the monitoring varies by institution.

24. Do stump pressures provide reliable cerebral perfusion information?

No. The stump pressure is the pressure in the portion of the internal carotid artery immediately cephalad to the carotid cross-clamp. This pressure is presumed to represent pressure transmitted from the contralateral carotid artery and vertebrals via the circle of Willis. In the past, it was believed that a stump pressure of 50 mmHg was indicative of adequte cerebral blood flow and perfusion. However, studies have shown that stump pressures have **no** correlation with flow. Some patients with stump pressures less than 50 mmHg are adequately perfused, whereas some patients with "adequate" stump pressures have suffered ischemic injury. Studies have also shown a lack of correlation between stump pressures and EEG and between stump pressures and neurologic exam in awake patients.

25. Does jugular venous or transconjunctival oxygen saturation correlate with cerebral perfusion?

No. There appears to be no correlation between transconjunctival oxygen saturation and regional cerebral blood flow. Jugular venous oxygen saturation is a reliable measure of global cerebral perfusion if cerebral metabolic oxygen consumption remains constant. However, significant alterations in regional blood flow and perfusion may occur with no change in jugular venous oxygen saturation; thus this monitoring technique is inadequate for detecting regional cerebral ischemia.

26. What is currently the most accurate method of evaluating cerebral perfusion during general anesthesia?

Tracer washout methods provide accurate information about regional cerebral blood flow but require highly sophisticated technical equipment and expertise. This method involves inhalation, intravenous or intracarotid injection of a radioactive tracer such as xenon-133 or krypton-85, and measurement of the tracer's washout from the brain via an external array of scintillation monitors. Another drawback to this method is that it provides instantaneous rather than continuous perfusion information.

27. Does intraoperative EEG provide clinically useful information during CEA?

No data show that EEG during CEA results in improved patient outcomes. Although the EEG is a highly sensitive and early indicator of global cortical ischemia, it is not highly specific and results in many false-positive (though few false-negative) warnings. It is also affected by multiple variables, including temperature, blood pressure, $PaCO_2$, PaO_2, serum glucose and sodium levels, anesthetic depth, and preexisting neurologic deficits. The value of the EEG may lie in myocardial protection. Monitoring of the EEG with the goal of maximally reducing blood pressure without producing EEG evidence of cerebral ischemia reduces myocardial afterload and the incidence of perioperative myocardial ischemia.

28. What are the common postoperative complications of CEA ?

Hypotension associated with decreased systemic vascular resistance is common and is believed to be caused by an intact carotid sinus responding to higher arterial pressures after removal of the atheromatous plaque. Such hypotension responds well to fluid administration and vasopressors and may be prevented by infiltration of the sinus with local anesthetic. Hypotension also may result from myocardial ischemia. The incidence of postoperative myocardial ischemia and infarction has already been discussed and obviously indicates a need for continued careful control of postoperative blood pressure, heart rate, and oxygenation. Therefore, a 12-lead ECG should be obtained soon after the patient arrives in the recovery room and leads II and V of the ECG should be continuously monitored.

Hypertension is also common but less understood. Obviously, the high incidence of preoperative hypertension, particularly when it is poorly controlled, may result from labile postoperative hypertension. It may also be the result of denervation of the carotid sinus or trauma to the sinus intraoperatively. Other causes of postoperative hypertension must also be sought, such as bladder distention, hypoxia, hyercarbia, and pain. Given the high association of postoperative hypertension with onset of new neurologic deficit, postoperative hypertension must be aggressively monitored and treated.

Cerebral hyperperfusion caused by increased cerebral blood flow is also a recognized postoperative complication It typically results from an increase in flow of not less than 35%, but the increase may approach 200%. Poorly controlled hypertension contributes to this complication. Symptoms and side effects of hyperperfusion are headache, face and eye pain, cerebral edema, nausea and vomiting, seizure and intracerebral hemorrhage. The blood pressure of such patients should be very carefully controlled, preferably without the use of cerebral vasodilators.

Respiratory difficulties may result from several different mechanisms. Hematomas may form postoperatively and lead to airway compromise and cranial nerve palsies. Treatment involves drainage of the hematoma followed by intubation of the patient as needed. Respiratory problems also may result from vocal cord paralysis due to intraoperative damage to laryngeal nerves. Depending on the severity of the respiratory compromise, intubation may be indicated. The chemoreceptor function of the carotid bodies is predictably lost in most patients after CEA, as evidenced by a complete loss of the respiratory response to hypoxia and an average increase in the resting pCO_2 of 6 mmHg. Thus, patients should receive supplemental oxygen postoperatively for at least 24 hours; adequate attention to pulmonary toilet is mandatory.

Most **strokes** associated with CEA occur postoperatively as a result of surgical factors involving carotid thrombosis and emboli from the surgical site.

BIBLIOGRAPHY

1. Brown DL: Atlas of Regional Anesthesia. Philadelphia, W.B.Saunders, 1992.
2. Chambers BR, Norris JW: Outcome in patients with asymptomatic neck bruits. N Engl J Med 315:860–865, 1986.
3. Frost EAM: The patient for carotid endarterectomy. Anesthesiol News, Dec 18–25, 1994.
4. Herrick JA, Gelb AW: Occlusive cerebrovascular disease: Anesthetic considerations. In Cottrell JE, Smith DS (eds): Anesthesia and Neurosurgery. St. Louis, Mosby, 1994, pp 481–494.
5. Jaffe RA, Samuels SI: Anesthesiologist's Manual of Surgical Procedures. New York, Raven Press, 1994, pp 76–80.
6. Lien CA, Poxnak AV: Carotid endarterectomy. In Yao FSF, Artusio JF (eds): Anesthesiology—Problem-Oriented Patient Management, 3rd ed. Philadelphia, J.B. Lippincott, 1993, pp 335–61.
7. North American Symptomatic Carotid Endarterectomy Trial Steering Committee: North American Symptomatic Carotid Endarterectomy Trial. Methods, patient characteristics, and progress. Stroke 22:711–720, 1991.
8. O'Donnell TF, Callow AD, Willet C, et al: The impact of coronary artery disease on carotid endarterectomy. Ann Surg 198:705–712, 1983.
9. Roederer GO, Langlois YE, Joger KA, et al: The natural history of carotid arterial disease in asymptomatic patients with cervical bruits. Stroke 15:605–613, 1984.
10. Roizen MF, Ellis JE: Anesthesia for vascular surgery. In Barash PG, Cullen BF, Stoelting RK (eds): Clinical Anesthesia, 2nd ed. Philadelphia, J.B. Lippincott, 1992, pp 1059–1072.
11. Smith JS, Roizen MF, Cahalan MK, et al: Does anesthetic technique make a difference? Augmentation of systolic blood pressure during carotid endarterectomy: Effects of phenylephrine versus light anesthesia and of isoflurane versus halothane on the incidence of myocardial ischemia. Anesthesiology 69:846, 1988.
12. Stoelting RK, Dierdorf SF: Anesthesia and Co-Existing Disease. New York, Churchill Livingstone, 1993, pp 202–207.
13. Sundt TM Jr, Whinant JP, Houser OW, et al: Prospective study of the effectiveness and durability of carotid endarterectomy. Mayo Clin Proc 65:625–635, 1990.
14. Wade JG, Larson CP, Hickey RF, et al: Effect of carotid endarterectomy on carotid chemoreceptor and baroreceptor function in man. N Engl J Med 282:823,1970.

44. REACTIVE AIRWAY DISEASE

Malcolm Packer, M.D.

1. Define reactive airway disease.

This term is used to describe a family of diseases that share an airway sensitivity to physical, chemical, or pharmacologic stimuli. This sensitivity results in a bronchoconstrictor response and is seen in patients with asthma, chronic obstructive pulmonary disease (COPD), emphysema, viral upper respiratory illness, and other disorders. COPD and emphysema are covered in chapter 46 and this chapter concentrates on asthma.

Asthma is defined by the American Thoracic Society as "a disease characterized by an increased responsiveness of the trachea and bronchi to various stimuli manifested by a widespread narrowing of the airways that changes in severity either spontaneously or as a result of therapy. Asthma is manifested by episodes of dyspnea, cough and wheezing." These symptoms are related to the increased resistance to airflow in the patient's airways.

2. What are the different types of asthma?

Although the common denominator lies in hyperreactivity of the airways, patients may fit into two subgroups: allergic (extrinsic) and idiosyncratic (intrinsic). Many believe that the terms extrinsic and intrinsic should be discarded. Underlying all asthma are airway hyperreactivity and inflammation, and the cause includes the interaction of allergic and nonallergic stimuli.

The allergic type of asthma is thought to result from an IgE-mediated response to certain antigens such as dust and pollen. Among the mediators released are histamine, leukotrienes, prostaglandins, bradykinin, thromboxane, and eosinophilic chemotactic factor. Their release leads to capillary leakage in the airways, along with mucous secretions and smooth muscle contraction surrounding the airway. Inflammation is a prominent feature.

The idiosyncratic type of asthma is not mediated by IgE but by nonantigenic stimuli, such as exercise, cold, pollution, and infection. Bronchospasm is caused by increased parasympathetic (vagal) tone. Patients in the idiosyncratic group also have release of the same mediators as the allergic group. Conversely, certain patients with allergic asthma have increased vagal tone.

3. How common is asthma? Is it inherited?

Population studies have shown that asthma affects 3–5% of adults and 7–10% of children. Among children, boys predominate 2:1, but this gender distinction disappears by age 30. Although children can "outgrow" their asthma, it may return in later life and adults with no previous history may become symptomatic. Asthma related to environmental factors is commonly seen in industrial areas, in homes of smokers, or where woodburning stoves are used.

Studies of families prove asthma is inherited. Data on twins show a concordance rate of 67% in monozygous twins and 34% in dizygous twins for airway hyperreactivity.

4. List the common pharmacologic and food additive causes of asthma.

Serious asthmatic responses have been associated with aspirin and nonsteroidal antiinflammatory agents. Beta-adrenergic blockers are contraindicated in asthmatics. Certain patients have severe reactions to ingestion of metabisulfite (food preservative) or tartrazine (food color). To define the degree of hyperreactivity of a patient's airway, a methacholine challenge test is performed under controlled conditions in the pulmonary function laboratory.

5. What diseases mimic asthma?

Upper and lower airway obstruction from tumor, aspirated foreign bodies, or stenosis may mimic asthma. Left ventricular failure (cardiac asthma) and pulmonary embolism both simulate airway hyperreactivity. Gastroesophageal reflux and aspiration also may produce airway hyperreactivity. Viral respiratory illnesses (e.g., respiratory syncytial virus) also produce bronchospasm. A careful history and physical exam help to define the cause.

6. What are the important historical features of an asthmatic patient?
A careful history allows a close estimate of the severity of disease. Questions should include:
  1. How and when the patient was first diagnosed.
  2. How often the patient has "attacks," what typically initiates them, and how long the illness has lasted.
  3. Whether the patient has been treated as an outpatient or inpatient.
  4. If the patient was an inpatient, ask for details of hospital stay, including length of admission, requirement of intensive care, and intubation.
  5. What medications the patient takes, including as-needed usage and over-the-counter medications. Has the patient ever taken steroids?

7. What physical findings are associated with asthma?
The most common physical finding is expiratory wheezing. Wheezing is a sign of obstructed airflow, and is often associated with a prolonged expiratory phase. As asthma progressively worsens, patients use accessory respiratory muscles. A significantly symptomatic patient with quiet auscultatory findings may signal impending respiratory failure because not enough air is moving to elicit a wheeze. Patients also may be tachypneic and probably are dehydrated; they prefer an upright posture and demonstrate pursed-lip breathing. Cyanosis is a late and ominous sign.

8. What preoperative tests should be ordered?
The patient's history guides the judicious ordering of preoperative tests. A mild asthmatic on as-needed medication who is currently healthy will not benefit from preoperative testing. Symptomatic patients with no recent evaluation deserve closer attention.

The most common test is a pulmonary function test, which allows simple and quick evaluation of the degree of obstruction and its reversibility. The important measures are FEV_1 (the amount of air forcefully expired in 1 second), FVC (the total amount of air expired or forced vital capacity), MMEFR (the flow rate noted while expiring 25–75% of the forced vital capacity), and PEFR (peak expiratory flow rate). A comparison of values obtained from the patient with predicted values helps to assess the degree of obstruction. Severe exacerbation correlates with a PEFR or FEV_1 less than 30 to 50% of predicted, which for most adults is a PEFR of less than 120 L/min and a FEV_1 of less than 1 L. Tests should be repeated after a trial of bronchodilator therapy to assess reversibility and response to treatment.

Arterial blood gases are usually not helpful. Hypoxia may be evaluated with a pulse oximeter, and hypercapnia is not noted until the FEV_1 is less than 25%. Electrocardiograms, chest radiographs, and blood counts are rarely indicated for evaluation of asthma unless particular features of the patient's presentation suggest alternative diagnoses (e.g., fever and rales suggesting pneumonia).

9. What specific medications and routes of delivery are used in asthma?
The mainstay of therapy remains inhaled beta agonists. Specific $beta_2$ agonists, such as albuterol, terbutaline and fenoterol, have become available over the last 10 years. They offer greater specificity for $beta_2$-mediated bronchodilation and fewer side effects (e.g., $beta_1$-associated tachydysrythmias and tremors). Albuterol can be administered orally or by metered dose inhaler (MDI). Terbutaline is effective via nebulizer, subcutaneously, or as a continuous intravenous infusion (beware of hypokalemia, lactic acidosis, and cardiac tachydysrhythmias with intravenous use). Epinephrine is available for subcutaneous use in severely asthmatic patients. Patients with coronary artery disease have difficulty with tachycardia and need the more $beta_2$-specific agents. The data about delivery of beta agonists delivery support the inhaled route over parenteral administration

for routine treatment. Fenoterol is not available in the U.S. at this time; adult dosages of commonly used drugs are as follows:

Albuterol: 2.5 mg in 3 ml of normal saline for nebulization or 2 puffs by MDI. Patients with active asthma may need repeat treatments.

Terbutaline: 0.3–0.4 mg subcutaneously; may repeat as required every 20 minutes for 3 doses.

Epinephrine: 0.3 mg subcutaneously; may repeat as required every 20 minutes for 3 doses.

The use of theophylline in asthma is controversial. Theophylline has some bronchodilatory effects and improves diaphragmatic action. Such benefits must be weighed against a long list of side effects: tremor, nausea and vomiting, palpitations, tachydysrhythmias, and seizures. Careful monitoring of serum levels is mandatory. Theophylline is the oral form, whereas aminophylline (its water-soluble form) is for intravenous use. Dosage for adults is as follows:

Theophylline: 5 mg/kg intravenously over 30 minutes (loading dose in patients not previously taking theophylline). After loading dose, start continous infusion of 0.4 mg/kg/hr. Check level in 6 hours. Beware of drug interactions and certain diseases that alter theophylline clearance.

The use of anticholinergic compounds has increased over the years. Atropine, glycopyrrolate, and ipratropium are useful in bronchospasm associated with chronic obstructive pulmonary disease and beta blockade. Anticholinergics also may be helpful in severe airway obstruction ($FEV_1 < 25\%$ predicted). Ipratroprium, glycopyrrolate, and atropine may be given via nebulizer; ipratroprium is available in an MDI. The following dosages are for adults:

Anticholinergics: ipratroprium, 0.5 mg by nebulization or 4–6 puffs by MDI; atropine, 1–2 mg per nebulization.

Corticosteroid medications reverse airway inflammation, decrease mucus production, and potentiate beta agonist-induced smooth muscle relaxation. Steroids should be considered seriously in patients with moderate-to-severe asthma or patients who have required steroids in the last 6 months. Onset of action is 1–2 hours after administration. Methylprednisolone is popular because of its strong antiinflammatory powers but weak mineralocorticoid effect. Side effects include hyperglycemia, hypertension, hypokalemia and mood alterations, including psychosis. Long-term steroid use or prolonged use with muscle relaxants is associated with myopathy. Steroids may be given orally, via MDI, or intravenously.

Cromolyn sodium is a mast cell stabilizer that is useful for long-term maintenance therapy in certain patients. Patients younger than 17 years of age and with moderate-to-severe exercise-induced asthma appear to benefit the most. Side effects include some minimal local irritation on delivery. Cromolyn sodium may be administered via multidose inhaler or as a powder in a turboinhaler. Cromolyn sodium is not effective and in fact is contraindicated in acute asthmatic attacks.

Patients with severe asthma may require methotrexate or gold salts. Both medications have undesirable side effect profiles and are reserved for patients who have major difficulties with corticosteroids. The following dosages are for adults:

Corticosteroids: methylprednisolone, 60–125 mg IV as required every 6 hours, or prednisone, 30–50 mg orally every day.

10. What is the best approach to preoperative medical management?
First the anesthesiologist should classify each patient in one of several groups. Asymptomatic patients with no recent bouts of asthma, no current medications and no history of serious illness usually require only careful observation. Currently, asymptomatic patients who have a history of recurrent asthma and use bronchodilators require optimization of pulmonary function. The dosing of beta agonists should be guided by symptoms and pulmonary function tests. Theophylline dosing may be adjusted if levels are inadequate or toxic. The decision to start corticosteroids is difficult, but in general they should be used to pretreat (1) patients with a history of moderate-to-severe asthma, especially with intensive care admissions and mechanical ventilation; (2) patients who required steroids in the last 6 months; and (3) patients at risk for adrenal insufficiency.

The final group is the symptomatic patient with ongoing bronchospasm. If at all possible, surgery should be delayed. If emergent surgery is required, treatment with beta agonists, up to and including continuous nebulizations, is useful. For patients who do not improve on this regimen, a trial of intravenous terbutaline or subcutaneous epinephrine should be made. Corticosteroids should be started early and continued. For patients taking theophylline, therapy should be optimized on the basis of serum levels. Consider whether regional anesthesia is possible.

11. Should theophylline be initiated in symptomatic patients?
Available data allow no definite recommendation. In some studies, patients taking theophylline show ventilatory improvement in the first 24 hours of use, whereas other studies show no benefit in patients with acute asthma. The use of theophylline increases the incidence of tremor, nausea, palpitations, and tachycardia. Until definite proof is available, many investigators suggest that theophylline therapy should be initiated only in patients with acute asthma who do not improve with maximal beta agonist and corticosteroid therapy.

12. What premedicants should be used or avoided?
Patients should be made comfortable and less anxious. Use of opioids (excluding morphine because of its histamine-releasing side effect) for pain and benzodiazapines for anxiolysis, with careful attention to avoid respiratory depression, is acceptable. Histamine-1 receptor antagonists may be useful, but only in conjunction with a histamine-2 receptor antagonist. Histamine-2 antagonists without a histamine-1 antagonist theoretically should be avoided.

13. What are the safe methods of inducing general anesthesia in asthmatic patients?
Intravenous induction agents used in asthmatic patients include oxybarbiturates, thiobarbiturates, ketamine, and propofol. Thiobarbiturates constrict airways in laboratory investigations and may have a loose association with clinical bronchospasm. The most common cause of bronchospasm is the stimulus of intubation, and large doses of barbiburates are required to block this effect successfully. Ketamine has well-known bronchodilatory effects secondary to the release of endogenous catecholamines with $beta_2$ agonism. Ketamine also has a small, direct relaxant effect on smooth muscles. In a recent study, propofol demonstrated no significant effect on peripheral airway tone. Intravenous lidocaine is a useful adjunct to the above induction agents in blunting the response to laryngoscopy and intubation.

Mask induction with halothane is an excellent method to block airway reflexes and to relax airway smooth muscles directly. Halothane as an induction agent is much more palatable to the airway than isoflurane or enflurane. Sevoflurane may compete with halothane as the induction agent of choice for asthmatic patients as it enters the U.S. market.

14. What agents may be used for maintenance anesthesia?
Inhaled anesthetics are excellent for maintenance anesthesia in asthmatic patients. Halothane, isoflurane, and enflurane appear equally effective in blocking airway reflexes and bronchoconstriction. Inhaled anesthetics have been used in the intensive care unit to provide broncodilation in intubated patients with severe asthma, improving indices of respiratory resistance (inspiratory and expiratory flows), decreasing hyperinflation, and lowering intrinsic positive end-expiratory pressure (PEEP).

Opioids at higher doses block airway reflexes but do not provide direct bronchodilation. Morphine remains controversial because of its histamine-releasing activity. Anesthetics relying primarily on opioids may cause problems with respiratory depression at emergence (particularly in patients with COPD that has an asthmatic component).

Neuromuscular blocking agents, such as d-tubocurarine, atracurium, and mivacurium, release histamine from mast cells upon injection. They also may bind directly to muscarinic receptors on ganglia, nerve endings, and airway smooth muscle. Both mechanisms theoretically may increase airway resistance. Pancuronium and vecuronium continue to be used safely in asthmatic patients. In patients with bronchospasm neuromuscular blocking agents improve chest wall compliance, but smooth muscle airway tone and lung compliance remain the same. Prolonged use of muscle relaxants in ventilated asthmatic patients is associated with increases in creatine kinase and clinically significant myopathy.

15. What are the complications of intubation and mechanical ventilation in asthmatic patients?

The stimulus of intubation causes significant increases in airway resistance. Lung hyperinflation occurs when diminished expiratory flow prevents complete emptying of the alveolar and small airway gas. Significant gas trapping may cause hypotension by increasing intrathoracic pressure and reducing venous return. Pneumomediastinum and pneumothorax are also potential causes of acute respiratory decompensation.

Several measurements of ventilator function may give some insight into a patient's improving or worsening status. Plateau pressures (the pressure measured at end inspiration and before expiration starts, averaged over an 0.4–second pause) correlate loosely with complications at pressures greater than 30 cm H_2O. Auto-PEEP is the measurement of end-expiratory pressure (taken at end expiration while the expiratory port is momentarily occluded) and may correlate with alveolar pressures in the bronchospastic patient. Auto-PEEP, however, does not specifically correlate with complication. Plateau pressure and auto-PEEP measurements require a relaxed patient.

Several strategies for mechanically ventilating bronchospastic patients have been developed:

1. Increase expiratory time by decreasing ventilator rate, increasing inspiratory flow rates to decrease inspiratory time; and directly increasing the inspiratory:expiratory ratio.
2. Avoid ventilator-applied PEEP.
3. Decrease minute volume, allowing controlled hypoventilation and permissive hypercapnea.

16. What are the causes of intraoperative wheezing and the correct responses to asthmatic patients with acute bronchospasm?

Airway secretions, foreign body, pulmonary edema (cardiac asthma), obstructed endotracheal tube, endotracheal tube at the carina or down a mainstem bronchus, allergic or anaphylactic response to drugs, and asthma cause wheezing in intubated patients. A number of medications cause wheezing in asthmatic patients, including beta blockers, muscle relaxants, and aspirin.

After carefully checking the endotracheal tube and listening for bilateral breath sounds, one should increase the inspired oxygen to 100% and deepen the anesthetic if hemodynamically tolerated by the patient. Provoking factors such as medication infusions, misplaced endotracheal tubes, or other causes of airway stimulation should be corrected. Manipulating the ventilator (see question 15) may help. Reversal of bronchospasm may be attempted with such medications as $beta_2$ agonists, and corticosteroids. Aminophylline and anticholinergics may be added for patients with poor response to $beta_2$ agonists and corticosteroids.

17. Describe the emergence techniques for asthmatic patients under general endotracheal anesthesia (GETA).

Awake and deep extubations are alternatives in patients under GETA. The endotracheal tube is a common cause of significant bronchospasm, and its removal under deep inhaled anesthetic in a spontaneously ventilating patient often leads to a smooth emergence. Deep extubations should be avoided in patients with difficult airways, morbidly obese patients, and patients with full stomachs.

18. Does regional anesthesia offer any advantages over general anesthesia?

Regional anesthesia should be considered for all patients amenable to such care. Regional anesthesia is considered advantageous compared with general endotracheal anesthesia because it avoids the provocative endotracheal tube. Regional anesthesia in conjunction with GETA may be helpful in alleviating the need for large doses of opioids and the risk of postoperative respiratory depression. Asthmatic patients undergoing high abdominal or thoracic procedures may benefit from a thoracic epidural block. Regional anesthesia does not obviate bronchospasm, and asthmatic patients under such care should receive the same aggressive care to avoid bronchospasm.

19. What new therapies are available to anesthesiologists treating asthmatic patients in bronchospasm?

Recently intensivists have administered magnesium sulfate to patients in status asthmaticus. Hypothetically magnesium interferes with calcium-mediated smooth muscle contraction and decreases acetylcholine release at the neuromuscular junction. Magnesium reduces histamine- and methacholine-induced bronchospasm in controlled studies, but so far clinical studies have failed to show a significant response.

Heliox, a blend of helium and oxygen, has been successful in reducing airway resistance, peak airway pressures, and $PaCO_2$ levels when administered to spontaneously and mechanically ventilated patients. The mixture contains 60–80% helium and 20–40% oxygen and is less dense than air. The decrease in density allows less turbulent flow and significant declines in resistance to flow. The device for heliox administration in intubated patients is cumbersome unless the anesthesia machine is already equipped.

A new endotracheal tube on the market, the Lita-Tube, allows intraoperative instillation of lidocaine at and below the cords of the intubated patient. This technique decreases airway stimulation from the endotracheal tube and may prevent reflex bronchospasm.

BIBLIOGRAPHY

1. Bishop MJ: Respiratory Disease: When to Delay Surgery and How to Proceed. Annual Refresher Course Lectures, American Society of Anesthesiologists, 1991.
2. Corbridge TC, Hall JB: The assessment and management of adults with status asthmatics. Am J Respir Crit Care Med 151:1296–1316, 1995.
3. Fung D, Smith NT: Anesthetic considerations in asthmatic patients. In Gershwin ME (ed): Bronchial Asthma. London, Grune & Stratton, 1986, pp 525–540.
4. Groeben H, Schwalen A, Irsfeld B, et al: High thoracic epidural does not alter airway resistance and attenuates the response to an inhalation provocation test in patients with bronchial hyperactivity. Anesthesiology 81: 868–874, 1994.
5. Hirshman CA: Anesthesia for Patients with Reactive Airways Disease. Annual Refresher Course Lectures, American Society of Anesthesiologists, 1993.
6. Hudgel DW: Bronchial asthma. In Baum GL, Wolinsky E (eds): Textbook of Pulmonary Diseases, 5th ed. Boston, Little, Brown, 1994, pp 647–685.
7. Kiu HK, Rook GA, Ryan-Dykes MA, Bishop MJ: Effect of prophylactic bronchodilator treatment on lung resistance after tracheal intubation. Anesthesiology 81:43–48, 1994.
8. Pizov R, Brown RH, Weiss YS, et al: Wheezing during induction of general anesthesia in patients with and without asthma. Anesthesiology 82:1111–1116, 1995.
9. Stoller JK, Wiedemann HP: Chronic obstructive lung diseases: Asthma, emphysema, chronic bronchitis, bronchiectasis and related conditions. In George RB (ed): Chest Medicine Essentials of Pulmonary and Critical Care Medicine, 2nd ed. New York, Churchill Livingstone, 1990, pp 161–203.
10. Yao FF: Asthma—Chronic obstructive pulmonary disease. In Yao FF, Artusio OF (eds): Anesthesiology: Problem-Oriented Patient Management. Philadelphia, J.B. Lippincott, 1993, pp 3–25.

45. ASPIRATION

Malcolm Packer, M.D.

1. What is aspiration?

Aspiration is the passage of material from the pharynx into the trachea. Aspirated material can originate from the stomach, esophagus, mouth, or nose. The materials involved can be particulate, such as food or a foreign body, or fluid, such as blood, saliva, or gastrointestinal contents. Aspiration of gastric contents may occur by vomiting, which is an active propulsion from the stomach up the esophagus, or by regurgitation, which is the passive flow of material along the same path.

2. Who first described aspiration associated with anesthesia?

Sir James Simpson described the death of a 15-year-old girl given chloroform for toenail removal in the mid 19th century. Simpson reasoned that she died from choking on her own secretions. In 1946 Curtis Mendelson reported 60 cases of aspiration associated with patients receiving general anesthesia for vaginal delivery. Mendelson performed an animal study describing the physiologic response to the different types of aspirates: liquid vs. particulate and acidic vs. neutral pH. This compilation of clinical and animal study data opened physicians' eyes to the serious sequence of events following the aspiration of gastric contents. This sequence is known as Mendelson's syndrome.

3. How often does aspiration occur?

The results of several different retrospective and prospective surveys place the incidence at 1–7 cases of significant aspiration per 10,000 anesthetics.

4. Name the risk factors for aspiration.

Extremes of age
Emergency cases
Type of surgery (most common in cases of esophageal, upper abdominal, or
    emergency laparotomy surgery)
Recent meal
Delayed gastric emptying and/or decreased lower esophageal sphincter tone (diabetes,
    gastric outlet obstruction, hiatal hernia, medications [e.g., narcotics, anticholinergics])
Trauma
Pregnancy
Pain and stress
Depressed level of consciousness
Morbid obesity
Difficult airway
Poor motor control (neuromuscular disease)
Esophageal disease (e.g., scleroderma, achalasia, diverticulum, Zenker's disease)

5. Describe the different clinical pictures caused by the three broad types of aspirate: acidic fluid, nonacidic fluid, and particulate matter.

Acidic aspirates with a pH less than 2.5 and volumes of more than 0.4 ml/kg immediately cause alveolar-capillary breakdown, resulting in interstitial edema, intraalveolar hemorrhage, atelectasis, and increased airway resistance. Hypoxia is common. Although such changes usually start within minutes of the initiating event, they may worsen over a period of hours. The first phase of the response is direct reaction of the lung to acid; hence the name chemical pneumonitis. The second phase, which occurs hours later, is due to leukocyte or inflammatory response to the original damage and may lead to respiratory failure.

Aspiration of **nonacidic fluid** destroys surfactant, causing alveolar collapse and atelectasis. Hypoxia is common. The destruction of lung architecture and the late inflammatory response are not as great as in acid aspiration.

Aspiration of **particulate food matter** causes both physical obstruction of the airway and a later inflammatory response related to the presence of a foreign body. Alternating areas of atelectasis and hyperexpansion may occur. Patients show hypoxia and hypercapnia due to physical obstruction of airflow. If acid is mixed with the particulate matter, damage is often greater and the clinical picture worse.

6. What is the incidence of clinical signs and symptoms after aspiration of gastric contents?
Fever occurs in over 90% of aspiration cases, with tachypnea and rales in at least 70%. Cough, cyanosis and wheezing occur in 30–40% of cases. Aspiration may occur "silently"—without the anesthesiologist's knowledge—during anesthesia. Any of the above clinical deviations from the expected course may signal an aspiration event. Patients undergoing anesthesia should be monitored according to the recommendations of the American Society of Anesthesiologists. Included are temperature, breath sound, and oxygenation monitoring, which ensure early detection of aspiration.

7. When is a patient suspected of aspiration believed to be out of danger?
The patient who shows none of the above signs or symptoms and has no increased oxygen requirement at the end of 2 hours should recover completely.

8. Describe the treatment of aspiration.
Supportive care remains the mainstay. Immediate suctioning should be instituted. Supplemental oxygen and ventilatory support should be initiated if respiratory failure is a problem. Patients with respiratory failure often demonstrate atelectasis with alveolar collapse and may respond to positive end-expiratory pressure (PEEP). Patients with particulate aspirate may need bronchoscopy to remove large obstructing pieces.

9. What are the major controversies in the treatment of aspiration?
Discussions about treating patients with prophylactic antibiotics and corticosteroids continue. Presently no evidence suggests that antibiotics are helpful unless intestinal obstruction causes the aspirated fluid to be fecally contaminated. Corticosteroids have not been shown to be helpful in human studies. Lastly, some practitioners advocate lavaging the trachea with normal saline or sodium bicarbonate in the case of acid aspiration. This procedure, however, has not been shown to be helpful and may actually worsen the patient's status.

10. What precautions prior to anesthetic induction are required to prevent aspiration or mollify its sequelae?
The main precaution is to recognize which patients are at risk. Patients should have an adequate fasting period to improve the chances of an empty stomach. Gastrokinetic medications such as metaclopramide immediately improve gastric emptying and increase esophageal sphincter tone. It is also helpful to increase gastric pH by either nonparticulate antacids such as sodium citrate or H_2 receptor antagonists, which decrease acid production.

The market now includes several H_2 antagonists, giving anesthesiologists a choice (e.g., cimetidine, ranitidine and famotidine). Cimetidine was first on the market and is still widely used. Although cimetidine increases gastric pH, it also has a significant side-effect profile, including hypotension, heart block, central nervous dysfunction, decreased hepatic blood flow, and significant retardation of the metabolism of many drugs. Ranitidine, a newer H_2 antagonist, is much less likely to cause side effects; only a few cases of central nervous dysfunction and heart block have been reported. Famotidine is equally as potent as cimetidine and ranitidine and has no significant side effects.

11. What are considered adequate fasting times?
In general, adults should have no solid food for 6–8 hours prior to surgery. Over the years anesthesiologists have shortened the time during which no oral ingestion (NPO) is permitted and currently allow clear liquid intake 3–4 hours before surgery. Infant NPO times are usually 4–6 hours for formula and 2–3 hours for clear liquids or breast milk.

12. Define rapid-sequence induction.
Patients with an airway that is by exam easy to intubate may receive a rapid-sequence induction, which consists of preoxygenating the patient and placing pressure over the cricoid cartilage (Sellick maneuver). This pressure prevents gastric contents from leaking into the pharynx by extrinsic obstruction of the esophagus. The cricoid cartilage is the only complete cartilaginous ring of the tracheal tree. After preoxygenation and cricoid pressure, general anesthesia is induced and a paralyzing dose of relaxant is administered. The patient's trachea is intubated, and the endotracheal balloon cuff is inflated. To ensure proper placement, breath sounds should be symmetrical and end-tidal carbon dioxide detected. Cricoid pressure should be released only after endotracheal tube placement is assured.

13. Which procedures are safer for patients at risk for aspiration?
Patients with airways thought to be difficult to intubate may require placement of an endotracheal tube while awake to allow spontaneous breathing and to protect the airway from aspiration. Awake intubations are facilitated by such devices as light wands, fiberoptic bronchoscopes, and retrograde intubation kits. Patient comfort is aided by the judicious use of sedation and topical local anesthetic. Oversedation as well as a topicalized airway may make the patient unable to protect the airway. Therefore, keeping the patient conscious and applying topical local anesthetic only to the airway above the glottis leads to safe intubation.

Endotracheal intubation does not guarantee that no aspiration will occur. Material may still slip past a deflated or partly deflated cuff. In pediatric patients less than 8 years old, an endotracheal cuff is not recommended; thus leakage of material into the lungs is common.

14. Describe the morbidity and mortality associated with pulmonary aspiration of stomach contents.
The average hospital stay is 21 days, much of which is in intensive care. Complications range from bronchospasm and pneumonia to acute respiratory distress syndrome, lung abscess, and empyema. The average mortality rate is 5%.

BIBLIOGRAPHY

1. Gibbs C, Modell J: Management of aspiration pneumonitis. In Miller R (ed): Anesthesia, 4th ed. New York, Churchill Livingstone, 1994, pp 1437–1464.
2. Kallar SK, Everett LL: Potential risks and preventive measures for pulmonary aspiration: New concepts in preoperative fasting guidelines. Anesth Analg 77:171–182, 1993.
3. Mecca RS: Postanesthesia recovery. In Barash PG, Cullen BF, Stoelting RK (eds): Clinical Anesthesia. Philadelphia, J.B. Lippincott, 1989, pp 1414–1415.
4. Mendelson CL: The aspiration of stomach contents into the lungs during obstetric anesthesia. Am J Obstet Gynecol 52:191–205, 1946.
5. Rout CC, Rocke A, Gouws E: Intravenous ranitidine reduces the risk of acid aspiration of gastric contents at emergency cesarean section. Anesth Analg 76:156–161, 1993.
6. Vaughan GG, Gryeko RJ, Montgomery MT: The prevention and treatment of aspiration of vomiting during pharmacosedation and general anesthesia. J Oral Maxillofac Surg 50:874–879, 1992.
7. Warner MA, Warner ME, Weber JG: Clinical significance of pulmonary aspiration during the perioperative period. Anesthesiology 78:56–62, 1993.

46. CHRONIC OBSTRUCTIVE PULMONARY DISEASE

Howard J. Miller, M.D.

1. Define chronic obstructive pulmonary disease (COPD).
COPD is a clinical spectrum of diseases including emphysema, chronic bronchitis, and asthmatic bronchitis. It is a common disorder characterized by progressive increased resistance to flow of gases in the airways. Airflow limitation (obstruction) may be due to loss of elastic recoil or obstruction of small or large (or both) conducting airways. The increased resistance may have some degree of reversibility. Cardinal symptoms are cough, dyspnea, and wheezing.

2. What are the features of asthma and asthmatic bronchitis?
Asthma
- A heterogeneous disorder characterized by reversible airway obstruction
- Asthma "attacks" may be gradual or sudden in onset and are associated with a variety of precipitating factors (i.e., exercise, dander, pollen, intubation)
- After treatment, complete or near-complete resolution of symptoms

Asthmatic bronchitis
- Consists of airway obstruction, chronic productive cough, and episodic bronchospasm
- It can result from progression of asthma or chronic bronchitis
- Major reversibility cannot be achieved in asthmatic bronchitis and some degree of airway obstruction exists at all times

Asthma, with the strict definition of reversibility, should not be included in the COPD spectrum, whereas asthmatic bronchitis should.

3. Describe chronic bronchitis and emphysema.
Chronic bronchitis is characterized by cough, sputum production, recurrent infection, and airway obstruction for many months to several years. Historically, chronic bronchitis has been defined as a chronic cough with sputum production for at least 3 months per year for 2 consecutive years. Chronic bronchitis consists of mucous gland hyperplasia, mucous plugging, inflammation and edema, peribronchiolar fibrosis, narrowing of airways, and bronchoconstriction. Decreased airway lumina owing to mucus and inflammation increase resistance to flow of gases.

Emphysema is characterized by progressive dyspnea and variable cough. Destruction of the elastic and collagen network of alveolar walls without resultant fibrosis leads to abnormal enlargement of air spaces. Additionally the loss of airway support leads to airway narrowing and collapse during expiration (air trapping).

4. List contributory factors associated with the development of COPD.
1. **Smoking:** Smoking impairs ciliary function, depresses alveolar macrophages, leads to increased mucous gland proliferation and mucus production, increases the inflammatory response in the lung leading to increased proteolytic enzyme release, reduces surfactant integrity, and causes increased airway reactivity.
2. **Occupational exposure:** animal dander, toluene and other chemicals, various grains, cotton.
3. **Environmental exposure:** air pollution in industrialized areas (e.g., sulfur dioxide and nitrogen dioxide).
4. **Recurrent infection:** viral or bacterial (or both), including human immunodeficiency virus (HIV), which can produce an emphysema-like picture.

5. **Familial and genetic factors:** A predisposition to COPD exists among family members and is more common in men than women. Also, alpha1-antitrypsin deficiency exists in heterozygous and homozygous forms. This disorder results in autodigestion of pulmonary tissue by proteases and should be suspected in younger patients with basilar bullae on chest x-ray. Smoking accelerates its presentation and progression.

5. What historical information should be obtained preoperatively?
1. Smoking history: number of packs per day (PPD) and duration
2. Presence and severity of dyspnea, especially exercise tolerance (for example, one would be reassured if the patient could climb two to three flights of stairs comfortably)
3. Productive cough and the patient's ability to produce a forceful cough
4. History of wheezing
5. Prior and most recent hospitalizations for COPD and length of stay
6. Prior intubations secondary to COPD/respiratory failure
7. Medications, including home oxygen therapy and steroids, either systemic or inhaled
8. Allergies
9. Recent pulmonary infections, exacerbations, or change in character of sputum
10. Weight loss in the absence of other factors suggests end-stage disease
11. Symptoms of right-sided heart failure, including peripheral edema, right upper quadrant pain from an enlarged liver, jaundice, and anorexia secondary to liver and splanchnic congestion
12. Problems with previous surgeries or anesthetics, including postoperative intubation and mechanical ventilation

6. What are "pink puffers" and "blue bloaters"?

Pink puffers	Blue bloaters
Usually older (> 60 years)	Relatively younger
Pink in color	Cyanotic
Thin	Heavier in weight
Have minimal cough	Frequently wheeze
Have predominantly emphysema	Have chronic productive cough
	Have predominantly chronic bronchitis or asthmatic bronchitis

7. List pertinent physical findings in patients with COPD.
- Breathing pattern, including respiratory rate, depth, use of accessory muscles
- Chest auscultation for presence of focally or unilaterally decreased breath sounds, wheezing, or rhonchi
- Presence of jugular venous distention (JVD), a hepatojugular reflux, and peripheral edema indicating right-sided heart failure
- Palpation of peripheral pulses, assessing stroke volume and ease of obtaining arterial blood samples if needed

8. What laboratory examinations are useful?
1. **White count and hematocrit:** Elevation suggests infection and chronic hypoxemia, respectively.
2. **Electrolytes:** Bicarbonate levels are elevated to buffer a chronic respiratory acidosis if the patient retains carbon dioxide. Hypokalemia can occur with repeated use of beta-adrenergic agonists.
3. **Chest x-ray:** Look for lung hyperinflation, bullae or blebs, flattened diaphragm, increased retrosternal air space, atelectasis, cardiac enlargement, infiltrate, effusion, cancer, or pneumothorax.
4. **Electrocardiogram:** Look for decreased voltage amplitude, signs of right atrial (peaked P waves in leads II and V_1) or ventricular enlargement (right axis deviation, R/S ratio in $V_6 \leq 1$,

increased R-wave in V_1 and V_2, right bundle-branch block), and arrhythmias. Atrial arrhythmias are common, especially multifocal atrial tachycardia and atrial fibrillation.

    5. **Arterial blood gas:** Hypoxemia, hypercarbia, and acid-base status, including compensation, can be evaluated.

    6. **Pulmonary function tests (PFTs):** Determine the degree of obstruction and bronchodilator response.

9. What are normal PFT values? How are these changed in COPD?

PFT	NORMAL	EMPHYSEMA	BRONCHITIS	ASTHMA
FVC	$\geq$ 3–4 L	Decreased	Normal to slightly decreased	Decreased
FEV_1	> 2–3 L	Decreased	Normal to slightly decreased	Decreased
TLC	5–7 L	Increased	Normal to slightly increased	Decreased
RV	1–2 L	Increased	Increased	Increased
$FEF_{25-75\%}$	60–70% predicted	Decreased	Normal to slightly decreased	Decreased
Hypoxemia/ hypercarbia		Late in disease	Early in disease	Acute attack only
Air trapping		Moderate to marked	Moderate, partly reversible	Mild, intermittent
Diffusion capacity		Decreased	Normal to slightly decreased	Normal

Key: FVC = forced vital capacity; FEV_1 = forced expiratory volume in 1 second; TLC = total lung capacity; RV = residual volume; $FEF_{25-75\%}$ = forced expiratory flow, midexpiratory phase at 25–75%. PFT values are based on sex, age, and height of the patient, not on weight.

10. How does a chronically elevated arterial carbon dioxide partial pressure ($PaCO_2$) affect the respiratory drive in a person with COPD?

Persons with COPD have a reduced ventilatory drive in response to carbon dioxide (CO_2). Chronically elevated $PaCO_2$ produces increased cerebrospinal fluid bicarbonate concentrations. The respiratory chemoreceptors at the medulla become "reset" to a higher concentration of CO_2. Thus, diminished ventilatory drive secondary to CO_2 exists. In these patients, ventilatory drive may be more dependent on oxygen. If given high concentrations of oxygen, these persons may hypoventilate because of the loss of the hypoxic stimulus and the relative insensitivity to hypercarbia.

    Additionally, inhalation of 100% oxygen may increase ventilation/perfusion (V/Q) mismatch by inhibiting hypoxic pulmonary vasoconstriction (HPV). HPV is an autoregulatory mechanism in the pulmonary vasculature that decreases blood flow to poorly ventilated areas of the lung. Therefore, more blood flow is available for gas exchange in better ventilated areas of the lung. Inhibition of HPV results in increased perfusion of poorly ventilated areas of lung contributing to hypoxemia and/or hypercarbia.

11. How do general anesthesia and surgery affect pulmonary mechanics?

Vital capacity (VC) is reduced by 25–50% and residual volume (RV) increases by 13% following many general anesthetics and surgical procedures. Expiratory reserve volume (ERV) decreases by 25% after lower abdominal surgery and 60% after upper abdominal and thoracic surgery. Tidal volume (V_T) decreases 20%, and pulmonary compliance (PC) and functional residual capacity (FRC) decrease 33%. Atelectasis, hypoventilation, hypoxemia, and pulmonary infection may result. Many of these changes require a minimum of 1–2 weeks to resolve.

PULMONARY FUNCTION	CHANGE WITH SURGERY
VC, ERV, V_T, PC, FRC	Decrease
RV	Increase

12. Does one site of surgery affect pulmonary mechanics more than another?
Upper abdominal incisions and thoracotomy affect pulmonary mechanics the greatest, followed by lower abdominal incisions and sternotomy. These changes are secondary to supine position, decreased diaphragmatic excursion, and decreased effective cough secondary to pain.

13. What factors are associated with an increased perioperative morbidity or mortality?

FACTOR	ABDOMINAL SURGERY	THORACOTOMY	LOBECTOMY/PNEUMONECTOMY
FVC	< 70% predicted	< 70%	< 50% or < 2L
FEV_1	< 70%	< 1L	< 1L
FEV_1/FVC	< 50%	< 50%	< 50%
$FEF_{25-75\%}$	< 50%	< 50%	
RV/TLC			> 40%
$PaCO_2$	> 45–50 mmHg	> 45–50 mmHg	

Increased morbidity includes hypoxemia, hypoventilation with elevated PCO_2, pulmonary infection, and the need for reintubation and mechanical ventilation. All of these can prolong intensive care unit and overall hospital stay as well as increase mortality. Additionally, an FEV_1 less than 800 ml in a 70-kg person is probably incompatible with life and is an absolute contraindication to lung resection because of the high incidence for prolonged or even lifetime mechanical ventilation.

Patients presenting for lung resection (lobectomy and pneumonectomy) must have pulmonary function and arterial blood gas values that are superior to the values in the table. If any of the aforementioned criteria are not satisfied, further preoperative testing is indicated to determine the risk-benefit ratio for lung resection. Further tests include split-lung function, regional perfusion, regional ventilation, regional bronchial balloon occlusion, and pulmonary artery balloon occlusion studies. Additionally, spirometry should yield a predicted postresection FEV_1 greater than 800 ml.

14. List the common pharmacologic agents used to treat COPD and their mechanism of action.

Agents Used to Treat COPD

AGENT	MECHANISM OF ACTION
Beta-adrenergic agonists Albuterol Metaproterenol Isoetharine Terbutaline Epinephrine	Stimulation of $beta_2$ receptors leads to an increase in adenylate cyclase, increasing intracellular cAMP, resulting in decreased smooth muscle tone (bronchodilation). Excessive use may lead to hypokalemia owing to $beta_2$-adrenergic stimulation that causes redistribution of potassium into cells. Typically inhaled in nebulized or metered dose inhaler forms.
Methylxanthines Aminophylline Theophylline	Inhibition of phosphodiesterase produces increased cAMP. Facilitates endogenous catecholamines. Improved contraction of respiratory muscles, e.g., the diaphragm. Respiratory system stimulant. Administered orally or intravenously.
Corticosteroids Cortisol Methylprednisolone Dexamethasone Prednisone	Anti-inflammatory. Membrane stabilization of mast cells reduces/prevents release of histamine and other vasoactive agents. Potentiate beta-adrenergic agonists. These agents are either inhaled or given systemically.

Table continued on next page.

Agents Used to Treat COPD (Cont.)

AGENT	MECHANISM OF ACTION

Anticholinergics
  Atropine
  Glycopyrrolate
  Ipratropium
	Inhibition of acetylcholine on postganglionic cholinergic receptors of airway smooth muscle, decreasing intracellular cGMP, producing smooth muscle relaxation. Ipratropium, administered as an aerosol, has the advantage of being poorly absorbed by the gastrointestinal tract. Therefore, if swallowed, systemic side effects (e.g., tachycardia and increased secretion viscosity) are reduced.

Membrane stabilizers
  Cromolyn sodium
  Corticosteroids
	Stabilizes mast cell membrane to prevent degranulization. Cromolyn is for prevention of bronchoconstriction only and must be given prophylactically.

15. What therapies are available to reduce perioperative pulmonary risk?

1. **Stop smoking**
   a. Cessation for 48 hours prior decreases carboxyhemoglobin levels. The oxyhemoglobin dissociation curve shifts to the right, allowing increased tissue oxygen availability.
   b. Cessation for 4–6 weeks before surgery has been shown to decrease the incidence of postoperative pulmonary complications.
   c. Cessation for 2–3 months before surgery results in all the above benefits plus improved ciliary function, improved pulmonary mechanics, and reduced sputum production.
2. Optimize pharmacologic therapy. Continue medications even on the day of surgery.
3. Recognize and treat underlying pulmonary infection.
4. Maximize nutritional support, hydration, and chest physiotherapy.
5. Institute effective postoperative analgesia allowing the patient to cough effectively, take large tidal volumes, and ambulate early after surgery.

16. Do advantages exist with regional anesthesia techniques in patients with COPD?

Regional anesthesia, such as extremity and neuraxial blockade, offers several advantages in certain surgical procedures and is an excellent choice for surgery involving the extremities, perineum, and lower abdomen. Under regional anesthesia, the patient breathes spontaneously and does not require intubation. Neuraxial techniques that produce surgical anesthesia at levels higher than a T-10 dermatome may reduce effective coughing secondary to abdominal muscle dysfunction, leading to decreased sputum clearance and atelectasis. Additionally, one must be careful with certain brachial plexus techniques, which may anesthetize the phrenic nerve or cause a pneumothorax. Sedatives may depress respiratory drive and should be titrated to effect.

Continuous regional anesthetic techniques can be used during the postoperative period as well. For example, continuous lumbar and thoracic epidurals, continuous brachial plexus catheters, and intrathecal narcotics can all be used for optimizing postoperative pain control, resulting in improved pulmonary mechanics. These techniques accomplish this goal with lower doses of narcotics than intramuscular or intravenous methods and with less sedation.

17. What agents can be used for induction of general anesthesia? Should certain drugs be avoided? Do certain agents offer any advantages?

Induction of general anesthesia can be accomplished with any of the common induction agents, including barbiturates, benzodiazepines, opioids, propofol, etomidate, or ketamine. One should be cautious with agents that are known to release histamine (i.e., morphine sulfate), which may cause bronchospasm. Ketamine has the advantage of producing bronchodilation secondary to its sympathomimetic effects and by direct antagonism of bronchoconstricting mediators. Ketamine may be the induction drug of choice if the patient does not have underlying cardiac disease or pulmonary hypertension.

Once induction of anesthesia has been accomplished, complete suppression of airway reflexes must be ensured before tracheal intubation. Muscle relaxants facilitate intubation. The patient is commonly mask ventilated with a volatile anesthetic to deepen the plane of anesthesia, thereby decreasing airway reflexes. Volatile anesthetics have the advantage of producing bronchodilation. Intravenous lidocaine given before intubation can help blunt airway reflexes.

18. What are the advantages and disadvantages of different agents for general anesthesia?
Volatile agents (halothane, isoflurane, enflurane, sevoflurane, and desflurane). All produce bronchodilation and are useful in patients with COPD. Most, especially desflurane, are quickly eliminated and produce little, if any, respiratory depression postoperatively. Halothane has the highest cardiac arrhythmogenic potential and should be used with extreme caution in the presence of sympathomimetics.

Muscle relaxants and their reversal agents. Depolarizing and nondepolarizing muscle relaxants are commonly used and include succinylcholine, vecuronium, rocuronium, and pancuronium. They facilitate endotracheal intubation and mechanical ventilation. They are skeletal muscle, not smooth muscle, relaxants. Agents that may cause histamine release (atracurium and d-tubocurarine) should be avoided or used with extreme caution.

Neuromuscular reversal agents (neostigmine and edrophonium). These agents reverse the effects of nondepolarizing relaxants. They may theoretically precipitate bronchospasm and bronchorrhea secondary to stimulation of postganglionic cholinergic and muscarinic receptors. Clinically, however, bronchospasm is rarely seen after administration of these agents, possibly because anticholinergic agents (atropine or glycopyrrolate) are concurrently administered with the reversal agents.

Opioids. Opioids blunt airway reflexes and deepen anesthesia. Morphine produces histamine release and should be used with caution. Fentanyl, sufentanil, and alfentanil do not cause histamine release. One must always consider the residual respiratory depressant affects of opioids at the end of surgery.

Nitrous oxide. Nitrous oxide increases the volume and pressure of blebs or bullae, thereby increasing the risk of barotrauma and pneumothorax. Additionally, nitrous oxide may increase pulmonary vascular resistance and pulmonary artery pressures. This would be especially deleterious in patients with coexisting pulmonary hypertension or cor pulmonale (or both). Therefore, nitrous oxide should be avoided or used with extreme caution in patients with COPD.

19. Discuss the use of mechanical ventilation during general anesthesia.
As discussed in question 11, pulmonary mechanics are greatly affected by general anesthesia. Mechanical ventilation of the lungs is employed to optimize oxygenation and ventilation. Extended expiratory time is needed in patients with COPD. Too short of an expiratory phase leads to air trapping and increased peak airway pressures.

20. Define auto-PEEP.
Air trapping is known as auto-PEEP (positive end-expiratory pressure) and results from "stacking" of breaths when full exhalation is not allowed to occur. Auto-PEEP results in impairment of oxygenation and ventilation as well as hemodynamic compromise by decreasing preload and increasing pulmonary vascular resistance. Increasing expiratory time, by increasing inspiratory flow and increasing tidal volume with decreasing respiratory rate, reduces the likelihood of auto-PEEP. All people have some degree of intrinsic PEEP (PEEPi); however, PEEPi may be higher in patients with COPD. One may use PEEP to improve oxygenation in patients with COPD; however, studies have shown that PEEP levels should not exceed 85% of PEEPi to avoid further hyperinflation, compromised hemodynamics, and impairment of gas exchange.

21. Form a differential diagnosis for intraoperative wheezing.
Bronchoconstriction can cause wheezing; however, it is not the only cause. Other causes may be considered before appropriate treatment can begin:

- Mechanical obstruction of the endotracheal tube by secretions or kinking
- Aspiration of gastric contents or of a foreign body (i.e., a dislodged tooth)
- Endobronchial intubation (most commonly right mainstem intubation)
- Inadequate anesthesia
- Pulmonary edema (cardiogenic and noncardiogenic)
- Pneumothorax

22. How would you treat intraoperative bronchospasm?
1. Administer 100% oxygen and manually ventilate with sufficient expiratory time.
2. Identify and correct the underlying condition.
    a. Relieve mechanical obstruction by suctioning or unkinking the endotracheal tube.
    b. Remove foreign bodies if present.
    c. Ensure that the endotracheal tube is not endobronchial or resting on the carina.
    d. Treat pulmonary edema.
    e. Relieve a pneumothorax.

Once bronchoconstriction is established as the diagnosis, pharmacologic therapy can be instituted. Options include:
- Deepening the anesthetic with volatile agents
- Beta-adrenergic agonists aerosolized via the endotracheal tube (e.g., albuterol), subcutaneously (e.g., terbutaline), or intravenously (e.g., epinephrine or terbutaline)
- Ketamine intravenously or intramuscularly
- Intravenous aminophylline
- Intravenous lidocaine
- Intravenous corticosteroids

Although controversial, extubation may be beneficial because the endotracheal tube may contribute to or be the stimulus causing bronchoconstriction.

23. Do patients with COPD need to have postoperative mechanical ventilation?
Every patient must be considered individually. Those patients that exhibit a resting $PaCO_2$ > 45–50, FEV_1 < 1 L, FVC < 50–70% of predicted, or FEV_1/FVC < 50% may require postoperative intubation and ventilation, especially for upper abdominal and thoracic surgeries. In addition, consider how well the patient was prepared preoperatively, the respiratory rate and observed work of breathing, the patient's spontaneous tidal volume, the negative inspiratory force generated by the patient, arterial blood gas parameters, and body temperature. Is the patient fully reversed from muscle relaxation or are residual anesthetic drugs affecting the patient? Does the patient have adequate pain control?

CONTROVERSIES

24. Should H_2-receptor antagonists be avoided in patients with COPD?
Two types of histamine receptors have been identified: H_1-receptor stimulation results in bronchoconstriction, and H_2-receptor stimulation results in bronchodilation. Theoretically, H_2-receptor antagonist administration would result in unopposed H_1-receptor stimulation causing bronchosconstriction. H_2-receptor antagonists have been safely used in patients with COPD; however, their administration should be determined individually based on a risk-benefit ratio. Because many patients with COPD take corticosteroids, which can cause gastritis or peptic ulcers, concomitant H_2-antagonists are prescribed as well.

25. At the conclusion of surgery, should a patient with COPD be extubated "deep" or awake?
"Deep" extubation involves removing the endotracheal tube while the patient remains in a deep plane of anesthesia, while airway reflexes are suppressed. Typically, deep extubation is accomplished with the patient breathing spontaneously, deeply anesthetized with a volatile agent. Deep

extubation, however, does not guarantee against bronchospasm while the patient awakens. Furthermore, many patients are not suitable for deep extubation. Patients at risk for aspiration and those with difficult airways usually require awake extubation. If awake extubation is required, attempts should be made to blunt airway reflexes. Appropriate interventions include intravenous or intratracheal lidocaine and aerosolized beta-adrenergic agonists for smooth muscle relaxation.

Preoperatively, alternatives to general endotracheal anesthesia should be considered, including regional anesthesia or general anesthesia by mask or laryngeal mask airway (LMA). Use of an LMA and mask anesthesia does not require placement of an endotracheal tube in the trachea, which may act as a bronchoconstriction stimulus. LMA use allows the anesthesiologist to have free hands to perform other tasks and can provide a conduit for positive pressure ventilation. Positive pressure ventilation via an LMA, however, is often limited secondary to an inadequate seal surrounding the glottic opening.

BIBLIOGRAPHY

1. Aubier M, Murciano D, Milic-Emili J, et al: Effects of the administration of O_2 on ventilation and blood gases in patients with chronic obstructive pulmonary disease during acute respiratory failure. Am Rev Respir Dis 122:747–754, 1980.
2. Beckers S, Camu F: The anesthetic risk of tobacco smoking. Acta Anaesthesiol Belg 42:45–56, 1991.
3. Egan TD, Wong KC: Perioperative smoking cessation and anesthesia: A review. J Clin Anesth 4:63–72, 1992.
4. Eisenkraft JB, Neustein SM, Cohen E: Anesthesia for thoracic surgery. In Barash PG, Cullen BF, Stoelting RK (eds): Clinical Anesthesia, 2nd ed. Philadelphia, J.B. Lippincott, 1992, pp 943–948.
5. Gateau O, Bourgain J, Gaudy J, Benveniste J: Effects of ketamine on isolated human bronchial preparations. Br J Anaesth 63:692–695, 1989.
6. Ingram RH: Chronic bronchitis, emphysema, and airways obstruction. In Isselbacher KJ, Braunwald E, Wilson JD, et al (eds): Harrison's Principles of Internal Medicine, 13th ed. New York, McGraw-Hill, 1993, pp 1197–1206.
7. Konrad FX, Schreiber T, Brecht-Kraus D, Georgieff M: Bronchial mucus transport in chronic smokers and nonsmokers during general anesthesia. J Clin Anesth 5:375–380, 1993.
8 Kroenke K, Lawrence VA, Theroux JF, Tuley MR: Operative risk in patients with severe obstructive pulmonary disease. Arch Intern Med 152:967–971, 1992.
9. Martin RJ: Reexamining theophylline for asthma. Contemp Intern Med 5:8–14, 1993.
10. Moorthy SS, Dierdorf SF: Anesthesia for patients with chronic obstructive pulmonary disease. In Kirby RR, Gravenstein N (eds): Clinical Anesthesia Practice. Philadelphia, W.B. Saunders, 1994, pp 963–968.
11. Pearce AC, Jones RM: Smoking and anesthesia: Preoperative abstinence and perioperative morbidity. Anesthesiology 61:576–584, 1984.
12. Pepe PE, Marini JJ: Occult positive end-expiratory pressure in mechanically ventilated patients with airflow obstruction. Am Rev Respir Dis 126:166–170, 1982.
13. Petty TL: Chronic obstructive pulmonary disease—can we do better? Chest 97:2s–5s, 1990.
14. Petty TL: Definitions in chronic obstructive pulmonary disease. Clin Chest Med 11:363–373, 1990.
15. Ranieri VM, Giuliani R, Cinnella G, et al: Physiologic effects of positive end-expiratory pressure in patients with chronic obstructive pulmonary disease during acute ventilatory failure and controlled mechanical ventilation. Am Rev Respir Dis 147:5–13, 1993.
16. Sassoon CSH, Hassell KT, Mahutte CK: Hyperoxic-induced hypercarbia in stable chronic obstructive pulmonary disease. Am Rev Respir Dis 135:907–911, 1987.
17. Stock MC, Harrison RA: Respiratory function in anesthesia. In Barash PG, Cullen BF, Stoelting RK (eds): Clinical Anesthesia, 2nd ed. Philadelphia, J.B. Lippincott, 1992, pp 938–939.
18. Stoelting RK, Deirdorf SF, McCammon RL: Obstructive airways disease. In Stoelting RK, Deirdorf SF, McCammon RL (eds): Anesthesia and Coexisting Disease, 2nd ed. New York, Churchill Livingstone, 1988, pp 195–225.
19. Warner MA, Divertie MB, Tinker JH: Preoperative cessation of smoking and pulmonary complications in coronary artery bypass patients. Anesthesiology 60:380–383, 1984.

47. PULMONARY HYPERTENSION AND VASODILATOR THERAPY

James Duke, M.D.

1. Define pulmonary hypertension.

Pulmonary hypertension (PH) exists when the pulmonary systolic pressure exceeds 25–30 mmHg and diastolic pressures exceed 12 mmHg.

2. List conditions that produce pulmonary hypertension.

PH may be primary or secondary. Pulmonary hypertension is said to be primary in the absence of secondary causes, such as pulmonary disease (congenital or parenchymal), cardiac disease (shunts, mitral stenosis, left ventricular failure), thromboembolic or obliterative pulmonary vascular disease, collagen vascular disease, exogenous vasoconstrictive substances, or portal hypertension.

3. Discuss the natural history of pulmonary hypertension.

The pulmonary circulation has high flow and low resistance. The right ventricle (RV) is thin-walled and accommodates changes in volume better than changes in pressure. To accommodate increases in flow, such as during exercise, unopened vessels are recruited, and patent vessels distended, and pulmonary vascular resistance (PVR) may decrease. Such normal adaptive mechanisms can accommodate threefold to fivefold increases in flow without significant increases in pulmonary artery (PA) pressures. Early in the evolution of PH, the pressure overload results in hypertrophy of the RV without significant changes in cardiac output (CO) or RV filling pressures either at rest or during exercise. As the disease progresses, the vessels become less distensible, and the actual cross-sectional area of the pulmonary circulation decreases. Initially with exercise, CO eventually declines despite modest increases in right ventricular end-diastolic pressures (RVEDP). In time, RV failure ensues, and the patient is symptomatic even at rest. RV myocardial blood flow becomes compromised, and tricuspid regurgitation develops secondary to RV distention, further increasing RVEDP and worsening failure. In addition, left ventricular (LV) diastolic function may deteriorate, and LV filling may be compromised by excessive septal incursion into the left ventricle, with a resultant decrease in cardiac output.

4. What is the prognosis for a patient with pulmonary hypertension?

Alhough life expectancy varies widely, right heart failure is clearly associated with poor outcome. Rozkovec et al. found that radiographic evidence of cardiac enlargement and ECG evidence of right heart strain predicted a survival of less than 5 years. Increased PVR was associated with a decreased survival, but increased PA pressures were not. Age of onset did not predict life expectancy. A large national prospective registry determined median survival in patients with PPH to be 2.8 years. Variables associated with poor survival included New York Heart Association (NYHA) functional class III or IV, presence of Raynaud's phenomenon, elevated mean right atrial pressures, elevated mean PA pressure (in contrast to Rozkovec's findings), and decreased cardiac index. The usual terminal events are progressive RV failure and sudden death. Hypoxemia and decreasing cardiac output lead to cardiogenic shock. Sudden death is postulated to be due to precipitous bradydysrhythmias and ventricular dysrhythmias often secondary to RV ischemia, pulmonary embolus, or massive pulmonary hemorrhage.

5. What are some electrocardiographic and radiologic features of the disease?

The **electrocardiogram** (ECG) commonly shows right axis deviation, right ventricular hypertrophy (tall R-waves in V1–V3), RV strain (T-wave inversion in V1–V3), S-wave in V6, and enlarged P-waves in II, III, and AVF. Although atrial fibrillation is rare, its presence should be viewed with concern because it suggests that the contribution of "atrial kick" to ventricular filling is unavailable. In the presence of stiff pulmonary vasculature and a noncompliant right ventricle, cardiac output may become significantly diminished. **Radiologic abnormalities** have been observed in over 90% of cases. Abnormalities on chest radiographs suggestive of PH include prominence of the right ventricle as well as the hilar pulmonary artery trunk, rapid tapering of vascular markings and a hyperlucent lung periphery.

6 What signs and symptoms suggest pulmonary hypertension?

Early findings

Increase in pulmonic component of S_2
Narrowly split S_2
Right-sided fourth heart sound (gallop)
Early diastolic murmur of tricuspid regurgitation
RV heave

Symptoms

Dyspnea, initially on exertion*
Angina (50% of patients)
Fatigue (20% of patients)
Syncope

Late findings

Jugular venous distention
Peripheral edema
Cyanosis
RV third heart sound

* Eventually, virtually all patients with PH become dyspneic.

7. Discuss the observed abnormalities on pulmonary function testing.

Pulmonary function tests demonstrate mild restrictive defects secondary to the effects of the noncompliant pulmonary vasculature. Arterial blood gases reveal varying degrees of hypoxemia.

8. What additional diagnostic tests are available for evaluating pulmonary hypertension? What results may be expected?

An **echocardiogram** is an excellent noninvasive method for following progression of the disease. Echocardiographic features of PH include enlarged RV dimension, small LV dimension, thickened interventricular septum, systolic mitral valve prolapse, and abnormal septal motion. Determination of pulmonary artery pressures and PVR by pulsed Doppler echocardiography correlates well with values determined at cardiac catheterization.

Perfusion lung scans are particularly important in patients in whom thromboembolic disease is suspected. Thromboembolic disease is remediable with thromboendarterectomy and anticoagulation, whereas PPH is not. Lung scan demonstrates segmental defects in patients with thromboemboli but not in patients with PPH. **Pulmonary angiography** is indicated in patients demonstrating segmental perfusion scan defects, but pulmonary angiography should be undertaken cautiously in patients with PH. Although they are not contraindications, the associated risks of this procedure, including hypotension, worsening oxygenation, and cardiac arrest, should be weighed carefully against the potential benefit. In particular, patients with RV failure and increased RVEDP tolerate this procedure poorly.

Finally, **cardiac catheterization** is mandatory for confirming the diagnosis of PH and ruling out intracardiac shunts as a cause. In PH, catheterization may prove to be technically demanding and require guide wire assistance. Detection of an elevated wedge pressure is an indication for left-sided heart catheterization to rule out mitral stenosis, congenital heart disease and left-sided heart failure as causes of PH.

9. Discuss standard therapies for patients suffering from pulmonary hypertension.

Supplemental oxygen therapy is common, the goal being to maintain saturations above at least 90%. **Diuretics** may be prescribed to patients with RV failure, hepatic congestion, and peripheral edema, although excessive diuresis may decrease RV preload and CO. Anticoagulation is often instituted (usually oral warfarin), because patients are at great risk for thromboembolic events (which may prove to be terminal). The use of cardiac glycosides is controversial; no studies clearly suggest a beneficial or detrimental effect. **Vasodilator therapy** is discussed in question 10.

Finally, **lung or heart-lung transplantation** must be considered a contemporary yet expensive option in selected patients with PH.

10. What medications are available to treat increased pulmonary artery pressures?

Virtually all classes of vasodilators have been investigated, including direct smooth muscle vasodilators, alpha-adrenergic antagonists, beta-adrenergic agonists, calcium channel blockers, prostaglandins, and angiotensin-converting enzyme (ACE) inhibitors. Intravenous medications available for intraoperative use and intensive care management include nitroglycerin, nitroprusside, prostaglandin E_1, prostacyclin (PGI_2), phentolamine, and isoproterenol. Calcium channel blockers are the current outpatient therapy of choice. Rich et al.[9] found that 20% reductions in PVR in patients taking nifedipine or hydralazine were associated with increased long-term survival. High doses of nifedipine or diltiazem have produced reductions in PA pressures and PVR as well as regression of RV hypertrophy.

11. Are there ways to prognosticate which patients with pulmonary hypertension may improve with therapy?

The decision to begin outpatient vasodilator therapy is influenced by the likelihood that the patient will respond to such management. In the early stages of PH, the pulmonary vasculature is reactive and may dilate or constrict, depending on the balance of vasodilatory and vasoconstrictive influences. At some point in the disease progression, the vasculature becomes "fixed" and unresponsive to vasodilator therapy. PA catheters may be inserted to attempt an acute vasodilator challenge. A positive response includes a decrease in PVR of greater magnitude than the associated decrease in systemic vascular resistance. Cardiac output improves, but because of the enhanced output, reductions in pulmonary artery pressures may not be observed. Reductions in PVR of at least 30% or more have been associated with improved long-term benefit.

Prostacyclin, a prostaglandin with vasodilator properties, is more commonly available in Europe than in the United States. Prostacyclin has been used to assess vasodilator potential in patients with PH when outpatient therapy with oral vasodilators is being considered.

12. A patient with a history of pulmonary hypertension presents for a surgical procedure. How should this patient be monitored intraoperatively?

In addition to the routine monitors for every general anesthetic (pulse oximetry, ECG, temperature, precordial or esophageal stethoscope, and noninvasive blood pressure), invasive monitoring is standard management for patients with PH. **Invasive arterial pressure** monitoring allows beat-to-beat assessment of blood pressure and frequent blood analysis. A **PA catheter** should be introduced preoperatively to allow direct monitoring of PA pressure and right atrial pressure, and indirect assessment of LV volume and performance through determination of pulmonary occlusion pressures. Other standard monitors of particular use include **end-tidal carbon dioxide** and **inspired oxygen concentrations. Transesophageal echocardiography** is particularly useful in assessing volume status, left and right ventricular performance and valvular regurgitation, and early detection of segmental wall motion abnormalities secondary to myocardial ischemia.

13. What intraoperative measures may lessen pulmonary hypertension?

1. As hypoxemia and hypercarbia increase PA pressures, optimize the patient's oxygenation and ventilation.

2. Assess myocardial performance; increasing PA pressures may be secondary to a failing left ventricle.

3. If ischemia is associated with a decreasing cardiac output (CO), consider infusing nitroglycerin to improve coronary perfusion. Inotropic drugs such as dobutamine or dopamine may enhance contractility and improve CO.

4. Assess volume status. Patients may be highly volume-dependent to maintain CO, yet hypervolemia may increase PA pressures.

5. Correct acid-base status, and ensure the patient is not becoming hypothermic. Both acid-base abnormalities and hypothermia may cause increased PA pressure.

6. Deepen the anesthetic.
7. Consider the use of direct-acting vasodilators.

14. What is nitric oxide?

Nitric oxide (NO), a small molecule produced by vascular endothelium, is also known as endothelium-derived relaxing factor (EDRF). Formed from the action of EDRF synthetase on arginine, EDRF crosses into vascular smooth muscle and stimulates guanylate cyclase, resulting in formation of cyclic 3'-5' guanosine monophosphate (cGMP). Subsequently, cGMP produces smooth muscle relaxation and vasodilation. Donation of NO groups is the mechanism of action of the nitrovasodilators. Awareness of the role of endothelium in vasoreactivity and identification of NO as the EDRF in 1987 stimulated further research in endothelial physiology and the role of NO in many physiologic processes.

15. Discuss therapeutic usefulness and limitations of nitric oxide in pulmonary hypertension.

A frequently associated complication of intravenous vasodilator therapy for PH is systemic hypotension. Nitric oxide is administered by inhalation and crosses the alveolar membrane to the vascular endothelium, producing smooth muscle relaxation. But when it crosses into the circulation, it is rapidly bound to hemoglobin (with an affinity 1,500 times greater than carbon monoxide) and deactivated; thus it has no vasodilator effect on the systemic circulation. Deactivation upon entering the circulation also limits the effectiveness of NO in reducing PA pressures substantially to the period in which it is administered by inhalation. Because storage in oxygen produces toxic higher oxides of nitrogen, especially nitrogen dioxide (NO_2), NO is stored in nitrogen and blended with ventilator gases immediately before administration. The potential for increased methemoglobin levels during NO administration should also be recognized.

16. Is nitric oxide useful in other conditions besides primary pulmonary hypertension?

Numerous reports document the efficacy of NO in improving oxygenation and PH in adult respiratory distress syndrome (ARDS). Nitric oxide has been shown to reverse hypoxic pulmonary vasoconstriction. PH associated with congenital diaphragmatic hernias, congenital heart disease and persistent PH of the neonate, PH associated with adult mitral valve disease, and PH after cardiopulmonary bypass have been successfully managed through inhalation of NO. Doses have ranged from as high as 80 parts per million (ppm) to as low as 2 ppm. Individual dose-response relationships should be determined for each patient, and the lowest dose that produces a satisfactory pulmonary vasodilator response should be used to ensure the smallest possible production of methemoglobin. Methemoglobin levels should be assessed regularly. What constitutes a satisfactory dose of NO may depend on the desired endpoint; for instance, improvement in oxygenation in ARDS or reduction in PA pressures in PH.

Nitric oxide is also thought to be a humoral neurotransmitter in the central and peripheral nervous systems and to have some effect on the cerebral circulation. In addition, NO is recognized as playing a role in platelet aggregation, vascular permeability, and secretion of insulin, to name a few. Nitric oxide may also play a role in pain modulation. Future investigations will continue to elaborate its role in these and other biologic functions.

17. Why might a patient with cirrhosis develop pulmonary hypertension?

Patients with cirrhosis and end-stage liver disease (ESLD) develop anatomic shunts that increase PA blood flow. In addition, the failing liver is unable to detoxify circulating substances that, in susceptible individuals, may produce pulmonary vascular injury. Pulmonary hypertension associated with ESLD has been observed with a greater incidence than in the normal population. Because early symptoms of developing PH are nonspecific and may be attributed to liver disease, PH is easily missed unless specifically addressed. Diagnosis is suggested by examination of the ECG and chest radiographs and confirmed by ultrasound and cardiac catheterization.

Management of PH in patients with ESLD and PH who undergo liver transplantation presents great challenges to the anesthesiologist. Well-described complicating events with the potential to increase PA pressures include air embolization to the pulmonary circulation, characteristic massive fluid shifts, and effects of reperfusion of the donor liver. Nitric oxide has been used effectively at 40 ppm during liver transplantation to treat PH. Liver transplantation does not reliably produce long-term reductions in PH.

CONTROVERSIES

18. Discuss the advantages and disadvantages of the intravenous nitrovasodilators.
Because of their ready availability, titratability, and common use, intravenous nitrovasodilators are popular in the acute management of increased PA pressures. Commonly used nitrovasodilators include nitroglycerin and sodium nitroprusside. **Nitroglycerin** has the advantage of providing coronary vasodilation. Principally a venodilator, nitroglycerin may excessively decrease preload. Nitroglycerin infusion is started at about 1 µg/kg/min and ordinarily produces a smooth reduction in vascular pressures. Above 3 µg/kg/min, venodilation may become excessive, decreasing preload and requiring intravenous fluid augmentation. **Sodium nitroprusside** (SNP) is an extremely potent, principally arterial vasodilator. Infusions begin about 0.5–1.0 µg/kg/min and are carefully adjusted upward to effect. SNP is extremely effective at afterload reduction. Despite its potency and potential for creating excessive hypotension, SNP is safe for short-term use. Long-term use is associated with tachyphylaxis and the potential for cyanide toxicity.

19. Are any anesthetic agents effective in lowering pulmonary artery pressures?
When used as part of a maintenance anesthetic, isoflurane, a volatile anesthetic agent, has been demonstrated to lower PA pressure and PVR and to improve CO in this setting. Its presumed mechanism is direct action on pulmonary vascular smooth muscle. Of the volatile anesthetics, isoflurane has probably the greatest effect on vascular smooth muscle.

Few data suggest a beneficial effect of other agents commonly used during general anesthesia. Muscle relaxants have no pulmonary vasodilator effect. Opioids do not have a direct vasodilator effect but may attenuate the vasoconstrictor effect of noxious pain stimuli. Studies suggest that nitrous oxide should be used cautiously if at all; it is best avoided in the presence of significant RV dysfunction. In children with intracardiac shunts, ketamine may prevent reversal of left-to-right shunts, because it increases systemic vascular resistance to a greater extent than PVR.

BIBLIOGRAPHY

1. Cheng DCH, Edelist G: Isoflurane and primary pulmonary hypertension. Anaesthesia 43:22–24, 1988.
2. D'Alonzo GE, Barst RJ, Ayres SM, et al: Survival in patients with primary pulmonary hypertension: Results from a national prospective registry. Ann Intern Med 115:343–349, 1991.
3. Mandell SM, Duke J: Nitric oxide reduces pulmonary hypertension during hepatic transplantation. Anesthesiology 81:1538–1542, 1994.
4. Moser KM, Page GT, Ashburn WL, Fedullo PF: Perfusion lung scans provide a guide to which patients with apparent primary pulmonary hypertension merit angiography. West J Med 148:167–170, 1988.
5. Palmer RMJ, Ferrige AG, Moncada S: Nitric oxide release accounts for the biological activity of endothelium-derived relaxing factor. Nature 327:524–526, 1987.
6. Reeves JT, Groves BM, Turkevich D: The case for treatment of selected patients with primary pulmonary hypertension. Am Rev Respir Dis 134:342–346, 1986.
7. Rich S, Brundage BH, Levy PS: The effect of vasodilator therapy on the clinical outcome of patients with primary pulmonary hypertension. Circulation 71:1191–1196, 1985.
8. Rich S, Martinez J, Lam W: Reassessment of the effects of vasodilator drugs in primary pulmonary hypertension: Guidelines for determining a pulmonary vasodilator response. Am Heart J 105:119–127, 1983.
9. Roissant R, Falke KJ, López F, et al: Inhaled nitric oxide for the adult respiratory distress syndrome. N Engl J Med 328:399–405, 1993.
10. Rozkovec A, Montanes P, Oakley CM: Factors that influence the outcome of primary pulmonary hypertension. Br Heart J 55:449–458, 1986.
11. Rubin LJ: Primary pulmonary hypertension (ACCP consensus statement). Chest 104:236–250, 1993.
12. Zapol WM, Rimar S, Gillis N, et al: Nitric oxide and the lung. Am J Respir Crit Care Med 49: 1375–1380, 1994.

48. ANESTHESIA AND PERIOPERATIVE HEPATIC DYSFUNCTION

M. Susan Mandell, M.D., Ph.D.

1. What is the rate of transmission for hepatitis B and hepatitis C following an accidental needlestick?

Anesthesiologists are at increased risk for acquiring hepatitis as shown by a prevalence of 19–49% for hepatitis B serum markers compared to 3–5% for healthy blood donors. Based upon information from the Centers for Disease Control, 30% of hepatitis B and 3% of hepatitis C exposed individuals will become infected following a needlestick from an infected patient.

2. What is recommended following a needlestick injury in a health care worker from a patient with hepatitis?

Hepatitis A. Immune globulin when given intramuscularly within 4 weeks of exposure provides passive immunity for 6 months. No vaccine is available.

Hepatitis B. High anti-hepatitis B surface antigen titer immune globulin (HBIG) is recommended following percutaneous exposure in health care workers who have no antibodies to hepatitis B surface antigen. This is followed by hepatitis B vaccine.

Hepatitis C. The effectiveness of immune globulin following exposure to hepatitis C virus is uncertain but offered in some institutions. No vaccine is available. Laboratory testing for virus and elevations of liver enzymes is performed at the time of injury and repeated at 3 and 6 months to detect infection. Treatment with alpha interferon may be recommended if viral infection is detected although the efficacy of treatment is unknown.

3. What is cirrhosis of the liver?

Cirrhosis of the liver is characterized by diffuse death of liver cells causing formation of fibrous tissue and nodular regeneration of hepatic tissue. The consequent distortion of the hepatic circulation further propagates cellular damage and results in a progressive reduction of liver cells which eventually manifests as impairment of liver function. Hepatic synthetic failure, indicated by a prolonged prothrombin time and fall in albumin or impairment of detoxification mechanisms resulting in encephalopathy, is often termed end-stage liver disease.

4. Describe the changes in the cardiovascular system of patients with cirrhosis.

As liver disease progresses, most patients develop a hyperdynamic circulatory state, characterized by a fall in total peripheral resistance and a compensatory rise in cardiac output. The circulating plasma volume increases in response to vasodilation, and peripheral blood flow is enhanced. The arteriovenous oxygen gradient narrows due to increased peripheral shunting. Consequently, the mixed venous oxygen saturation of blood is higher than normal.

5. What pulmonary changes occur in a patient with cirrhosis?

Arterial hypoxemia with compensatory hyperventilation occurs in liver disease and is multifactorial in origin. Intrinsic and extrinsic pulmonary venous shunts form in response to portal hypertension and neovascularization. Deoxygenated blood that does not participate in pulmonary exchange is returned to the arterial circulation and reduces oxygen content.

Circulating vasoactive substances normally metabolized by the liver inhibit hypoxic pulmonary vasoconstriction, the mechanism responsible for optimal matching of ventilation and perfusion. Inhibition may be so profound that the patient becomes short of breath in the upright position (platypnea) due to gravity-induced pooling within the lung. Encephalopathy, pleural effusion, and reduced functional capacity from ascites also worsen arterial hypoxemia.

Anesthesia in cirrhotic patients is complicated by an increased risk of hypoxemia. Oxygen supplementation and positive pressure ventilation may improve ventilation and perfusion mismatch intraoperatively. However, pulmonary shunt and alveolar hypoventilation are generally worsened by anesthesia and postoperative narcotic analgesics.

6. What is hepatorenal syndrome? How does it differ from acute tubular necrosis?

Both types of acute renal failure occur in patients with cirrhosis and are characterized by increases in serum creatinine and oliguria. Differentiation is important, as treatment and prognosis vary.

Hepatorenal syndrome occurs in cirrhotic patients with portal hypertension and ascites. Intense vasoconstriction of the afferent arteriole reduces renal blood flow and impairs glomerular filtration. Abnormalities in the renin-angiotensin system, prostaglandins, catecholamines, and other endogenous factors probably contribute to vasoconstriction.

Acute tubular necrosis (ATN) is caused by renal tubular injury from ischemic or toxic injury. Tubular debris produces high intraluminal pressures and glomerular vasoconstriction. ATN may respond to diuretics, dopamine, calcium channel blockers, or angiotensin-converting enzyme inhibitors, and is often reversible. In contrast, hepatorenal failure is minimally responsive to the above drug therapy and only reversible by normalization of hepatic function. The onset of hepatorenal syndrome is indicative of a poor prognosis.

7. How can hepatorenal syndrome be differentiated from acute tubular necrosis by urinalysis?

The two conditions can be differentiated by the clinical pattern of onset and the laboratory values listed in the table.

8. Describe volume assessment and fluid management in patients with hepatorenal syndrome.

Differential Diagnosis of Renal Failure in Liver Disease

MEASUREMENT	HEPATORENAL	ATN
Onset	Slow	Acute
Urine sodium concentration	< 10 mmol/L	50–70 mmol/L
Urine/plasma creatinine	> 10	< 10
Urine specific gravity	> 1.010	1.010–1.015
Casts in urine	Seldom	Frequent

Optimization of renal blood flow by correction of hypovolemia may prevent further renal injury during anesthesia and surgery in patients with liver disease. Volume assessment, however, can be misleading as central venous pressures are often elevated despite relative hypovolemia due to increased back pressure in the inferior vena cava from hepatic enlargement or scarring. The pressure profiles of a pulmonary artery catheter are often required for accurate volume assessment.

A trial of volume expansion should be undertaken as the initial treatment of low urine output. Although immediate improvement occurs in more than one-third of patients treated, hepatorenal syndrome leads to progressive renal failure unless hepatic function improves.

9. Which liver function tests are used to detect hepatic cell damage?

The cytosolic enzymes alanine aminotransferase (ALT) and aspartate aminotransferase (AST) are released into the blood as a result of increased membrane permeability or cell necrosis. They tend to rise and fall in parallel, although AST is cleared more rapidly from the circulation by the reticuloendothelial system. Their levels are not affected by changes in renal or biliary function. In contrast to ALT, which is mainly confined to hepatocytes, AST is found in heart and skeletal muscle, pancreas, kidney, and red blood cells. Therefore AST lacks specificity as a single diagnostic test. Alanine aminotransferase is more specific but less sensitive for hepatic disease detection.

10. Briefly describe the laboratory tests used to assess hepatic synthetic function and their limitations.

All clotting factors except factor VIII are synthesized by the liver. Prothrombin time (PT) indirectly determines the amount of clotting factors available and therefore is used to assess hepatic synthetic function. Elevation in PT is not specific for liver disease, and is altered, for instance, by the hemophilias and disseminated intravascular coagulation. Vitamin K deficiency due to gastrointestinal diseases and anticoagulant therapy can also prolong PT. Once other disease processes have been excluded, PT becomes a sensitive prognostic indicator for acute hepatocellular injury.

Albumin is made only by the liver and reflects hepatic synthetic ability. However, renal and gastrointestinal losses can affect plasma levels as can vascular permeability changes in critically ill patients. A reduction in synthesis due to liver disease may require 20 days to detect changes in serum levels because of the long plasma half-life. Low serum albumin levels are therefore indicators of chronic liver disease.

11. What laboratory enzyme assays are used in the diagnosis of cholestatic liver disease

Alkaline phosphatase (ALP), gamma-glutamyl transferase (GGT) and 5'nucleotidase are commonly used to assess biliary tract function. These enzymes are located in the biliary epithelial cell membranes. ALP occurs in a wide variety of tissues and is elevated in a number of conditions, notably bone disease and pregnancy. Hepatic origin of an elevated ALP can often be suggested by clinical context and simultaneous elevations of GGT and 5'nucleotidase.

12. How can laboratory results be used to predict outcome in liver disease?

In acute liver disease such as viral hepatitis, plasma transaminase concentrations often reach levels 10 to 100 times normal. The higher plasma concentrations are associated with greater hepatocyte death and therefore an increased mortality rate. Relatively normal plasma levels can also be found in patients with acute liver disease, signifying massive cellular necrosis and associated with a very high mortality. PT is usually grossly prolonged and correlates with hepatic synthetic ability. Albumin levels are often normal. The mortality for intraabdominal surgery in patients with severe acute hepatic disease approaches 100%.

Liver function tests have also been used to predict outcome following surgery in patients with chronic hepatic impairment. Child's scoring system (see Table below) was originally used to stratify risk in patients undergoing portosystemic shunting procedures. Using this method, mortality rates of 10%, 31%, and 76% were identified in Child's class A, B, and C, respectively. This scoring system has been tested and found to have predictive value for operative outcome of hepatobiliary procedures. This classification is generally associated with outcome for nonoperative patients, but specific survival and mortality rates for each category are unknown.

Child's Classification of Liver Failure*

GROUP	A	B	C
Serum bilirubin (mg/dl)	Below 2.0	2.0–3.0	Over 3.0
Serum albumin (g/dl)	Over 3.5	3.0–3.5	Under 3.0
Ascites	None	Easily controlled	Poorly controlled
Encephalopathy	None	Minimal	Advanced
Nutrition	Excellent	Good	Poor

* The Pugh modification replaces nutrition with prothrombin time prolongation (A: 1–4 seconds; B: 5–6 seconds; C: > 6 seconds).

13. What risk factors for liver disease can be identified by medical history?

The following table lists risk factors for liver disease easily obtained in a brief medical history. Patients with these problems, previous jaundice, or a history of liver disease should have liver function tests evaluated before anesthesia and surgery.

Risk Factors for Liver Disease

RISK FACTOR	EXAMPLE
Viral hepatitis	Intravenous drug abuse, transfusion, tattoos, contact with infected person
Drugs	Alcohol, prescription medications (e.g., acetaminophen, haloperidol, tetracycline, isoniazid, hydralazine, captopril, and amiodarone)
Autoimmune disease	Systemic lupus erythematosus, sarcoidosis, mixed connective tissue disorder
Metabolic disease	Hemochromatosis, Wilson's disease, cystic fibrosis, alpha-1 antitrypsin deficiency, and glycogen storage disease
Inflammatory bowel disease	Crohn's disease and ulcerative colitis

14. What is jaundice?
Jaundice is a visible yellow or green discoloration, usually first observed in the sclera, caused by elevation of the total serum bilirubin. Levels of 2.0–2.5 mg/dl (normal 0.5–1.0 mg/dl) result in jaundice. The oxidation of bilirubin to biliverdin gives the green hue often observed on physical exam.

15. What are the common causes of jaundice?
The distinction between unconjugated and conjugated hyperbilirubinemia is essential to the differential diagnosis of jaundice. Elevations in the serum unconjugated bilirubin fraction are usually related to changes in the turnover of red blood cells and their precursors. Conjugated hyperbilirubinemia always signifies dysfunction of the liver or biliary tract.

16. List the common causes of increases in unconjugated bilirubin.
Unconjugated hyperbilirubinemia is defined as an elevation of the total serum bilirubin of which the conjugated fraction does not exceed 15%. The causes are listed in the table below.

Causes of Increased Unconjugated Bilirubin

CAUSE	EXAMPLE
Hemolysis	Incompatible blood transfusion, arterial/venous bypass circuit, congenital or acquired defects (autoimmune and drug-induced hemolytic anemia, glucose-6-phosphatase deficiency)
Hematoma resorption	Retroperitoneal or pelvic hematoma
Enzymatic deficiencies	Congenital deficiency (Gilbert's syndrome) to complete absence (Crigler Najjar syndrome) of hepatic uridine diphosphate glucuronlytransferase

17. List the common causes of biliary obstruction.
Elevations of conjugated bilirubin are due to hepatocyte dysfunction and intrahepatic or extrahepatic stasis. A differential diagnosis of biliary stasis is listed below.

Causes of Biliary Obstruction

EXTRAHEPATIC OBSTRUCTION	INTRAHEPATIC OBSTRUCTION
Tumor (bile duct, pancreas and duodenum)	Primary biliary cirrhosis
Cholecystitis	Drugs (estrogens, anabolic steroids, tetracycline, and valproic acid)
Biliary stricture	Total parenteral nutrition
Ascending cholangitis	Pregnancy
Sclerosing cholangitis	Sclerosing cholangitis

18. What are the main causes of hepatocyte injury?

Causes of Hepatocyte Injury

CAUSE	EXAMPLE
Infectious	Hepatitis A, B, C, D, and E, cytomegalovirus, Epstein-Barr
Drugs	Acetaminophen, isoniazid, phenytoin, hydralazine, alpha methyldopa, sulfasalazine
Sepsis	
Total parenteral nutrition	Abnormal liver function tests in 68–93% of patients given TPN for longer than 2 weeks
Hypoxemia	Low arterial oxygen or interference with peripheral use as in cyanide and carbon monoxide poisoning
Ischemic	Increased venous pressure (congestive heart failure, pulmonary embolus, and positive pressure ventilation) Decreased arterial pressure (hypovolemia, vasopressors and aortic cross-clamp)

19. How do inhalational anesthetic gases produce liver dysfunction?

Though rare, all inhalational agents can cause inflammation or death of hepatocytes by direct toxicity. Adverse reactions are caused by metabolic products of inhalational agents. Halothane, the most extensively metabolized agent, is associated with mild liver dysfunction in up to 30% of individuals exposed, reflected as an asymptomatic transient elevation of hepatic AST and ALT.

20. What is halothane hepatitis?

Anesthetic exposure to halothane results in severe hepatic impairment in approximately 1/30,000 individuals. This is termed an idiosyncratic reaction and is immunologically mediated. Halothane is metabolized by the liver and produces acyl chloride, which acts as a hapten. This results in trifluoroacetylation of hepatocyte membranes. The membrane–hapten complex induces an immune response resulting in hepatic necrosis. Risk factors associated with halothane hepatitis include obesity, female gender, familial factors, and prior exposure.

21. How is halothane hepatitis diagnosed?

Unfortunately, because there is no specific test for halothane-induced hepatitis, it has been considered a diagnosis of exclusion once other etiologies for perioperative hepatic dysfunction have been excluded. Careful screening of the history and laboratory results, however, will help diagnose halothane hepatitis. Most patients will have at least one of the risk factors cited in question 20. In addition, since this is an immunologically-mediated reaction, there is usually a delay of 7–28 days in the development of hepatic dysfunction. Associated findings include pyrexia, arthralgia, rash, eosinophilia, autoantibodies, and circulating immune complexes.

If halothane hepatitis is strongly suspected, there are several centers in the United States and Europe that test for immune-modified hepatocyte complexes that are diagnostic for this condition.

22. Do any other inhalational anesthetic agents cause immune-mediated hepatitis?

Enflurane has rarely been associated with immune-based hepatitis with a documented incidence of 1/800,000. There have also been only a few case reports of isoflurane hepatitis. In general, the potential of an inhalational anesthetic agent to induce immune complexes is related to the extent of metabolism. Generally the degree of metabolism of agents is: halothane > enflurane > isoflurane > desflurane.

23. How do inhalational anesthetic agents alter hepatic blood flow?

All these agents vasodilate the hepatic artery and preportal blood vessels. This decreases mean hepatic artery pressure and increases venous pooling in the splanchnic vessels. Portal flow decreases. Overall the result is suboptimal perfusion of the liver. In addition, autoregulation of the hepatic artery is abolished and blood flow becomes pressure dependent. This is usually tolerated well in patients with normal hepatic function, as metabolic demand is also decreased by these drugs. Patients with hepatic disease are more susceptible to injury secondary to preexisting impaired perfusion.

24. Why is drug metabolism altered in cirrhosis of the liver?

Cirrhosis generally leads to a decrease in blood flow through the liver due to fibrotic changes, leading to ischemia in regions most distant from branches of the hepatic artery. The cytochrome P450 system is concentrated in these regions and is responsible for the metabolism of a wide variety of drugs. Damage to this area causes a decrease in the rate of drug metabolism and leads to a prolonged plasma half-life.

BIBLIOGRAPHY

1. Allardyce D, Salvian A, Quenville N: Cholestatic jaundice during total parenteral nutrition. Can J Surg 21:332–339, 1978.
2. Berry AJ, Issacson IJ, Kane MA, et al: A multicenter study of the prevelance of hepatitis B viral serological markers in anesthesia personnel. Anesth Analg 63:738–742, 1984.
3. Brown B: Anesthetic management in the patient with abnormal liver function.Washington D.C., In American Society of Anesthesiologist Annual Refresher Course Lectures, 1993, 241, pp 1–6.
4. Cade R, Wagenmaker H, Vogel S, et al: Hepatorenal syndrome: Studies of the effect of vascular volume and intraperitoneal pressure on renal and hepatic function. Am J Med 82:427–438, 1987.
5. Centers for Disease Control: Protections against viral hepatitis: Recommendation of the Immunization Practices Advisory Committee (ACIP). MMWR 39 (RR-2):1, 1990.
6. Conn HO: A peek at the Child-Turcotte classification. Hepatology 1:673–676, 1981.
7. Epstein M, Berk DP, Hollenber NK, et al: Renal failure in patients with cirrhosis. Am J Med 49:175–185, 1970.
8. Furukawa T, Hara N, Yasumoto K, Inokuchi K: Arterial hypoxemia in patients with hepatic cirrhosis. Am J Med Sci 287: 10–13, 1984.
9. Hawker F: Liver function tests. In Hawker F (ed): The Liver. Philadelphia W.B. Saunders, 1993, pp 43–70.
10. Kenna J, Van Pelt F: The metabolism and toxicity of inhaled anaesthetic agents. Anaesth Pharmacol Rev 2:29–42, 1994.
11. Maze M: Anesthesia and the liver. In Miller RD (ed): Anesthesia, 4th ed. New York, Churchill Livingstone, 1994, pp 1969–1980.
12. Stoelting RK, Blitt CD, Cohen PJ, et al: Hepatic dysfunction after isoflurane anesthesia. Anesth Analg 66:147–151, 1987.

49. RENAL FUNCTION AND ANESTHESIA

James Duke, M.D.

1. Describe the anatomy of the kidney.

The kidneys are paired organs lying retroperitoneally against the posterior abdominal wall. Although their combined weight is only 300 grams (about 0.5% of total body weight), they receive 20–25% of total cardiac output. The renal arteries are branches of the aorta, originating below the superior mesenteric artery. There are numerous arterial anastomoses with the mesenteric and suprarenal vessels. The renal veins drain into the inferior vena cava. Nerve supply is abundant; sympathetic constrictor fibers originate from the fourth thoracic to first lumbar spinal segments and are distributed via celiac and renal plexuses. There is no sympathetic dilator or

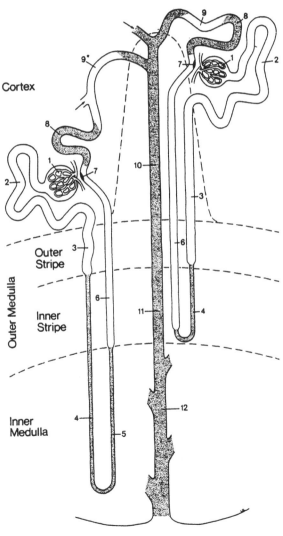

This scheme depicts a short-looped and a long-looped nephron together with the collecting system. Not drawn to scale. Within the cortex a medullary ray is delineated by a dashed line. 1, Renal corpuscle including Bowman's capsule and the glomerulus (glomerular tuft); 2, proximal convoluted tubule; 3, proximal straight tubule; 4, descending thin limb; 5, ascending thin limb; 6, distal straight tubule (thick ascending limb); 7, macula densa located within the final portion of the thick ascending limb; 8, distal convoluted tubule; 9, connecting tubule; 9*, connecting tubule of the juxtamedullary nephron that forms an arcade; 10, cortical collecting duct; 11, outer medullary collecting duct; 12, inner medullary collecting duct. (From Kriz W, Bankir I: A standard nomenclature for structures of the kidney. Am J Physiol 254:F1, 1988, with permission.)

parasympathetic innervation. Pain fibers, mainly from the renal pelvis and upper ureter, enter the spinal cord via splanchnic nerves.

On cross-section of the kidney, three zones are apparent: cortex, outer medulla, and inner medulla. Eighty percent of renal blood flow is distributed to cortical structures. Each kidney contains about one million nephrons. Nephrons are classified as superficial (about 85%) or juxtamedullary, depending on location and length of tubules. The origin of all nephrons is within the cortex, where abundant glomerular capillary networks (continuations of interlobular arteries) surround the Bowman's capsule of each nephron.

The glomerulus and capsule are known collectively as the renal corpuscle. Each Bowman's capsule is connected to a proximal tubule that is convoluted within its cortical extent but becomes straight-limbed within the outer cortex; at this point the tubule is known as the loop of Henle. The loop of Henle of superficial nephrons descends only to the intermedullary junction, where it makes a hairpin turn, becomes thick-limbed, and ascends back into the cortex, where it approaches and touches the glomerulus with a group of cells known as the juxtaglomerular apparatus (JGA). The superficial nephrons form distal convoluted tubules that merge to form collecting tubules within the cortex. About five thousand tubules join to form collecting ducts. Ducts merge at minor calyces, which in turn merge to form major calyces. The major calyces join and form the renal pelvis, the most cephalic aspect of the ureter. The renal corpuscles of juxtamedullary nephrons are located at juxtamedullary cortical tissue. They have long loops of Henle that descend deep into medullary tissue; the loops also reascend into cortical tissue, where they form distal convoluted tubules and collecting tubules. These nephrons (15% of the total) are responsible for conservation of water.

2. List the major functions of the kidney.
1. Regulation of body fluid volume and composition
2. Acid-base balance
3. Detoxification and excretion of nonessential materials, including drugs
4. Elaboration of renin, which is involved in extrarenal regulatory mechanisms
5. Endocrine and metabolic functions, such as erythropoietin secretion, vitamin D conversion, and calcium and phosphate homeostasis.

3. Discuss glomerular and tubular function.
Glomerular filtration results in production of about 180 L of glomerular fluid each day. Filtration does not require the expenditure of metabolic energy; rather it is due to a balance of hydrostatic and oncotic forces. The glomerular membrane possesses negatively charged pores that allow passage of water, ions, and negatively charged ions of less than approximately 40Å (molecular weight < 15,000). Substances between 40 and 80Å (molecular weight ~40,000) ordinarily pass if they are neutrally charged; substances > 80Å are unfiltered. Normal glomerular filtration rate (GFR) is 125 ml/min.

Tubular function reduces the 180 L/day of filtered fluid to about 1 L/day of excreted fluid, altering its composition through active and passive transport. Transport is passive when it is the result of physical forces, such as electrical or concentration gradients. When transport is undertaken against electrochemical or concentration gradients, metabolic energy is required and the process is termed active.

Substances may be either reabsorbed or secreted from tubules; both processes may be active or passive. Substances may move bidirectionally, taking advantage of both active and passive transport. The direction of transit for reabsorbed substances is from tubule to interstitium to blood, whereas the direction for secreted substances is from blood to interstitium to tubule. Secretion is the major route of elimination for drugs and toxins, especially when they are plasma protein-bound.

4. How is urine concentrated or diluted?
Loops of Henle allow formation of urine that is hypertonic relative to plasma. The greater the length of the loops, the more concentrated the urine can become. Throughout the animal kingdom, production of hypertonic urine requires the presence of loops of Henle.

The most energetically efficient manner for concentrating tubular fluid involves active transport of ions and osmotic equilibration of water. The passive transport of water is known as countercurrent multiplication of concentration.

Beginning at the glomerulus, the balance of hydrostatic and oncotic forces favors filtration of plasma at the rate of about 180 L/day. At the proximal convoluted tubule (PCT), sodium passively moves down a concentration gradient into the sodium-poor milieu of the cells lining the PCT. Chloride passively follows to maintain electrical neutrality, and water moves into the cells passively as well in response to osmotic gradients. Sodium is then transported **against** a concentration gradient into the renal interstitium. This energy dependent process (active transport) uses the intracellular Na-K-ATPase–driven sodium pump, exchanging intracellular sodium for extracellular potassium. Again, chloride and water passively follow. About 75% of the filtered tubular fluid is then taken back up into the circulation via peritubular capillaries with no net change in osmotic activity.

At the level of the thin descending loop of Henle the nephron reaches medullary tissue with its hypertonic interstitium. Water moves along its osmotic gradient, but the cells are poorly permeable to sodium and incapable of active transport; sodium remains intratubular. By the time of reversal of flow at the ascending loop of Henle, the volume of tubular fluid has decreased and its osmolality has increased substantially. The thin ascending loop is impermeable to water, but some diffusion and active transport of sodium and chloride take place. The thick ascending loop is also impermeable to water but allows active transport of chloride and passive movement of sodium. This active transport of chloride is the driving force for urinary concentration and dilution.

By the time tubular fluid reaches the distal convoluted tubule (DCT), its volume is only about 15% of the originally filtered fluid, and it is hypotonic relative to the interstitium. The cells of the DCT and collecting ducts are hormonally responsive; when antidiuretic hormone (ADH)

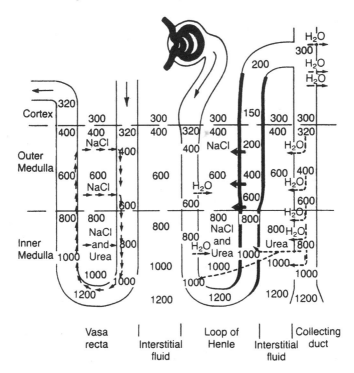

The countercurrent mechanism for concentrating the urine. Numerical values are in mOsm/L. (From Guyton AC: Textbook of Medical Physiology, 8th ed. Philadelphia, W.B. Saunders, 1991, with permission.)

levels are high, water moves out of the tubules and back into the circulation. What remains is a fluid rich in urea. By the time tubular fluid has reached the midpoint of the PCT, the tubule is once again cortical; the osmotic difference between tubule and cortical interstitium is small. Active transport of sodium and passive movement of water continue, leaving only 5–8% of the original filtered fluid within the tubules.

Entering the ADH-responsive collecting tubules and again descending into medullary tissue, water moves into the hypertonic interstitium. The tubular fluid that finally enters the renal pelvis is only about 0.5% of the originally filtered fluid.

5. Discuss diuresis and the site of action of commonly used diuretics.

An appreciation of the site and mode of diuretic action reinforces understanding of nephronal function. For instance, diuretics such as acetazolamide, which act on the PCT, do not significantly affect urine volume or concentration because the majority of sodium and water reabsorption occurs in the loop of Henle. On the other hand, diuretics that interfere with the active transport of chloride within the loop of Henle affect urine formation greatly. With the exception of osmotic diuretics, all diuretics interfere with sodium conservation.

Diuretics

DRUG	SITE OF ACTION	ACTIONS/SIDE EFFECTS
Carbonic anhydrase inhibitors (acetazolamide)	Proximal convoluted tubule	Inhibits sodium reabsorption Interferes with H^+ excretion Hyperchloremic, hypokalemic acidosis
Thiazides (hydrochlorothiazide)	Cortical diluting segment (between ascending limb and aldosterone-responsive DCT)	Inhibits sodium reabsorption Accelerates sodium-potassium exchange—hypokalemia Decreases GFR in volume-contracted states
Potassium-sparing diuretics (spironolactone, triamterene)	Competitive inhibition of aldosterone in DCT	Inhibiting aldosterone prevents sodium reabsorption and sodium-potassium exchange Modest diuretic that often supplements thiazides
Loop diuretics (furosemide, bumetanide, ethacrynic acid)	Inhibit Cl^- reabsorption at thick ascending loop of Henle	Potent diuretic, acts on critical urine concentrating process Renal vasodilation, significant hypokalemia Can produce significant volume contraction
Osmotic diuretics (mannitol, urea)	Filtered at glomerulus but not reabsorbed; creates osmotic gradient into tubules; excretion of water and some sodium	Hyperosmolality reduces cellular water Limited ability to excrete sodium Renal vasodilator

6. Describe the unique aspects of renal blood flow (RBF) and control. How does RBF affect urine concentration?

RBF of about 1200 ml/min is well maintained (autoregulated) at blood pressures of 80–180 mmHg. Blood flow to cortex, outer medulla, and inner medulla has a distinct relationship to function. The cortex requires about 80% of blood flow to achieve its excretory and regulatory functions, and the outer medulla receives 15%. The inner medulla receives a small percent of blood flow; a higher flow would wash out solutes responsible for the high tonicity (1200 mOsm/kg) of the inner medulla. Without this hypertonicity, urinary concentration would not be possible.

Control of RBF is through extrinsic and intrinsic neural and hormonal influences; a principal goal of blood flow regulation is to maintain GFR. As mentioned, the potential sympathetic vasoconstrictor capacity is extensive, but the euvolemic, nonstressed state has little baseline sympathetic tone. Under mild-to-moderate stress, RBF decreases slightly, but efferent arterioles constrict, maintaining GFR. During periods of severe stress (hemorrhage, hypoxia, major surgical procedures) both RBF and GFR decrease secondary to sympathetic stimulation. This phenomenon is also observed when high concentrations of epinephrine or norepinephrine are infused.

The renin-angiotensin-aldosterone axis also has an effect on RBF. A proteolytic enzyme formed at the macula densa of the juxtaglomerular apparatus, renin acts on angiotensinogen within the circulation to produce angiotensin I. Enzymes within lung and plasma convert angiotensin I to angiotensin II, a potent pressor and renal vasoconstricting agent (especially of the efferent arteriole) as well as a factor in the release of aldosterone. Stimuli for renin release include tubular sodium content, catecholamine levels, sympathetic stimulation, and afferent arteriolar tone. During periods of stress levels of angiotensin are elevated and contribute (along with sympathetic stimulation and catecholamines) to decrease RBF.

Prostaglandins are also found within the kidney. PGE_2 and PGE_3 are intrinsic mediators of blood flow, producing vasodilation.

Blood flows to the medulla through the vasa recta, which are continuations of juxtamedullary glomerular efferent arterioles. Bundles of vasa recta do not descend deeply into the medulla, and the inner medulla receives only 1–3% of RBF. The hairpin arrangement of the vasa recta functions as a countercurrent exchanger. Water leaves the descending limb and enters the more hypertonic ascending limb, thus bypassing the inner medulla. Medullary solute travels in the opposing direction, leaving the hypertonic ascending limb and entering the less tonic descending limb. An osmotic gradient is thus maintained; the tip of the renal papilla has a osmolality of 1200 mOsm/kg.

7. Describe the sequence of events associated with decreased RBF.
The initial response to decreased RBF is to preserve ultrafiltration through redistribution of blood flow to the kidneys, selective afferent arteriolar vasodilation, and efferent arteriolar vasoconstriction. Renal hypoperfusion also results in active absorption of sodium and passive absorption of water in the ascending loop of Henle; paradoxically, oxygen demand is increased in an area particularly vulnerable to decreased oxygen delivery (75–80% of the energy expended in the kidney is for active sodium transport). Compensatory sympathoadrenal mechanisms redistribute blood flow from outer cortex to inner cortex and medulla. If renal hypoperfusion persists or worsens despite early compensatory mechanisms, and as sodium is resorbed in the ascending loop, increased sodium is delivered to the macula densa, producing afferent arteriolar vasoconstriction and decreasing glomerular filtration. Because GFR is decreased, less solute is delivered to the ascending loop. Because less solute is delivered, less is resorbed (an energy-requiring process); thus less oxygen is needed, and the net effect is that afferent arteriolar vasoconstriction decreases oxygen-consuming processes. The result, however, is oliguria. **Oliguria is a symptom of decreased RBF and oxygen delivery and a result of compensatory mechanisms designed to prevent ischemic renal injury.**

8. What preoperative risk factors are associated with postoperative renal failure?
Variability in the definition of renal failure (impaired glomerular function as measured by blood urea nitrogen [BUN], creatinine or GFR or impaired tubular function as measured by urine specific gravity, osmolality, or fractional excretion of sodium), nonuniformity of statistical methods, and inconsistent criteria for establishing risk factors have made metaanalysis of published studies impossible. Nonetheless, a few patterns emerge. Preoperative renal risk factors (increased BUN and creatinine and a history of renal dysfunction), left ventricular dysfunction, advanced age, jaundice, and diabetes mellitus are predictive of postoperative renal dysfunction. Patients undergoing cardiac or aortic surgery are particularly at risk for developing postoperative renal insufficiency.

9. How are jaundice and acute renal failure (ARF) related?

The increased incidence of ARF associated with jaundice is most likely related to the degree of bilirubin elevation. Sepsis and preexisting renal dysfunction are also predisposing factors. Although bilirubin itself is not thought to be nephrotoxic, patients with hyperbilirubinemia are prone to hypotension due to decreased peripheral vascular resistance and have an exaggerated decrease in blood pressure associated with hemorrhage. Endotoxemia also may predispose jaundiced patients to ARF.

10. Discuss the relationship between aortic surgery and renal dysfunction.

The incidence of ARF associated with aortic surgery is about 8%; the mortality rate in such cases is about 60%. The most common cause of ARF is ischemic injury leading to acute tubular necrosis. An association with preexisting renal insufficiency (creatinine > 2.3 mg/dl) is particularly worrisome. Complicated aneurysms (e.g., expanding, ruptured, suprarenal, thoracic, and pararenal aneurysms) have a higher incidence of ARF (10–30%) than uncomplicated infrarenal aneurysms (5%). When ARF accompanies repair of an expanding or ruptured aneurysm, the mortality rate ranges between 75 and 95%. Suprarenal cross-clamping carries a higher incidence of ARF compared with infrarenal cross-clamping. The higher incidence may be associated with enhanced atheromatous embolization to renal vessels; curiously, *supraceliac* cross-clamping and infrarenal cross-clamping have a nearly equal incidence of ARF.

11. What is the effect of cardiopulmonary bypass (CPB) on renal blood flow?

CPB decreases RBF and GFR by 30%. Nonpulsatile CPB appears more detrimental to renal blood flow. The correlation between length of CPB and ARF is linear. Hemolysis associated with CPB and pigment nephrotoxicity may be a cause of ARF, although renal ischemia associated with CPB is by far the leading cause. Valvular surgical procedures have twice the incidence of ARF compared with coronary artery bypass grafting.

12. What is the impact of renal dysfunction on perioperative mortality and morbidity rates?

Variation in patient populations and definition of renal failure have led to great disparity in the reported incidence of perioperative renal failure, which ranges from 0.1 to 50%. But once established, acute renal failure still has a mortality rate between 20 and 90%, despite advances in technology. The number of other malfunctioning organ systems correlates with mortality. Isolated renal failure has a mortality rate of only 10%, but the rate increases to 60% and 90%, respectively, when two or three organ systems fail. Perioperative renal failure accounts for one-half of all patients requiring acute dialysis.

13. Discuss the major causes of perioperative acute renal failure.

Acute renal failure (ARF) is defined as a significant decrease in GFR over a period of 2 weeks or less. Renal failure, or azotemia, can be categorized broadly into prerenal, renal, and postrenal etiologies. Prerenal azotemia is due to decreased blood flow to the kidney and accounts for about 60% of all cases of ARF. Causes include renal vascular disease and renal ischemia. In the perioperative setting, ischemia is most likely due to inadequate perfusion from blood and volume losses. Other mechanisms of prerenal azotemia include hypoperfusion secondary to myocardial dysfunction and congestive heart failure or shunting of blood away from the kidneys, as in sepsis.

Renal causes account for 30% of all cases of ARF. Acute tubular necrosis is the leading cause and may be due to either ischemia or toxins. Nephrotoxins include radiocontrast media, aminoglycosides, and fluoride associated with volatile anesthetic metabolism. Hemolysis or muscular injury (producing hemoglobinuria and myoglobinuria) are also causes of intrinsic ARF.

Postrenal causes (10% of cases) are due to obstructive nephropathy and may be observed in men with prostatism, women with pelvic malignancies, diabetes-associated neuropathy that affects bladder function, ureteral obstruction, and anticholinergic-associated bladder dysfunction from anesthetic agents or antihistamines.

14. Discuss the utility of urine output in assessing renal function.

Urine output is easily measured through insertion of an indwelling Foley catheter and connection to a urimeter. A daily output of 400–500 ml of urine is required to excrete obligatory nitrogenous wastes. In adults, an inadequate urine output (oliguria) is often quoted as < 0.5 ml/kg/hour. In the absence of preexisting renal disease and urinary obstruction, oliguria is usually a manifestation of diminished renal perfusion and glomerular filtration, either from hypovolemia or renal vaso-constriction. As discussed in question 7, oliguria is both a symptom and a compensatory mecha-nism in the setting of renal perfusion. GFR also may be decreased by the effects of anesthesia, sympathetic activity, hormonal influences, and surgical procedure via redistribution of blood away from outer cortical nephrons.

Despite reliance on urine output to gauge adequacy of volume resuscitation and renal func-tion, numerous studies show no correlation between urine volume and histologic evidence of acute tubular necrosis, GFR, creatinine clearance, or perioperative changes in the levels of BUN or creatinine. This lack of correlation has been noted in patients with burns, trauma, shock states, or cardiovascular surgery.

Finally, a normal urine output does not rule out renal failure. Nonoliguric renal failure is not uncommon perioperatively. Levels of renin, aldosterone, and antidiuretic hormone (ADH) may affect tubular secretion of water and solute independent of GFR. At best, urinary flow rate and volume are indirect measures of the adequacy of renal function.

15. If oliguria is both a symptom of acute renal failure and a compensatory mechanism, what additional information is available to differentiate the two?

The following tests may be of further usefulness in assessing renal function: urine specific grav-ity, urine osmolality, serum BUN and creatinine, fractional excretion of sodium, free water clear-ance, creatinine clearance, ratio of urine to plasma creatinine, ratio of urine to plasma urea, urine sodium, and renal blood flow.

16. How useful are urine specific gravity and osmolality in assessing perioperative renal function?

Specific gravity (SpGr), a measure of the kidney's concentrating ability, is determined by com-paring the mass of 1 ml of urine to 1 ml of distilled water. Normal values range between 1.010 and 1.030. In prerenal azotemia, the kidney's attempts to conserve sodium and water are reflected in a concentrated urine with SpGr > 1.030; loss of concentrating ability, as in acute tubular necro-sis, is reflected by SpGr < 1.010. However, many factors can change SpGr, including protein, glucose, mannitol, dextran, diuretics, radiographic contrast, extremes of age, and thyroid, parathyroid, adrenal, or pituitary disease. Hence, measurement of specific gravity is a nonspe-cific measure of renal function.

The same factors that render SpGr nonspecific also affect the reliability of urine osmolality as an assessment of renal function. Traditionally, an osmolality > 500 mOsm/kg H_2O has been used as a guideline to identify prerenal azotemia and an osmolality < 350 mOsm/kg H_2O to iden-tify acute tubular necrosis, but these values are not particularly predictive.

17. What are the limitations in using serum creatinine and BUN to assess renal function?

Many nonrenal variables may be responsible for elevation of BUN and creatinine, including increased nitrogen absorption, hypercatabolism, hepatic disease, diabetic ketoacidosis, hematoma resorption, gastrointestinal bleeding, hyperalimentation, and many drugs (e.g., steroids). In addition, elevation of serum creatinine is a late sign of renal dysfunction. GFR may be reduced as much as 75% before abnormal elevation is observed. Because creatinine production is proportionate to muscle mass, settings in which substantial wasting has already occurred (e.g., chronic illness, advanced age) may have "normal" creatinine levels despite markedly reduced GFR. Postoperative creatinine measurements are not particularly predictive of renal dysfunction.

18. Are estimates of urine-to-plasma ratios of creatinine or urea predictive of renal dysfunction?

Urine-to-plasma creatinine ratios are neither sensitive nor specific for renal dysfunction. Only at extremes do they indicate renal dysfunction (may indicate acute tubular necrosis if < 10 or prerenal azotemia if > 40). Because so many nonrenal variables may influence BUN levels, the urine-to-plasma urea ratio is also neither sensitive nor specific for renal dysfunction.

19. Is measurement of urinary sodium useful in assessing renal function? What factors influence urinary sodium excretion?

Urinary sodium levels appear to correlate more with the amount and type of resuscitation fluid than with renal function. Factors that influence urinary sodium levels include secretion of aldosterone and ADH, diuretic therapy, saline content of IV fluids, sympathetic tone, and coexisting sodium avid states, such as cirrhosis and congestive heart failure.

20. How is the fractional excretion of sodium (FeNa) determined? Is it of value in assessing renal function?

FeNa represents the fraction of all filtered sodium that is excreted:

$$\text{FeNa} = \text{excreted Na/filtered Na} \times 100 = U_{Na} \times P_{Cr}/U_{Cr} \times P_{Na}) \times 100$$

where U_{Na} is urinary sodium, U_{Cr} is urinary creatinine, P_{Cr} is plasma creatinine, and P_{Na} is plasma sodium.

Numerous retrospective and prospective investigations demonstrated a high sensitivity and specificity in differentiating prerenal azotemia (FeNa < 1%) from acute tubular necrosis (FeNa > 1%), but more recent reports dispute the earlier studies, noting that the determination is not particularly accurate early in the course of renal impairment, when it would be most useful. Conditions other than acute tubular necrosis that may have an FeNa > 1% include normal renal function with high salt intake and volume depletion with preexisting chronic renal disease. Other conditions that may have an FeNa < 1% include congestive heart failure, acute glomerulonephritis, myoglobinuric and hemoglobinuric renal failure, acute urinary tract obstruction, renal transplant rejection, and contrast nephrotoxicity.

21. What is free water clearance (C_{H_2O})? Is it predictive of renal dysfunction?

$$C_{H_2O} = UV - \{(U_{osm}/P_{osm}) \times UV\}$$

where UV is urine volume, U_{osm} is urinary osmolality and P_{osm} is plasma osmolality. Free water clearance is a measure of the kidney's ability to dilute or concentrate urine. Because numerous nonrenal factors may affect urine osmolality, this determination is often not likely to have value. Free water clearance is not as useful as determination of creatinine clearance.

22. How is creatinine clearance (CrCl) determined? What does it measure? What is its usefulness in assessing acute renal dysfunction?

Creatinine clearance approximates glomerular filtration and measures the ability of the glomerulus to filter creatinine from plasma:

$$\text{CrCl} = (\text{Urine Cr} \times UV)/\text{Plasma Cr}$$

where Urine Cr is urinary creatinine, UV is urine volume, and Plasma Cr is plasma creatinine.

CrCl is the most efficient test available for assessing glomerular filtration. A significant limitation is the necessity for 24-hour urine collection, clearly an obstacle if an immediate assessment of renal function is needed. Creatinine clearance estimated from 2-hour urine collections has been shown to be reasonably valid if urine is collected conscientiously, although longer collection periods always provide more accurate assessments.

23. Given the preceding discussions about methods that *may* be useful in assessing perioperative renal dysfunction, can any generalizations be made?

The majority of renal function tests are neither sensitive nor specific in predicting perioperative renal dysfunction. Currently we rely on a number of indirect variables that do not reliably correlate with glomerular filtration. Creatinine clearance is the most sensitive test available but is limited by the need for prolonged urine collection; in the operative setting it is clearly not practical.

In daily anesthetic practice, considerable attention continues to be given to urine output. In most patients, an output of 0.5–1.0 ml/kg/hr reassures the anesthesiologist that renal function is probably intact. However, an "adequate" urine output should be considered only in the context of preexisting renal disease or other conditions associated with increased renal morbidity, recent or ongoing renal insults (e.g., surgical procedure, renal toxins, volume losses, resuscitation), and medications (e.g., osmotic diuretics, volatile anesthetics, anticholinergics, nonsteroidal antiin-flammatory drugs).

24. Discuss dopamine and its effect on renal blood flow.

Dopamine is a precursor in the synthetic pathway of norepinephrine and epinephrine. When in-fused in low concentrations, norepinephrine and epinephrine produce an increase in systemic blood pressure accompanied by a decrease in total RBF with maintenance of GFR; when they are infused in higher concentrations, GFR also decreases.

In contrast, low-dose dopamine increases RBF, GFR, and urinary sodium excretion sec-ondary to intracortical redistribution of blood flow. This effect is observed when dopamine recep-tors are differentially activated. Infusion rates of 0.5–2.0 µg/kg/min (some say 1–3 µg/kg/min) stimulate primarily dopaminergic receptors (DA_1 and DA_2). Infusion of 2–5 µg/kg/min stimulate beta-adrenergic receptors, whereas rates above 5 µg/kg/min stimulate alpha-adrenergic receptors. Some clinicians fail to appreciate the significant variability within patients due to receptor activa-tion and binding affinities as well as up- and downregulation of receptors. Thus, it is at best diffi-cult to characterize an observed effect as purely dopaminergic. It is also likely that dopamine is not a usual modulator of renal hemodynamics and function.

In euvolemic adults with normal renal function, dopamine is natriuretic, because it inhibits reabsorption at the proximal convoluted tubule. But in most critically ill patients, natriuresis is not often seen because of multiple influences; the goal of the kidney is sodium conservation. In fact, when baseline GFR is < 70 ml/min, low-dose dopamine is not likely to increase GFR, per-haps because blood flow in chronic renal dysfunction has already been redistributed toward inner cortex and medulla. Marik observed that in a group of critically ill, oliguric patients only those with low plasma renin responded with an improved urine output.

Dopamine, in combination with loop diuretics, increases urine output in patients with acute oliguric renal failure who were previously unresponsive to volume expansion or furosemide; however, this effect may not be due to dopamine's effect on GFR but rather to its effect on RBF, which enhances delivery of furosemide to its site of action. In conclusion, dopamine increases urine output in healthy, hydrated patients and in **some** oliguric patients.

25. Describe the effects of anesthetics on renal function.

It is difficult to separate the effects of anesthetic agents on renal function from the effects of sur-gical stress. Likewise, the indirect effects of general anesthesia on renal hemodynamics, sympa-thetic activity, and humoral regulation confound interpretation of direct anesthetic effects, although it appears that the indirect effects of anesthetic agents have a greater influence on RBF and GFR.

General anesthesia temporarily depresses renal function as measured by urine output, GFR, RBF, and electrolyte excretion. Renal impairment is usually short-lived and completely re-versible. Maintenance of systemic blood pressure and especially preoperative hydration lessen the effect on renal function. Spinal and epidural anesthesia also appear to depress renal function, but not to the same extent as general anesthesia. In this setting decrements in renal function par-allel the magnitude of sympathetic blockade.

Agents that produce myocardial depression (such as volatile anesthetics) are associated with an increase in renal vascular resistance to maintain blood pressure; RBF and GFR decrease. The effects of volatile anesthetics on renal autoregulation are conflicting, but their indirect effects of renal hemodynamics are probably of greater significance.

Methoxyflurane is no longer used because its significant degree of biotransformation (50%) produced toxic amounts of fluoride (peak concentrations > 50 μmol). **Enflurane**, also through production of fluoride, is potentially nephrotoxic, but the duration of exposure necessary to produce toxic levels is far beyond normal limits (although transient impairment in renal concentrating ability has been noted). In any case, with the introduction of newer volatile anesthetics, clinical use of enflurane appears to be declining. A recently introduced volatile anesthetic, **sevoflurane**, is metabolized to fluoride ions; about 3.5% of a dose appears in the urine as inorganic fluoride. Peak concentrations of about 25 μmol appear within 2 hours of discontinuing the agent. The safety of sevoflurane in patients with baseline creatinine > 1.5 mg/dl has not been fully assessed; its use cannot be recommended at this time.

Opioids, barbiturates, and **benzodiazepines** also reduce GFR and urine output. When **droperidol** is administered in combination with opioids to produce general anesthesia (neuroleptanesthesia), its alpha-adrenergic blocking properties maintain the normal distribution of blood flow within the kidney and may result in somewhat smaller changes in renal hemodynamics. **Anticholinergic agents** may predispose patients with obstructive uropathies to postrenal azotemia.

Ketorolac is a nonsteroidal antiinflammatory drug and anesthetic adjuvant that may be administered intramuscularly or intravenously. As a prostaglandin inhibitor, ketorolac interferes with prostaglandin-associated intrinsic renal vasodilation and is a well known cause of drug-induced acute renal failure. In patients at risk and in patients with preexisting renal dysfunction, its use must be avoided.

In conclusion, preexisting cardiovascular and renal function, extent of surgery, and intravascular volume status appear to be the major determinants of the duration and extent of renal impairment associated with anesthetic agents.

26. What muscle relaxants have substantial renal excretion?

Because virtually all relaxants have some degree of renal excretion, their duration of action is prolonged in patients with renal insufficiency. Atracurium undergoes spontaneous degradation under physiologic conditions (Hofmann degradation and ester hydrolysis) and may be preferred in patients with significant renal impairment. Because atracurium is water-soluble, patients with altered body water composition may require larger initial doses to produce rapid paralysis but smaller and less frequent doses to maintain paralysis.

Muscle Relaxants and Renal Excretion

Gallamine > 90%	Doxacurium 30%
Tubocurarine 45%	Vecuronium 15%
Metocurine 43%	Atracurium 10%
Pancuronium 40%	Rocuronium 10%
Pipecuronium 38%	Mivacurium < 10%

27. Does mechanical ventilation affect renal function?

Increases in intrathoracic pressure may decrease urine volume and sodium excretion. Because the magnitude of increased pressure is influential in depressing renal function, ventilatory techniques that use only partial ventilatory support (intermittent mandatory ventilation, pressure support ventilation, continuous positive airway pressure with spontaneous ventilation) are less deleterious. Increases in ADH secretion are noted during controlled ventilation but may be attenuated by volume loading. Decreases in intrathoracic blood volume and changes in transmural pressures do not appear to have a major direct influence on renal function. However, reduced systemic pressures may produce reflex increases in renal sympathetic neural tone. Activation of the renin-angiotensin-aldosterone system by mechanical ventilation also probably acts to reduce renal function.

28. Describe management strategies to prevent renal failure in high-risk patients.

In patients with elevated creatinine or suspected renal insufficiency with "normal" creatinine, determining the creatinine clearance is useful in adjusting the doses of renally excreted and renally toxic drugs, such as aminoglycosides. When radiocontrast must be given, the dose should be limited to the minimum needed, and the patient should be hydrated. Laboratory studies should be appropriate to the patient group. Before surgery, the patient must be euvolemic; pulmonary artery catheterization may be indicated to guide fluid management and to optimize hemodynamics and therefore RBF. Medications that may be nephrotoxic (e.g., amphotericin, nonsteroidal antiinflammatory drugs, aminoglycosides) or produce an obstructive uropathy (anticholinergics, antihistamines) should be avoided if possible.

29. Do diuretics have a role in preventing renal failure in high-risk patients?

Mannitol may be of use because (1) it is a renal vasodilator, increasing cortical blood flow; (2) it increases tubular flow, clearing tubules of necrotic cellular debris that may contribute to acute tubular necrosis; (3) as an oxygen scavenger, it may be of benefit in preventing ischemia-reperfusion injuries. However, with the exception of contrast nephrotoxicity, no controlled prospective studies clearly demonstrate the benefit of mannitol in preventing acute renal failure in high-risk patients. Diuretics may convert oliguric renal failure to nonoliguric renal failure; management may be easier but prognosis is not improved. Mannitol may also potentiate acute renal failure if it precipitates congestive heart failure and produces renal hypoperfusion. Finally, like mannitol, furosemide has been shown to be of benefit in high-risk groups only anecdotally.

30. How are patients with chronic renal failure best managed perioperatively?

The surgical mortality rate for patients with end-stage renal disease (ESRD) is about 4%, but when such patients require emergency procedures, the rate increases to 20%. Clearly preoperative preparation is of benefit. Primary causes of death include sepsis, dysrhythmias, and cardiac dysfunction.

The morbidity rate is substantial, approaching 50%. Hyperkalemia is the most common cause of morbidity, although infections, hemodynamic instability, bleeding, and arrhythmias are extremely common and problematic. Renal causes for increased morbidity include decreased ability to concentrate and dilute urine, decreased ability to regulate extracellular fluid and sodium, impaired handling of acid loads, hyperkalemia, and impaired excretion of medications. Renal impairment is confounded by anemia, uremic platelet dysfunction, arrhythmias, pericardial effusions, myocardial dysfunction, chronic hypertension, neuropathies, malnutrition, and susceptibility to infection. Of note, patients with chronic renal failure who are not yet on dialysis are at greater risk for developing acute renal failure.

Preoperatively patients must be euvolemic, normotensive, normonatremic, and normokalemic, not acidotic or severely anemic, and without significant platelet dysfunction. Suggested laboratory values include complete blood count, electrolytes, arterial blood gases, and template bleeding time. Bleeding time measured at the thigh rather than the arm is a better predictor of bleeding in the perioperative period. Dialysis usually corrects uremic platelet dysfunction and is best performed within the 24-hours before surgery. Administration of 1-deamino-8-D-arginine vasopressin (DDAVP) or cryoprecipitate is also of benefit.

Other indications for acute dialysis include uremic symptoms, pericardial tamponade, bleeding, hypervolemia, congestive heart failure, hyperkalemia, and severe acidosis.

Patients with ESRD who have left ventricular dysfunction or undergo major procedures with significant fluid shifts require pulmonary artery monitoring to guide fluid therapy. Sterile technique should be strictly followed when inserting any catheters. In minor procedures, fluids should be limited to replacement of urine and insensible losses. Hypotension and drugs with substantial renal excretion must be avoided. Succinylcholine increases extracellular potassium. Meperidine has a renally excreted, active toxic metabolite (normeperidine). As in the operative phase, postoperative potassium restriction and close monitoring of potassium levels is a must. Hyperkalemia should be considered in patients with ESRD who develop ventricular arrhythmias and experience a cardiac arrest. Rapid administration of calcium chloride temporizes the cardiac effects of hyperkalemia until further measures (administration of glucose and insulin, hyperventilation, administration of sodium bicarbonate, and potassium-binding resins, and dialysis) can be taken to shift potassium intracellularly and to decrease total body potassium.

CONTROVERSY

31. What recent developments may produce better "real-time" assessment of renal function?
The fundamental parameters that most accurately characterize renal function are GFR and RBF.
Rigorous assessment of GFR requires measurement of a filtration marker that is filtered but not
reabsorbed or secreted; this method proves technically difficult. Alternatively, GFR may be calculated by measuring the rate of disappearance from plasma of a specific substance after a single
IV injection. A radiolabelled tracer monitored by a portable detector, known as the ambulatory
renal monitor (ARM), is currently under investigation in the perioperative setting. A major limitation is that ARM measures only total RBF.

　　If the redistribution of RBF from outer to inner cortex and medulla could be appreciated, it
would herald the earliest events in renal dysfunction. Recently, contrast ultrasonography has
proved feasible for intraoperative determination of regional RBF; further studies are needed to
demonstrate its usefulness as a direct on-line monitor of renal function in the perioperative setting.

BIBLIOGRAPHY

  1. Amoroso P, Lanigan C: Renal dysfunction and anesthesia. Curr Opin Anesth 8:267–270, 1995.
  2. Aronson S: Monitoring renal function. In Miller RD (ed): Anesthesia, 4th ed. New York, Churchill
     Livingstone, 1993, pp 1293–1317.
  3. Aronson S: Controversies: Should anesthesiologists worry about the kidney? Review Course Lectures.
     Anesth Analg 80(Suppl):68–73, 1995.
  4. Aronson S, Thisthelwaite R, Walke R, et al: Safety and feasibility of renal blood flow determination
     during kidney transplant surgery with perfusion ultrasonography. Anesth Analg 80:353–359, 1995.
  5. Burchardi H, Kaczmarczyk: The effect of anaesthesia on renal function. Eur J Anaesth 11:163–168,
     1994.
  6. Charlson ME, MacKenzie CR, Gold JP, et al: Postoperative changes in serum creatinine: When do they
     occur and how much is important? Ann Surg 209:328–333, 1989.
  7. Cullen DJ: Monitoring of renal function. In Miller RD (ed): Anesthesia, 4th ed. New York, Churchill
     Livingstone, 1993, pp 1165–1184.
  8. Guyton AC: Textbook of Medical Physiology, 8th ed. Philadelphia, W.B. Saunders, 1991.
  9. Hock R, Anderson RJ: Prevention of drug-induced nephrotoxicity in the intensive care unit. J Crit Care
     10:33–43, 1995.
 10. Kellen M, Aronson S, Roizen MF, et al: Predictive and diagnostic tests of renal failure: A review. Anesth
     Analg 78:134–142, 1994.
 11. Kellerman PS: Perioperative care of the renal patient. Arch Intern Med 154:1674–1688, 1994.
 12. Kriz W, Bankir I: A standard nomenclature for structures of the kidney. Am J Physiol 254:F1, 1988.
 13. Marik PE: Low-dose dopamine in critically ill oliguric patients: The influence of the renin angiotensin
     system. Heart Lung 22:171–175, 1993.
 14. Mazze RI: Renal physiology. In Miller RD (ed): Anesthesia, 3rd ed. New York, Churchill Livingstone,
     1990, pp 601–619.
 15. Rabito C, Moore R, Bougas C, et al: Noninvasive, real-time monitoring of renal function: The ambula-
     tory renal monitor. J Nucl Med 34:199–207, 1993.
 16. ter Wee PM, Smit AJ: Effects of intravenous infusion of low-dose dopamine on renal function in normal
     individuals and in patients with renal disease. Am J Nephrol 6:42–46, 1986.

50. INCREASED INTRACRANIAL PRESSURE

William D. Sefton, M.D.

1. Define elevated intracranial pressure.
Elevated intracranial pressure (ICP) is usually defined as a sustained pressure of 20 mmHg or greater within the subarachnoid space. The normal ICP is 10–20 mmHg.

2. What are the determinants of ICP?
The space-occupying contents of the skull—i.e., brain, cerebrospinal fluid (CSF), extracellular fluid, and blood perfusing the brain—are contained in the virtually fixed volume of the cranium. If any of these contents increases in volume, the ICP will increase.

3. How is ICP measured?
Various techniques are available. The standard method is a ventriculostomy, in which a burr hole is made in the cranium and a soft plastic catheter is introduced into the lateral ventricle. Saline-filled tubing is attached, and an external transducer measures the pressure in the fluid column of the tubing. Another common method is the subarachnoid bolt, which is also placed via a burr hole but does not require insertion through brain tissue or identification of the position of the ventricle. Pressure is transduced via saline-filled tubing. A third technique involves the insertion of a fiber-optic bundle through a small burr hole. The fiberoptic bundle senses changes in the amount of light reflected off a pressure-sensitive diaphragm at its tip. This system, commonly called a Camino (it is manufactured by Camino Laboratories), has recently gained popularity because of ease of placement and avoidance of difficulties associated with the fluid-filled transducing systems.

4. Summarize the conditions that commonly cause elevated ICP. 5. Describe the symptoms of increased ICP.

Common Causes of Elevated ICP

CSF DISORDERS	MASSES	HEAD TRAUMA	MIXED CAUSES
Communicating hydro-cephalus Obstructing hydro-cephalus (e.g., from a posterior fossa lesion)	Neoplasm Hematoma (epidural or subarachnoid) Cysts	Contusion Cerebral edema Cerebral lacerations	Bleeding from cerebral aneurysm or arteri-ovenous malforma-tion Hepatic encephalopathy Malignant hypertension Cerebrovascular acci-dent with edema

Symptoms associated with increased ICP alone include headache, vomiting, papilledema, drowsiness, loss of consciousness, and behavioral changes. Several other symptoms, such as pathologic (decerebrate) posturing, oculomotor nerve palsy, abnormalities of brainstem reflexes, and abnormal respiratory patterns (including apnea), are probably caused by brainstem distortion or ischemia secondary to elevated ICP. The classic Cushing reflex, consisting of hypertension and bradycardia, is probably due to medullary ischemia and generally occurs when ICP approaches systemic arterial pressure.

6. Discuss the possible consequences of increased ICP.
In addition to producing the above symptoms, the ultimate danger of increased ICP is a decrease in cerebral perfusion pressure, which may result in regional or global cerebral ischemia and

possible irreversible neurologic damage. In addition, sufficient elevation of ICP may result in herniation of brain contents (across the falx cerebri or tentorium or inferiorly from the foramen magnum).

7. What are the determinants of cerebral perfusion pressure?

Cerebral perfusion pressure is defined as the difference between mean arterial pressure (MAP) and either ICP or central venous pressure (CVP), whichever is higher.

8. What is intracranial elastance? Why is it clinically significant?

Intracranial elastance, commonly misnamed intracranial compliance, refers to the variation in intracranial pressure in accordance with intracranial volume. Because intracranial components can shift their volumes to an extent (for example, CSF movement from the intracranial compartment to the spinal compartment), intracranial pressure remains somewhat constant over a certain range of volume. However, when compensatory mechanisms are exhausted, ICP rises rapidly with further increases in volume.

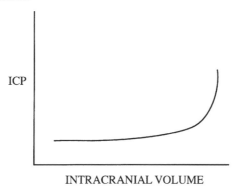

Intracranial elastance.

9. How is cerebral blood flow regulated?

Cerebral blood flow (CBF) is coupled to cerebral metabolic rate by an as yet uncharacterized mechanism. In general, increases in the cerebral metabolic rate for oxygen ($CMRO_2$), lead to increases in CBF, although the increase in flow is delayed by 1–2 minutes. Several other parameters influence flow. Specifically, an increase in the partial pressure of carbon dioxide in arterial blood ($PaCO_2$) is a powerful vasodilator that increases flow. Similarly, a decrease in the partial pressure of oxygen (PaO_2) in arterial blood below 50 mmHg greatly increases flow. Variations in mean arterial pressure (MAP) also may result in large increases or decreases in flow, but over a broad range flow is nearly constant. When the brain has been injured, as in stroke, tumor accompanied by edema, or trauma, autoregulation may not be intact. Systemic hypertension may result in precipitous increases in flow, with secondary increases in ICP leading to regional ischemia elsewhere.

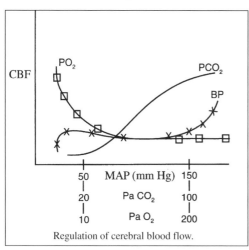

Regulation of cerebral blood flow.

10. Should premedication be given to patients with elevated ICP?

Neurologic assessment should be performed in all patients before administering premedication. Some patients with elevated ICP are asymptomatic, and premedication may help to prevent further elevations due to systemic hypertension related to preoperative anxiety or pain associated with placement of intravascular lines. However, all patients with the potential for increased ICP should be premedicated judiciously, because respiratory depression with resultant increases in $PaCO_2$ may have deleterious effects. In addition, supplementary oxygen is recommended to prevent decreases in PaO_2 and secondary increases in CBF.

11. What is the goal of anesthetic care for patients with elevated ICP?

Because patients with elevated ICP may be located on the elbow of the elastance curve, wherein a small change in volume leads to a large increase in ICP and probable decrease in cerebral perfusion, the goal of anesthetic care is to use all possible measures to reduce intracranial volume.

12. Can this goal be aided by preoperative interventions?

Traditionally, several techniques have been used to decrease intracranial volume before surgery, particularly when the volume is already increased by local edema surrounding brain tumors. Mild fluid restriction (intake of one-third to one-half of daily maintenance requirements) may decrease ICP over a period of several days. Corticosteroids are particularly effective in decreasing edema associated with tumors.

13. How is the goal of reduced intracranial volume achieved at induction of anesthesia?

Generally, the measures used at induction of anesthesia are geared specifically to reduce cerebral blood volume. If conscious and cooperative, the patient is encouraged to hyperventilate during preoxygenation to reduce $PaCO_2$. Most commonly used intravenous anesthetics, such as the barbiturates (usually thiopental), propofol, benzodiazepines, and etomidate lower CBF either by reducing cerebral metabolic rate or by direct cerebral vasoconstriction. Narcotics appear to have little effect on CBF but are commonly used to blunt the sympathetic response to laryngoscopy and tracheal intubation. Common adjuncts include intravenous lidocaine, which is also a cerebral vasoconstrictor, and may blunt the response to intubation, and short-acting beta blockers such as esmolol, which blunt systemic hypertension due to laryngoscopy. Ketamine is to be avoided, because it increases CBF and ICP via sympathomimetic effects.

14. How is ICP moderated during maintenance of anesthesia?

Most intraoperative maneuvers for controlling ICP rely on reduction of cerebral blood volume or total brain water content. Blood volume is minimized by hyperventilation to lower $PaCO_2$ (25–30 mmHg), which results in cerebral vasoconstriction, and by using anesthetic agents that decrease CBF. Maintaining the patient in a slightly head-up position promotes venous drainage. To shrink brain water content acutely, furosemide and mannitol are commonly used to promote diuresis. In addition, intravenous fluids are limited to the minimal amount necessary to maintain cardiac performance. The surgeon may drain CSF directly from the surgical field or use spinal drainage to decrease total intracranial volume. If oxygenation is not problematic, positive end-expiratory pressure should be avoided, because it can be transmitted to the intracranial compartment. Lastly, moderate hypothermia (approximately 35° Celsius) decreases $CMRO_2$ and thus CBF.

15. Which intravenous fluids are used during surgery to minimize ICP?

This is an area of some controversy. In general, hypotonic crystalloid infusions should be avoided, because they may increase brain water content. Glucose-containing solutions are avoided because of evidence of worsened neurologic outcome if ischemia occurs in the setting of hyperglycemia. Therefore, hyperglycemia (serum glucose > 180 mg/dl) should be treated with insulin. Whether colloid solutions are better than isotonic crystalloid is debatable. However, glucose-free isotonic crystalloid appears to be the standard infusion in neurosurgical cases. For cases that involve significant blood loss, some authorities believe that colloid solutions, such as hetastarch or albumin, are preferable because they replete intravascular volume more quickly without increasing brain water content. Hetastarch, however, has been associated with an elevation of prothrombin and partial thromboplastin times when given in volumes > 1 L. Others argue that fractionated blood products are the most physiologic replacement possible for intraoperative blood loss. However, because of infectious risk, this option should be reserved for patients with physiologically significant anemia.

16. What are the effects of volatile anesthetics on CBF?
All of the commonly used inhaled anesthetics—halothane, isoflurane, enflurane, and desflurane—have been noted to increase CBF and to uncouple $CMRO_2$ and CBF in the presence of normocapnia. However, because the response of CBF to $PaCO_2$ is preserved with the volatile anesthetics (most reliably with isoflurane), hyperventilation may prevent this increase in CBF.

17. How do neuromuscular blocking agents affect ICP?
Succinylcholine has been reported to increase ICP, but the clinical significance of this transient increase remains doubtful. The increase also appears to be attenuated by pretreatment with a defasciculating dose of a nondepolarizing relaxant. Therefore, in cases of emergent surgery in patients with a full stomach, rapid-sequence induction with succinylcholine is acceptable. Commonly used nondepolarizing agents, such as vecuronium, atracurium, and the newer rocuronium, have no effect on ICP and can be used safely. Pancuronium has not been definitively shown to increase ICP or CBF, but theoretically its vagolytic effects may increase heart rate and blood pressure, leading to increased ICP in patients with decreased intracranial elastance. The ability of curare to release histamine, which causes decreased blood pressure and increased ICP, makes it an undesirable neuromuscular blocking agent in neurosurgical patients.

18. Discuss strategies for controlling ICP at emergence from anesthesia.
The usual strategy is control of systemic blood pressure to prevent elevation above the level of autoregulation, in which case blood flow (and possibly ICP) increases in linear fashion with elevations in blood pressure. Autoregulation in the operative site may be impaired; that is, blood flow may increase dramatically at lower-than-usual blood pressures. Usually beta blockers such as esmolol and labetalol are given in divided doses to attenuate the increased sympathetic tone present at emergence. Nitroprusside, a direct-acting vasodilator, is also useful in controlling blood pressure when administered by infusion. In addition, as at induction, normo- or hypocarbia is preferred.

19. If the above measures fail to control ICP, what other measures are available?
Barbiturate coma has been used in patients refractory to other methods of ICP control. Typical doses of pentobarbital are 10 mg/kg given over 30 minutes to load, followed by three hourly doses of 5 mg/kg. This regimen usually provides a therapeutic serum level of 30–50 µg/ml. Maintenance is usually achieved by dosing of 1–2 mg/kg/hr. Pentobarbital has been shown to reduce ICP, probably by reducing CBF. Systemic blood pressure, however, may drop enough to decrease cerebral perfusion pressure and require the use of vasopressors.

20. In a patient with traumatic head injury, how should fluid resuscitation be prioritized?
As a general rule, hemodynamic stability takes precedence over concern for further elevation of ICP by fluid administration. Initial resuscitation, particularly in the face of hemorrhagic hypovolemia, is best achieved with blood products, ideally fresh whole blood. Because fresh whole blood is rarely available, fractionated blood products, particularly packed red blood cells, are the second choice. Isotonic crystalloid solutions are the third choice. They are both inexpensive and effective at increasing intravascular volume rapidly, but they may increase cerebral edema compared with blood products. Hetastarch is probably best avoided because of its ability to produce coagulopathy when given in larger volumes. A 5% solution of albumin is also useful, but it is expensive and has not been shown to reduce formation of cerebral edema compared with isotonic crystalloid.

21. Discuss fluid resuscitation strategies in burn victims with head injury.

Burn victims with head injury pose a somewhat more complicated problem than trauma victims. Frequently the burn victim's fluid deficit is due to loss of free water rather than hemorrhage. For this reason, crystalloid solutions are the fluid of choice, although the need to use hypoosmolar solutions in some burn cases and the need to limit cerebral edema are somewhat mutually incompatible goals. The use of colloid products, particularly 5% albumin, to replace protein losses may help to limit cerebral edema, although colloid fluids do not replace free water loss. In patients with blood loss and physiologically significant anemia, blood products are the ideal choice.

BIBLIOGRAPHY

1. Bendo A, Kass I, Hartung J, Cotrrell JE: Neurophysiology and Neuroanesthesia. In Barash PG, Cullen BF, Stoelting RK (eds): Clinical Anesthesia, 2nd ed. Philadelphia, J.B. Lippincott, 1992, pp 876–891.
2. Cucchiara RF, Mahla ME: Anesthesia in patients with elevated intracranial pressure. In Barash PG, Deutsch S, Tinker J (eds): Refresher Courses in Anesthesiology, vol 21. Philadelphia, J.B. Lippincott, 1993, pp 177–188.
3. Gopinath SP, Robertson CS: In Cottrell JE, Smith DS (eds): Anesthesia and Neurosurgery, 3rd ed. St. Louis, Mosby, 1994, pp 676–677.
4. Michenfelder JD: Intracranial pressure. In Cucchiara RF, Michenfelder JD (eds): Clinical Neuroanesthesia. New York, Churchill Livingstone, 1990, pp 81–82.
5. Minton MD, Stirt JA, Bedford RF, Haworth C: Intracranial pressure after atracurium in neurosurgical patients. Anesth Analg 64:1113–1116, 1985.
6. Minton MD, Stirt JA, Bedford RF: Vecuronium: Effect on ICP and hemodynamics in patients with brain tumors. Anesth Analg 65:S101, 1986.
7. Shapiro HM, Drummond JC: Neurosurgical anesthesia. In Miller RD (ed): Anesthesia, 4th ed. New York, Churchill Livingstone, 1994, pp 1909–1917.
8. Zornow MH, Scheller MS: Intraoperative fluid management during craniotomy. In Cottrell JE, Smith DS (eds): Anesthesia and Neurosurgery, 3rd ed. St. Louis, Mosby, 1994, pp 254–257.

51. MUSCULAR DISORDERS AND NEUROPATHIES

Timothy Fry, D.O.

1. What are major clinical features of muscular dystrophy?

The most severe form of muscular dystrophy, Duchenne's muscular dystrophy, is associated with painless degeneration and atrophy of skeletal muscle. Muscular dystrophy is a sex-linked recessive disease with signs and symptoms presenting between 2 and 5 years of age. Death is typically due to congestive heart failure or pneumonia.

2. Name the important systems involved with muscular dystrophy.

Degeneration of cardiac muscle, as demonstrated by progressive decrease in R wave amplitude on ECG, may lead to a decrease in contractility and mitral regurgitation secondary to papillary muscle dysfunction. The respiratory system also may be affected with degeneration of ventilatory muscles. A restrictive pattern is observed on pulmonary function testing. Patients are more prone to aspiration of secretions, which may lead to pneumonia. Bedside vital capacity testing is easily performed and gives an objective indicator of pulmonary function.

3. What are the anesthetic considerations in patients with muscular dystrophy?

Patients with muscular dystrophy may be more sensitive to the myocardial depressant effects of inhaled anesthetics. Succinylcholine should not be used because of the possibility of massive rhabdomyolysis, hyperkalemia, and subsequent cardiac arrest. In fact, cardiac arrest has been reported in patients with unrecognized muscular dystrophy. One should be aware of this possibility and have calcium readily available as an antidote. Nondepolarizing relaxants are acceptable but may be associated with longer than normal recovery times. Because smooth muscle may be affected, patients may have gastrointestinal tract hypomotility, delayed gastric emptying, and impaired swallowing, which may lead to increased risk of aspiration.

4. What is myotonic dystrophy?

Myotonic dystrophy, an autosomal dominant disease that usually presents in the second or third decade, is characterized by persistent contraction of skeletal muscle after stimulation. The contractions are not relieved by regional anesthetics, nondepolarizing muscle relaxants, or deep anesthesia. Deterioration of skeletal, cardiac, and smooth muscle function is progressive.

5. How does myotonic dystrophy affect the cardiopulmonary system?

The cardiac conduction system (mostly the His-Purkinje system) deteriorates more rapidly than myocardial systolic function. Heart failure is rare, but dysrhythmias and atrioventricular block are common. Mitral valve prolapse occurs in 20% of patients. Restrictive lung disease, with mild hypoxia on room air and a weak cough, may lead to pneumonia.

6. What are the important anesthetic considerations with myotonic dystrophy?

Management of patients with myotonic dystrophy must include careful consideration of cardiac and respiratory muscle dysfunction. Succinylcholine produces exaggerated contraction of skeletal muscles, possibly making ventilation of the lungs and tracheal intubation difficult or impossible. The response to nondepolarizing muscle relaxants is normal.

7. What are the clinical manifestations of Guillain-Barré syndrome?

Guillain-Barré syndrome usually presents as a postinfectious state with sudden onset of weakness or paralysis, typically in the legs, that spreads cephalad over several days. The symptoms may involve the skeletal muscles of the arms, trunk, and head. Patients may have dysphagia due to pharyngeal muscle weakness and impaired ventilation due to intercostal muscle paralysis. Complete spontaneous recovery may occur within weeks. Mortality (3–8%) is typically due to sepsis, adult respiratory distress syndrome, pulmonary embolism, or cardiac arrest.

8. How is the autonomic nervous system affected?

Autonomic dysfunction is a common finding. Patients may experience wide fluctuations in blood pressure, profuse diaphoresis, peripheral vasoconstriction, tachycardia, cardiac conduction abnormalities, and orthostatic hypotension.

9. What are the major anesthetic considerations for patients with Guillain-Barré syndrome?

Because compensatory cardiovascular responses may be absent, patients may become hypotensive with changes in posture, mild blood loss, or positive pressure ventilation. On the other hand, laryngoscopy may produce exaggerated increases in blood pressure. Succinylcholine should not be used because of the potential for exaggerated potassium release in the presence of lower motor neuron lesions. Postoperative ventilation may be necessary and should be explained to the patient preoperatively.

10. What are the pathophysiologic features of Parkinson's disease?

Parkinson's disease, an adult-onset degenerative disease of the extrapyramidal system, is characterized by the loss of dopaminergic fibers and dopamine depletion in the basal ganglia. The results are diminished inhibition of the extrapyramidal motor system and unopposed action of acetylcholine.

11. Define Lewy body.

Lewy bodies are cytoplasmic eosinophilic inclusions found in the substantia nigra and locus ceruleus neurons. They are one of the pathologic features of Parkinson's disease.

12. What are the clinical manifestations of Parkinson's disease? How is it commonly treated?

Patients with Parkinson's disease display increased rigidity of the extremities, facial immobility, shuffling gait, rhythmic resting tremor, dementia, depression, diaphragmatic spasms, and occulogyric crisis. Oculogyric crisis is a form of dystonia in which the eyes are deviated in a fixed position for minutes to hours. Parkinson's disease is commonly treated with levodopa, which crosses the blood-brain barrier, where it is converted to dopamine. Carbidopa is often combined with levodopa to inhibit the activity of dopa decarboxylase.

Patients with mild symptoms may be treated with amantadine or anticholinergic agents such as benztropine and procyclidine. Anticholinergic treatment is limited by autonomic side effects such as urinary retention and dry mouth.

Some patients with moderate-to-severe disease may be treated with direct-acting dopaminergic agents, such as bromocriptine, to limit exposure to levodopa.

13. Why is orthostatic hypotension a common side effect in patients treated with levodopa?

Increased levels of dopamine may increase myocardial contractility and heart rate. Renal blood flow is likely to increase, causing an increase in glomerular filtration rate and excretion of sodium. Intravascular fluid volume is therefore decreased, and the renin-angiotensin aldosterone system is depressed. Orthostatic hypotension is a common finding. High concentrations of dopamine may cause negative feedback for norepinephrine production, which also causes orthostatic hypotension.

14. Describe the complications that may occur when patients with Parkinson's disease need anesthesia.

1. Abrupt withdrawal of levodopa may lead to skeletal muscle rigidity that interferes with adequate ventilation. Levodopa should be administered on the morning of surgery throughout the perioperative period.

2. Orthostatic hypotension, cardiac dysrhythmias, and even hypertension may occur.

3. Phenothiazines (e.g., chlorpromazine, promethazine, fluphenazine, prochlorperazine) and butyrophenones (e.g., droperidol) may antagonize the effects of dopamine in the basal ganglia. Metoclopramide inhibits dopamine receptors in the brain. These medications should be avoided.

4. Patients may be intravascularly volume-depleted; therefore, aggressive administration of crystalloid or colloid solutions may be required before induction of anesthesia.

15. What surgical method is used to treat Parkinson's disease?
Fetal tissue transplantation is used with increasing frequency in the United States and Europe. Dopamine-rich neurons taken from the ventral mesencephalon of a fetus are implanted into the dopamine-innervated striatum of the patient. Grafting of Schwann cells and fetal adrenal medullar tissue also has been performed. Survival and long-term function of fetal tissue transplantations continue to be evaluated. Some studies have shown only marginal symptomatic improvement, and all patients still require levodopa therapy. Other studies have shown significant longstanding improvements. Ethical concerns have focused on the concern that grafting fetal tissue may encourage elective abortions.

Advances in molecular biology may provide transplantation of genetically engineered cells or modification of existing brain cells by transfection with viral vectors.

16. What are the clinical signs and symptoms of Alzheimer's disease?
Alzheimer's disease accounts for 60% of the severe cases of dementia in the United States. The disease follows an insidious onset with progressive worsening of memory despite a normal level of consciousness. CT shows ventricular dilation and marked cortical atrophy.

17. What is the most significant anesthetic problem associated with Alzheimer's disease?
The inability of some patients to understand their environment or to cooperate with providers of medical care becomes an important anesthetic consideration. Sedative drugs may exacerbate confusion and probably should be avoided in the perioperative period. Regional techniques may be used with the understanding that the patient may be frightened or confused by the operating room environment. However, they avoid administration of volatile anesthetics and reduce opioid administration, which may be of benefit.

18. What are the hallmark features of multiple sclerosis?
The corticospinal tract neurons of the brain and spinal cord show random and multiple sites of demyelination, which result in visual and gait disturbances, limb paresthesias and weaknesses, and urinary incontinence. The onset of disease is typically between the ages of 15 and 40. The cause appears to be multifactorial, including viral and genetic factors. The course of multiple sclerosis is characterized by periods of exacerbations and remissions of symptoms. Residual symptoms eventually persist.

19. Do steroids have a role in the treatment of multiple sclerosis?
Steroids may shorten the duration of an attack but probably do not influence progression of the disease.

20. How do patient temperature and stress play a role in exacerbation?
It is thought that elevated temperature causes complete blocking of conduction in demyelinated neurons. Emotional stress and excessive fatigue should be avoided, because they may exacerbate symptoms.

21. What perioperative problems must be anticipated in patients with multiple sclerosis?
Surgical stress most likely will exacerbate the symptoms of multiple sclerosis. Even modest increases in body temperature (> 1°C) must be avoided. Spinal anesthesia has been implicated in

postoperative exacerbation of symptoms. The mechanism is unknown, but epidural or peripheral nerve blocks may be a better choice for regional techniques. There are no known unique interactions between multiple sclerosis and drugs selected for general anesthesia, although succinylcholine may cause an exaggerated release of potassium.

22. Describe the neuropathies associated with diabetes.
  1. Autonomic neuropathy. The diabetic patient with an autonomic neuropathy may manifest with one or all of the entities in the table below. A patient with autonomic neuropathy may not have angina pectoris in the presence of ischemic heart disease. Once an autonomic neuropathy develops, the mortality rate exceeds 50% over a 5-year period. Gastroparesis may place such patients at an increased risk of aspiration due to delayed gastric emptying.
  2. Peripheral neuropathies. Diabetic patients may complain of sensory discomfort of the lower extremities or carpal tunnel syndrome. They also may develop segmental demyelination of the cranial, median, and ulnar nerves; numbness and tingling or burning and itching of the lower extremities; and skeletal muscle weakness of the upper and lower extremities.

Manifestations of Diabetic Autonomic Neuropathy

Orthostatic hypotension	Gastroparesis
Resting tachycardia	Bladder atony
Cardiac dysrhythmias	Impotence
Sudden death syndrome	Hypoglycemia

23. What neurologic disorders are associated with human immunodeficiency virus (HIV)?
As many as 50% of patients infected with HIV may display peripheral neuropathy in the form of paresthesias, weakness, and sensory loss. They also may develop encephalitis, myelopathies (spastic paresis, incontinence), and aseptic meningitis.

24. What are the manifestations of alcoholic neuropathy?
Symptoms of alcoholic neuropathy typically begin with pain and numbness in the feet. Patients also may have weakness of foot muscles along with decreased Achilles tendon reflexes. Alcoholic neuropathy is usually due to a nutritional deficiency. Proper diet, multivitamins, and abstinence from alcohol may resolve the neuropathy.

25. Describe postpoliomyelitis syndrome.
Postpoliomyelitis syndrome (postpolio syndrome) is characterized by progressive weakness that begins years after a severe attack of poliomyelitis. The syndrome typically presents many years after the acute disease as a progression of weakness in the originally affected muscles. Normal muscles are less often affected. Common signs and symptoms include fatigue, cold intolerance, joint deteriorations, muscle pain, atrophy, respiratory insufficiency, dysphagia, and sleep apnea. One study revealed that patients with postpolio syndrome who complain of dysphagia demonstrate some degree of vocal cord paralysis. Some patients have decreased lung function; considerable cardiorespiratory deconditioning also may be present.

26. What are the anesthetic considerations for patients with postpoliomyelitis syndrome?
Because postpolio syndrome may affect several different muscle groups, involved areas of the body must be carefully assessed. Patients may have respiratory insufficiency demonstrated by pulmonary function testing. Patients should be informed about the possibility of postoperative mechanical ventilation after general anesthesia. If sleep apnea is present, the patient may have coexisting pulmonary hypertension. Dysphagia and vocal cord paralysis may place patients at increased risk for aspiration. If progressive skeletal muscle weakness is present, succinylcholine should be avoided because of the possibility of exaggerated potassium release.

BIBLIOGRAPHY

1. Ackerman MS: The patient with parkinson's disease. In Frost EAM (ed): Preanesthetic Assessment 2. Boston, Birkhauser, 1989, pp 289–302.
2. Ahlskog JE: Cerebral transplantation for Parkinson's disease: Current progress and future prospects. Mayo Clin Proc 68:578–591, 1993.
3. Boer GJ: Ethical guidelines for the use of human embryonic or fetal tissue for experimental and clinical neurotransplantation and research. J Neurol 242:1–13, 1994.
4. Dierdorf SF: Rare and coexisting diseases. In Barash PG, Cullen BF, Stoelting RK (eds): Clinical Anesthesia. Philadelphia, J.B. Lippincott, 1992, pp 563–587.
5. Driscoll BP, Gracco C, Coelho C, et al: Laryngeal function in postpolio patients. Laryngoscope 105:35–41, 1995.
6. Eriksson LI: Neuromuscular disorders and anaesthesia. Curr Opin Anesthesiol 8:275–281, 1995.
7. Fahn S: The extrapyramidal disorders. In Wyngaarden JB, Smith LH Jr (eds): Cecil's Textbook of Medicine, 18th ed. Philadelphia, W.B. Saunders, 1988, pp 2141–2152.
8. Jubelt B, Drucker J: Post-polio syndrome: An update. Semin Neurol 13:283–290, 1993.
9. Katzman R: Alzheimer's disease. N Engl J Med 314:964–973, 1983.
10. Lindvall O: Clinical application of neuronal grafts in Parkinson's disease. J Neurol 242(1 Suppl 1):S54–S56, 1994.
11. Mitchell MM, Ali HH, Savarese JJ: Myotonia and neuromuscular blocking agents. Anesthesiology 49:44–48, 1978.
12. Price R: Poliomyelitis. In Wyngaarden JB, Smith LH Jr (eds): Cecil's Textbook of Medicine, 18th ed. Philadelphia, W.B. Saunders, 1988, pp 2198–2200.
13. Redman DE Jr, Roth RH, Spencer DD, et al: Neural transplantation for neurodegenerative diseases: Past, present, and future. Ann N Y Acad Sci 695:258–266, 1993.
14. Stanghelle JK, Festvag L, Aksnes AK: Pulmonary function and symptom-limited exercise testing in subjects with late sequelae of poliomyelitis. Scand J Rehabil Med 25(3):125–129, 1993.
15. Stoelting RK, Dierdorf SF: Diseases of the nervous system. In Anesthesia and Co-Existing Diseases, 3rd ed. New York, Churchill Livingstone, 1993, pp 181–250.
16. Stoelting RK, Dierdorf SF: Skin and musculoskeletal diseases. In Anesthesia and Co-Existing Diseases, 3rd ed. New York, Churchill Livingstone, 1993, pp 427–457.
17. Stoelting RK, Miller RD: Endocrine and nutritional disease. In Basics of Anesthesia, 3rd ed. New York, Churchill Livingstone, 1994, pp 315–329.
18. Zhang WC, Ding YJ, Cao JK, et al: Intracerebral co-grafting of Schwann's cells and fetal adrenal medulla in the treatment of Parkinson's disease. Chin Med J 107:583–588, 1994.

52. ANESTHETIC CONCERNS IN PATIENTS WITH SPINAL CORD INJURY

Andrew A. Shultz, M.D., and Kenneth Niejadlik, M.D.

1. How common are spinal cord injuries?

There are approximately 10,000 new spinal cord injuries (SCIs) in the United States each year. Of patients with new injuries, approximately 50% die; of these, 80% die before reaching medical evaluation, and 20% die during hospitalization. The incidence of spinal cord injuries is approximately 28–50/1,000,000 people. As of 1980, there were approximately 200,000 persons in the U.S. with some degree of spinal cord injury.

2. What are the more common causes of SCIs?

Motor vehicle accidents are the most common cause of acute SCIs, followed by falls and sports injuries (especially diving accidents). It is estimated that cervical SCIs occur in approximately 1.5–3% of all major traumatic accidents. The most common nontraumatic cause of spinal cord transection is multiple sclerosis. Rheumatoid arthritis of the spine may cause subluxation of the C1 on the C2 vertebra, leading to progressive quadriparesis. In major urban regions, gunshot wounds are a major cause of SCIs. Lastly, vascular, infectious, and developmental abnormalities may cause damage to the spinal cord with neurologic sequelae.

3. Describe the blood supply to the spinal cord.

The superior cervical spinal cord derives the majority of its blood supply from the anterior spinal artery (ASA) and posterior spinal artery (PSA). The ASA originates from a medial branch of the vertebral arteries at the level of the foramen magnum and courses inferiorly along the anterior median fissure of the spinal cord, supplying approximately two-thirds of the anterior spinal cord. The paired PSAs originate from the intracranial portions of either the vertebral arteries or the posterior inferior cerebellar arteries and run down the posterior region of the spinal cord, supplying the posterior one-third of the spinal cord.

From the inferior cervical spinal cord caudally, the ASA and paired PSAs are joined by the radicular arteries, which form a plexus surrounding the cord. In the cervical regions, the radicular arteries originate from the vertebral, cervical, and inferior thyroid arteries. In the thoracic and lumbar regions, the radicular arteries originate from the intercostal, lumbar, or lateral sacral arteries.

4. What is the artery of Adamkiewicz?

The artery of Adamkiewicz is any one of a number of anterior radicular arteries from either an intercostal or lumbar branch of the aorta that supply the lumbar region of the spinal cord.

5. Which region of the spinal cord seems most predisposed to ischemia? Why?

The lower cervical spinal cord, specifically C5–C8, seems most predisposed to ischemic injury. This region is supplied almost exclusively by the small anterior and posterior spinal arteries and is deficient of the radicular artery plexus that supplies the more caudal regions of the spinal cord. Of note, manipulation of the head and neck during surgical positioning may further compromise blood flow to this already vulnerable area of the spinal cord.

6. What is the approximate range of autoregulation of blood supply to the spinal cord?

Recent investigation has demonstrated that, at least in animals, autoregulation of spinal cord perfusion is similar to autoregulation of cerebral blood flow; that is, blood flow between mean arterial pressures (MAPs) of 60–120 mmHg is held relatively constant. In contrast, blood flow above or below these values becomes flow-dependent. This information is especially important in patients with an acute ischemic insult to the spinal cord, in whom prolonged hypotensive periods may further damage an already compromised spinal cord. Conversely, MAPs greater than 120 mmHg may cause extensive hemorrhagic insult.

7. Describe the function and innervation of the diaphragm and accessory muscles of respiration.

To initiate inspiration, the diaphragm contracts, causing it to descend. This action increases the intrathoracic volume and decreases the intrathoracic pressure below atmospheric pressure, allowing air to enter the lungs down its pressure gradient. Each hemidiaphragm is supplied by the ipsilateral phrenic nerve, which originates principally from the fourth cervical nerve (C4) with lesser contributions from the C3 and C5 segments.

Accessory Muscles of Respiration

MUSCLE	FUNCTION	INNERVATION
Sternocleidomastoid	Lifts sternum during inspiration	Accessory (cranial nerve XI)
Anterior serrati	Lift ribs during inspiration	Long thoracic
Scaleni	Lift the first two ribs during inspiration	Ventral rami of the cervical nerves
External intercostal	Lifts the ribs during inspiration	Intercostal or thoracoabdominal
Rectus abdominis	Used during forced expiration and coughing	Thoracoabdominal or subcostal
Internal intercostal	Pulls the ribs downward during expiration	Intercostal or thoracoabdominal

8. Describe the respiratory sequelae of acute SCI.

The major cause of death in patients with acute SCI is respiratory failure secondary to paralysis of the respiratory muscles. The level of SCI dictates the degree of ventilatory compromise.

Pentaplegia describes a state of SCI at the junction of the brainstem and spinal cord. Voluntary diaphragmatic contraction is not possible because of phrenic nerve paralysis. In addition, accessory muscles of respiration, including those controlled by cranial nerves (sternocleidomastoid, trapezius, pharyngeal), are no longer under voluntary control. As a result, the patient is chronically ventilator-dependent.

Respiratory quadriplegia results from cervical lesions at approximately C2–C3, sparing the cranial and uppermost cervical nerves. Because of paralysis of the phrenic nerves and the nerves that innervate the accessory muscles of respiration, this condition also results in chronic ventilator dependence.

Cervical lesions below C4 permit partial functioning of the phrenic nerve, resulting in at least some degree of voluntary control of respiration. Vital capacities, however, are approximately 20–25% of normal.

Cervical lesions at or below C6 allow full diaphragmatic control. However, accessory muscles of respiration are affected, depending on the level of the spinal cord lesion. Expansion of the rib cage via the accessory muscles contributes to approximately 60% of tidal volume in healthy people.

Of note, acute reactions to injury may extend several segments superiorly and inferiorly from the level of the original lesion. This phenomenon may resolve, leading to eventual improvement of respiratory function.

9. Are other pulmonary complications seen in the quadriplegic patient?

Accessory muscle weakness or paralysis may result in absent or weak cough, predisposing to retained secretions, atelectasis, and hypoxia. Hypoxia, superimposed on acute gastric dilatation, may result in conditions ideal for regurgitation and aspiration, especially in pentaplegics with ineffective upper airway reflexes.

10. Which position facilitates ventilation in the quadriplegic patient—supine or upright? Why?

In the person without spinal injury, the upright position facilitates respiration, because the caudal migration of abdominal contents results in greater excursion of the diaphragm and lower end-expiratory volumes. In contrast, the supine position greatly improves ventilation in the quadriplegic patient. During inspiration, diaphragmatic contraction leads to compression of abdominal contents, which results in anterior displacement of the abdominal wall. Conversely, return of the diaphragm during expiration is facilitated by the elastic recoil of the abdominal wall as well as the cephalad movement of the abdominal contents. The net result of the supine position is decreased end-expiratory volume and greater excursion of the diaphragm.

The beneficial effects of gravity and abdominal wall recoil are lost when the quadriplegic patient assumes the upright position, in which the abdominal wall protrudes and the abdominal contents move toward the pelvis. In addition, the resting position of the diaphragm is lower. These factors result in decreased excursion and greater end-expiratory volumes. The anatomic advantages of the supine position should be exploited whenever the patient is breathing spontaneously in the ICU or operating room.

11. What derangements in pulmonary function tests are seen in quadriplegics?

Vital capacity (VC) is reduced by 36–91% and is affected by the patient's posture (VC is greater in the supine and Trendelenburg positions than in the upright position).

Forced vital capacity (FVC) and forced expiratory volume at 1 second (FEV_1) are surprisingly not found to be lower in quadriplegics than in patients with lumbar lesions.

Total lung capacity (TLC) and **expiratory reserve volume** (ERV) are lower. **Reserve volumes** are higher, and **functional residual capacity** (FRC) is normal.

FEV_1/FVC ratio is normal, indicating no significant degree of airway obstruction.

Pulmonary function in quadriplegics generally tends to deteriorate from the time of acute injury to approximately day 4, at which time a gradual improvement through the second and third weeks is seen. Early deterioration in PFTs is thought to be secondary to the acute and transient upward spread of the spinal cord lesion due to edema and hemorrhage. Resolution of these acute processes and return of motor function result in improvement of PFTs.

12. What is Ondine's curse? Why is it seen in patients with acute SCI?

Ondine's curse, also called idiopathic or primary alveolar hypoventilation syndrome, is a condition in which spontaneous ventilation occurs only with voluntary effort and ceases during periods of inattention to breathing or sleep. This condition was named by Severinghaus and Mitchell after the 1939 play entitled *Ondine,* in which a knight, Hans, is unfaithful to a sea nymph, Ondine. In a jealous rage, Ondine places a curse on Hans whereby he must pay constant attention to his breathing.

Although mostly idiopathic, Ondine's curse also may occur after surgical or traumatic injury to the brainstem and high cervical regions of the spinal cord (especially the anterolateral region of C2–C4). Studies have demonstrated that the greatest danger of sleep apnea occurs during the first 5 nights after an acute SCI. Therefore, close observation of patients with high cervical lesions is warranted during this period.

13. Describe the nature and cause of neurogenic pulmonary edema.

A condition seen immediately after SCI, neurogenic pulmonary edema (NPE) is secondary to central nervous system insult, such as trauma to the spinal cord, stroke, increased intracranial pressure, seizures, tumors, or intracerebral hemorrhage. As the name implies, there must be a complete absence of concurrent cardiac or pulmonary disease.

The cause of NPE is controversial, but two mechanisms have been postulated. Animal studies have shown an acute increase in sympathetic activity after mechanically induced SCI, resulting in increased mean arterial pressure (MAP), systemic vascular resistance (SVR), and pulmonary vascular resistance (PVR). The mediators of this response act at the pulmonary vascular bed to increase vascular permeability to proteins, leading to a pulmonary alveolar exudate and fluid accumulation. An alternative proposal suggests that increased hydrostatic forces in the pulmonary capillary secondary to transient afterload-induced left ventricular failure lead to NPE.

14. What hemodynamic changes can be seen in patients with acute SCI?

The initial hemodynamic findings, described as "spinal shock," may persist for 1–3 weeks after acute injury. Profound systemic hypotension may result from loss of vascular tone and consequent diminished preload. The extent of hypotension is directly related to the level of the spinal cord lesion and is more pronounced in cervical than lumbar lesions.

A broad spectrum of cardiac dysrhythmias is observed in the patient with acute SCI, including sinus bradycardia, P-wave changes, increased P-R interval, ectopic beats, and complete heart block. Supraventricular arrhythmias such as atrial fibrillation and multifocal atrial tachycardia may occur. Ventricular arrhythmias such as premature ventricular contractions (PVCs) and ventricular tachycardia (VT) are also observed. Bradycardia is also noted in cervical lesions because of a predominance of vagal tone at the sinoatrial (SA) node of the heart. This predominance results from a lack of sympathetic input (so-called cardioaccelerator fibers, T1–T4) to the heart.

The significance of such circulatory derangements is that the patient with acute spinal cord injury compensates poorly for sudden changes in posture, blood loss, or anesthetics with cardiodepressant or vasodilating properties.

15. Define autonomic hyperreflexia. What are its clinical manifestations?

Autonomic hyperreflexia (AH) is a syndrome of massive, disinhibited reflex sympathetic discharge in response to cutaneous or visceral stimulation below the level of a spinal cord lesion in paraplegic and quadriplegic patients. Autonomic hyperreflexia is seen only after the resolution of spinal shock and the return of spinal cord reflexes (approximately 1–3 weeks after injury). In AH, the sympathetic nervous system below the level of spinal cord transection is functionally isolated from all inhibiting influences of the brainstem and hypothalamus. Therefore, any afferent cutaneous or visceral stimulus that enters the spinal cord below the level of the lesion has the potential to trigger a widespread reaction called a "mass reflex" below the level of the lesion.

In general, the clinical manifestations of AH are a result of SNS stimulation below the spinal cord lesion and compensatory parasympathetic nervous system stimulation above the spinal cord lesion. The classic syndrome includes paroxysmal hypertension and compensatory bradycardia. Below the transection, sympathetically mediated pallor, pilomotor erection, somatic and visceral muscle contraction, and increased spasticity may be seen. Above the lesion, the PNS mediates internal vasodilation, resulting in flushing of the face and mucous membranes. Sweating and mydriasis are also common. If left untreated, severe hypertension may lead to confusion, seizures, encephalopathy, retinal and cerebral bleeds, subarachnoid hemorrhage, strokes, or death. Cardiac manifestations include left ventricular failure secondary to acute increased SVR, pulmonary edema, and myocardial ischemia. ECG findings may include atrioventricular dissociation, premature atrial contractions, PVCs, and acute atrial fibrillation.

16. What factors provoke autonomic hyperreflexia?

In short, almost anything. Bladder distention seems to be the most common eliciting factor. However, almost any genitourinary stimulus may elicit AH, e.g., bladder catheterization, urinary tract infections, testicular torsion, or cystoscopy. The second most common cause of AH is gastrointestinal insults, including sigmoidoscopy, enemas, acute appendicitis, or perforated duodenal ulcers. Almost any stimulus below the level of the spinal cord lesion may cause AH, including temperature extremes, decubitus ulcers, sunburn, and tight clothing.

17. Which factors affect the severity and incidence of autonomic hyperreflexia?

For any given spinal cord lesion, the more caudad the peripheral stimulus, the greater the sympathetic response. In other words, the severity of the response is proportional to the number of spinal cord segments interposed between the spinal cord lesion and the stimulus level. Therefore, the maximal SNS response results from stimulation of the anorectal area (S2–S4).

The critical level of spinal cord lesion for development of AH seems to be midthoracic, approximately T7. In fact, AH in some form is observed in 85% of patients with spinal cord lesions at or above T7. Lesions between T6 and T10 seem to produce minimal hemodynamic changes. Lesions at or below T10 produce no consistent hemodynamic changes consistent with AH. Such data indicate that the lower the spinal cord lesion, the greater the potential for compensatory vasodilation above the lesion; therefore, the lesser the hemodynamic response.

18. Discuss the prevention and treatment of autonomic hyperreflexia.

Prevention of AH incorporates good comprehensive medical care of patients with spinal cord injury. In the operating room one must provide appropriate anesthesia even for operative procedures on insensate parts of the body; AH is an autonomic phenomenon independent of the patient's perception of pain.

Topical anesthetics are unreliable in preventing AH. Their inability to effectively block afferent transmissions from the deeper underlying muscle layers is the proposed explanation.

Subarachnoid blocks are highly effective in preventing AH in procedures involving the lower abdomen, pelvis, and lower extremities. Epidural anesthesia also may be effective; however, the most intense stimuli provoking AH originate from the S2–S4 segments, an area sometimes missed with epidural blocks. All regional techniques are plagued by technical difficulties secondary to vertebral column distortion, positioning, determining the level of blockade, and ruling out subarachnoid injection with epidural anesthesia. General anesthetics (GAs) are effective if a deep plane of anesthesia is achieved before the surgical stimulus is begun.

Autonomic hyperreflexia, once suspected, should be treated immediately and aggressively. The stimulus should immediately be discontinued. Deepening the plane of anesthetic during a GA or raising the level of epidural anesthesia may prove to be effective.

Pharmacologic intervention includes several options. Sodium nitroprusside seems to be the drug of choice because of its titratability with sudden blood pressure changes; an arterial line is recommended. Calcium channel blockers are increasing in popularity, and nifedipine and nicardipine have been successfully used. Calcium channel blockers may be used both for prophylaxis (given 30 minutes before the procedure) and for an acute crisis. Alpha-adrenergic blocking agents have been used with limited efficacy, because they are most effective on receptors susceptible to circulating levels of norepinephrine (NE) (i.e., adrenal release) rather than to NE released at nerve terminals, which is thought to be the mechanism of AH.

19. Discuss the issues to consider in the preoperative evaluation of persons with SCI.

Associated injuries are seen in 25–60% of patients with spinal cord injuries. Head trauma should be suspected in cases of cervical spine injuries. Chest trauma, including rib fractures, flail segments, pneumothorax, or hemothorax, may be seen with thoracic spine injuries. Respiratory assessment should include physical exam, bedside spirometry, arterial blood gas assessment, and chest radiograph to assess possible aspiration, pulmonary edema, and central line placement. Renal function can be evaluated via urine output and levels of blood urea nitrogen, creatinine, and electrolytes. Myocardial function should be assessed by EKG, chest radiograph, and invasive monitoring values, if available. Baseline neurologic function should be documented carefully for comparison with postanesthetic function in the event of possible intraoperative neurologic damage. In general, preoperative medications should not be used in patients with associated head injuries or high cervical/thoracic spinal cord lesions because of their ventilatory-depressant effects. Atropine may be given preoperatively for significant bradycardia.

20. What problems may be predicted during the induction phase in patients with acute SCI?

The induction phase of patients with SCIs involves two basic considerations: airway management and hemodynamic control.

Patients with high cervical lesions have probably been intubated early in the course of treatment, either in the field or in the emergency department. Patients who present to the operating room (OR) in acute respiratory distress, unconscious, or uncooperative should be managed with oral intubation; direct laryngoscopy should follow general anesthesia with a rapid-sequence technique. All patients should be presumed to have a cervical spine injury. Manual in-line stabilization is used to counter extension or flexion during laryngoscopy and tracheal intubation. Elective intubation in the OR should be performed in an awake patient to allow neurologic evaluation both before and after intubation. After adequate topical anesthesia of the pharynx, transtracheal and superior laryngeal nerve blocks (contraindicated in patients with a full stomach) may be performed in preparation for fiberoptic oral or nasal tracheal intubation. Blind nasotracheal intubation is an acceptable alternative in an awake patient for practitioners without expertise or access to a fiberoptic bronchoscope.

In terms of hemodynamic derangements, patients have low basal sympathetic outflow (spinal shock), which results in decreased SVR; increased venous capacitance; and decreased preload. Together these elements produce the potential for catastrophic cardiovascular collapse with induction. Therefore, the placement of arterial and pulmonary artery catheters before induction is useful. If the patient is not a candidate for awake intubation, a rapid-sequence induction with preoxygenation, cricoid pressure, and manual in-line stabilization is indicated. Commonly used induction agents include opiates, etomidate, and ketamine. Unlike etomidate and opiates, ketamine acts to increase cerebral blood flow and intracranial pressure, making its use contraindicated if a closed head injury is suspected. Succinylcholine may be used safely within the first 48 hours of an acute SCI (see question 22). Hypotension upon induction should be treated aggressively with fluids, as guided by hemodynamic indices, and small doses of direct-acting sympathomimetics (e.g., phenylephrine).

21. What are the intraoperative goals for patients with SCI?
One goal of the intraoperative stage of anesthesia is maintainence of spinal cord perfusion to prevent further damage. Both intravenous and inhalational agents may be used, but inhalational agents have the advantage of greater titratability in the face of intraoperative changes in blood pressure. At least in theory, the spinal cord circulation is similar to the cerebral circulation. Therefore, hypocapnia via hyperventilation may lead to vasoconstriction and the potential for ischemia. Thus normocapnia or only mild hypocapnia is recommended. Nondepolarizing muscle relaxants are safe to use and are selected on the basis of duration, route of metabolism, and hemodynamic stability. Meticulous attention to positioning is mandatory in preventing skin breakdown and peripheral nerve injuries. Maintaining normothermia via warming blankets, heated and humidified gases, increased ambient temperature, and warmed intravenous fluids is essential.

22. What about the use of succinylcholine in patients with SCI?
Within 48–72 hours after acute SCI, the denervated muscles respond with proliferation of extrajunctional acetylcholine receptors along the muscle cell membrane. Depolarization in response to administration of succinylcholine (SCh) involves both the neuromuscular junction and extrajunctional receptors. A large release of potassium into the circulation may result in ventricular fibrillation and cardiac arrest. Prior administration of a nondepolarizing muscle relaxant does not reliably decrease the potassium release associated with SCh administration in patients with SCI. Peak release of potassium in response to SCh occurs when the injury is approximately 2 weeks old. The duration of exaggerated potassium release is unknown, but it is thought to be reduced in 3–6 months. However, some authors advocate waiting at least 8 months after SCI to use SCh.

BIBLIOGRAPHY

1. Albin MS: Spinal cord injury. In Cottrell JE, Smith DS (eds): Anesthesia and Neurosurgery. St. Louis, Mosby, 1994, pp 713–743.
2. Amzallag M: Autonomic hyperreflexia. Int Anesthesiol Clin 31:87–102, 1993.
3. Ditunno JF, Formal CS: Chronic spinal cord injury. N Engl J Med 330:550–556, 1994.
4. Erickson RP: Autonomic hyperreflexia: Pathophysiology and medical management. Arch Phys Med Rehabil 61:431–440, 1980.
5. Lam AM: Acute spinal cord injury: Monitoring and anaesthetic implications. Can J Anaesth 38:R60–73, 1991.
6. Stoelting RK, Dierdorf SF: Anesthesia and Coexisting Disease. New York, Churchill Livingstone, 1993, pp 226–230.

53. ANESTHETIC MANAGEMENT OF MYASTHENIA GRAVIS

James Duke, M.D.

1. Describe the clinical presentation of myasthenia gravis (MG).

Myasthenic patients present with generalized fatigue and weakness of striated muscles that worsen with repetitive muscular use and improve with rest. Very commonly, extraocular muscles are the first affected and the patient complains of diplopia or ptosis. Of particular concern are myasthenic patients who develop weakness of their respiratory muscles or the muscles controlling swallowing and the ability to protect the airway from aspiration. Depending on whether extraocular, airway, or respiratory muscles are affected, MG may be described as ocular, bulbar, or skeletal, respectively.

2. What is the pathophysiologic process that leads to MG?

Myasthenia gravis is an autoimmune disease of the neuromuscular junction (NMJ). Antibodies to the acetylcholine receptor (see #3) may reduce the absolute number of functional receptors by direct destruction of the receptor, blockade of the receptor, or by complement-mediated destruction. Antibodies are found in about 90% of all myasthenics. Additionally, when all myasthenics are compared, the absolute level of antibody correlates poorly with disease severity, though changes in antibody levels within individual patients may correlate with disease progression.

3. Discuss the anatomy and physiology of the NMJ.

The NMJ is a nicotinic cholinergic receptor at the synaptic juncture of a motor neuron and striated muscle. The small area of skeletal membrane known as the junction is chemically sensitive to acetylcholine (ACh). Vesicles containing about 10,000 molecules of ACh congregate along thickened patches of axonal membrane known as "active zones." Across from the active zones on the postjunctional membrane are invaginations known as "junctional folds," which are the location of the ACh receptors. An action potential reaches the terminal neuron, stimulates binding of the vesicles with the membrane with the release of ACh. Diffusing across the synapse, ACh binds to and depolarizes the receptors, eventually producing an action potential that propagates along the muscular membrane, leading to the excitation-contraction mechanisms that result in muscular contraction. The action of ACh is terminated either through hydrolysis by the enzyme acetylcholinesterase (AChE) or by diffusion away from the NMJ.

4. Besides the abnormalities at the NMJ, can MG be pathologically associated with any other tissue?

Abnormalities of the thymus gland are associated with MG. The thymus is derived primarily from the third and fourth branchial arches and tends to be four-lobed, residing posterior to the sternum, although thymic tissue may be found throughout the mediastinum. Thymic hyperplasia, defined as a greater abundance of germinal centers in affected vs. unaffected individuals, is more often seen in younger patients with MG. The typical patient is a female in the third decade of life. Thymomas are also associated with MG. These neoplasias of thymic epithelial cells are found in older myasthenics, often males in their fifth or sixth decade. Myasthenia gravis is also associated with other autoimmune diseases, including hyperthyroidism, diabetes mellitus, rheumatoid arthritis, and collagen vascular diseases. Malignancies are also noted with greater incidence in myasthenics.

5. How is MG diagnosed?

The very characteristic pattern of progressive fatigue that improves with rest suggests the diagnosis. Once suspected, careful electromyographic evaluation or provocative testing substantiates the clinical impression. Repetitive stimulation of muscle groups of myasthenic or normal individuals results in progressive diminution of motor action potentials. Nonmyasthenic individuals, with their normal complement of motor end plates, do not clinically manifest any signs that the motor action potentials are declining with repetitive stimulation. Myasthenics, with their markedly reduced population of receptors, manifest the diminution in action potentials electromyographically. The diminution is known as "fade." If at least three muscle groups are tested in myasthenics, 95% of these individuals demonstrate fade electromyographically. Provocative testing is undertaken by intravenously administering dilute solutions of the neuromuscular relaxant curare into an extremity isolated with a blood pressure cuff. A positive response is considered a 10% decrement in electromyographic testing from baseline values. Edrophonium chloride, a short-acting AChE agent, is also useful in diagnosing MG. An intravenous dose of 2–10 mg produces a transient improvement in strength in most myasthenics tested.

6. Describe immunosuppressant therapy for MG.

As MG is an autoimmune process, corticosteroids and other immunosuppressants (azathioprine and cyclophosphamide) have long been used in medical management. Rarely are they first-line therapy, as patients develop the sequelae of long-term steroid use, such as hypertension, hyperglycemia, poor wound healing, fluid and electrolyte disturbances, gastric erosions, and impaired immunity, as well as the potential for steroid-induced myopathy and enhanced weakness. Plasmapheresis may be of transient benefit in profoundly weakened myasthenics who have failed medical management and are awaiting thymectomy.

7. Discuss the pros and cons of anticholinesterase therapy. Where else in the practice of anesthesia are anticholinesterases used?

Anticholinesterase agents have been employed in the therapy of MG for more than 50 years. Their mechanism of action is through reversible inhibition of AChE, the enzyme that metabolizes ACh. Because of its prolonged duration of effect, pyridostigmine is most commonly prescribed. A sustained-release preparation is available for myasthenics so profoundly affected that they may experience difficulty swallowing their morning doses. Anticholinesterases are used daily by anesthesiologists to reverse the residual effects of nondepolarizing muscle relaxants. By inhibiting ACh breakdown, anticholinesterases essentially overcome the competitive antagonism of the nondepolarizing relaxants at the NMJ. Doses to reverse motor blockade are much greater then are needed to treat myasthenic symptoms.

8. What is the role of surgery in the treatment of MG?

Numerous studies document that thymectomy arrests progress of the disease, decreases mortality, and accelerates remission. The exact indications, timing of surgery, and surgical approach are matters of controversy. Thymomas, generalized MG, and the necessity to administer steroids to control symptoms are considered indications for surgery. Formerly, surgery was undertaken only if the patient failed medical management, but it is now recognized that thymectomy early in the clinical course of the disease favors greater postoperative symptomatic improvement and possibly even remission. The alternative surgical approaches are transcervical and transsternal thymectomy. Surgeons who favor the former approach believe there is less postoperative embarrassment in respiration, whereas those who favor the latter approach believe that mediastinal exentration is necessary to obliterate all embryologic remains of thymic tissue.

9. What are some of the principal anesthetic concerns in the management of a myasthenic patient for any operative procedure?

Principal concerns include the degree of pulmonary impairment produced by the disease, the magnitude of bulbar involvement with attendant impairment in handling oral secretions and the risk of pulmonary aspiration, and adrenal suppression from long-term steroid use. As patients electively scheduled for surgery undertake an overnight fast, myasthenics who have profound dysphagia on awakening may require intravenous supplementation with anticholinesterase medication. Hence, it is best to continue oral anticholinesterases the morning of surgery. Although uncommon, cardiac disease that is MG-related should be considered in the preoperative evaluation. Because symptoms are primarily related to arrhythmias, an electrocardiogram should be evaluated. Symptoms of congestive heart failure should be sought as well.

10. Can the likelihood of postoperative ventilation be predicted?

Postoperative mechanical ventilation has been required in up to 30% of all myasthenic patients studied. As the potential need for ventilatory assistance is significant, attempts have been made to identify predictors of postoperative ventilation. Leventhal et al. identified four risk factors that correctly identified the need for ventilatory support in 91% of those studied:

1. Duration of disease longer than 6 years
2. History of chronic respiratory disease
3. Pyridostigmine dose 48 hours preoperatively of greater than 750 mg/day
4. Preoperative vital capacity of less than 2.9 liters.

Eisenkraft et al. found this scoring system greatly overestimated the number of myasthenic patients requiring postoperative ventilation. His group found advanced, generalized disease, a previous history of MG-related respiratory failure, and associated steroid therapy more predictive. Perhaps the utility of any scoring system is to draw attention to the significant clinical features which may portend ventilatory failure.

11. Describe the altered responsiveness of myasthenic patients to muscle relaxants.

Because of the decreased number of functional NMJs, understanding the altered responsiveness of myasthenic patients to relaxants is absolutely fundamental. Depolarizing and nondepolarizing relaxants have been administered safely, although at altered doses, to myasthenic patients. But consideration should always be given to alternatives to muscle relaxants. The inhalational anesthetics are well known to facilitate muscular relaxation and intubation. Perhaps the surgical procedure contemplated could be performed under a regional anesthetic or nerve block, eliminating the need for relaxation altogether. Muscle relaxants sometimes may be indicated, however, and understanding the pharmacodynamic principles is essential.

Like ACh, succinylcholine (SCh), a *depolarizing* muscle relaxant, is dependent upon binding to the NMJ, where under normal situations it depolarizes the NMJ for a prolonged period, relative to ACh. Numerous case reports have demonstrated that in MG, where there are fewer functional receptors, patients actually have been *resistant* to SCh. When nonmyasthenic and myasthenic persons were given SCh by a cumulative dose plus infusion technique, Eisenkraft et al. demonstrated resistance to the depolarizing relaxant. However, the degree of resistance did not appear to be of great clinical significance. Myasthenic patients, when given 2 mg/kg (still considered a normal acceptable dose), instead of 1 mg/kg of SCh, experienced satisfactory intubating conditions only seconds after nonmyasthenic persons.

Myasthenic patients are *more sensitive* than nonmyasthenic persons to the *nondepolarizing* relaxants. Numerous case reports have demonstrated that vecuronium, atracurium, and mivacurium may be safely used in MG. Dosing should start at about one-tenth of usual recommended doses. Recovery time for these reduced doses is quite variable but may be quite prolonged. Relaxation should be reversed at case conclusion and the patient carefully evaluated for return of strength.

Patients in remission should be presumed to persist in their sensitivity to the nondepolarizing relaxants. A case report describes a physically vigorous myasthenic patient, 9 years post-thymectomy, on no medications, who experienced prolonged paralysis after receiving a normal intubating dose of 0.1 mg/kg of vecuronium. One might say, "once a myasthenic, always a myasthenic."

12. Are there any medications (besides the relaxants) that might potentiate the weakness found in MG?

Aminoglycosides, magnesium, lithium, calcium channel blockers, and antiarrhythmics all have been reported to exacerbate myasthenic symptoms. The effects may be prejunctional (decreasing

ACh release), postjunctional (decreasing sensitivity of the receptor), or secondary to intrinsic weak relaxant properties.

13. Do intravenous anesthetic agents have altered effects in persons with MG?

Intravenous agents do not appear to offer significant disadvantages in myasthenic individuals. Opioids and sedatives do have the potential to depress respiratory drive, could become problematic in a myasthenic patient with respiratory impairment, and are best titrated to effect. The action of ester anesthetics may be prolonged, as they are metabolized by plasma cholinesterases, enzymes that may be impaired by anticholinesterase medications.

14. How might a myasthenic patient respond to volatile anesthetic agents?

Potent inhaled agents have muscle relaxant properties in general and may be used to advantage in myasthenic patients. Often they are the sole agent used to facilitate muscular relaxation. Neuromuscular transmission may by impaired through inhibition of ACh release and by desensitization of the postjunctional receptor.

15. What are the postanesthetic concerns in a patient with MG?

Assessing whether the patient has adequate respiratory capabilities is a primary concern prior to extubation. Neuromuscular function should be assessed electromyographically. If relaxants were given, they should be reversed with an appropriate anticholinesterase, most probably the agent most familiar to the anesthesiologist. Strength should be assessed. The patient should be able to demonstrate a sustained head-lift for 5 seconds. Vital capacity should be at least 15 ml/kg and the patient should generate a negative inspiratory force of 25 cm water. As these patients can have weakness of upper airway musculature, be wary of the patient who may generate apparently adequate respiratory activity while still intubated but suffer upper airway collapse and obstruction after extubation. At least 3 hours of clinical stability should be observed in a postoperative care unit (PACU) if consideration is being given to discharging a recovering myasthenic patient to a routine surgical floor. Otherwise, in a patient who was significantly compromised prior to surgery or whose immediate recovery period has proved somewhat problematic, postoperative disposition should be made to an intermediate care or intensive care unit. Anticholinesterase agents are usually introduced orally once the patient is awake and strong enough to swallow.

16. What are myasthenic and cholinergic crises, and how might they be differentiated?

Receptors responsive to ACh are described as cholinergic and further subclassified as nicotinic or muscarinic. The NMJ is a nicotinic receptor. Ganglionic receptors are muscarinic. Efforts to increase nicotinic (NMJ) receptor stimulation, a goal in myasthenic therapy, run the risk of overstimulation of the muscarinic, cholinergic receptors, producing a cholinergic crisis. Cholinergic crises result from relative overdosing of anticholinesterases. Should a patient's myasthenic symptoms improve, either spontaneously, after thymectomy, or from corticosteroid administration, a "usual" dose of anticholinesterase may prove excessive, precipitating a cholinergic crisis. Patients with ocular myasthenia may be particularly at risk, as extraocular muscles tend to be resistant to the effects of anticholinesterases. Adequate doses to improve ptosis and diplopia may produce generalized muscarinic symptoms and weakness of other muscle groups.

Signs and symptoms of muscarinic overstimulation include excessive salivation, lacrimation, urinary incontinence, diarrhea, bronchorrhea, pulmonary edema, miosis and paralysis of accommodation (blurred vision), as well as weakness. Collectively, this is known as the **SLUDGE syndrome**.

The hallmark of a myasthenic crisis is acute respiratory insufficiency and may be precipitated by infections, exertion, menstruation, emotional stress or acute illness, or underdosing of anticholinesterase medication. Pupils tend to be mydriatic. As both crises involve weakness and acute respiratory failure, recognition and differentiation depend on review of historical information, searching for SLUDGE symptoms, and examination of the pupils. Edrophonium chloride, given cautiously in 1-mg doses, should improve a myasthenic crisis. Anticholinesterases are withheld if a cholinergic crisis is likely. In either case, the airway should be protected and the patient ventilated.

BIBLIOGRAPHY

1. Adams SL, Matthews J, Grammer LC: Drugs that may exacerbate myasthenia gravis. Ann Emerg Med 13:532–538, 1984.
2. Baraka A: Anaesthesia and myasthenia gravis. Can J Anaesth 39:476–486, 1992.
3. Duke J: Anesthetic management of myasthenia gravis. In Eisenkraft JB (ed): Progress in Anesthesiology. San Antonio, Dannemiller Memorial Educational Foundation, 1992, pp 273–288.
4. Drachman DB: Myasthenia gravis. New Engl J Med 330:1797–1810, 1994.
5. Eisenkraft JB, Book WJ, Mann SM, et al: Resistance to succinylcholine in myasthenia gravis: a dose-response study. Anesthesiology 69:760-763, 1988.
6. Eisenkraft JB, Papatestas AE, Kahn CH, et al: Predicting the need for postoperative mechanical ventilation in myasthenia gravis. Anesthesiology 65:79–82, 1986.
7. Leventhal SR, Orkin FK, Hirsh RA: Prediction of the need for postoperative mechanical ventilation in myasthenia gravis. Anesthesiology 53:26–30, 1980.
8. Lumb AB, Calder I: "Cured" myasthenia gravis and neuromuscular blockade. Anaesthesia 44: 828–830, 1989.
9. Nilsson E, Meretoja OA: Vecuronium dose-response and maintenance requirements in patients with myasthenia gravis. Anesthesiology 73:28–32, 1990.

54. MALIGNANT HYPERTHERMIA

Lee Weiss, M.D.

1. Define malignant hyperthermia.

Malignant hyperthermia (MH) is an inherited myopathy characterized by a hypermetabolic state when the patient is exposed to an appropriate triggering agent. A defect at the sarcoplasmic reticulum leads to decreased calcium reuptake. Specifically, the ryanodyne receptor (a calcium release channel) fails, and intracellular calcium increases 500-fold, leading to sustained muscle contractions, glycolysis, and heat production. Oxidative phosphorylation uncouples, with resulting membrane instability and rhabdomyolysis. The incidence is 1:15,000 pediatric anesthetics and 1:50,000 adult anesthetics.

2. Name the MH triggers.

Malignant hyperthermia is an anesthetic-related disease. Medications definitely identified as triggers include:

- Depolarizing muscle relaxants (e.g., succinylcholine)
- Potent inhalational agents (e.g., halothane, isoflurane, enflurane, desflurane, sevoflurane)

3. Which anesthetic agents are safe?

The following agents have been found safe in patients susceptible to MH:

- Benzodiazepines (e.g., midazolam, diazepam, lorazepam)
- Barbiturates (e.g.,thiopental, methohexital)
- Local anesthetics (e.g., lidocaine, bupivacaine)
- Nondepolarizing muscle relaxants (e.g., pancuronium, rocuronium, vecuronium)
- Propofol
- Ketamine

Ketamine and pancuronium should be used with caution in MH-susceptible patients, because the resulting tachycardia may mask the onset of MH.

4. Describe the clinical syndrome and intraoperative diagnosis.

The initial signs are an increase in end-tidal carbon dioxide and decrease in arterial oxygen saturation, tachycardia and dysrhythmias, rigidity (despite the use of a muscle relaxant), and tachypnea (in spontaneously breathing patients). An unexplained tachycardia, however, is usually the first sign. Other findings are hyperthermia and cyanosis. When clinical signs are suggestive of MH, several laboratory tests may lead to a presumptive diagnosis. A blood gas analysis may be obtained to determine whether metabolic acidosis is present (venous blood is better than arterial blood to observe the immense production of carbon dioxide). Other possible metabolic abnormalities include hyperkalemia, hypercalcemia, hyperphosphatemia, creatinine kinase levels > 1000 IU, and myoglobinuria. All of these tests are suggestive of the diagnosis, but a caffeine and halothane contracture test performed postoperatively is more definitive.

5. Define masseter muscle rigidity. What is its relationship to malignant hyperthermia?

After an intubating dose of succinylcholine with loss of twitches on neuromuscular stimulation, difficulty in opening the mouth represents masseter muscle rigidity (MMR). Such patients may be susceptible to MH; a full-blown episode typically occurs 20–30 minutes after the onset of MMR. The incidence of MMR is 1% in children induced with halothane and succinylcholine and 2.8% in children having strabismus surgery. Such patients are prone to an increase in creatinine kinase, myoglobinuria, tachycardia, and dysrhythmias independent of MH. It is controversial whether to proceed with an anesthetic if the patient develops MMR. Some anesthesiologists elect to cancel the scheduled procedure, whereas others continue the case using an anesthetic that does not involve triggering agents.

6. How is MH diagnosed?

The diagnosis of MH is immensely more difficult than its treatment. A suspicion that testing is needed is based on patient history, positive family history, or use of an anesthetic remarkable for clinical diagnosis of MH. Key features in the patient's history include strabismus, myalgias on exercise, tendency to fever, myoglobinuria, muscular disease, and intolerance of caffeine. Patients requiring a more definitive diagnosis are referred for muscle biopsy. A caffeine and halothane contraction test (the gold standard) is performed on muscle obtained by biopsy. Caffeine and halothane decrease the threshold for muscle contraction and therefore facilitate diagnosis. This test is 85% specific and 100% sensitive. Creatine phosphokinase is elevated in 70 % of susceptible patients. A genetic test of the ryanodyne receptor may eventually be developed.

7. How is MH treated?

1. Call for help; management is involved and difficult for one person.
2. Discontinue triggering agents.
3. Hyperventilate the patient with 100% oxygen.
4. Expedite or abort procedure.
5. Administer dantrolene (2.5 mg/kg bolus; may repeat 2 mg/kg every 5 minutes, then 1–2 mg/kg/hr).
6. Cool patient (cold intravenous normal saline, cold body cavity lavage, ice bags to body, cold nasogastric lavage, cooling blanket).
7. Change to a clean circuit not exposed to volatile agents.
8. Monitor and treat acidosis (follow serial arterial blood gases and administer sodium bicarbonate).
9. Promote urine output (maintain > 2 ml/kg/hr urine output with conscientious fluid management; furosemide, 0.5–1.0 mg/kg IV; and 20% mannitol, 1gm/kg IV).
10. Treat hyperkalemia (0.1–0.2 U/kg regular insulin + 500 mg/kg dextrose IV).
11. Treat dysrhythmias with procainamide and calcium chloride, 2–5 mg/kg IV (calcium chloride is used to treat the hyperkalemia-associated dysrhythmias).
12. Monitor creatinine kinase, urine myoglobin, and coagulation for 24–48 hours.

8. Why is procainamide the drug of choice for dysrhythmias?

Most antiarrhythmic agents can be used without difficulty. However, in addition to controlling multiple arrhythmias, procainamide inhibits abnormal drug-induced contraction in MH-susceptible muscle in vitro. On the other hand, calcium channel blockers should not be used; in combination with dantrolene, they may cause hyperkalemia and cardiovascular collapse.

9. Describe the mechanism of action of dantrolene.

Dantrolene impairs calcium-dependent muscle contraction. Side effects are muscle weakness, hyperkalemia, gastrointestinal upset, and thrombophlebitis. The solution is prepared by mixing 20 mg of dantrolene with 3 gm of mannitol in 60 ml of water. Preparation is tedious and time-consuming, requiring several people to mix the dantrolene into solution; this is one reason to call for help.

10. Describe the preparation of an anesthetic for MH-susceptible patients.

1. Clean machine; remove vaporizers; and replace CO_2 canisters, bellows, and gas hose.
2. Flush the machine for 20 minutes with 10 L/min.
3. Have the MH cart in the operating room (this cart contains all the supplies needed to resuscitate a patient with MH).
4. Schedule the patient as the first case of the day, and notify the postanesthesia care unit to be prepared to provide the necessary manpower.

5. Consider dantrolene and sedation for premedication.

6. Check creatinine kinase and complete blood count preoperatively.

7. Consider anesthetic alternatives; monitored anesthetic care with sedation and local anesthesia, regional anesthesia, or a general anesthetic using nontriggering agents (e.g., oxygen, propofol, and vecuronium).

8. After surgery check laboratory values and monitor patient in an appropriate setting (intensive care unit vs. step-down unit, depending upon the need for invasive monitoring).

11. What syndromes are associated with MH?

There is a strong correlation between central core disease (a sarcoplasmic myopathy characterized by proximal muscle weakness) and MH. Other syndromes with decreasing risk include Duchenne's dystrophy (an X-linked myopathy), King-Denborough syndrome (characterized by short stature, musculoskeletal abnormalities, and mental retardation), myoadenylate deaminase deficiency, Fukuyama's muscular dystrophy, and Becker's muscular dystrophy.

12. Compare neuroleptic malignant syndrome with MH.

Neuroleptic malignant syndrome (NMS), which may be confused with MH, may appear 24–72 hours after administration of a psychotropic drug (e.g., haloperidol, fluphenazine, clozapine, perphenazine, thioridazine). The cause of NMS is related to dopamine receptor blockade in the hypothalamus and basal ganglia. NMS is characterized by akinesia, muscle rigidity, hyperthermia, tachycardia, cyanosis, autonomic dysfunction, sensorium change, diaphoresis, and elevated levels of creatinine kinase. NMS has a mortality rate of 10%. Treatment is with dantrolene or bromocriptine (a dopamine receptor agonist). Patients with NMS are not prone to MH.

CONTROVERSY

13. Should patients with MH be pretreated with dantrolene?

MH can be prevented by giving dantrolene preoperatively. However, many problems are associated with its use. Dantrolene may mask or delay the diagnosis of MH. Pretreatment depletes the supply of this expensive medication and may induce or worsen muscle weakness; dantrolene is synergistic with muscle relaxants. The anesthesiologist still needs to prepare a nontriggering anesthetic.

BIBLIOGRAPHY

1. Gronert GA, Antognini JF: Malignant hyperthermia. In Miller RD (ed): Anesthesia, 4th ed. New York, Churchhill Livingstone, 1994, pp 1075–1094.
2. Levitt RC: Prospects for the diagnosis of malignant hyperthermia susceptibility using molecular approaches. Anesthesiology 76:1039–1048,1992.
3. Maclennan DH, Phillips MS: Malignant hyperthermia. Science 256:789–794,1992.
4. Miller JD, Lee C: Muscle diseases. In Katz J, Benumof JL, Kadis LB (eds): Anesthesia and Uncommon Diseases, 3rd ed. Philadelphia, W.B. Saunders, 1990, pp 590–644.
5. Rosenberg H: Understanding Malignant Hyperthermia. Westport, CT, Malignant Hyperthermia Association of the United States, 1992.

55. ALCOHOLISM

Andrew M. Veit, M.D., and Kevin Fitzpatrick, M.D.

Ninety percent of Americans consume alcohol at some point in their lives. Alcoholism affects 15% of the American population: 200,000 deaths per year are attributed to alcohol, and one-third of all adults have medical problems related to alcohol use. Because of the high prevalence of alcoholism and alcohol use in the U.S., it is important to understand the pharmacologic and physiologic effects of alcohol and how they affect the delivery of an anesthetic.

1. Is alcohol a drug?

Yes. Alcohol (ethanol) behaves like many other pharmacologic agents. Its pharmacokinetics are well understood, including absorption, distribution, metabolism, and excretion. Ethanol is a two-carbon hydrocarbon molecule.

Molecular structure of ethanol.

2. How is alcohol absorbed and metabolized?

Alcohol is absorbed across the gastrointestinal mucosa by simple diffusion. Absorption is greater in the small intestine than in the stomach. The volume of distribution (Vd) of alcohol is that of body water, which is equal to approximately 80% of total body weight. The distribution of alcohol to the tissues is related directly to tissue blood flow, and alcohol easily crosses the blood-brain barrier. Five to ten percent of consumed alcohol is excreted unchanged in the breath and urine. Alcohol **excretion** follows first-order kinetics: the rate of excretion is directly proportional to the concentration of alcohol in the blood. Arterial blood levels of alcohol correlate well with concentrations in lung alveoli; hence the basis of the breathalyzer test used by law enforcement officers.

Alcohol is **metabolized** primarily in the liver. The majority of consumed alcohol is metabolized to acetaldehyde by the enzyme alcohol dehydrogenase. Alcohol metabolism follows Michaelis-Menten zero-order kinetics. When alcohol dehydrogenase is saturated with ethanol, the rate of metabolism is constant, although alcohol concentration may increase. Nicotinamide adenine dinucleotide [NAD] acts as a cofactor in the oxidation of alcohol to acetaldehyde by accepting a hydrogen molecule. The hepatic conversion of reduced NAD to NAD is the rate-limiting step in alcohol metabolism. When the liver can no longer keep up with the demand for production of NAD, normal liver function is impaired. In addition, an insignificant amount of alcohol is also metabolized during first-pass through the gastric mucosa and in the microsomes of endothelial cells.

An average adult is able to metabolize approximately 10 ml of alcohol per hour. Four ounces of whiskey or 1.2 L of beer require approximately 5–6 hours for metabolism. At this slow rate it is not difficult to envision how blood alcohol levels rise to intoxicating levels quite quickly. The maximal amount of alcohol that an average adult can metabolize in a 24-hour period is 450 ml.

Oxidation of alcohol to acetaldehyde.

3. What is the mechanism of action of alcohol?

The exact mechanism of action of alcohol is unknown. Alcohol is thought to have a widespread disordering effect on cell membranes, which, in turn, alters the action of membrane-bound proteins. Centrally, the inhibitory action of alcohol, thought to be mediated by gamma-aminobutyric acid [GABA] receptors, results in disinhibition.

4. Is alcohol sexist?

Yes. Alcohol affects men and women differently. The Vd of alcohol is greater in men than in women. Thus, a woman who consumes the same amount of alcohol as a man of similar height and weight has a higher plasma level of alcohol. In simple terms, less alcohol is required to reach intoxicating blood levels in women. This fact provides the physiologic and economic basis of tavern-sponsored drink specials for women.

In addition, laboratory studies have demonstrated that the first-pass metabolism of alcohol in the gastric mucosa is less pronounced in nonalcoholic women than in their male counterparts. The ability of the gastric mucosa to metabolize alcohol is reduced in alcohol-habituated men and nonexistent in alcohol-habituated women.

5. How much alcohol is required to produce intoxication?

A plasma level of 25 mg/dl is associated with impaired cognition and incoordination. A level > 100 mg/dl is associated with vestibular, cerebellar, and autonomic dysfunction. A level > 500 mg/dl is associated with respiratory depression and death.

Undoubtedly, anyone who has spent time in the emergency department has met a member of the "500 Club," a patient who is alert and oriented yet demonstrates a blood alcohol level (BAL) > 500 mg/dl. How can this be? The answer is simple: chronic abuse leads to tolerance of physiologic effects, allowing the patient to appear quite sober despite an otherwise lethal BAL.

6. What are the acute and chronic effects of alcohol on the nervous system?

In **acute** terms, alcohol depresses the central nervous system by inhibiting polysynaptic function. Disorder of polysynaptic pathways is manifested by generalized blunting and loss of higher motor, sensory, and cognitive function. Although the behavioral effects of alcohol consumption may seem excitatory or stimulating to observers and users, this impression is probably due to a depressive effect on inhibitory pathways (disinhibition).

Chronic alcohol use is associated with peripheral nerve and neuropsychiatric disorders, many of which—such as Wernicke's encephalopathy, Korsakoff's psychosis, and nicotinic acid deficiency encephalopathy—may be linked to nutritional dificiencies. Alcohol-related neuropathy usually involves pain and numbness in the lower extremities, often with concomitant weakness of the intrinsic muscles of the feet. Patients may exhibit hypalgesia in a stocking-foot distribution, and the Achilles tendon reflex may be absent. Finally, generalized weakness in the proximal limb musculature also may be seen with chronic alcohol use.

7. What are the effects of alcohol on the cardiovascular system?

Moderate **acute** ingestion of alcohol produces no significant changes in blood pressure (BP) or myocardial contractility. Cutaneous vasodilatation occurs and heart rate increases via sympathetic reflex. At toxic levels of acute alcohol ingestion, a decrease in central vasomotor activity causes respiratory and cardiac depression.

The leading cause of death in **chronic** users of alcohol is cardiac dysfunction. Consumption of 60 ounces of ethanol/month (8 pints of whiskey or 55 cans of beer) may lead to the development of alcohol-induced hypertension. An intake > 90 ounces/ month over a 10-year period may lead to the development of congestive cardiomyopathy. The cardiomyopathy of alcoholism is associated with pulmonary hypertension, right-heart failure, and dysrhythmias. The most common dysrhythmias are atrial fibrillation and premature ventricular contractions. Patients with left ventricular disease, however, are subject to ventricular tachydysrhythmias, ventricular fibrillation, and sudden death.

8. How does alcohol affect the respiratory system?

Acute alcohol intake may cause hyperventilation via disinhibition of central respiratory regulation centers. Hyperventilation increases dead-space ventilation (ventilation of the bronchial airspace as opposed to the alveolar air spaces); the result is a reduction in arterial oxygen saturation. Despite hyperventilation, alcohol depresses the ventilatory response to carbon dioxide. The most significant danger to the respiratory tract associated with acute alcohol intoxication is chemical pneumonitis caused by the aspiration of gastric contents.

Chronic alcohol use may lead to dysfunction of the cilia lining the respiratory tract, inhibition of macrophage mobility, and reduction in surfactant production. Chronic alcohol users are more susceptible to pulmonary infection, often by staphylococci or gram-negative organisms. Chronic alcohol users with concurrent liver and heart disease may have pulmonary hypertension and pulmonary congestion as well as a generalized decrease in all lung capacities: vital capacity, functional residual capacity, and inspiratory capacity.

9. How does alcohol affect the gastrointestinal and hepatobiliary systems?

Phrenohepatology is a historical technique defined as the study of determining a patient's alcohol history by palpating the bumps on his liver. Acute alcohol use may cause esophagitis, gastritis, and pancreatitis. Chronic alcohol use leads to delayed gastric emptying and relaxation of the lower esophageal sphincter. This, in turn, increases the risk of gastric acid aspiration.

The liver undergoes transient and reversible fatty infiltration during acute alcohol use. Although such changes resolve with abstinence and the cycle can repeat itself many times, prolonged alcohol exposure leads to chronic infiltration of fat, which over time progresses to necrosis and fibrosis of liver tissue. The initial presentation of fatty liver changes is hepatomegaly. When necrosis, fibrosis, and cirrhosis become apparent, the liver regresses in size. Consumption of 90 ounces of ethanol/day over a 10-year period leads to irreversible cirrhosis, and 10–15% of such patients later suffer from alcohol-induced hepatitis. Alcohol-induced hepatitis is a serious complication of cirrhosis and carries a 30% mortality rate.

In addition to structural changes, the synthetic function of the liver is also impaired. Production of albumin and coagulation factors II, V, VII, X, and XIII is decreased. Reduction of albumin results in lower intravascular oncotic pressure and may lead to tissue edema. A reduction in circulating coagulation factors may predispose to bleeding, which is evidenced by a prolonged prothrombin time (PT).

10. How is the blood supply to the liver altered by cirrhosis?

The blood supply to the liver is derived from the portal vein and hepatic artery. The portal vein provides 75% of hepatic blood flow and 55% of hepatic oxygen supply. The structural changes that occur with cirrhosis reduce portal blood flow, making the liver more dependent on the hepatic artery for blood supply. Blood from the splanchnic beds, no longer able to pass through the liver, is diverted through portosystemic collateral channels: the esophageal venous plexus, splenic vein, epigastric venous plexus, perineal venous plexus, and mediastinal veins. Over time the collateral vessels dilate and undergo varicose changes.

11. Is ethanol part of a balanced diet?

Alcohol is not a member of the four food groups. Gastric irritation, poor absorption, and poor nutritional habits lead to a generalized state of malnutrition in many chronic alcohol users.

12. Which nutritional deficiencies are seen in chronic alcohol users?

Chronic alcohol use leads to deficiencies of thiamine and folic acid. Beriberi (thiamine deficiency), which is commonly seen in third-world countries where milled rice is a dietary staple, presents as Wernicke's encephalopathy, polyneuropathy, and cardiac failure. The cardiac failure in thiamine deficiency is characterized by high cardiac output, low systemic vascular resistance, and loss of vasomotor tone. Folic acid deficiency causes bone marrow depression and leads to thrombocytopenia, leukopenia, and anemia.

13. Does a single episode of acute intoxication have permanent effects?

No. For the most part, the effects of alcohol on many of the organ systems are reversible with abstinence. Fatty infiltration of hepatic tissue resolves within 1–2 days of acute ethanol ingestion. The metabolic and pharmacokinetic tolerance to ethanol that develops with 1–2 weeks of daily use resolves with an equal period of abstinence. With prolonged abuse, the cellular adaptation to chronic ethanol exposure may require from several weeks to months to return to normal.

14. What are the effects of alcohol on inhalational anesthetics?

In acutely intoxicated, nonhabituated patients the requirement for inhalational anesthetics is decreased. In other words, the minimal alveolar concentration (MAC) of inhalational agents is reduced. By definition, MAC describes the alveolar concentration of inhalational anesthetic that prevents 50% of patients from moving away from surgical stimulation. The alveolar concentration of an inhalational anesthetic necessary to provide adequate analgesia in healthy patients is close to the lethal level in intoxicated patients. Studies demonstrate that the concentration of halothane required to produce respiratory arrest in nonhabituated, intoxicated patients is not significantly different from the concentration that causes cardiac arrest. For chronic users of alcohol, the MAC for inhalational agents is increased. This is evidenced by the fact that chronic alcohol exposure leads to the development of tolerance to the pharmacodynamic and central nervous system depressant effects of inhalational agents.

15. What are the effects of alcohol ingestion on intravenous narcotics such as barbiturates, benzodiazepines, and opioids?

Acutely intoxicated patients are more sensitive to the effects of barbiturates, benzodiazepines, and opioids. Cross-tolerance develops to intravenous agents with chronic alcohol exposure.

16. How does alcohol affect muscle relaxants?

The choice of muscle relaxant in **nonhabituated** acutely intoxicated patients should be based more on the requirements of the surgical procedure than the physiologic state of the patient. Most acutely intoxicated patients require rapid-sequence induction for intubation and a rapid-acting muscle relaxant (succinylcholine, rocuronium). Choice of a particular muscle relaxant should be based on the duration of the procedure and medical history of the patient. The pharmacokinetics of muscle relaxants is not affected by acute alcohol intoxication in nonhabituated patients.

The pharmacodynamic profile of muscle relaxants is altered in **alcohol-habituated** patients. In healthy patients, succinylcholine is rapidly hydrolyzed and thus inactivated by plasma cholinesterases produced in the liver. Patients with liver disease may have decreased levels of circulating plasma cholinesterase; therefore, the effects of succinylcholine may be prolonged in alcoholic patients. Cirrhotic patients with poor liver function have a greater Vd for injected drugs and thus require a larger dose of nondepolarizing relaxants. Relaxants that rely on hepatic clearance may have a prolonged duration of action. Muscle relaxants that are metabolized independently of organ function (e.g., atracurium) are good choices in patients with liver disease.

17. Describe special considerations in the preoperative assessment of alcohol-abusing patients.

A complete history and physical exam should be performed for all patients before they receive an anesthetic. Special consideration must be given to the cardiovascular system of chronic alcohol users. Tachycardia, dysrythmias, or cardiomegaly may indicate alcohol-related cardiac dysfunction. A 12-lead electrocardiagram (ECG) should be evaluated for dysrythmias and signs of cardiomegaly and ischemia. Useful laboratory studies include measurement of serum electrolytes to check for hypokalemia and hypoglycemia, complete blood count to evaluate the anemia associated with chronic alcohol use, and coagulation studies (PT, partial prothrombin time, platelet count) to evaluate propensity toward a bleeding diathesis secondary to hepatic disease. Ten percent of intoxicated trauma patients have a cervical spine injury; a lateral cervical spine radiograph should be evaluated before manipulation of the neck and intubation.

18. What are the special monitoring considerations in alcohol-abusing patients?

All patients brought to the operating theater should be monitored in accordance with standards of practice outlined by the American Society of Anesthesiology: noninvasive blood pressure measurement, continuous ECG, pulse oximetry, and temperature monitoring. Invasive monitoring should be considered on an individual basis. Chronic alcohol abusers with hepatic dysfunction and well-developed portosystemic collateral circulation rely on hepatic arterial blood flow for hepatic perfusion. Inhalational agents may cause vasodilatation of preexisting hepatic shunts and increase the liver's dependence on arterial flow. Placement of an arterial catheter in such patients maintains beat-to-beat control of systemic blood pressure and reduces the risk of hypotensive hepatic ischemia. In addition, an arterial catheter provides access for blood gas sampling. Because acutely intoxicated patients are subject to hypoglycemia, serum glucose levels should be followed closely.

Volume status may be assessed by placement of an indwelling bladder catheter and central venous catheter. Patients with alcohol-induced cardiac disease are less sensitive to endogenous or parenteral catecholamines and may benefit from pulmonary artery catheterization and close monitoring of cardiac filling pressures and cardiac output.

Instrumentation of the esophagus should be avoided in patients with known liver disease because of the possibility of rupturing esophageal varices. Patients have been known to exsanguinate and die as a result of bleeding from esophageal varices. A precordial stethoscope and cutaneous temperature probe are safe alternatives to the esophageal stethescope.

19. Is premedication necessary in alcohol-abusing patients?

Special premedication is not necessary for sober chronic alcohol abusers scheduled for routine elective surgery. Acutely intoxicated patients, to a certain degree, have provided their own premedication. Alcohol is, after all, a sedative. Acutely intoxicated patients should also be premedicated with oral sodium citrate (Bicitra or Alka-Seltzer Gold) to neutralize gastric acid and with metoclopramide to enhance gastric motility and facilitate gastric emptying. Pretreatment with an H_2-receptor blocker also may assist in reducing the acidic output from the gastric mucosa.

20. How does one anesthetize sober chronic alcohol abusers?

No one anesthetic technique is safer than another. As previously mentioned, sober chronic alcohol users may demonstrate tolerance to many intravenous and inhalational anesthetic agents. Isoflurane is thought by many to be the best inhalational agent for maintaining hepatic blood flow and should be considered in patients with hepatic disease. An opioid-based anesthetic may be more appropriate in patients with cardiac disease because of its minimal effects on myocardial contractility and heart rate. Anesthetic techniques for patients with severe organ dysfunction are discussed elsewhere in this text. In general, a balanced anesthetic technique using amnestics, opioids, nitrous oxide, and an inhalational agent will suffice.

21. How does one anesthetize intoxicated patients?

One must first determine whether the operation is elective or emergent. An elective procedure should be postponed until the patient is sober and meets the fasting (NPO) guidelines for elective surgery. In an emergent situation, rapid-sequence induction and general endotracheal anesthesia are usually indicated. Rapid-sequence induction involves adequate preoxygenation with 100% oxygen via face mask at high flow rates for 3–5 minutes of normal breathing, or 4 full vital-capacity breaths. This regimen adequately denitrogenates the lungs. The next step is to administer an induction dose of an intravenous anesthetic, followed by a rapid-acting muscle relaxant. During this step, an assistant applies firm downward pressure over the cricoid cartilage to compress and occlude the esophagus (Sellick's maneuver). This maneuver prevents passive regurgitation of gastric contents. The trachea is then intubated with a cuffed endotracheal tube. Position of the tube in the trachea is confirmed by ascultating breath sounds bilaterally, visualizing bilateral chest wall movement with respiration, and noting the presence of end-tidal carbon dioxide on the capnograph. Once correct placement of the tube is confirmed, cricoid pressure may be released.

22. What special criteria apply to extubation of acutely intoxicated, postsurgical patients?
Extubation of the acutely intoxicated is not without risk; the patient must be fully awake and able to protect the airway.

23. What are the signs and symptoms of alcohol withdrawal?
Alcohol withdrawal syndrome presents as anorexia, insomnia, weakness, combativeness, tremors, disorientation, auditory and visual hallucinations, and convulsions. The peak onset is 10–30 hours after abstinence from alcohol. The symptoms may last for 40–50 hours. Prolonged abstinence may lead to delirium tremens or hyperactivity of the autonomic nervous system that manifests as tachycardia, diaphoresis, fever, anxiety, and confusion. Delirium tremens carries a 10% mortality rate. Alcohol withdrawal syndrome may occur in anesthetized patients in the operating theater. Under anesthesia it can present as uncontrolled tachycardia, diaphoresis, and hyperthermia. The treatment for alcohol withdrawal syndrome is the administration of benzodiazepines or intravenous infusion of ethanol. Often chronic alcohol abusers receive benzodiazepines as prophylaxis against withdrawal. This treatment should be continued during anesthesia or may be initiated during induction.

24. How do the experts feel regarding alcohol use and operative procedures?
"I'd rather have a bottle in front of me than a frontal lobotomy."—W.C. Fields

BIBLIOGRAPHY

1. Fiamengo SA: Alcoholism. In Yao FS, Artusio JF (eds): Anesthesiology Problem-Oriented Patient Management, 3rd ed. Philadelphia, J.B. Lippincott, 1993, pp 680–692.
2. Gaiser R: Airway evaluation and management. In Davison JK, Eckhardt WF, Pelese DA (eds): Clinical Anesthesia Procedures of the Massachusetts General Hospital, 4th ed. Boston, Little, Brown, 1993, p 184.
3. Gilman AG, Rall TW, Nies AS, et al (eds): Goodman and Gilman's The Pharmacological Basis of Therapeutics, 8th ed. New York, Pergamon Press, 1990, pp 371–372 and 807–808.
4. Schuckit MA: Alcohol and alcoholism. In Braunwald E, Isselbacher KJ, Petersdorf RG, et al (eds): Harrison's Principles of Internal Medicine, 11th ed. [international]. New York, McGraw-Hill, 1987, pp 2106–2111.
5. Stoelting RK: Pharmacology and Physiology in Anesthetic Practice, 2nd ed. Philadelphia, J.B. Lippincott, 1991, pp 783–785.
6. Stoelting RK, Dierdorf SF: Anesthesia and Co-existing Disease, 3rd ed. New York, Churchill Livingstone, 1993, pp 223, 262–268, 445, and 526–528.

56. DIABETES MELLITUS

Robert H. Slover, M.D., and Robin B. Slover, M.D.

1. Describe the two principal types of diabetes mellitus.
Type I diabetes mellitus is an autoimmune disorder in which destruction of the pancreatic islet cells results in the inability to produce insulin. Type I diabetes is common in children, adolescents, and young adults. Onset is typically between infancy and the early twenties, although occasionally adults in their early thirties develop the disease. Type I diabetes is also commonly called insulin-dependent diabetes mellitus (IDDM). Type II diabetes mellitus is a disorder in the body's ability to use insulin. Early in the course of the disease the patient is able to make sufficient insulin, but cell receptor impairment results in high blood glucose levels despite normal or high insulin levels. Type II diabetes is usually a disease of older adults. Onset in the thirties and forties is unusual; onset in the sixth decade and beyond is more common. Type II diabetes is also called non–insulin-dependent diabetes mellitus because, at least early in the disease, most adults can be managed with diet and oral hypoglycemic agents alone.

2. Why should glucose be controlled during surgery?
Macrovascular disease in older patients with diabetes involves an increased risk of mortality and morbidity. Sustained hyperglycemia results in increased risk for infection, impaired wound healing, and increased length of postsurgical hospitalization. The underlying insulin deficiency associated with hyperglycemia may lead to ketogenesis, acidosis, and protein catabolism. Specific complications include:
 1. Hyperglycemia producing osmotic diuresis
 2. Hyperosmolar states with hyperviscocity, thrombogenesis, and cerebral edema
 3. Ketogenesis and the risk of diabetic ketoacidosis
 4. Proteolysis and decreased amino acid transport, resulting in retarded wound healing
 5. Loss of polymorphonuclear cell phagocytic function

3. What factors affect metabolic decompensation?
The following factors favor metabolic decompensation—a shift from glucose homeostasis toward catabolism—in patients with poorly controlled diabetes:
 1. Insulin deficiency
 2. Increased counterregulatory hormones (epinephrine, cortisol, glucagon growth hormone)
 3. Fasting states (glycogen depletion)
 4. Dehydration

4. Describe glucose metabolism in the setting of surgery.
Insulin enhances glucose uptake, glycogen storage, protein synthesis, amino acid transport, and fat formation. The counterregulatory hormones promote glycogenolysis, gluconeogenesis, proteolysis, and lipolysis. Basal insulin secretion is essential even in the fasting state to maintain glucose homeostasis. The potential consequences of insulin deficiency and excessive counterregulatory hormones in diabetic patients are far-reaching in the acute operative period as well as during recovery.

Surgery leads to increased stress and high counterregulatory hormone activity with a decrease in insulin secretion. In diabetic patients this leads to lipolysis, gluconeogenesis, and glycogenolysis—and thus to increased glucose production and decreased utilization. In diabetics, especially patients with type II diabetes, peripheral insulin resistance is also significant. Therefore, in diabetics without adequate insulin replacement, the combination of insulin deficiency and excessive counterregulatory hormones may lead to severe hyperglycemia and diabetic ketoacidosis, which are associated with hyperosmolarity, and increases in protein catabolism, fluid loss, lipolysis, and protein breakdown.

5. What other complications are associated with diabetes mellitus?
1. Hypertension is seen in 40% of poorly controlled diabetics who undergo surgery. The effect of potassium-wasting diuretic agents must be closely monitored, because even mild acidosis results in total body potassium loss.
2. Diabetic autonomic neuropathy may compromise neuroreflexic control of cardiovascular and pulmonary function, manifesting as orthostatic hypotension and loss of variations in cardiac rhythm with deep breathing and the Valsalva maneuver as well as urinary retention, ileus, and gastric retention.
3. Disturbances in renal function are common, including increased blood urea nitrogen and creatinine, protein loss and hypoalbuminemia, and electrolyte disturbances.
4. Occult infections are present in 17% of diabetics.

6. Describe the goals of diabetic therapy in the perioperative state.
Given the potential and demonstrable complications in patients with diabetes, certain reasonable goals should be kept in mind:
1. Avoid hypoglycemia, severe hyperglycemia, protein catabolism, electrolyte imbalance, and ketoacidosis.
2. Anticipate, prevent, and treat imbalances of potassium, magnesium, and phosphate.
3. Avoid significant glycosuria and osmotic diuresis.

7. What preoperative considerations influence the management of diabetes?
First, the type of diabetes and previous therapy must be considered. For example, a patient with type I diabetes certainly requires insulin, usually as an intravenous infusion during surgery. On the other hand, a patient with type II diabetes who does not normally require insulin should be well managed with dietary control only. A patient with type II diabetes who requires daily insulin will require insulin on the day of surgery. If the procedure is short or minimally invasive, the patient is not likely to require an insulin infusion. The second consideration is obviously the nature of the surgery. Control of postoperative infection should be considered. If the procedure involves a significant risk of postoperative infection, insulin infusion may be considered to establish tighter glucose control. Underlying fluid and electrolyte imbalances should be corrected and severe hyperglycemia or ketosis should be controlled. Diabetic complications mentioned earlier, such as hypertension or neuropathy, should be kept in mind, along with the fact that insulin requirements are increased by infection, hepatic disease, obesity, steroids, stress (including pain), and cardiovascular surgery. Consider the following questionnaire for a surgical patient with diabetes:
1. Type of diabetes and duration of disease
2. Daily therapy at home: amount of insulin dose, diet, oral hypoglycemics
3. Underlying diabetic complications
   • Renal disease
   • Neuropathy (early satiety and reflux suggest gastroparesis)
   • Retinopathy
   • Hypertension and medications
   • Hepatic disease
   • Infections, skin disease, foot disease, vaginitis
   • Cardiac disease, silent ischemia
4. Evidence of overt infectious disease
5. Status of electrolytes, phosphate, and magnesium
6. Blood glucose, ketones, acidosis
7. Does the procedure involve high risk of postoperative infection or pain?

8. Describe effective preoperative management for the diabetic patient.

Patients undergoing more serious and invasive procedures have higher levels of counterregulatory hormones and require closer attention to good glucose control. Blood glucose levels under 200 mg/dl in the days preceding surgery are ideal and ensure adequate glycogen stores and insulin sufficiency. In major procedures it may be prudent to observe the patient's glucose, electrolytes, blood pressure, and hydration for 24–48 hours before surgery. Insulin requirements may be lower during prolonged preoperative hospitalization than at home because of inactivity. If the patient is hospitalized, it is possible to control the diet (with cooperation, of course, the same control is possible at home) to help in achieving glucose control. On the day before surgery glucose should be monitored at bedside before each meal, at bedtime, and in the early morning. The goal is to have most glucose levels under 200 mg/dl. Underlying complications should be managed, and electrolytes, phosphate, magnesium, and hydration should be normal. A baseline electrocardiogram is important in adult patients.

9. A patient has been admitted for a lengthy procedure with the anticipation of significant postoperative recovery time and risk of infection. How should this patient's diabetes be managed during surgery?

It is ideal, especially in children with type I diabetes, to schedule the surgery early in the day. This allows a subcutaneous insulin injection on the night before the procedure and initiation of insulin infusion on the morning of surgery. The patient should fast for 12 hours before surgery.

At least 1 hour before surgery a combined insulin-dextrose infusion should be initiated. The infusion is made by adding 0.32 units of insulin per gram of glucose (32 units of insulin to 1000 ml of 10% dextrose [D10] in water or 16 units of insulin to 1000 ml of 5% dextrose [D5] in water). Ensure that electrolytes and phosphate are normal. Glucose should be under 200 mg/dl. No parenteral insulin is given on the morning of surgery.

Glucose and potassium should be checked hourly during surgery and in the postanesthetic care unit, using rapid bedside monitoring of glucose levels. The recommended infusion of insulin is 32 units with 20 mEq/L of potassium in 1000 ml of D10 at 100 ml/hr. The infusion may be increased or decreased by 4-unit increments. Potassium should be omitted if the blood level is > 5.5 mEq/L or increased to 40 mEq/L if the blood level is < 4 mEq/L.

10. Describe the postoperative management of the same patient.

In significant procedures with prolonged recovery time and a period of decreased intake, it is easier to manage the patient by continuing the insulin and glucose infusion for up to 48 hours, matching increased or decreased insulin needs with changes in rate of concentration of the infusate. The following guidelines are recommended:

1 Continue bedside monitoring of glucose, electrolytes, and fluids.

2. Using the insulin-glucose infusion, alter the rate or concentration as needed.

3. A glucose goal of 100–250 mg/dl is reasonable.

4. With the resumption of oral feeding, insulin is given subcutaneously according to the patient's preoperative schedule. If pain or stress is still significant, it will be necessary to increase the dose by as much as 20%. Monitor glucose at bedside before meals, at bedtime, and early in the morning, adjusting doses as necessary.

5. Monitor nutrition! If total parenteral nutrition is used, the insulin rate may need to increase and should be adjusted based on glucose monitoring.

11. Describe the management of diabetic patients who require emergency surgery.

If at all possible, electrolyte and glucose imbalance should be corrected before surgery. Sufficient rehydration, electrolyte replacement, and insulin treatment can be achieved in 4–6 hours to improve hyperglycemia and to suppress ketogenesis and acidosis. Rehydration is initiated with 10–20 ml/kg normal saline. Insulin infusion at 0.1U/kg/hr, using 0.45 normal saline (NS) (or D10 in 0.45 NS if glucose is < 150 mg/dl). If the patient is in ketoacidosis and immediate surgery is imperative, the following guidelines may be useful.

Insulin Infusion Rate for Emergency Surgery

BLOOD GLUCOSE (MG/DL)	RATE (ML/HR)	INSULIN RATE (U/HR)*	
		A	B
0–50	5	.25	.50
50–100	10	.50	1.00
100–150	15	.75	1.50
150–200	20	1.00	2.00
200–250	25	1.25	2.50
250–300	30	1.50	3.00
300–350	35	1.75	3.50
350–400	40	2.00	4.00
> 400	50	3.00	6.00

* Solution A is used for patients with an insulin requirement of < 50 units/day and is made with 50 units of insulin in 1000 ml NS with potassium, 20 mEq/L. Solution B is used for patients with an insulin requirement > 50 units/day and is made with 100 units insulin in 1000 ml NS with potassium 20 mEq/L. Pediatric patients require 0.1 unit/kg/hr of insulin for ketoacidosis and 0.05 unit/kg/hr for maintenance.

12. What type of insulin should be used during surgery?

During the preoperative period and after the patient has returned to subcutaneous insulin postoperatively, both long-acting insulin (NPH, lente) and short-acting insulin (regular) are used. However, during the operative period only regular insulin is used. All of the infusion suggestions in this chapter refer to human regular insulin. Given subcutaneously, regular insulin has an onset of action within 20–30 minutes and a duration of up to 2–3 hours. Given intravenously, regular insulin acts within 3–5 minutes and has a duration of 20–30 minutes.

13. What specific assessments should be performed during the anesthetic evaluation of an insulin-dependent diabetic?

A major task during the preoperative evaluation of an insulin-dependent diabetic should be the search for major end-organ damage. The risk of significant end-organ damage increases with the time that the patient has been diabetic, although the quality of glucose control is more important than the length of the disease. Cardiovascular, renal, and autonomic and peripheral nervous systems may be affected. A diligent search should be made for signs and symptoms of congestive heart failure or myocardial ischemia. Frequently, myocardial ischemia is silent in diabetics, even without signs of associated neuropathy. A preoperative electrocardiogram (ECG) should be performed on all diabetics. Because myocardial infarction carries a higher risk of morbidity and mortality in diabetic patients, myocardial ischemia should be minimized in the perioperative period. Congestive heart failure and valvular heart disease are significant risk factors for perioperative cardiac complications in diabetic patients. Decisions about intraoperative monitoring should be individualized, recognizing the increased risk such patients for silent perioperative myocardial ischemia. Because diabetics have an increase in small vessel disease throughout the body, cerebrovascular or peripheral vascular disease also may be present. Proteinuria is an early manifestation of diabetic nephropathy. Preoperative evaluation should include measurement of elecrolytes, serum blood urea nitrogen and creatinine, and urinalysis. Quantitative urinary protein determination is usually not necessary; the results would not change intraoperative management. In patients with end-stage renal disease on dialysis, the type of dialysis and schedule of dialysis in relationship to the date of surgery should be determined. Optimally, surgery should occur the day after dialysis. Peripheral neuropathies are common in diabetics; they should be documented carefully preoperatively. Diabetic patients may be more susceptible to iatrogenic peripheral nerve injuries. Visual acuity also should be assessed in a general fashion; patients with decreased vision appreciate additional explanations of the perioperative experience. Autonomic neuropathy may affect cardiovascular (silent ischemia), gastrointestinal (gastroparesis with increased risk of aspiration), thermoregulatory (decreased ability to alter blood vessel flow to conserve temperature), and neuroendocrine systems (decreased catecholamine production in response to stimulation). Patients with autonomic neuropathy should receive aspiration prophy-laxis: an H_2-blocking agent, a gastric stimulant to decrease gastroparesis, and a nonparticulate antacid. Autonomic neuropathy can be assessed by simple exams. The first two tests examine the sympathetic nervous system; the last two tests examine the parasympathetic nervous system.

1. A normal response is a change of at least 16 mmHg; an affected patient has a response of < 10 mmHg.

2. A larger change in postural systolic blood pressure (from lying to standing). A normal decrease is < 10 mmHg; an affected patient has a decrease of at least 30 mmHg.

3. Decreased heart rate response to deep breathing. Normal patients increase heart rate by at least 15 beats per minute. Affected patients have an increase of 10 or fewer beats per minute.

4. If the ECG is recorded, the R-R ratio can be determined with a Valsalva maneuver. A normal ratio is > 1.20; an abnormal response is < 1.10.

Oral intubation may be difficult in some diabetic patients because of stiff joint syndrome, with decreased mobility at the atlantooccipital joint. The remainder of the airway exam may be normal. Stiff joint syndrome is suggested by the inability to approximate the palmar pharyngeal joints (touch the palmar aspects of the fingers together when the palms are together—the prayer sign) and correlates with duration of insulin-dependent diabetes and microvascular complica-tions. Atlantooccipital joint mobility can be evaluated radiographically. If decreased mobility is documented or stiff joint syndrome is suspected clinically, an awake intubation may be required.

14. What additional operative concerns are associated with diabetic patients?
The most important monitoring for insulin-dependent diabetics is to check blood glucose meas-urements frequently during the perioperative period, at least once an hour. Patients should be positioned carefully, recognizing the increased risk of iatrogenic nerve injuries. Hypoglycemia may be difficult to detect in an anesthetized patient; blood glucose levels should be kept above 100 mg/dl. Hyperglycemia also should be avoided; blood glucose levels above 300 mg/dl may lead to osmotic diuresis, making volume status difficult to determine and leading to hypovolemia. In patients with an elevated blood glucose during surgery, the level should be decreased gradually by additional small doses of intravenous insulin or by changing the insulin infusion rate. If the blood glucose level is decreased too rapidly (> 200 mg/dl/hr), cerebral edema may result. Brief vasopressor therapy may be needed after induction of general anesthesia, because catecholamine production and response may be impaired.

15. Are regional anesthetics helpful in insulin-dependent diabetics?
Regional anesthetic techniques (epidural anesthetics, spinal anesthetics, and peripheral nerve blocks) decrease the stress response of the patient. In insulin-dependent diabetics, this can help to maintain a more stable blood glucose as well as decrease stress on the cardiovascular system. Epinephrine should not be used in peripheral nerve blocks (e.g., ankle blocks) because of the risk of decreasing blood flow to the area; insulin-dependent diabetics often already have dis-eased microcirculation. In blocks with high systemic absorption, such as brachial plexus or in-tercostal blocks, low-dose epinephrine may be used.

BIBLIOGRAPHY

1. Gavin LA:Management of diabetes mellitus during surgery. West J Med 151:525–529, 1989.
2. George K, Alberti MM, Gill GV, Elliott MJ: Insulin delivery during surgery in the diabetic patient. Diabetes Care 5(S1):65–75, 1982.
3. Hirsh IB, McGill JB: The role of insulin in management of surgical patients with diabetes mellitus. Diabetes Care 13:980–991, 1990.
4. MacKenzie CR, Charlson ME: Assessment of perioperative risk in the patient with diabetes mellitus. Surg Obstet Gynecol 167:293–299, 1988.
5. Rosenstock J, Raskin P: Surgery! Practical guidelines for diabetes management. Clin Diabetes 5:49–61, 1987.
6. Schade DS: Surgery and diabetes. Med Clin North Am 72:1531–1543, 1988.
7. Schuman CR, Podolsky S: Surgery in the diabetic patient. In Podolsky S (ed): Clinical Diabetes: Modern Management. New York, Appleton-Century-Crofts, 1980, pp 509–535.
8. Wissler RN: The patient with endocrine disease. Probl Anesth 6(1):61–89, 1992.

57. THYROID AND ADRENAL DISEASE

Kenneth M. Swank, M.D., and Christopher A. Mills, M.D.

1. Describe four steps involved in thyroid hormone synthesis.

Step 1: Uptake of iodide. Iodide from the bloodstream is concentrated in thyroid cells by an active transport mechanism.

Step 2: Iodination of thyroglobulin. Thyroglobulin, a large glycoprotein rich in tyrosine, is enzymatically iodinated and stored in the thyroid follicles.

Step 3: Coupling reactions. The monoiodotyrosine and diiodotyrosine moieties within the thyroglobulin molecule are coupled to one another to form triiodothyronine (T_3) and thyroxine (T_4).

Step 4: Release of hormones. T_3 and T_4 are enzymatically cleaved from thyroglobulin within the follicular cell and released into the bloodstream.

2. How much T_3 and T_4 is produced? What regulates their production?

Approximately 8 μg of T_3 and 90 μg of T_4 are produced daily. Additional T_3 is formed from the peripheral conversion of T_4 to T_3. T_3 is approximately four times more potent than T_4 but has a much shorter half-life; therefore the contribution of each to total thyroid activity is approximately equal. Thyroid-stimulating hormone (TSH) (produced by the anterior pituitary gland) acts on thyroid tissue to increase the rates of all steps involved in thyroid hormone synthesis and release. Thyrotropin-releasing hormone (TRH) (produced by the hypothalamus), in turn, regulates the amount of TSH produced by the pituitary. T_3 and T_4 inhibit release of TSH and to a much smaller degree the release of TRH, thus establishing a negative feedback control mechanism.

3. List the common thyroid function tests and their use in assessment of thyroid disorders.

Total T_4 level, total T_3 level, TSH level, resin T_3 uptake (T_3RU). The T_3RU is useful in conditions that alter levels of thyroid binding globulin, which would alter total T_4 results.

Utility of Thyroid Function Tests in the Diagnosis of Hypothyroid or Hyperthyroid States

DISEASE	T4	T3	TSH	T3RU
Primary hypothyroidism	−	−	+	−
Secondary hypothyroidism	−	−	−	−
Hyperthyroidism	+	+	0	+
Pregnancy	+	0	0	+

+, Increased; −, decreased; 0, no change.

4. What is the Wolff-Chaikoff effect?

Large doses of iodine cause an acute temporary paradoxical decrease in the production of thyroid hormones because of an inhibitory effect on all of the steps involved in hormone production, but especially on the iodination of thyroglobulin and coupling reactions. This effect can be used in the management of hyperthyroidism.

5. Discuss some common signs, symptoms, and causes of hypothyroidism.

Symptoms	**Signs**
Fatigue	Bradycardia
Cold intolerance	Hypothermia
Constipation	Deep tendon reflex relaxation
Dry skin	phase prolongation
Hair loss	Hoarseness
Weight gain	Periorbital edema

The signs and symptoms observed in patients with mild hypothyroidism are nonspecific, and therefore detection of this situation on a clinical basis alone is extremely difficult. Patients with severe long-term untreated hypothyroidism may progress to myxedema coma, which is frequently fatal. Myxedema coma is characterized by hypoventilation, hypothermia, hypotension, hyponatremia, hypoglycemia, obtundation, and adrenal insufficiency.

Factors that may lead to myxedema coma in hypothyroid patients include cold exposure, infection, trauma, and administration of central nervous system depressants.

The most common cause of hypothyroidism is surgical or radioiodine ablation of thyroid tissue used for the treatment of hyperthyroidism, most commonly Graves' disease. Other causes of hypothyroidism include chronic thyroiditis (Hashimoto's thyroiditis), drug effects, iodine deficiency, and pituitary or hypothalamic dysfunction.

6. Of the numerous manifestations of hypothyroidism, which are most important in relation to anesthesia?

With regard to the **cardiovascular system**, hypothyroidism causes depression of myocardial function owing to protein and mucopolysaccharide deposition within the myocardium and owing to depression of intracellular myocardial metabolism. Hypothyroidism causes decreased cardiac output as a result of decreased heart rate and stroke volume. Decreased blood volume, baroreceptor reflex dysfunction, and pericardial effusion may accompany hypothyroidism as well. All of these effects make the hypothyroid patient sensitive to the hypotensive effects of anesthetics. The **respiratory system** can be affected, causing hypoventilation; in severe hypothyroidism, respiratory failure can be present. The ventilatory responses to both hypoxia and hypercarbia are significantly impaired, making the hypothyroid patient sensitive to drugs that cause respiratory depression. Hypothyroidism also decreases the hepatic and renal clearance of drugs. These patients are also prone to hypothermia because of lowered metabolic rate and consequent lowered heat production.

7. How does hypothyroidism affect minimum alveolar concentration (MAC) of anesthetic agents?

Animal studies show that MAC is not affected by hypothyroidism. Clinically, it has been noted that hypothyroid patients have increased sensitivity to anesthetic agents. This is due not to a decrease in MAC per se but to the patient's metabolically depressed condition.

8. How is hypothyroidism treated?

Treatment consists of supplementation with exogenous thyroid hormones, most frequently levothyroxine because its long half-life results in a more constant serum level. The principal risk with treatment is in patients with coronary artery disease (CAD). These patients are at risk for developing worsening in their status owing to increased demand placed on the ischemic myocardium because of an increase in the basal metabolic rate.

Suggested Thyroid Supplementation Protocol for Hypothyroid Patients:
- Patients without CAD: T_4 50 µg/day increasing monthly by 50 µg/day increments until a euthyroid state is reached.
- Patients with CAD: T_4 25 µg/day increasing monthly by 25 µg/day increments until a euthyroid state is achieved.
- In urgent situations, thyroid supplementation may be cautiously given intravenously. Recommended dose is T_4 300 µg/m^2 by slow infusion.

Hypothyroid patients receiving intravenous supplementation must be monitored closely for signs and symptoms of cardiac ischemia as well as adrenal insufficiency.

9. Under what circumstances should elective surgery be delayed for a hypothyroid patient?

Patients with **mild to moderate hypothyroidism** are not at increased risk undergoing elective surgical procedures. Some authors suggest that elective surgery in patients who are symptomatic should be delayed until the patient is rendered euthyroid. Other authorities recommend against delaying surgery if thyroid replacement can begin before surgery (in patients without CAD). In patients with **severe hypothyroidism**, elective surgery should be delayed until they have been rendered euthyroid. This may require 2–4 months of replacement therapy for complete reversal of cardiopulmonary effects. Normalization of the patient's TSH level reflects reversal of hypothyroid-induced changes. In patients with CAD who are unable to tolerate replacement therapy, coronary artery bypass grafting has been performed successfully.

10. List common signs, symptoms, and causes of hyperthyroidism.

Signs	Symptoms	Causes
Goiter	Anxiety	Graves' disease
Tachycardia	Tremor	Toxic multinodular goiter
Proptosis	Heat intolerance	
Atrial fibrillation	Fatigue	
	Weight loss	
	Muscle weakness	

11. How is hyperthyroidism treated?
There are three approaches to treatment.

1. **Antithyroid drugs** such as propylthiouracil (PTU) inhibit iodination and coupling reactions in the thyroid gland, thus reducing production of T_3 and T_4. PTU also inhibits peripheral conversion of T_4 to T_3. **Iodine** in large doses not only blocks hormone production, but also decreases the vascularity and size of the thyroid gland, making iodine useful in preparing hyperthyroid patients for thyroid surgery.

2. **Radioactive iodine**, I^{131}, is actively concentrated by the thyroid gland, resulting in destruction of thyroid cells and thus a decrease in the production of hormone.

3. **Surgical subtotal thyroidectomy**

All of these approaches may render the patient hypothyroid. In the short term, beta-adrenergic blockers control symptoms of hyperthyroidism.

12. Which effects of hyperthyroidism are the most important with regard to anesthesia?
In hyperthyroidism, the metabolic rate of the body is increased, causing significant changes in the **cardiovascular system**, the magnitude of which are proportional to the severity of the thyroid dysfunction. Because of the elevated oxygen consumption, the cardiovascular system is hyperdynamic. Tachycardia and elevated cardiac output are present, and tachyarrhythmias, atrial fibrillation, left ventricular hypertrophy, and congestive heart failure may develop. Hyperthyroid patients with **proptosis** are more susceptible to ocular damage during surgery because of difficulty with taping their eyelids closed.

13. How is minimum alveolar concentration (MAC) affected by hyperthyroidism?
As in hypothyroidism, MAC is not affected by hyperthyroidism, although clinically hyperthyroid patients appear to be resistant to the effects of anesthetic agents. Induction with volatile agents is slowed by the increased cardiac output. The rate of drug metabolism is increased, giving the appearance of resistance. Hyperthyroidism-induced hyperthermia may indirectly elevate MAC.

14. Define thyrotoxicosis.
Also known as **"thyroid storm,"** this is an acute exacerbation of hyperthyroidism usually caused by a stress such as surgery or infection. It is characterized by extreme tachycardia, hyperthermia, and possibly severe hypotension. Perioperatively, it usually occurs 6–18 hours after surgery but can occur intraoperatively and can be confused with malignant hyperthermia.

15. How is thyrotoxicosis treated?
Intraoperative treatment must be immediate, consisting of careful beta-adrenergic blockade, infusion of intravenous fluids, and temperature control if hyperthermia is present. Corticosteroids

should be considered for refractory hypotension because hyperthyroid patients may have a relative deficiency of cortisol due to increased demand. Antithyroid drugs should be added postoperatively.

16. What complications may occur after a surgical procedure involving the thyroid gland?
Because of the close proximity of the thyroid gland to the trachea and larynx, many of the complications that occur (such as laryngeal edema or cervical hematoma) can cause airway obstruction. Chronic pressure on the trachea from a goiter, for example, can lead to tracheomalacia, which may lead to tracheal collapse and airway obstruction following extubation. Inadvertent resection of the parathyroid glands, in turn, can lead to hypocalcemia, which may produce laryngospasm. Innervation to the vocal cord musculature may be compromised by surgical damage to the recurrent laryngeal nerves (RLN). Bilateral RLN injury can result in the vocal cords being passively drawn together during inspiration, leading to severe obstruction that necessitates emergent tracheostomy. Unilateral injury results in dysfunction of the ipsilateral vocal cord. Damage to the nerve fibers innervating the vocal cord adductors results in unopposed abduction of the ipsilateral vocal cord, increasing the risk of aspiration. Damage to the innervation of the abductor muscles results in an abnormally adducted vocal cord, which can cause hoarseness. Vocal cord function may be assessed following surgery with direct laryngoscopy or via a fiberoptic laryngoscope.

17. Why is levothyroxine given to organ donors?
Hypotension in the donor before organ donation decreases organ perfusion, which adversely affects the viability and function of the donor organs after transplantation. This hypotension may be due to cardiac dysfunction from a hypothyroid state induced by failure of the hypothalamic-pituitary axis. Infusion of levothyroxine appears to improve donor hemodynamics, thus improving the quality of the donated organs.

18. Describe the functions and regulation of the adrenal gland.
The adrenal gland can be functionally divided into the adrenal cortex and the adrenal medulla. The **adrenal cortex** principally produces the steroid hormones cortisol and aldosterone. Production of cortisol is regulated by adrenocorticotropic hormone (ACTH) produced by the anterior pituitary. The release of ACTH is promoted by corticotropin-releasing hormone (CRH) derived from the hypothalamus. Cortisol inhibits release of both CRH and ACTH, establishing negative feedback control. Ectopic ACTH can be produced by various neoplasms, such as small cell lung carcinomas. Aldosterone secretion is regulated by the renin-angiotensin system. The **adrenal medulla** secretes epinephrine and norepinephrine. Their release is governed by the sympathetic nervous system.

19. Define pheochromocytoma.
A pheochromocytoma is a neoplasm arising from the adrenal medulla or paravertebral chromaffin tissue. Ninety percent of these tumors arise from the adrenal medulla, and 10% are bilateral. Pheochromocytomas may secrete norepinephrine, epinephrine, or other catecholamines. The ratio of secreted norepinephrine to epinephrine is higher than that found in normal adrenal medullary tissue. Most extra-adrenal pheochromocytomas secrete only norepinephrine.

20. How much cortisol is produced by the adrenal cortex?
Normally, approximately 20–30 mg of cortisol per day is produced. This amount increases dramatically as a response to a stress, such as infection or surgery. Under stressful conditions, 75–150 mg per day may be produced, with the increase in production being generally proportional to the severity of the stress.

21. What is the most common cause of hypothalamic-pituitary-adrenal (HPA) axis disruption?
Exogenous steroids (glucocorticoids) result in HPA axis suppression. Conditions for which steroids are given include many autoimmune diseases, organ transplants, reactive airways disease, and inflammatory bowel disease.

Short-term steroid administration—no longer than 7–10 days—results in suppression of CRH and ACTH release, which usually returns to normal about 5 days after discontinuation of steroid therapy. Long-term administration of exogenous steroids results in adrenocortical atrophy secondary to a lack of ACTH. This results in prolonged adrenocortical insufficiency, which can last a year or more following steroid discontinuation. Therefore, long-term steroid administration should not be abruptly terminated; rather it should be gradually tapered off over a period of 1–4 weeks.

22. What is addisonian crisis?

Also referred to as acute adrenocortical insufficiency, an addisonian crisis is caused by a relative lack of cortisol or other glucocorticoid in relation to a stress such as surgery. It is a shocklike state characterized by refractory hypotension, hypovolemia, and electrolyte disturbances. Causes of adrenocortical insufficiency include

- HPA axis suppression by exogenous corticosteroid administration
- Autoimmune adrenalitis
- Adrenal hemorrhage
- Adrenal tuberculosis
- Septic shock

23. How is addisonian crisis treated?

Treatment must be immediate and consists of intravenous cortisol, fluid replacement, physiologic monitoring, and correction of electrolyte abnormalities.

CONTROVERSY

24. Is perioperative stress steroid supplementation for patients on steroid therapy necessary?

Few documented cases of acute perioperative adrenal insufficiency, addisonian crisis, exist. Studies have shown that patients who have been on long-term steroid therapy undergoing even major surgery rarely become hypotensive because of glucocorticoid deficiency. If observed, hypotension is usually due to one or more of the more common causes, such as hypovolemia or cardiac dysfunction. Such hypotension is responsive to therapies other than the administration of glucocorticoids. The possible side effects of perioperative steroid supplementation include

- Hyperglycemia
- Aggravation of hypertension
- Impaired wound healing
- Fluid retention
- Gastric ulceration
- Immunosuppression

One answer to this question might be that no supplementation is required unless hypotension refractory to standard tratment occurs. However, although considerable data exist regarding the problems associated with long-term steroid therapy, few data indicate any significant side effects or problems related to short-term perioperative steroid supplementation. Despite its rarity, acute adrenal insufficiency is associated with significant morbidity and mortality. Therefore, another answer to the question could be that, because perioperative steroid supplementation is associated with few risks in itself and because acute adrenal insufficiency can potentially lead to death, supplemental steroids should be given. Currently, this seems to be the view of most authors.

25. If supplemental corticosteriods are to be administered perioperatively, how much should one give?

The dosage is highly dependent on the amount of stress that the surgery is likely to cause. **For minor surgery**, no supplementation or minimal supplementation, such as hydrocortisone 25 mg, may suffice. **For major surgery**, a variety of dosages have been suggested, with none being shown to be superior to the rest. One regimen consists of hydrocortisone 25 mg intraoperatively followed by an infusion of hydrocortisone 100 mg over the immediate 24 hours postoperatively. Another is to give 200–300 mg/70 kg in divided doses each day. The goal of these regimens is to give the lowest dose that provides sufficient supplementation while avoiding potential side effects.

BIBLIOGRAPHY

1. Graber AL, Ney RL, Nicholson WE, et al: Natural history of pituitary-adrenal recovery following long-term suppression with corticosteroids. J Clin Endocrinol Metab 25:11–16, 1965.
2. Knudsen L, Christiansen A, Lorentzen JE: Hypotension during and after operation in glucocorticoid-treated patients. Br J Anaesth 53:295–300, 1981.
3. Lampe GH, Roizen MF: Anesthesia for patients with abnormal function at the adrenal cortex. Anesthiol Clin North Am 5:245–267, 1987.
4. Murkin JM: Anesthesia and hypothyroidism: A review of thyroxine physiology, pharmacology, and anesthetic implications. Anesth Analg 61:371–383, 1982.
5. Napolitano LM, Chernow B: Guidelines for corticosteroid use in anesthetic and surgical stress. Int Anesthesthiol Clin 26:226–232, 1988.
6. Orlowski JP: Evidence that thyroxine (T_4) is effective as a hemodynamic rescue agent in management of organ donors. Transplantation 55:959–960, 1993.
7. Roizen MF: Anesthetic implications of concurrent diseases. In Miller RD (ed): Anesthesia, 4th ed. New York, Churchill Livingstone, 1994, pp 916–928.
8. Stehling LC: Anesthetic management of the patient with hyperthyroidism. Anesthesiology 41:585–595, 1974.
9. Stoelting RK, Dierdorf SF: Endocrine diseases. In Anesthesia and Coexisting Disease, 3rd ed. New York, Churchill Livingstone, 1993, pp 347–367.
10. Streck WF, Lockwood DH: Pituitary adrenal recovery following short-term suppression with corticosteroids. Am J Med 66:910–914, 1979.
11. Wartofsky L, Ingbar SH: Diseases of the thyroid. In Wilson JD, Braunwald E, Isselbacher KJ, et al (eds): Harrison's Principles of Internal Medicine, 13th ed. New York, McGraw-Hill, 1994, pp 1930–1952.
12. Weatherill D, Spence AA: Anaesthesia and disorders of the adrenal cortex. Br J Anaesth 56:741–749, 1984.
13. Wenning GK, Wietholter H, Schnauder G, et al: Recovery of the hypothalamic-pituitary-adrenal axis from suppression by short-term, high-dose intravenous prednisolone therapy in patients with MS. Acta Neurol Scand 89:270–273, 1994.
14. Williams GH, Dluhy RG: Diseases of the adrenal cortex. In Wilson JD, Braunwald E, Isselbacher KJ, et al (eds): Harrison's Principles of Internal Medicine, 13th ed. New York, McGraw-Hill, 1994, pp 1953–1979.

58. OBESITY

Lisa Leonard, C.R.N.A., M.H.S., and Elizabeth Ward, C.R.N.A.

1. Define obesity and morbid obesity.
Obesity is defined as body weight 20% greater than ideal weight. Approximately 20% of males and 30% of females are obese. Morbid obesity is defined as body weight more than two times ideal weight or greater than 100 lbs over ideal weight. In morbidly obese men, aged 23–34 years, the death rate is increased 12 times, primarily because of cardiovascular impairments.

2. What are the causes of morbid obesity?
Obesity is caused primarily by environmental and societal factors as well as psychopathologic alterations that lead to excessive caloric intake and inadequate activity. Researchers speculate that genetic factors such as an inherited metabolic defect may be influential. Endocrine dysfunction also may result in obesity, including hypothalamic disorders, diabetes mellitus, Cushing's syndrome, hypothyroidism, hypogonadism, and hypopituitary syndrome.

3. How is ideal body weight calculated?
The Broca index is a practical way to determine ideal body weight:

Height (cm) – 100 = ideal weight (kg) for males
Height (cm) – 105 = ideal weight (kg) for females
For example, a male 6 feet tall (72 in) 180 cm – 100 = 80 kg ideal body.

Body mass index (BMI) is another method of determining ideal body weight:

$BMI = weight (kg) / height (m^2)$
Ideal body weight = BMI of 22–28
Obesity = BMI of 28–35
Morbid obesity = BMI > 35

4. What systems are affected by morbid obesity? What disease processes are associated with obesity?
The systems most profoundly affected by obesity include the respiratory, cardiovascular, gastrointestinal, endocrine, and hepatic systems. Other disease processes associated with obesity include osteoarthritis, sciatica, varicose veins, thromboembolism, ventral and hiatal hernias, cholelithiasis, hyperuricemia, and gout.

5. Do obese patients have an altered response to CO_2?
Obesity per se has not been found to decrease the respiratory center's sensitivity to CO_2. Yet approximately 5–10% of obese patients experience an apparent decreased ventilatory response to CO_2, resulting in one or more of the following syndromes.

1. Obstructive sleep apnea syndrome (OSAS)—defined as 30 apneic periods of > 20 seconds over 7 hours;

2. Obesity hypoventilation syndrome (OHS)—decreased ventilatory response to CO_2 and O_2, resulting in sleep apnea, hypoventilation, hypercapnea, pulmonary hypertension, and hypersomnolence;

3. Pickwickian syndrome—first named in 1956 by Burwell, who believed that the syndrome was described in 1837 by a Charles Dickens' character in the *Posthumous Papers of the Pickwick Club*. Symptoms include OHS, hypoxemia, hypercarbia, pulmonary hypertension, polycythemia, and biventricular failure.

6. Discuss the respiratory changes that occur in morbidly obese patients.

Obesity is typically accompanied by hypoxemia, the mechanisms of which include:

1. An increased work of breathing 2–4 times greater than normal. An increased chest wall mass decreases chest wall compliance and diaphragmatic excursion.

2. The large tissue mass increases total oxygen (O_2) consumption and increases carbon dioxide (CO_2) production.

3. Changes in lung volumes result in closure of small airways during tidal respiration and ventilation/perfusion (V/Q) mismatch. An altered response to CO_2 is seen in some obesity syndromes. The pulmonary function tests of obese patients show a restrictive pattern of lung disease.

Changes in Pulmonary Volumes and Function Tests Associated with Obesity

LUNG VOLUMES	CHANGES WITH OBESITY
Tidal volume (V_T)	Normal or increased
Inspiratory reserve volume (IRV)	Decreased
Expiratory reserve volume (ERV)	Greatly decreased
Residual volume (RV)	Normal
Functional residual capacity (FRC = RV + ERV)	Greatly decreased
Vital capacity (VC) (VC = IRV + V_T + ERV)	Decreased
Total lung capacity	Decreased
Forced expiratory volume at 1 second (FEV_1)	Normal or slightly decreased
Maximal midexpiratory flow rate (MMEF)	Normal or slightly decreased

7. What arterial blood gas changes are common in obese patients?

The most common alteration is hypoxemia due to ventilation/perfusion mismatching. Pulmonary perfusion is increased because of increased cardiac output, circulating blood volume and pulmonary hypertension. Alveolar ventilation is decreased secondary to airway closure. Closing capacity is the lung volume at which small airways begin to close. Because closing capacity is unchanged in obesity, reduced functional residual capacity may result in lung volumes below closing capacity during normal tidal ventilation.

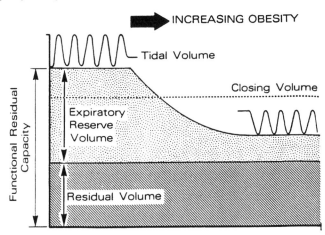

Changes in ventilation associated with weight gain. (From Fox GS: Anaesthesia for intestinal short circuiting in the morbidly obese with reference to the pathophysiology of gross obesity. Can Anaesth Soc J 22:307, 1975, with permission.)

8. Describe the changes in the cardiovascular system of obese patients.
Cardiac output (CO) and stroke volume (SV) increase in proportion to oxygen consumption and weight gain. An increase in CO of 100 ml/min accompanies each kilogram increase in adipose tissue. Circulating blood volume is also increased proportionately with increasing weight. Systemic hypertension is 10 times more prevalent in obese patients because of the increases in CO and blood volume. Pulmonary hypertension is present in Pickwickian patients as a result of increased CO and hypoxic pulmonary vasoconstriction (the reflex constriction of pulmonary arterioles in areas of atelectasis). Right and left end-diastolic pressures may be elevated. Ventricular hypertrophy and biventricular failure are common; as many as 10% of obese patients develop congestive heart failure.

9. What changes in gastrointestinal and hepatic function can be expected in obese patients?
The large tissue mass in obese patients increases intraabdominal and intragastric pressures. Hiatal hernias and gastric reflux are common. Several studies have shown that, despite an 8-hour fast, 85–90% of morbidly obese patients have gastric volumes >25 ml and gastric pH <2.5, greatly increasing their risk for pulmonary aspiration. Obese patients typically have fatty infiltration of the liver and may have hepatic inflammation, focal necrosis, and cirrhosis. At present no causal relationship between fatty infiltration and cirrhotic changes is known. Hepatic enzymes are generally elevated, especially after jejunoileal bypass operations.

10. Do obese patients metabolize anesthetic drugs differently from nonobese patients?
Alterations in drug metabolism in obese patients may be unpredictable. Obesity increases the biotransformation rate of methoxyflurane, enflurane, and halothane, resulting in increased serum levels of flouride ions. Prolonged exposure to increased concentrations of flouride ions is associated with renal toxicity. Isoflurane and desflurane have not been associated with significant increases in the rate of biotransformation in obese patients and are therefore the volatile agents of choice. Lipophilic or fat-soluble drugs such as opioids, benzodiazipines, and barbiturates have an increased volume of distribution and decreased elimination half-life, resulting in lower serum drug concentrations and decreased clearance. Exceptions include fentanyl, a lipophilic opioid that shows similar pharmacokinetics in obese and nonobese patients. In obese patients, hydrophilic, water-soluble drugs generally have similar volumes of distribution, elimination half-lives, and rates of clearance in obese and nonobese patients. Pseudocholinesterase activity is increased with obesity, and larger doses of succinylcholine are required (1.2–1.5 mg/kg). Nondepolarizing muscle relaxants show variability in dosing, duration, and recovery and should be followed closely with a peripheral nerve stimulator for return of neuromuscular function.

11. Discuss the relationship between obesity and diabetes mellitus.
Adult-onset diabetes mellitus occurs 7 times more frequently in obese than in nonobese patients. Insulin resistance is a prominent feature of both obesity and non–insulin-dependent diabetes mellitus (NIDDM). Several studies have shown a relationship between obesity and impairment of insulin action in NIDDM. Insulin action in obese patients is impaired by decreasing insulin suppression of hepatic glucose production and decreasing glucose utilization at the muscle. Obese patients, therefore, are at increased risk for hyperglycemia and hyperinsulinemia.

12. What factors should be considered in preparing an obese patient for surgery?
   1. **History.** A thorough medical history should include incidence of sleep apnea, snoring, somnolence, and periodic breathing as well as assessment of hypertension, congestive heart failure, and coronary artery disease. Obese patients are frequently inactive, and determination of impaired cardiac performance may be difficult. Questions involving symptoms of gastroesophageal reflux, hiatal hernia, diabetes mellitus, and deep vein thrombosis should also be asked.
   2. **Physical examination.** Airway evaluation is extremely important and should include cervical and mandibular range of motion, thyromental distance, and oral airway assessment.

Subjective evaluation of chest and neck fat may suggest difficulties with intubation. If the airway examination suggests a potentially difficult intubation, the patient should be counseled on the procedure and benefits of an awake, sedated fiberoptic intubation. Adequacy of arterial and venous access also should be evaluated.

3. **Preoperative tests.** An electrocardiogram should be obtained for all obese patients to look for increased voltage, signs of atrial or ventricular enlargement, and arrhythmias. Ventricular arrhythmias are common. Chest radiographs are necessary and may reveal atelectasis, cardiac enlargement, infiltrates, effusion, or pneumothorax. A complete blood count and electrolytes should be obtained. Elevations in the white cell count and hematocrit may suggest infection and chronic hypoxemia, respectively. Bicarbonate levels are elevated to buffer a chronic respiratory acidosis if the patient retains carbon dioxide. Hypokalemia may occur with repeated use of diuretics. A room-air arterial blood gas analysis helps to identify baseline hypoxemic and hypercarbic patients and to determine acid/base status. Pulmonary function tests characterize pulmonary impairment. Liver function tests may prove valuable if hepatic dysfunction is suspected.

13. Is preoperative medication of an obese patient desirable?

An obese patient's increased risk of pulmonary aspiration should be prophylactically treated with H2-receptor antagonists, such as cimetidine or ranitidine, combined with metoclopramide and nonparticulate antacids. Current recommendations suggest that ranitidine, 150 mg orally on the night before surgery and 1–2 hours before surgery, may be preferable to cimetidine. The side effects of cimetidine include inhibition of hepatic microsomal enzymes and decreased liver blood flow, which may decrease the metabolism of certain drugs.

14. What are the primary operative concerns in morbidly obese patients?

1. **Airway and ventilatory management.** Before induction of anesthesia, preparation for a difficult airway should be completed. A fiberoptic bronchoscope, cricothyrotomy equipment, a variety of laryngoscope blades, endotracheal tubes, and oral and nasal airways should be available. Preoxygenation and denitrogenation of the patient are critical, using three minutes of spontaneous breathing with 100% oxygen. If the airway exam suggests that laryngoscopy and intubation are not problematic, rapid-sequence induction and intubation with cricoid pressure may be used. Otherwise, awake, sedated fiberoptic intubation is the technique of choice. Rarely can the awake obese patient tolerate a supine position, and a head-elevated position of at least 30° may be necessary for induction of anesthesia. Careful attention to airway positioning before induction greatly facilitates intubation. A wedge under the patient's shoulder blades, combined with good head extension, is frequently helpful. Capnography is necessary to help verify endotracheal tube placement, because auscultation through the thick chest wall can be difficult. Pulse oximetry is mandatory for detection of hypoxemia in obese patients, and an inspired oxygen of greater than 50% is strongly recommended once intubation is obtained. Positive-pressure ventilation is necessary, because spontaneous ventilation may predispose the patient to atelectasis and hypoxemia. Adequate ventilation may require the addition of positive end-expiratory pressure (PEEP) to maintain arterial oxygenation; increases in tidal volume may worsen oxygenation if high peak pressures impair return of blood to the chest, decreasing cardiac output and producing V/Q mismatch.

2. **Cardiovascular management.** Cardiovascular monitoring in obese patients can be difficult. Large blood pressure (BP) cuffs (the bladder of the cuff encloses 70% of the arm) are used to avoid false readings. A small cuff falsely elevates BP readings, whereas an excessively large cuff gives falsely low readings. Despite an appropriate cuff size, an invasive arterial line may be necessary to follow blood pressure closely and offers the option of serial arterial blood gas analysis for monitoring of ventilatory status. Monitoring of central venous pressure (CVP) and pulmonary artery pressure (PAP) may be advantageous to follow volume status and cardiac function, but catheters are difficult to place because landmarks and pulses may be obscured. Generally PAP catheter placement is unnecessary unless the patient is undergoing extensive surgery or shows evidence of cardiac or pulmonary disease, especially pulmonary hypertension or cor pulmonale.

3. **Positioning.** The operating table may be of inadequate width to accommodate an obese patient. Care must be taken to protect and pad all pressure points. It may become necessary to secure two operating tables together for extremely obese patients.

15. What criteria should be used for extubation of an obese patient?
Before extubation the obese patient should be awake, alert, and able to sustain a head-lift for 5 seconds. Muscle relaxants should be adequately reversed, as indicated by peripheral nerve stimulator findings (sustained tetanus with no posttetanic facilitation of twitches). The patient should have a respiratory rate of less than 30 breaths/minute. Arterial blood gases on 40–50% oxygen should be equal to or better than preoperative values; the PaO_2 should be greater than 80 torr and the $PaCO_2$ less than 45–50 torr if no preoperative values are available. A maximal inspiratory force of at least 25–30 cm H_2O, a vital capacity of 10–15 ml/kg, and a tidal volume greater than 5 ml/kg lean body weight are acceptable for extubation. The patient must be stable hemodynamically.

16. Discuss the postoperative course of morbidly obese patients.
Morbidly obese patients are at increased risk for hypoxemia for 4–7 days postoperatively. Therefore, supplemental oxygen is mandatory with the patient in a sitting or semirecumbent position. Aggressive pulmonary care with incentive spirometry, cough, deep breathing, and early ambulation is advised. Admission to an intensive care unit postoperatively may be necessary for close monitoring. An increased incidence of deep vein thrombosis in obese surgical patients necessitates early ambulation, which may be difficult because of relative postoperative immobility. Low-dose heparin and leg compression stockings are suggested. Postoperative pain control is important for both improved pulmonary function and early ambulation. Opioids may be used cautiously with adequate monitoring for respiratory depression. Intramuscular injections are likely to be subcutaneous and demonstrate unpredictable blood levels; therefore, intravenous narcotics are preferable; patient controlled analgesia (PCA) is a desirable option. Studies have shown that epidural opioids and local anesthetics facilitate earlier ambulation and decrease pulmonary complications as well as hospital stay compared with intramuscular narcotics. Epidural local anesthetic and opioid doses are similar to those for nonobese patients. In all patients, opioid epidural analgesia has the potential for unpredictable delayed respiratory depression and requires adequate monitoring at all times.

BIBLIOGRAPHY

1. Aker J, Biddle C: Current reviews for nurse anesthetists 8: 58–63, 1990.
2. Buckley FP: Anesthetizing the morbidly obese patient. ASA Refresher Course 151:1–6, 1993.
3. Campbell PJ, Carlson MG: Impact of obesity on insulin action in NIDDM. Diabetes 42:405–410, 1993.
4. Cork RC: General anesthesia for the morbidly obese patient—An examination of postoperative outcomes. Anesthesiology 54:310–313, 1981.
5. Everhart JE, Pettit DJ, Bennett PH, Knowler WC: Duration of obesity increases the incidence of NIDDM. Diabetes 41:235–240, 1992.
6. Fox GS: Anaesthesia for intestinal short circuiting in the morbidly obese with reference to the pathophysiology of gross obesity. Can Anaesth Soc J 22:307, 1975.
7. Fox G: Anesthesia for the morbidly obese, experience with 110 patients. Br J Anaesth 53:811–815, 1981.
8. Fox DJ: Obesity. In Bready LL, Smith RB (eds): Decision Making in Anesthesiology, 2nd ed. St. Louis, B.C. Decker, 1992, pp 116–117.
9. Klein SL: A Glossary of Anesthesia and Related Terminology. New York, Medical Examination, 1985, pp 365–366.
10. Lee J: Airway maintenance in the morbidly obese. Anesthesiol Rev 7:33–36, 1980.
11. Polk SL: Anesthesia for the morbidly obese patient. Trends Anesthesiol 6: 3–9, 1987.
12. Roizen MF: Anesthetic implications of concurrent diseases. In Miller RD: Anesthesia, 4th ed. New York, Churchill Livingstone, 1994, pp 903–1014.
13. Snyder DS, Humphrey LS: Evaluation of the obese patient. In Rogers MC, Covino BG, Tinker JH, Longnecker DE (eds): Principles and Practice of Anesthesiology. St. Louis, Mosby, 1993, pp 514–532.
14. Stoelting RK, Dierdorf SF: Anesthesia and Co-Existing Disease, 3rd ed. New York, Churchill Livingstone, 1993, pp 384–388.
15. Yao FF, Artusio JF: Anesthesiology: Problem-Oriented Patient Management, 3rd ed. Philadelphia, J.B. Lippincott, 1993, pp 715–766.

59. ANESTHESIA FOR TRAUMA

Laurel Mahonee, M.D., and Matt Flaherty, M.D.

1. Compare the death rate and years of potential life lost (YPLL) for trauma, heart disease, and cancer.

Trauma causes devastating loss of life; it is encountered by anesthesiologists throughout the world. Trauma death rates in the United States are surpassed only by death from heart disease, cancer, and stroke. The years of potential life lost before age 65 (YPLL-65) for trauma is generally larger than the combined YPLL-65 for heart disease and cancer. These statistics emphasize the fact that victims of trauma are often young.

2. Name the more common conditions that predispose trauma patients to increased anesthetic risk.

Trauma is highly variable in its pattern of injury. However, many common conditions in trauma victims pose increased anesthetic risk. **Depressed level of consciousness** may lead to hypoventilation, loss of protective airway reflexes, inappropriate behavior, and decreased ability to examine and obtain a history from the patient. **Full stomachs** increase the risk of pulmonary aspiration of gastric contents. **Hypothermia and major blood loss**, either obvious or concealed internally, are common. **Alcohol and drug ingestion** is often associated with major trauma, particularly with death from trauma. All of the above conditions require specific anesthetic management strategies to optimize patient outcome.

3. At what times is trauma most common?

Although trauma is unpredictable, most trauma centers in the U.S. report the highest incidence of trauma at night, on weekends, and in summer months.

4. What is the golden hour?

The golden hour is the first hour after injury. Death from trauma has a trimodal distribution. About 50% of victims die in the first seconds to minutes, usually of injuries that are not treatable by current surgical techniques. Another 30% die in the next few hours, usually of major hemorrhage. The remainder of deaths occur days to weeks later as a result of sepsis or multiple organ failure. Anesthesia has its greatest effect in initial treatment and early surgical therapy for patients who survive the immediate injury. If resuscitation from severe hypovolemic shock occurs within 30 minutes, 50% of patients survive acutely; after 60 minutes only 10% survive. Early, aggressive resuscitation also may improve late outcome.

5. Paramedics aboard an air ambulance notify the trauma center that an incoming patient has a Glasgow Coma Scale (GCS) score of 3. What is the significance of this score?

The GCS is a system for assessment of patients with brain injury. It is frequently cited in the literature as a means of comparing patients or groups of patients with head injury. The actual score is composed of scores for best eye opening and best motor and verbal responses. The scores range from 3–15, with higher scores indicating higher levels of consciousness. The GCS can be used to document state of central nervous system dysfunction before and after anesthesia. Generally the GCS for severe head injury is 9 or less; for moderate injury, 9–12; and for minor injury, 12 and higher. The incoming patient has the lowest possible score, which indicates no eye opening and no motor or verbal responses. The Advanced Trauma Life Support (ATLS) protocol calls for immediate tracheal intubation for airway protection and ventilation of all patients with a GCS ≤ 8.

6. Describe the likely vital signs of a patient who has lost 10% and then 30% of blood volume.

Healthy patients who acutely lose 10–15% of blood volume may experience mild (if any) anxiety and pain associated with the trauma. Changes in blood pressure, heart rate, pulse pressure, urine output, and respiratory rate are usually minimal. As the loss increases to 20–25% of blood volume, the vital signs become deranged. A patient with an acute loss of 30% of blood volume typically has a systolic blood pressure of 70–90 mmHg and a diastolic blood pressure > 50–60 mmHg; in addition, the heart rate usually increases to 120–130 beats per minute, the pulse pressure narrows to 20–30 mmHg, urine output falls to 5–15 ml/hr, and the respiratory rate increases to 30–40 breaths per minute.

7. What is the initial therapy for hypovolemic shock?

Hypovolemia shock occurs when the vascular tree is inadequately filled; blood returning to the heart (preload) is insufficient to sustain cardiac output and blood pressure. Blood leaving the heart is shunted to organs critical for survival. The brain and heart are perfused at the expense of low perfusion states in the muscles, skin, and abdominal viscera. Initial therapy for hypovolemia is replacement of the lost volume with crystalloid infusion. The volume administered is 3 times the estimated blood loss. Patients who have lost more than 25–30% of blood volume are likely to require transfusion with packed red blood cells.

8. How should the hypovolemic patient be monitored?

The standard noninvasive monitors are blood pressure, electrocardiogram, pulse oximetry, esophageal stethoscope, temperature, urinary catheter, and end-tidal CO_2. Arterial catheters are often placed to monitor blood pressure continuously and to draw frequent blood samples. Central venous and possibly pulmonary artery pressures are also monitored, particularly when the patient fails to respond as expected to volume resuscitation.

9. Outline the initial management of a an unconscious 70-kg patient who has lost 2000 ml of blood.

As in all types of resuscitation, the airway and breathing must be addressed first. All trauma patients are assumed to have full stomachs. For protection of the airway against pulmonary aspiration of gastric contents and for maintenance of oxygenation and ventilation, the patient must undergo immediate tracheal intubation and ventilation with 100% oxygen. The rapid-sequence intubation technique is frequently used (see question 11). The patient has lost approximately 40% of blood volume. The replacement of volume with crystalloid and lost blood cells with packed red blood cells (PRBCs) is the next priority. If cross-matched blood is not available, the transfusion of O-negative PRBCs may support the circulation until type-specific or cross-matched PRBCs are available. If more than 2 units of O-negative whole blood are given, further transfusion also should be with O-negative blood. O-negative whole blood (whole blood contains significantly more plasma and therefore more antibody than PRBCs) contains antibodies to A,B, and Rh antigens and may lead to hemolysis of red blood cells carrying these antigens. Hemolysis of the patient's remaining red cells also may occur if the patient carries the A, B, or Rh antigens.

10. What is the significance of lactic acidosis in a trauma patient?

Lactate is a product of anaerobic metabolism at the cellular level. Any tissue experiencing inadequate oxygen delivery may be a source of lactate in trauma patients. When significant lactic acidosis is present, the patient's circulatory status must be optimized. Treatment of lactic acidosis with sodium bicarbonate infusion in the presence of hypoperfusion may mask the true condition of tissues that are marginally perfused and has not been shown to improve outcome.

11. Why is the rapid-sequence induction frequently used for airway management in trauma patients?

The rapid-sequence induction is used because it minimizes the time between onset of loss of airway reflexes and protection of the airway with a cuffed endotracheal tube. All trauma patients are considered to have a full stomach, which places them at increased risk for aspiration. Other factors that increase the risk of pulmonary aspiration of gastric contents include decreased gastric motility, air swallowing and gastric distention, decreased gastric pH, and decreased esophageal tone secondary to ethanol. The usual rapid-sequence induction begins with preoxygenation of the patient for 3–5 minutes. Intravenous anesthetics used to produce immediate unconsciousness include midazolam, thiopental, ketamine, or etomidate. Reduced doses are used in trauma patients because of contracted blood volume. The muscle relaxant of choice is succinylcholine, which has the fastest onset of paralysis sufficient for intubation. After administration of the anesthetic and succinylcholine, pressure is applied firmly over the cricoid ring (Sellick maneuver) to prevent regurgitation of gastric contents. In 50% of adults studied, 10 pounds of pressure is required to seal the esophagus. The patient is intubated as soon as adequate muscle relaxation is achieved (usually around 45–60 seconds). The endotracheal tube cuff is immediately inflated. The presence of end-tidal CO_2 is confirmed, and breath sounds are auscultated over the chest before the cricoid pressure is released. Positive pressure ventilation is usually avoided during the rapid-sequence induction to minimize the risk of aspiration.

12. What are the alternatives to rapid-sequence induction?
Patients who are conscious and can protect their airway may be intubated awake. Local anesthetics, topical or injected at the superior laryngeal nerves, provide airway anesthesia and facilitate awake intubation. Modified rapid-sequence inductions are also commonly used. This technique is similar to rapid-sequence induction but uses ventilation by facemask and cricoid pressure. If succinylcholine is contraindicated, a nondepolarizing muscle relaxant is chosen; typically it is administered in a large dose (2–3 times the usual intubating dose) for rapid onset of action. Modified rapid-sequence inductions are also useful when interruption of ventilation during the traditional rapid-sequence induction would be detrimental. When the airway is so grossly distorted by trauma that conventional direct laryngoscopy is likely to be difficult, the options of awake fiberoptic intubation and awake cricothyrotomy with local anesthetic are sometimes used.

13. How does trauma to the cervical spine modify the approach to the airway?
The ideal technique for intubating patients with a cervical spine fracture is awake intubation with the flexible fiberoptic bronchoscope while the patient's neck is immobilized in a cervical collar. Conditions favoring this technique include a spontaneously breathing and cooperative patient and the absence of blood and debris in the upper airway. Some anesthesiologists use awake nasal intubations with the patient in the cervical collar. This approach can be technically difficult and is contraindicated in patients with basilar skull fractures. Also commonly used is oral intubation with manual in-line stabilization. The anterior half of the cervical collar is removed, cricoid pressure is applied, and rapid-sequence or modified rapid-sequence induction is initiated. As the anesthesiologist begins laryngoscopy, stabilization is applied by an assistant to minimize cervical extention. Consultation with a neurosurgeon is advised, and the stabilization may be performed by the neurosurgeon. The **Bullard laryngoscope** is a rigid fiberoptic laryngoscope that significantly decreases cervical spine mobility during intubation. Bullard laryngoscopy causes less extension at the atlantooccipital, atlantoaxial, and C3–C4 joints. In addition, evidence suggests that Bullard laryngoscopy allows better visualization of the larynx than either the Miller or Macintosh laryngoscope.

14. The patient's trachea is intubated and mechanically ventilated, but a tension pneumothorax suddenly develops. What are the common findings?
Pneumothoraces may develop quickly with positive pressure ventilation. On inspection the chest may rise unevenly with inspiration. The breath sounds become unequal. Percussion of the chest over the pneumothorax is tympanitic. The trachea may shift away from the affected side. Neck veins may become distended. The patient becomes progressively more hypotensive, and peak airway pressures progressively rise. Immediate treatment for tension pneumothorax is the placement of a large-bore needle through the chest wall in the second intercostal space in the midclav-

icular line. The needle should be left in place until a tube thoracostomy is performed. Tension pneumothorax is a clinical diagnosis; **do not delay treatment for radiologic confirmation** of this life-threatening condition.

15. How may a pulmonary contusion manifest during general anesthesia?
Blunt chest trauma may result in pulmonary contusion, a major cause of posttraumatic morbidity and mortality. Often associated with pulmonary contusion are multiple rib fractures. Pulmonary contusions decrease the ability of the lung to exchange gas. Hematoma and edema are often progressive. During mechanical ventilation peak airway pressures gradually rise, whereas oxygen saturation falls. Alveolar membranes in contused lung tissue lose integrity and begin to leak. Pulmonary edema develops, often aggravated by massive fluid resuscitation. Therapeutic measures include increased inspired oxygen concentration, positive end-expiratory pressure, and assessment of volume status. Optimal pain management also may help to improve gas exchange.

16. The patient becomes hypoxemic and peak airway pressures have doubled over 1 hour. How is tension pneumothorax differentiated from pulmonary contusion?
Both conditions may be caused by blunt chest trauma; penetrating trauma is more likely to cause tension pneumothorax.

Pulmonary Contusion vs. Tension Pneumothorax

SIGN	PULMONARY CONTUSION	TENSION PNEUMOTHORAX
Hypoxemia	+	+
Increased airway pressure	+	+
Tympany on percussion	–	+
Differential chest rise on inspiration	–	+
Tracheal shift	–	+
Bilateral breath sounds	+	–
Pulmonary edema, rales	+	–

17. Describe the presentation of a cardiac contusion under general anesthesia.
Blunt chest trauma may cause cardiac contusion. Associated injuries include sternal fractures, multiple rib fractures, and pulmonary contusion. Because it lies immediately posterior to the sternum, the contused myocardium is most often the right ventricle. After contusion cardiac muscle may recover or progress to complete infarction. The function of the right heart and electrical conduction system may be compromised. Under general anesthesia the primary electrocardiographic manifestations are atrial and ventricular dysrhythmias. The right ventricle may fail, causing the central venous pressure to rise and the pulmonary artery pressure and cardiac output to fall. Initial therapy for cardiac contusion involves treatment of arrhythmias, ensuring the absence of cardiac tamponade, and increasing central venous pressure to optimize right ventricular output.

18. What is Beck's triad?
Beck's triad consists of hypotension, distant heart sounds, and distended neck veins, the classic signs associated with cardiac tamponade. Central venous pressure is increased, because right atrial filling is impaired. Stroke volume decreases, and tachycardia may compensate for decreased cardiac output. Some patients have electrical alternans, a rhythmic variation in ECG voltage that originates as the heart begins to float more freely in the expanded pericardium, causing axis shifts.

19. A patient with undetected cardiac tamponade undergoes general anesthesia for laparotomy. What happens to cardiac filling as positive pressure ventilation begins?
Cardiac tamponade may arise from either blunt or penetrating trauma. When bleeding into the pericardial space causes pericardial pressures to equal or exceed right atrial pressures, cardiac

filling is impaired. Positive pressure ventilation further decreases venous return and may greatly exacerbate the reduction in cardiac output.

20. A patient with blunt chest trauma develops hypotension and increased central venous pressure (CVP) during emergency left thoracotomy. Differentiate cardiac tamponade from cardiac contusion.

Either condition may arise after blunt chest trauma, or the two may coexist.

Cardiac Contusion vs. Cardiac Tamponade

SIGN	CARDIAC CONTUSION	CARDIAC TAMPONADE
Elevated central venous pressure	+	+
Hypotension	+	+
Distant heart sounds	−	+
Dysrhythmias	Common	Uncommon
Hypotension exacerbated by positive pressure ventilation	Minimal	+
Pulsus paradoxus (spontaneous ventilation)	−	+

In addition, the pericardium can be visualized during thoracotomy; if tamponade is present, the pericardium is tense.

21. What risks are incurred when trauma patients are given analgesia and/or sedation?

Analgesia may mask undiagnosed conditions. Hypovolemic patients maintain vascular tone through massive secretion of catecholamines. Analgesia may decrease the catecholamine release and precipitate cardiovascular collapse. Sedation may cause hypoventilation, loss of airway reflexes, pulmonary aspiration of gastric contents, hypotension, disorientation, combativeness, vomiting, and increased intracranial pressure. Sedation of trauma patients, if done at all, should be accompanied by continuous monitoring of vital sign and mental status. The patient should remain conscious and oriented at all times.

22. Which induction agents are best for trauma patients?

Far more important than the particular drug is the dose given. Thiopental and propofol are appropriate for some trauma patients if given in reduced dosages. The intravascular volume is much smaller in hypovolemic patients; thus usual doses may result in higher-than-expected plasma concentrations. Some hypotensive, conscious patients benefit from induction with ketamine, which may increase both blood pressure and heart rate. Ketamine, however, may depress the myocardium in severely hypovolemic patients or when endogenous catecholamines are depleted. Fentanyl has minimal cardiac depressive action but may cause a drop in endogenous catecholamine output. Patients with massive blood loss may be unconscious; little or no induction agent is required. Etomidate is often used in hemodynamically unstable patients because of its minimal effect on hemodynamic variables.

Most trauma patients are intubated with succinylcholine during a rapid-sequence induction. It is generally wise to avoid muscle relaxants associated with histamine release, such as curare or atracurium. Nondepolarizing muscle relaxants with minimal hemodynamic changes, such as rocuronium and vecuronium, are commonly used in trauma (see question 12).

23. Is regional anesthesia used for trauma?

Major conduction blockade causes extensive sympathetic nervous system blockade and consequently extensive vasodilation. Spinal and epidural anesthesia may lead to hypotension if vasodilation occurs in patients with insufficient intravascular volume. Regional extremity anesthesia, such as brachial plexus blockade, may be appropriate for limited extremity trauma. Trauma patients are also prone to coagulopathies, which may increase the risk of hematoma after needle insertion.

24. When are trauma patients prone to coagulopathy?

Coagulopathies often begin after transfusion of approximately 1 blood volume (10–12 units of packed red blood cells). Dilutional thrombocytopenia is most common, because packed red blood cells have no functioning platelets. After 1 blood volume of transfusion the platelet count usually falls to less than 100,000. Plasma coagulation factors are also decreased (~ 40% of normal) after transfusion of 1 blood volume. This level of coagulation factors may or may not be adequate; plasma transfusion should be guided by laboratory assay of coagulation. Diffuse intravascular coagulopathy and fibrinolysis may occur after massive transfusion. Patients with increasing shock and tissue ischemia are particularly at risk. Hypothermia induces coagulopathy through alterations in platelet number and function, inhibition of coagulation enzymes, and possibly increased fibrinolytic activity.

25. What is the best intravenous line for fluid resuscitation?

The antecubital veins are easily accessible and accept almost any flow rate of infusion. The catheter should be the largest standard intravenous line available, commonly 14 gauge. The Hagen-Poiseuille equation relates flow directly to the radius to the fourth power. The length of a catheter is inversely related to the flow; therefore the shortest catheter is preferable. Systems for rapid delivery of warm intravenous fluids include the Level 1 System (delivers 500 ml/min at 35°C) and the Rapid Infusion System (delivers 1500 ml/min at 35°C).

26. Describe management of the pregnant trauma patient.

The patient should be positioned with left uterine displacement. Immediate consultation with an obstetrician to ascertain the viability of the fetus is advised. If fetal distress occurs, an emergency cesarean section may be required. If ultrasound or fetal heart tones indicate fetal demise and cesarean section is not indicated, all efforts are directed toward resuscitation of the mother. If the fetus is viable. fetal heart tones should be monitored continuously throughout resuscitation and surgery. After surgery the patient may experience premature labor. Monitoring for uterine contractions may detect premature labor and allow intervention, if necessary.

Regional anesthesia may be preferable to avoid airway complications. Inability to intubate the edematous pregnant airway and aspiration during attempted intubation are the most common complications associated with anesthesia during pregnancy. Desaturation occurs more quickly during pregnancy because of decreased functional residual capacity and increased oxygen consumption. Epidural or continuous spinal anesthesia may achieve an adequate block more slowly and thus allow replacement of intravascular volume. Pregnant patients experience a dilutional anemia with hematocrit levels at a nadir (usually in the low 30s) during the sixth month.This fact should be kept in mind during assessment of initial blood loss and volume status.

27. Why is it important to keep trauma patients euthermic?

As body temperature drops, a number of pathologic events occur. Shivering may increase oxygen consumption by up to 400%. Patients with marginal oxygen delivery may not tolerate shivering without arterial oxygen desaturation. Coagulopathy tends to develop with decreased core temperature. An increase in plasma catecholamine compromises peripheral circulation, as does a fall in cardiac output. As temperatures fall below 33°C, supraventricular dysrhythmias are common. Below 28°C, ventricular dysrhythmias and fibrillation are common. Heat loss occurs through radiation, evaporation, convection, and conduction. Radiation is most significant, causing 60% of total heat loss. Warming the OR is the most effective means of minimizing heat loss in surgical patients. Warm intravenous fluids, lower fresh gas flow rates, heat-moisture exchange devices in the breathing circuit, and warming blankets also help to maintain euthermia.

BIBLIOGRAPHY

1. Abrams K: Preanesthetic evaluation. In Grande CM: Textbook of Trauma Anesthesia and Critical Care. St Louis, Mosby, 1993, pp 421–431.
2. Ginsberg B, et al: Onset and duration of neuromuscular blockade following high-dose vecuronium administration. Anesthesiology 71:201–205, 1989.
3. Hastings RH, Vigil AC, Hanna R, et al: Cervical spine movement during laryngoscopy with Bullard, Macintosh, and Miller laryngoscopes. Anesthesiology 82:859–869, 1995.
4. Landow L, Shahnarian A: Efficacy of large bore intravenous fluid administration sets designed for rapid volume resuscitation. Crit Care Med 18:540, 1990.
5. Majernick TG, Bieniek R, Houston JB, et al: Cervical spine movement during orotracheal intubation. Ann Emerg Med 15:417–420, 1986.
6. Mizock BA, Falk JL: Lactic acidosis in critical illness. Crit Care Med 20:80–91, 1992.
7. Pavlin EG: Hypothermia in traumatized patients.In Grande CM: Textbook of Trauma Anesthesia and Critical Care. St Louis, Mosby, 1993, pp 1131–1139.
8. Priano L: Trauma. In Barash PG, Cullen BF, Stoelting RK (eds): Clinical Anesthesia. Philadelphia, J.B. Lippincott, 1989, pp 1365–1378.
9. Ryder IG, Brown D: Anesthetic risks for trauma patients. In Grande CM: Textbook of Trauma Anesthesia and Critical Care. St Louis, Mosby,1993, pp 445–452.
10. Schumaker PT, Cain SM: The concept of critical oxygen delivery. Intens Care Med 13:223–229, 1987.
11. White PF, Way WI, Trevor AJ: Ketamine—its pharmacology and therapeutic uses. Anesthesiology 56: 119–136, 1982.
12. Velanovich V: Crystalloid versus colloid fluid resuscitation: A meta analysis of mortality. Surgery 105:65–71, 1990.

60. ANESTHESIA AND BURNS

Alma N. Juels, M.D.

1. Who gets burned?

Approximately 70,000 people are hospitalized in the United States for thermal injury; one-half are children. Over 2 million burns require medical attention. Of thermal-related deaths, one-third are children younger than 15 years of age. The highest incidence occurs in children younger than 5 years of age. The majority of burns are thermal injuries. Electrical burns usually cause tissue destruction by thermal injury and associated injuries. In chemical burns, the degree of injury depends on the particular chemical, its concentration, and duration of exposure.

2. What systems are affected by burns?

All physiologic functions can be affected by burns, including the cardiovascular and respiratory systems, metabolism, gastrointestinal tract, kidney, endocrine glands, immune system, coagulation response, and liver.

3. How is the cardiovascular system affected?

A transient decrease in cardiac output is followed by a hyperdynamic response. In the acute phase organ and tissue perfusion decrease because of hypovolemia, depressed myocardial function, increased blood viscosity, and release of vasoactive substances. The acute phase starts immediately after injury; the second phase of burn injury, termed the metabolic phase, begins about 48 hours after injury and involves increased blood flow to organs and tissues. Geriatric patients may have a delayed or nonexisting second phase. Hypertension of unknown cause develops and may be quite extensive.

4. What is the cause of respiratory failure?

Respiratory problems can be due to inhalation of flames, smoke, steam, or toxic gases. Injury to the respiratory tract is identified by facial burns, singed facial or nose hairs, sooty sputum, and respiratory distress or wheezing. Steam or chemical inhalation may present with tracheobronchial edema, ulceration, or bronchospasm, which may cause alveolar damage. Heat from the inhalation injury damages the airways, especially the upper portion, and causes swelling, even to the extent of complete glottic closure and obstruction. Patients develop symptoms of hoarseness, stridor, and tachypnea. Carbon monoxide poisoning is the most common immediate cause of death from a fire. The clinical course of the pulmonary insult is characterized by acute pulmonary insufficiency during the first 36 hours. Pulmonary edema may develop 6–72 hours after injury as a result of fluid shifts and massive fluid resuscitation. Pulmonary complications can be reduced by early diagnosis, high index of suspicion, and aggressive treatment; therefore, early intubation or tracheostomy is appropriate.

5. What problems occur with the gastrointestinal tract?

Adynamic ileus may occur at any time after a burn injury. Acute ulceration of the stomach or duodenum, referred to as Curling's ulcer, may lead to gastrointestinal bleeding. The small and large intestine may develop acute necrotizing enterocolitis with abdominal distention, hypotension, and bloody diarrhea. During the second and third week after injury acalculous cholecystitis is common.

6. How is renal function affected?

Renal blood flow and glomerular filtration diminish immediately, activating the renin-angiotensin-aldosterone system and causing release of antidiuretic hormone. Results include retention of sodium and water and loss of potassium, calcium, and magnesium.

7. What is the endocrine response to a burn?

The endocrine response to a thermal burn involves massive release of catecholamines, glucagon, adrenocorticotropic hormone, antidiuretic hormone, renin, angiotensin, and aldosterone. Glucose levels are elevated, and patients are susceptible to nonketotic hyperosmolar coma.

8. How is the blood affected?

Blood viscosity is increased. Clotting factors and platelets decline during the first 24–48 hours after burn injury because of dilutional factors. The body responds with increased production of clotting factors, and patients develop a hypercoagulable state that usually gives rise to disseminated intravascular coagulation. Suppression of erythrocyte production with decreased erythrocyte survival may require transfusion around the fifth day after injury. Erythrocyte hemolysis may result from direct heat damage. Red blood cells may have a decreased half-life for up to 2 weeks after the burn because of microangiopathic hemolytic anemia. If surgical procedures are required, they should be done within the first 24 hours or delayed until the platelet and coagulation tests start to increase, if possible. The average patient with 50% burn requires 10–20 units of blood during hospitalization. An attempt should be made to keep the hematocrit over 35%.

9. What are the consequences of skin damage?

The skin is the largest organ of the human body. It has three principal functions, all of which are disrupted by burn injury: (1) it is an important sensory organ; (2) it performs a major role in thermoregulation for the dissipation of metabolic heat; and (3) it acts as a barrier to protect the body against the entrance of microorganisms in the environment. As different layers of skin are injured, a burn patient may have extensive evaporative heat and water loss, and loss of thermoregulation may lead to hypothermia. Such patients have a profound risk of infection and sepsis.

10. How are burns classified?

A general rule of thumb is that the size of the hand is equal to 1% of body surface area (BSA); more commonly the extent of injury is estimated with the rule of nines. The head and neck are 9% of the total body surface area (TBSA), the arms and hands are 9%, and the thighs and legs are 18%. The anterior trunk and posterior trunk (including the buttocks) are 18%, respectively, and the perineum is 1%. In infants and young children, estimations are different because of growth changes and relatively larger head.

The severity of the burn is graded by its depth, which depends on the extent of tissue destruction. **First-degree burns** involve the upper layers of the epidermis, the skin is painful and appears red and slightly edematous, much like a sunburn. **Second-degree burns** occur when tissue damage extends into the dermis, which is still lined with intact epithelium that proliferates and regenerates new skin. Second-degree burns develop blisters and have red or whitish areas that are very painful. **Third-degree burns** are due to the destruction of all layers of skin, including the nerve endings; therefore, there is no sensation. Skin will not regenerate, because part of the dermis with hair follicles, sweat glands, and other adnexal structures are required for reepithelialization. The skin appears charred. **Fourth-degree burns** involve destruction of all layers of skin and extend into the subcutaneous tissue, muscle, and fascia—even as far as the bone.

11. How are patients with burns resuscitated?

Burns cause a generalized increase in capillary permeability with loss of fluid and protein into interstitial tissue; this loss is greatest in the first 12 hours. Several formulas are recommended for treating burn shock in the first 24 hours. The **Parkland formula** involves giving 4 ml of lactated Ringer solution (LR) per kg body weight per percent of total body surface area burned; one-half of the calculated amount is given during the first 8 hours and the remainder over the next 16 hours, in addition to daily maintenance fluid. The **Brooke formula** requires 3 ml of LR per kg body weight per percent of BSA burned; one-half of the calculated amount is given in the first 8 hours and one-half in the next 16 hours On the second day after injury, capillary integrity is restored, and the amount of required fluid is decreased. Further administration of an electrolyte-containing solution may result in undesired edema. Infusion of crystalloid is decreased after the first day, and colloids are administered. The endpoint of fluid therapy is hemodynamic stability and urine output at a rate of 1 ml/kg/hr.

12. What is important in the preoperative history?
It is important to know at what time the burn occurred for fluid replacement. The type of burn is also important to assess airway damage, associated injuries, and the possibility of more extensive tissue damage than initially appreciated (electrical burns). A standard preoperative anesthetic history also must be taken, including present medical conditions, medications, allergies, anesthetic history, and other relevant information.

13. What should the anesthesiologist look for on the preoperative physical exam?
Most important to the anesthesiologist is the status of the patient's airway. Excessive sputum, wheezing, and diminished breath sounds may suggest inhalation injury to the lungs. Burns produce intestinal ileus, which increases the risk of aspiration; therefore, a nasogastric tube should be placed preoperatively. One should make note of all lines already placed and access areas where more may be placed if needed. The airway should be evaluated completely for associated signs of trauma.

14. What preoperative tests are required before induction?
Special emphasis should be placed on correcting the acid-base disturbance and electrolyte imbalance during the acute phase. Therefore, an arterial blood gas analysis and a chemistry panel are required. A chest radiograph also should be obtained in patients suspected of smoke inhalation, although a normal chest radiograph does not preclude significant injury. In the presence of carbon monoxide (CO) poisoning the pulse oximeter may overestimate the saturation of hemoglobin; therefore, a carboxyhemoglobin level, determined by cooximetry, may be helpful to assess the degree of CO poisoning and to guide treatment. Coagulation tests are also helpful, because such patients often have bleeding diathesis.

15. What monitors are needed to give a safe anesthetic?
Access for monitoring may be difficult. Needle electrodes or ECG pads sewn on the patient may be required for the ECG monitor and nerve stimulator. A blood pressure cuff may be placed on a burned area, but an arterial catheter may be better and allows frequent blood analysis. Temperature measurement is a must because of exaggerated decreases in body temperature. Invasive monitors are placed as deemed necessary, taking into account the patient's previous baseline medical condition. If the procedure involves a large amount of blood loss, central venous pressure (right atrial pressure) should be monitored through an introducer sheath. If the patient becomes unstable, a pulmonary artery catheter should be inserted to measure pulmonary artery pressures, pulmonary capillary wedge pressure, cardiac output, systemic vascular resistance, and pulmonary vascular resistance and to manage the patient with the proper pressors or fluid bolus.

16. Are drug responses altered?
Drugs administered acutely by any route other than intravenously have delayed absorption, whereas intravenous and inhaled drugs have increased effects on the brain and heart. After 48 hours the plasma albumin concentration is decreased, and albumin-bound drugs, such as benzodiazepines and anticonvulsants, have an increased free fraction and therefore a prolonged effect. The effect of drugs metabolized in the liver by oxidative metabolism (phase-I reaction) is prolonged (e.g., diazepam). However, drugs metabolized in the liver by conjugation (phase II) are not affected (e.g., lorazepam). Opioid requirements are increased, most likely because of habituation since pharmacokinetics seem to be unaltered. Ketamine may cause hypotension secondary to hypovolemia and depleted catecholamine stores, exerting its direct cardiodepressant effect. Thiopental, propofol, and etomidate may cause hypotension secondary to hypovolemia in the acute phase.

17. How are muscle relaxants affected?

From about 24 hours after injury until the burn has healed, succinylcholine may cause hyperkalemia, leading to cardiac arrest, because of proliferation of extrajunctional neuromuscular junction receptors. On the other hand, burned patients tend to be resistant to the effects of nondepolarizing muscle relaxants for the same reasons and may need 2–5 times the normal dose.

18. What drugs are good for burn patients?

Ketamine is especially good for dressing changes and escharatomies, because it provides good somatic analgesia. All anesthetic drugs may be used, but opioids must be considered because of the excruciating pain; long-acting opioids are best.

19. Describe specific features of electric burns.

Care of electrical burns is similar to care of thermal burns, except that the extent of injury may be misleading. Areas of devitalized tissue may be present under normal-appearing skin. The extent of superficial tissue injury may result in underestimation of initial fluid requirements. Myoglobinuria is common, and urine output must be kept high to avoid renal damage. The development of neurologic complications after electrical burns is common, including peripheral neuropathies or spinal cord deficits. Many believe that regional anesthesia is contraindicated. Cataract formation may be another late sequela of burn injury. Cardiac dysrhythmias and ventricular fibrillation or asystole may occur up to 48 hours after injury. Apnea may result from tetanic contraction of respiratory muscles or cerebral medullary injury.

20. How is myoglobinuria treated?

Renal blood flow may be affected by damage to renal parenchyma from myoglobinuria following rhabdomyonecrosis and hemoglobinuria due to hemolysis. Fresh-frozen plasma contains haptoglobin, which binds free hemoglobin, and may protect renal function. Vigorous fluid resuscitation as well as maintenance of urine output with osmotic diuretics (mannitol) and administration of bicarbonate to alkalinize the urine also help to protect the kidneys.

21. Describe carbon monoxide (CO) poisoning.

CO poisoning results from inhalation of CO produced by fires, exhaust from internal combustion engines, cooking stoves, and charcoal stoves. Its affinity for hemoglobin is 200 times that of oxygen. When CO combines with hemoglobin, it forms carboxyhemoglobin (COHb), and the pulse oximeter may overestimate saturation of hemoglobin with oxygen. Symptoms are due to tissue hypoxia, shift in the oxygen-hemoglobin dissociation curve, direct cardiovascular depression, and inhibition of the cytochrome system. Signs and symptoms depend on the carboxyhemoglobin concentrations, with 0% producing no symptoms and 70% leading to death. All systems may be affected. Treatment is initiated with 100% oxygen, which decreases the serum half-life of COHb. Hyperbaric oxygen therapy is recommended in severe cases. Indications for hyperbaric oxygen include coma, myocardial ischemia, persistent symptoms after 4 hours of 100% oxygen, or acidosis; hyperbaric oxygen is also indicated in neonates.

BIBLIOGRAPHY

1. Baxter W: Emergency treatment of burn injury. Ann Emerg Med 12:1305–1315, 1988.
2. Braen RG: Thermal injuries (burns). In Rosen P, Baker FJ, Braen GR, et al (eds): Emergency Medicine, Concepts and Clinical Practice, 2nd ed. St. Louis, Mosby, 1988, pp 573–584.
3. Dimick AR.: Burns and electrical injuries. In Tintinalli JE., Krome RL, Ruiz E (eds): Emergency Medicine: A Comprehensive Study Guide, 2nd ed. New York, McGraw-Hill, 1988, pp 796–801.
4. Firestone LL, Lebowitz PW, Cook CE.: Clinical Anesthesia Procedures of the Massachusetts General Hospital, 3rd ed. Boston, Little, Brown, 1988, pp 447–469.
5. Herndon DN, et al: Pulmonary injury in burn patients. Surg Clin North Am 67:31–46, 1987.
6. Martyn J: Clinical pharmacology and drug therapy in the burned patient. Anesthesiology 65:67–75, 1986.
7. Meyer AA, Trunkey DD: Shock and trauma. In Schrock TR: Handbook of Surgery, 8th ed. Greenbrae, CA, Jones Medical Publications, 1982, pp 1–29.
8. Stoelting RK, Dierdorf SF: Anesthesia and Co-existing Disease, 3rd ed. New York, Churchill Livingstone, 1993, pp 619–627.

61. HIV-RELATED DISEASE

Stuart G. Rosenberg, M.D.

1. Why is it important for the anesthesiologist to be familiar with human immunodeficiency virus (HIV)-related disease?

It is estimated that over one million people in the U.S. are infected with the human immunodeficiency virus (HIV). The worldwide estimate is approximately 10 million. Well over 400,000 cumulative cases of acquired immunodeficiency syndrome (AIDS, the full-blown syndrome caused by HIV) have been reported in the U.S. alone. Thus, HIV is widespread and continues to spread rapidly in certain high-risk populations. In fact, among adults aged 25–44, HIV-related disease has become the leading cause of death for men and the fourth leading cause of death for women in the U.S. As the numbers continue to increase, more and more patients will present for surgery and anesthesia. Their surgical problems may be related directly or indirectly or even totally unrelated to HIV. In many urban hospitals, especially on trauma services, the prevalence exceeds 10%. As HIV affects all organ systems, it is imperative to understand not only the types of surgical and medical problems that develop but also the physiologic and pharmacologic implications of administering an anesthetic. It is of equal importance to understand the risks of occupational transmission of the virus from patients to health care workers. The anesthesiologist must ensure that appropriate preventive measures are meticulously followed.

2. What is the cause of AIDS?

HIV, the etiologic agent for AIDS, belongs to the family of human retroviruses and the subfamily of lentiviruses. The four recognized human retroviruses belong to two distinct groups: human T-lymphotropic viruses (HTLV) I and II and HIV viruses 1 and 2. The most common cause of HIV disease is HIV-1.

3. How is AIDS defined?

AIDS is the syndrome caused by HIV-1. The Centers for Disease Control (CDC) definition is quite complex and comprehensive; designed for surveillance purposes, it has been modified several times. The anesthesiologist is best served by viewing HIV-related disease/AIDS as a spectrum of disease ranging from primary infection (with or without an acute HIV syndrome) through asymptomatic infection, to advanced disease with characteristic profound immunosuppression.

4. What are the transmission patterns of HIV?

HIV is a blood-borne virus that is transmitted most commonly through sexual intercourse and parenteral inoculation or from mothers to infants perinatally or via breast-feeding. Blood and its constituents are the most infectious bodily fluids. The more cellular the fluid, the more infectious it is. Other bodily fluids that have been documented to transmit HIV include semen, vaginal secretions, cerebrospinal fluid, and pleural and peritoneal fluid. Reports of isolation of the virus in body fluids such as tears, sweat, saliva, and urine are conflicting; however, none of these has been implicated in transmission. Transfusion of infected blood yields about a 90% infectious rate to the recipient. Blood transfusion in the U.S. is generally safe because of screening of donors. Because some donors with early disease may not have a detectable antibody when blood is donated, a small risk of transmission, estimated between 1:50,000 and 1:100,000 per transfused unit, still exists. Transmission from infected persons to health care workers is a major concern (see question 18).

5. What is the natural history of HIV disease?

Shortly after HIV infection an acute retroviral syndrome associated with a high plasma viral concentration is likely. This syndrome resembles mononucleosis, with fever, malaise, diarrhea, myalgias, sore throat, headache, lymphadenopathy, rash, and oral ulcerations. The syndrome precedes seroconversion to HIV antibody (+) by several weeks to months. The virus predominantly infects white blood cells, most notably CD_4 (helper) lymphocytes. Over a period of years, the virus progressively destroys immune function, ultimately resulting in characteristic opportunistic infections, malignancies, neurologic disease, wasting, and death. The CD_4 lymphocyte counts generally decline over time and correlate well with certain disease processes. For example, *Pneumocystis carinii* pneumonia (PCP), the most common pulmonary infection in AIDS patients, generally does not occur until the CD_4 count decreases below 200. The CD_4 count is useful preoperatively to stage the patient clinically; it indicates disease progression and immune compromise. Early disease is defined as a CD_4 count > 500 cells/ml, intermediate disease as 200–500, late symptomatic disease as 50–200, and advanced AIDS as < 50. Patients with advanced AIDS have a high likelihood of serious infections, malignancies, and death within 12–24 months, even with therapy. Such patients are severely immunocompromised and frequently quite ill (American Society of Anesthesiologists physical status 3 and above), with multisystem organ dysfunction that requires meticulous care by the anesthesiologist.

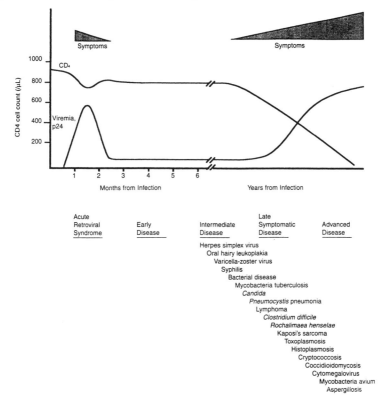

Natural history of HIV disease. Schematic of the natural history of HIV-1 disease over time. The curve labeled viremia, p24 shows the relative viral burden at different stages of disease. Below the figure are the associated opportunistic disease of the relative CD4 cell counts. (From Fischl MA, Volberding PA: HIV disease. In Goldman L (ed): American College of Physicians Medical Knowledge Self-Assessment Program. Philadelphia, American College of Physicians, 1994, p 6, with permission.)

6. When should the anesthesiologist suspect HIV?

History, physical exam, and laboratory data should help to alert one to the possibility of HIV-related disease. Certain medical as well as surgical problems are seen with increasing frequency in the HIV population (see questions 9–15). Of note, most persons currently infected with HIV in the U.S. are asymptomatic. Significant controversy surrounds routine preoperative testing. Some physicians advocate preoperative testing of all patients. Testing for HIV should be obtained in patients with risk factors for the disease or with compatable clinical or laboratory abnormalities. From an occupational risk standpoint, all patients should be treated as if they are infectious, whether from viral hepatitis or HIV. Universal precautions must constantly be observed, especially in a high-risk area such as the operating room (see question 18). The anesthesiologist must maintain a high index of suspicion of HIV-related disease.

When to Suspect HIV Infection

History
  High-risk behaviors or exposures
    Unsafe or promiscuous sex
      Prostitution
      Sex with prostitutes
      Sex with persons at risk for HIV
    Injection drug use
    Blood or blood product transfusion between 1977 and April 1985
    Blood clotting factor concentrate(s) transfusion prior to Januray 1985
  Sexually transmitted disease
  Tuberculosis
  Racial and ethnic minority populations in high-incidence areas of HIV disease
  Homeless persons in high-incidence areas of HIV disease
Symptoms and signs
  Acute retroviral syndrome
    Heterophile antibody-negative mononucleosis syndromes
    Viral syndrome with truncal maculopapular rash
    Aseptic meningitis
  Constitutional symptoms
    Fatigue, malaise, fever, night sweats, anorexia, weight loss
  Generalized lymphadenopathy
  Dermatologic manifestations
    Xerosis, seborrhea, psoriasis, folliculitis, pruritic eruptions, herpes zoster, superficial dermato-
      phytoses, molluscum contagiosum, warts
  Mucous membrane manifestations
    Thrush, aphthous stomatitis, oral hairy leukoplakia, necrotizing gingivitis, severe or frequently
      recurrent orolabial herpes simplex, genital candidiasis, severe or frequently recurrent genital
      herpes, condyloma acuminata, cervical intraepithelial neoplasia
Laboratory findings
  Anemia, leukopenia, lymphocytopenia, atypical lymphocytosis, thrombocytopenia
  CD_4 lymphocytopenia
  Polyclonal hyperglobulinemia
  Elevated lactate dehydrogenase
  Hypocholesterolemia and hypertriglyceridemia

From Fischl MA, Volberding PA: HIV disease. In Goldman L (ed): American College of Physicians Medical Knowledge Self-Assessment Program. Philadelphia, American College of Physicians, 1994, p 4, with permission.

7. What diagnostic tests are done in patients with an increased likelihood of HIV?
Enzyme immunoassay (EIA) for detection of antibodies is the most widely used method for screening for HIV infection. This test is highly sensitive and specific, but false positives do occur, especially in low-risk populations. The Western blot assay is used to confirm positive EIA tests. Additional tests include detection of HIV antigen (P24 antigen), polymerase chain reaction (PCR) techniques, culture of HIV from blood, and HIV-2 Western blot testing.

8. What medications are commonly prescribed to HIV patients? What are their major side effects?

Common Medications for HIV Infection, Indications, and Toxicities

MEDICATION	INDICATION	TOXICITIES
Zidovudine (AZT)	Antiretroviral	Anemia, leukopenia, myopathy
Didanosine (DDI)	Antiretroviral	Pancreatitis, peripheral neuropathy
Zalcitabine (DDC)	Antiretroviral	Pancreatitis, peripheral neuropathy
Stavudine (D4T)	Antiretroviral	Hepatitis, peripheral neuropathy
TMP/SMX	Prophylaxis and treatment of PCP	Rash, fever, neutropenia
Pentamidine	Prophylaxis and treatment of PCP	Intravenous—pancreatitis, hyperkalemia, hypotension, nephritis, hyper- and hypo-glycemia. Aerosolized form may cause bronchospasm
Fluconazole	Candidal infections	Hepatotoxicity
Amphotericin B	Fungal infections	Nephrotoxicity, fever/chills
Acyclovir	Herpes	Nephrotoxicity
Ganciclovir	Cytomegalovirus (CMV)	Neutropenia, increased liver function tests (LFTs), thrombocytopenia
Foscarnet	Herpes, CMV, anti-retroviral	Interstitial nephritis, seizures, hypocalcemia, increased LFTs, diabetes insipidus (DI), fever, electrolyte imbalance (decreased magnesium, potassium, and phosphorus)
Rifabutin	Prophylaxis of *Mycobacterium avium-intracellulare*	Bone marrow depression, increased LFTs, renal failure, diarrhea
Dapsone	PCP prophylaxis	Hemolysis, rash, nephrotic syndrome

TMP/SMX = trimethoprim-sulfamethoxazole, PCP = *Pneumocystis carinii* pneumonia.

9. What are the more common reasons for HIV patients to present for surgery and anesthesia?

Long-term vascular access catheters are frequently required for prolonged parenteral antibiotic administration and chemotherapy. Catheters are routinely placed under conditions of maximal sterility in the operating room, because of the increased incidence of infection. The anesthesiologist ensures optimal monitoring.

Abdominal surgery is also common. Gastrointestinal (GI) symptoms occur in 20–30% of HIV-infected patients, and diagnosis of the acute abdomen may be difficult. Delays in recognition and treatment increase the rate of complications. Of all acute surgical abdomens in the U.S., 2–4% are HIV-infected. The more common conditions requiring emergent surgery in HIV disease include GI tract perforation or obstruction, cholecystitis, cholangitis, acute appendicitis (twice as common as in the general population), inflammatory bowel disease, anorectal disease, hemorrhage, and neoplasia (especially lymphoma and Kaposi's sarcoma).

Open-lung biopsy for the diagnosis of pulmonary infiltrates is occasionally performed, although use has declined because of improved fiberoptic bronchoscopic biopsy techniques. Open-lung biopsy is still indicated when bronchoscopy is contraindicated (e.g., patients with high ventilatory requirements) and the diagnosis is not clear. Such patients are usually critically ill with severely compromised pulmonary function and generally have high ventilatory requirements, such as high minute volume, fractional concentration of oxygen in inspired gas (FiO_2), and positive end-expiratory pressure. Anesthetizing such patients for a thoracotomy may be challenging, because further decrements in pulmonary function from positioning, one-lung anesthesia, volume shifts, or surgery may worsen hypoxemia.

Pulmonary deterioration and the need for tracheal intubation and mechanical ventilation are common. Standard principles of airway management apply, with close attention to aseptic technique and universal precautions. Many patients refuse intubation and mechanical ventilation, and their primary care physician must establish advance care directives before they become critically ill. There also may be an increased role for noninvasive ventilation—such as continuous positive airway pressure (CPAP) by mask, Bi-PAP, or pressure support by mask—to avoid endotracheal intubation.

10. What are the important respiratory complications of HIV?
Virtually every patient with HIV develops pulmonary involvement at some point in the course of disease. Infections, malignancies, and direct HIV effects are common. Early in the disease course, one sees an increased incidence of community-acquired bacterial pneumonias. Over time, as immunity wanes, mycobacterial and other opportunistic infections occur. In late disease, pulmonary function and gas exchange are most assuredly abnormal. The anesthesiologist must pay meticulous attention to optimizing pulmonary function throughout the perioperative period.

Pneumonia secondary to *Pneumocystis carinii* (PCP) is the most common pulmonary pathogen as the CD_4 count falls to 200 and below. Various medical prophylactic regimens have decreased its incidence. The onset is usually insidious with dry cough, dyspnea, fever, and chest pain. Bronchospasm and hypoxemia may occur. PCP also may cause cavitary lung disease, predisposing the patient to pneumothoraces, especially with positive pressure ventilation. Chest radiography usually reveals diffuse interstitial infiltrates, but atypical infiltrates are also seen. The diagnosis is usually easily confirmed with a Giemsa stain of induced sputum or bronchoalveolar lavage. Occasionally patients require lung biopsy. The use of steroids in addition to antibiotics has decreased the incidence of respiratory failure, but when it occurs, the mortality rate is extremely high (80–90%). Severe PCP may produce hemodynamic changes similar to septic shock. Multiple organ failure also may occur.

Many other pulmonary infections also occur. Tuberculosis must always be kept in mind, and appropriate respiratory precautions should be taken in the operating and recovery rooms.

Malignancies such as Kaposi's sarcoma (KS) and lymphoma affect the lung. Adenopathy may cause tracheobronchial compression, leading to airway obstruction under anesthesia. Upright and supine flow-volume loops may show evidence of obstruction related to position. Pleural effusions may compromise pulmonary function, and endobronchial KS may cause massive hemoptysis.

Human immunodeficiency virus directly affects the lungs, causing a destructive pulmonary syndrome similar to emphysema. This syndrome can be diagnosed by pulmonary function testing, which typically shows an increase in lung volumes and decreased flows. Pulmonary artery hypertension resembling primary pulmonary hypertension has been reported. Prognosis is poor.

Upper airway pathology may be infectious or malignant. Of interest, the incidence of infections of the pharynx, supraglottic structures, glottic structures, and trachea is similar to that in the general population. Laryngeal tuberculosis in an HIV-infected patient has been reported to cause airway obstruction. Lymphoma and extensive pharyngeal and tracheobronchial KS also have been reported to cause upper airway obstruction. Emergent tracheotomy has resulted in severe airway hemorrhage and death due to the vascularity of the lesions. Therefore, it may be advisable to attempt orotracheal intubation, if possible.

11. What are the cardiac complications of HIV?
Cardiac involvement in the course of HIV disease is quite common but often clinically silent and may become manifest only during the stress of an anesthetic and surgical procedure. Cardiac involvement usually portends a poor, short-term prognosis. Myocarditis, pericarditis, endocarditis, left ventricular dysfunction, and various dysrhythmias have been reported. Up to 50% of patients with HIV may have abnormal echocardiographic findings at some point in their disease. Approximately 25% have pericardial effusions. Tamponade is rare but has been reported with KS and tuberculosis. Myocarditis, which is more common in advanced AIDS, may be caused by tox-

oplasmosis, disseminated cryptococcosis, group B coxsackievirus, CMV, lymphomas, *Nocardia sp.,* and *Aspergillus sp.* HIV per se may cause a lymphocytic myocarditis. Myocarditis produces a dilated cardiomyopathy. Affected hearts have little reserve. Pulmonary artery catheter monitoring is recommended for operative procedures associated with significant stress and volume shifts. Inotropic or vasodilator therapy should be instituted and cardiodepressant drugs avoided. Preoperative echocardiography may be of value in determining ventricular function, valvular competence, and the hemodynamic significance of pericardial effusions. Large or hemodynamically significant effusions may be drained under local anesthesia before induction. Preoperative treatment of the underlying cause of cardiomyopathy is rarely gratifying and largely anecdotal.

12. What is the differential diagnosis of hypotension in the HIV-infected patient?

In addition to the usual considerations in the differential diagnosis of hypotension, such as a low cardiac output state, sepsis, malnutrition, and hypovolemia, adrenal insufficiency also occurs in HIV-infected patients. Adrenalitis is commonly seen at autopsy, and approproximately 10% of patients with late-stage disease have evidence of adrenal insufficiency. Cytomegalovirus is the most common cause of adrenal gland disease in HIV infection. Other causes include mycobacterial infections, KS, histoplasmosis, cryptococcus, and ketoconazole toxicity. The presence of low serum sodium and high serum potassium should alert one to the possibility of adrenal insufficiency. Treatment consists of exogenous glucocorticords and occasionally mineralocorticoids.

13. What are the pertinent GI complications of HIV?

The majority of patients with HIV disease develop some type of GI distress during their illness. Many develop an acute abdomen, which brings them to surgical attention. Nausea, vomiting, and diarrhea are commonplace and contribute to hypovolemia, malnutrition, electrolyte disturbances, and aspiration. Hepatobiliary involvement, pancreatitis, and esophagitis with reflux is also quite common. Of note, many such patients are achlorhydric; this condition may improve the acid aspiration syndrome but worsen the potential infectious complications of pulmonary aspiration due to bacterial overgrowth. Appropriate aspiration precautions, such as cricoid pressure, rapid sequence induction, or awake intubation, should be considered. Metoclopramide may increase gastroesophageal sphincter tone and gastric motility. Small and large bowel pathology frequently lead to diarrhea with attendant fluid and electrolyte losses.

14. How may HIV neurologic involvement affect an anesthetic?

Neurologic disease, a major component of HIV infection, ranges from AIDS dementia to infectious and neoplastic involvement. Neoplasms such as lymphoma or KS and other focal processes, such as toxoplasmosis or progressive multifocal leukoencephalopathy (PML), may increase intracranial pressure (ICP). Increased ICP may preclude major conduction anesthesia because of the potential for brainstem herniation and necessitate ICP monitoring during general anesthesia. Major conduction anesthesia has been shown to be safe in a prospective study of patients with asymptomatic HIV infection. Many of the above conditions also lead to seizures. Treatment consists of standard antiseizure medications. Spinal cord involvement, peripheral neuropathy, and myopathy are primarily related to the HIV virus. The use of succinylcholine must be carefully evaluated in the face of spinal cord or skeletal muscle involvement to avoid a hyperkalemic response. Serum potassium may already be elevated from renal or adrenal dysfunction.

15. What hematologic abnormalities are seen with HIV?

Anemia is the most common hematologic abnormality in HIV-infected patients. Approximately 75% of patients with AIDS are anemic. Medications such as AZT may be a major contributor to the anemia. Systemic fungal and mycobacterial infections, lymphoma, malnutrition, and parvovirus infection may depress the bone marrow. Neutropenia may be drug-induced or related to infection. Because neutropenic patients are at extremely high risk for nosocomial infections, attention to sterile technique during invasive procedures must be meticulous. A coagulopathy may develop from thrombocytopenia (from idiopathic thrombocytopenic purpura, medications, or bone marrow invasion), liver disease, or malnutrition. Prolongation of the partial thromboplastin time may reflect the presence of a lupuslike anticoagulant and increase the risk for postoperative thromboembolic complications.

16. What about the pharmacology of anesthetic drugs in HIV-infected patients?

Renal and hepatic dysfunction are common. HIV-associated nephropathy may occur early in the disease and progresses to end-stage renal disease requiring dialysis in approximately 1 year. Hepatobiliary disease is also widespread. Drug metabolism is clearly altered during such states. Anesthetic agents must be carefully titrated to effect, because the pharmacokinetics and pharmacodynamics may be significantly altered. Protein binding may be decreased by malnutrition, thus increasing the amount of free active drug. Volume of distribution may be altered in conditions with increased third spacing of fluid such as ascites, pleural effusions, and peripheral edema. Larger initial doses of drugs such as muscle relaxants may be required to attain a given effect. Inhalation agents may demonstrate abnormal uptake and distribution because of underlying pulmonary and cardiac disease. Patients may be more susceptible to cardiovascular depression. Brain involvement with altered mental status renders a patient more susceptible to the central depressant effect of an anesthetic. In addition, neuroleptic anesthetics produce extrapyramidal side effects more frequently.

17. What are the infectious risks to the patient perioperatively?

Although it is generally accepted that the rate of postoperative infectious complications is increased in advanced AIDS, data are scant and conflicting. Data about HIV-positive asymptomatic hemophiliacs has not shown an increased infection rate or drastic change in postoperative CD_4 counts. Asymptomatic HIV-positive patients with orthopedic trauma (especially open fractures) have significantly increased rates of wound and nonwound infections postoperatively. The rate of infections of central venous catheters placed for long-term use in HIV-positive patients is 10 times that of the non-HIV population, even with tunneled catheters. Even patients with early asymptomatic HIV disease have immune dysfunction. Numerous studies indicate that general anesthesia and opiates may have an adverse effect on immune function. Alterations in the composition of circulating lymphocyte subsets, including a reduction in T-helper cells, may occur after an anesthetic. An increase in infectious postoperative complications is therefore not surprising. The anesthesiologist must minimize the risk of postoperative infections by minimizing invasive procedures, using meticulous sterile technique, and ensuring that appropriate prophylactic antibiotics have been given in a timely manner.

18. What are the risks of transmission to the anesthesiologist?

There is a small but definite risk to any health care worker who cares for HIV-infected patients. The risk of transmission following parenteral exposure from a contaminated hollow-bore needle is estimated to be approximately 0.3% compared with hepatitis B and C transmission rates of about 30% and 2%, respectively. The risk of transmission from a skin puncture from a solid-bore suture needle is estimated to be less than that of a hollow-bore needle. Reports of HIV transmission from body fluids such as saliva, tears, sweat, and urine are conflicting. (It appears that the more cellular the fluid, the greater the infectivity.) Patients with higher levels of plasma virus also may be more infective.

The key to decreasing the transmission rate is prevention. Adherence to universal precautions as described by the CDC in 1987 should minimize the risk of HIV infection. Universal precautions mandate that each and every specimen and bodily fluid should be handled as if it contained a blood-borne pathogen. Gloves should be worn, and the health care provider's mucous membranes and skin lesions should be protected. Sharps and spills should be disposed of properly. Recapping of needles should be avoided. Needleless intravenous additive systems and shielded needle systems have great appeal for potentially decreasing the risk of needlestick injury and thus transmission of the virus.

Postexposure management is controversial. All wounds should receive first aid and be documented. Postexposure chemoprophylaxis with AZT is accepted care, but positive data are lacking. Health care workers treated with AZT after an exposure have still seroconverted. Animal models suggest little protection when AZT is given after an exposure. In any event, if postexposure treatment with AZT is chosen, it should be started early, within hours of the exposure.

Again, prevention is key. All health care providers must be educated about the magnitude of risks, mechanisms of transmission, prevention strategies, and postexposure management.

BIBLIOGRAPHY

1. Berkowitz ID: Evaluation of the patient with AIDS and other serious infections. In Rogers MC, Tinker JH, et al (eds): Principles and Practice of Anesthesiology. St. Louis, Mosby, 1993, pp 410–418.
2. Case Records of the Massachusetts General Hospital (Case 34-1993). N Engl J Med 329:645–653, 1993 [review of respiratory failure and PCP in AIDS].
3. Case Records of the Massachusetts General Hospital (Case 44-1992). N Engl J Med 327:1370–1376, 1992 [HIV related myocarditis].
4. Fauci AS, Lane HC: HIV disease: AIDS and related disorders. In Isselbacher KJ, Braunwald E, et al (eds): Harrison's Principles of Internal Medicine,13th ed. New York, McGraw-Hill, 1994, pp 1566–1617.
5. Fischl MA, Volberding PA: HIV disease. In Goldman L (ed): American College of Physicians Medical Knowledge Self-Assessment Program. Philadelphia, American College of Physicians, 1994.
6. Hawley PH, Ronco JJ, et al: Decreasing frequency but worsening mortality of acute respiratory failure secondary to AIDS-related PCP. Chest 106:1456–1459, 1994.
7. Henderson DK: HIV and the Health-Care Worker. American Society of Anesthesiology Refresher Courses 331, 1993.
8. Hughes S, Dailey P, et al: Parturients infected with HIV and regional anesthesia. Anesthesiology 82:32–37, 1995.
9. Ognibene FP: Upper and lower airway manifestations of human immunodeficiency virus infection. ENT J 69:424–431, 1990.
10. Paiement GD, Hymes RA, et al: Postoperative infections in asymptomatic HIV- seropositive orthopedic trauma patients. J Trauma 37:545–551, 1994.
11. Shapiro H, Grant I, Weinger M: AIDS and the central nervous system: Implications for the anesthesiologist. Anesthesiology 80:187–200, 1994.
12. Simpson DM, Tagliati M: Neurologic manifestations of HIV infection. Ann Intern Med 121:769–785, 1994.
13. Tonnesen E, Wahlgreen C: Influence of extradural and general anesthesia on natural killer cell activity and lymphocyte subpopulations in patients undergoing hysterectomy. Br J Anaesth 60:500–507, 1988.
14. Wilson SE: Vascular problems in patients with HIV infection. In Wilson SE, Williams RA (eds): Surgical Problems in the AIDS Patient. New York, Igaku-Shoin, 1994, pp 119–128.

VII. Special Anesthetic Considerations

62. NEONATAL ANESTHESIA

Rita Agarwal, M.D.

1. Why are neonates and preterm infants at increased anesthetic risk?

1. **Pulmonary factors.** Differences in the neonatal airway, including large tongue and occiput, floppy epiglottis, small mouth, and short neck, predispose infants to upper airway obstruction. The more premature the infant is, the higher the incidence of airway obstruction. The carbon dioxide response curve is shifted further to the right in neonates than in adults; that is, infants have a decreased ventilatory response to hypercarbia. Newborn vital capacity is about one-half of an adult's vital capacity, respiratory rate is twice that of an adult, and oxygen consumption is 2–3 times greater. Consequently, opioids, barbiturates, and volatile agents have a more profound effect on ventilation in neonates than in adults.

2. **Cardiac factors.** Newborn infants have relatively stiff ventricles that function at close to maximal contraction. Cardiac output is heart rate-dependent, and neonates are highly sensitive to the myocardial depressant effects of many anesthetic agents, especially those that may produce bradycardia. Inhalational agents and barbiturates should be used cautiously.

3. **Temperature.** Infants have poor central thermoregulation, thin insulating fat, increased body surface area to mass ratio, and high minute ventilation. These factors make them highly susceptible to hypothermia in the operating room. Shivering is an ineffective mechanism for heat production because infants have limited muscle mass. Nonshivering thermogenesis uses brown fat to produce heat, but it is not an efficient method to restore body temperature and increases oxygen consumption significantly. Cold-stressed infants may develop cardiovascular depression and hypoperfusion acidosis.

2. Do neonates have normal renal function?

Glomerular function of the kidneys is immature, and the concentrating ability is impaired. Renal clearance of drugs may be delayed.

3. Why is it important to provide infants with exogenous glucose?

Neonates have low stores of hepatic glucose, and mechanisms for gluconeogenesis are immature. Infants who have fasted may develop hypoglycemia. Symptoms of hypoglycemia include apnea, cyanosis, respiratory difficulties, seizures, high-pitched cry, lethargy, limpness, temperature instability, and sweating.

4. What are the differences in the gastrointestinal or hepatic function of neonates?

Gastric emptying is prolonged, and the lower esophageal sphincter is incompetent; thus the incidence of reflux may be increased. Elevated levels of bilirubin are common in neonates. Kernicterus, a complication of elevated levels of bilirubin, may lead to neurologic dysfunction and even death in extreme cases. Commonly used medications such as furosemide and sulfonamide may displace bilirubin from albumin and increase the risk of kernicterus. Diazepam contains the preservative benzyl alcohol, which also may displace bilirubin. Hepatic metabolism is immature, and hepatic blood flow is less than in older children or adults. Drug metabolism and effect may be prolonged.

5. What is retinopathy of prematurity?

Retinopathy of prematurity is a disorder that occurs in premature and occasionally full-term infants who have been exposed to high inspired concentrations of oxygen. Proliferation of the retinal vessels, retinal hemorrhage, fibroproliferation, scarring, and retinal detachment may occur, with decreased visual acuity and blindness. Premature and full-term infants should have limited exposure to high concentrations of inspired oxygen. Oxygen saturation should be maintained between 92–95%, except during times of greater risk for desaturation.

6. How is volume status assessed in neonates?

Blood pressure is not a reliable measure of volume in neonates. If the anterior fontanelle is sunken, skin turgor is decreased, and the infant cries without visible tears, the diagnosis is dehydration. Capillary refill after blanching of the big toe should be less than 5 seconds. The extremities should not be significantly cooler than the rest of the body. Finally, the skin should look pink and well perfused—not pale, mottled, or cyanotic.

7. What problems are common in premature infants?

Common Problems in Premature Infants

PROBLEM	SIGNIFICANCE
Respiratory distress syndrome (RDS)	Surfactant, which is produced by alveolar epithelial cells, coats the inside of the alveolus and reduces surface tension. Surfactant deficiency causes alveolar collapse. BPD occurs in about 20% of cases.
Bronchopulmonary dysplasia (BPD)	Interstitial fibrosis, cysts, and collapsed lung impair ventilatory mechanics and gas exchange.
Apnea and bradycardia (A and B)	Most common cause of morbidity in postoperative period. Sensitivity of chemoreceptors to hypercarbia and hypoxia is decreased. Immaturity and poor coordination of upper airway musculature also contribute. If apnea persists > 15 sec, bradycardia may result and worsen hypoxia.
Patent ductus arteriosus (PDA)	Incidence of hemodynamically significant PDA varies with degree of prematurity but is high. Left-to-right shunting through the PDA may lead to fluid overload, heart failure, and respiratory distress.
Intraventricular hemorrhage (IVH)	Hydrocephalus usually results from IVH. Avoiding fluctuations in blood pressure and intracranial pressure may reduce the risk of IVH.
Retinopathy of prematurity (ROP)	See question 5.
Necrotizing enterocolitis (NEC)	Infants develop distended abdomen, bloody stools, and vomiting. They may go into shock and require surgery.

8. What special preparations are needed before anesthetizing a neonate?

1. Routine monitors in a variety of appropriately small sizes should be available.

2. The room should be warmed at least 1 hour before the start of the procedure to minimize radiant heat loss. A warming blanket and warming lights also help to decrease heat loss. Covering the infant with plastic decreases evaporative losses. Temperature should be monitored carefully, because it is easy to overheat a small infant.

3. At least 2 pulse oximeter probes are helpful in measuring preductal and postductal saturation. Listening to heart and breath sounds with a precordial or esophageal stethoscope is invaluable.

4. Placing 25–50 ml of balanced salt solution in a buretrol prevents inadvertent administration of large amounts of fluid.

5. Five percent albumin and blood should be readily available.

6. Calculate estimated blood volume and maximal acceptable blood loss.

9. What intraoperative problems are common in small infants?

Common Intraoperative Problems in Infants

PROBLEM	POSSIBLE CAUSES	SOLUTION
Hypoxia	1. Short distance from cords to carina; ETT easily dislodged or displaced into bronchus. 2. Pressure on abdomen or chest by surgeons may decrease FRC and vital capacity.	1. After intubation, place ETT into right mainstem and, carefully listening to breath sounds, pull tube back. Tape ETT 1–2 cm above level of carina. 2. Inform surgeons when they are interfering with ventilation. Hand ventilation helps to compensate for changes in peak pressure.
Bradycardia	1. Hypoxia 2. Volatile agents 3. Succinylcholine	1. Preoxygenate before intubation or extubation; all airway manipulations should be performed expeditiously. 2. Minimize amount of volatile agent administered, especially halothane. 3. Give atropine before administering succinylcholine.
Hypothermia	See question 1.	Warm operating room, warming blanket, warming lights, humidifier; keep infant covered whenever possible. Warming fluids may be helpful.
Hypotension	1. Bradycardia 2. Volume depletion	1. Treat bradycardia with anticholinergics and ensure oxygenation. 2. Many neonatal emergencies are associated with major fluid loss. Volume status should be carefully assessed, with replacement as needed.

ETT = endotracheal tube, FRC = forced residual capacity.

10. What are the most common neonatal emergencies?

Tracheoesophageal fistula (TEF)   Gastroschisis
Congenital diaphragmatic hernia (CDH)   Patent ductus arteriosus (PDA)
Omphalocele   Intestinal obstruction

11. Discuss the incidence and anesthetic implications of congenital diaphragmatic hernia.

1. The incidence is 1–2:5000 live births.

2. The diaphragm fails to close completely, allowing the peritoneal contents to herniate into the thoracic cavity. Abnormal lung development and hypoplasia usually occur on the side of the hernia but may be bilateral.

3. The majority of hernias occur through the left-sided foramen of Bochdalek.

4. Cardiovascular abnormalities present in 23% of patients.

5. Patients present with symptoms of pulmonary hypoplasia. The severity of symptoms and prognosis depend on the severity of the underlying hypoplasia.

6. Mask ventilation may cause visceral distention and worsen oxygenation. The infant should be intubated while awake. Low pressures must be used for ventilation to prevent barotrauma. Pneumothorax of the contralateral (healthier) lung may occur when high pressures are needed. Some patients may require high-frequency ventilation or extracorporeal membrane oxygenation (ECMO).

7. A nasogastric tube should be used to decompress the stomach.

8. A transabdominal approach is used for the repair.

9. Good intravenous access is mandatory. An arterial line may be necessary if the infant has significant lung or cardiac abnormalities.

10. Pulmonary hypertension may complicate management by impairing oxygenation and decreasing cardiac output. Most patients need to remain intubated in the postoperative period.

11. Opioids and muscle relaxants should be the primary agents used. Inhalational agents may be used to supplement the anesthetic if tolerated by the infant.

12. Which congenital anomalies are associated with tracheoesophageal fistula (TEF)?

TEFs may occur alone or as part of a syndrome. The two most common syndromes are the VATER and the VACTERL syndromes. Patients with VATER have vertebral anomalies, imperforate anus, tracheoesophageal fistula and renal or radial abnormalities. Patients with VACTERL have all of the above in addition to cardiac and limb abnormalities.

13. How should patients with TEF be managed?

1. Patients usually present with excessive secretions, inability to pass a nasogastric tube, and regurgitation of feedings. Respiratory symptoms are uncommon.

2. Positive pressure ventilation may cause distention of the stomach. In a spontaneously breathing patient, either an awake intubation or inhalational induction may be carried out.

3. The endotracheal tube should be placed into the right mainstem and gradually withdrawn until bilateral breath sounds are heard. The stomach should be auscultated to ensure that it is not overinflated. If the infant has significant respiratory distress because of overinflation of the stomach, it may be necessary to perform a gastrostomy before anesthetizing the patient.

4. An arterial line is frequently not necessary in an otherwise healthy infant with no other congenital anomalies. In selected patients, it may be helpful to monitor blood gas values.

5. Pulse oximetry is invaluable. Probes should be placed at a preductal (right hand or finger) and postductal site (left hand or feet).

6. Once the airway has been secured, the infant is placed in the left lateral decubitus position. Placing a precordial stethoscope on the left chest helps to detect displacement of the ETT.

7. A right-sided thoracotomy is made, and the fistula is divided. If possible, the esophagus is reanastomosed; if not, a gastrostomy tube is placed.

8. It is desirable to extubate the infant as soon as possible to prevent pressure on the suture line.

14. What are the differences between omphalocele and gastroschisis?

1. An omphalocele is a hernia within the umbilical cord caused by failure of the gut to migrate into the abdomen from the yolk sac. The bowel is completely covered with chorioamnionic membranes but otherwise usually normal. Patients with omphalocele frequently have associated cardiac, urologic, and metabolic anomalies.

2. The exact cause of gastroschisis is unknown; it may be due to vascular occlusion of blood supply to the abdominal wall or fetal rupture of an omphalocele. The bowel is often covered with an inflammatory exudate and may be abnormal. There are usually no associated anomalies.

15. How are patients with omphalocele or gastroschisis managed in the perioperative period?

1. It is important to prevent evaporative and heat loss from exposed viscera. The exposed bowel should be covered with warm, moist saline packs and saran wrap until the time of surgery. The operating room should be warmed before the arrival of the infant. Warming lights and a warming blanket help to decrease conductive and radiation loss. Covering the head and extremities with plastic prevents evaporative loss.

2. Respiratory distress is uncommon; therefore, infants usually arrive in the operating room breathing spontaneously. Awake intubation or rapid-sequence induction quickly establishes airway control.

3. Ventilation is controlled with muscle relaxants to facilitate return of the bowel into the abdomen.

4. After intubation a nasogastric tube should be placed if not already present.

5. Patients need good IV access to replace third-space and evaporative losses. An arterial line is frequently unnecessary.

6. Once the surgeons begin to put the viscera into the abdomen, the ventilatory requirements change. Hand ventilation during this phase allows the anesthesiologist to feel peak airway pressures and changes in airway pressures. If peak airway pressures are greater than 40 cm H_2O, the surgeons must be notified.

7. The abdominal cavity may be too small for the viscera. Venous return from or blood flow to the lower extremity may be compromised. A pulse oximeter on the foot helps to detect such changes. Renal perfusion may decrease and manifest as oliguria.

8. If primary closure is not possible, the surgeons choose either to do a fascial (skin) closure or to place a synthetic mesh silo over the defect. Both approaches necessitate return trips to the operating room for the final corrective procedure.

9. Patients usually remain intubated after surgery.

BIBLIOGRAPHY

1. Gregory GA (ed.): Pediatric Anesthesia, 3rd ed. New York, Churchill Livingstone, 1994.
2. Diaz JH (ed): Perinatal Anesthesia and Critical Care. Philadelphia, W.B.Saunders, 1991.
3. Coté CJ, Ryan JF, Todres ID, Goudsouzian NG (eds): A Practice of Anesthesia for Infants and Children., 2nd ed. Philadelphia, W.B. Saunders, 1993.
4. Klaus MH, Fanaroff AA (eds): Care of the High Risk Neonate, 3rd ed. Philadelphia, W.B. Saunders, 1986.

63. PEDIATRIC ANESTHESIA

Rita Agarwal, M.D.

1. What are the differences between the adult and pediatric airway?

Differences between the Adult and Pediatric Airway

DIFFERENCES IN INFANT AIRWAY	SIGNIFICANCE
Obligate nose breathers, narrow nares	Infants can breathe only through their nose, which can become easily obstructed by secretions
Large tongue	May obstruct airway and make laryngoscopy and intubation more difficult
Large occiput	Sniffing position achieved with roll under shoulder
Glottis located at C3 in premature babies, C3–C4 in newborns, and C5 in adults	Larynx appears more anterior; cricoid pressure frequently helps with visualization
Larynx and trachea are funnel-shaped	Narrowest part of the trachea is at the cricoid; the patient should have an ETT leak of < 30 cm H_2O to prevent excessive pressure on the tracheal mucosa, barotrauma
Vocal cords slant anteriorly	Insertion of ETT may be more difficult

ETT = endotracheal tube.

2. Are there any differences in the adult and pediatric pulmonary system?

Differences in the Pediatric and Adult Pulmonary System

DIFFERENCE IN PEDIATRIC PULMONARY SYSTEM	SIGNIFICANCE
Decreased, smaller alveoli	13-fold growth in number of alveoli between birth and 6 yr; 3-fold growth in size of alveoli between 6 yr and adulthood
Decreased compliance Decreased elastin	Increased likelihood of airway collapse
Increased airway resistance Smaller airways	Increased work of breathing and vulnerability to disease affecting small airways
Horizontal ribs, more pliable ribs and cartilage	Inefficient chest wall mechanics
Less type-1, high-oxidative muscle	Babies tire more easily
Decreased total lung capacity (TLC), faster respiratory and metabolic rate	Faster desaturation
Higher closing volumes	Increased dead-space ventilation

3. How does the cardiovascular system differ in a child?

1. Newborns are unable to increase cardiac output (CO) by increasing contractility; they can increase CO only by increasing heart rate.

2. Babies have an immature baroreceptor reflex and limited ability to compensate for hypotension by increasing heart rate. They are more susceptible, therefore, to the cardiac depressant effects of volatile anesthetics.

3. Babies and infants have increased vagal tone and are prone to bradycardia. The three major causes of bradycardia are hypoxia, vagal stimulation (laryngoscopy), and volatile anesthetics. **Bradycardia is bad!**

4. What are normal vital signs in children?

Normal Vital Signs in Children

AGE (YR)	HR	RR	SBP	DBP
< 1	120–160	30–60	60–95	35–69
1–3	90–140	24–40	95–105	50–65
3–5	75–110	18–30	95–110	50–65
8–12	75–100	18–30	90–110	57–71
12–16	60–90	12–16	112–130	60–80

HR = heart rate, RR = respiratory rate, SBP = systolic blood pressure, DBP = diastolic blood pressure. A good rule of thumb is: normal BP = 80 mmHg + 2 × age.

5. When should a child be premedicated? Which drugs are commonly used?

Children may have a great deal of fear and anxiety when they are separated from their parents and during induction of anesthesia. Vetter recommends premedicating children who are 2–6 years old and have had previous surgery or no preoperative tour and education or who fail to interact positively with health care providers in the preoperative area.

Commonly Used Preoperative Medications and Routes of Administration

DRUG	ROUTE OF ADMINISTRATION	ADVANTAGES	DISADVANTAGES
Midazolam	po, pr, in, iv, sl	Quick onset, minimal side effects	Tastes bad when given orally, burns intranasally
Ketamine	po, pr, in, iv, sl	Quick onset, good analgesia	May slow emergence, tastes bad, burns intranasally
Fentanyl	otfc	Tastes good, good analgesic, onset at 45 min.	Possible hypoxemia, nausea
Diazepam	po, pr, im	Cheap, minimal side effects	Long onset time, may prolong emergence

po = by mouth, pr = per rectum, iv = intravenous, sl = sublingual, im = intramuscular, in = intranasal, otfc = oral transmucosal fentanyl citrate.

6. Describe the commonly used induction techniques in children.

1. **Inhalational induction:** the most commonly used induction technique in children younger than 10 years. The child is asked to breathe 70% nitrous oxide and 30% oxygen for approximately 1 minute; halothane is then turned on slowly. The halothane concentration is increased 0.5% every 3–5 breaths. If the child coughs or holds the breath, the concentration of halothane is not increased until the coughing or breath-holding resolves.

2. **Rapid inhalational or "brutane" induction:** used in an uncooperative child. The child is held down, and a mask containing 70% nitrous oxide, 30% oxygen, and 3–5% halothane is placed on the child's face. This unpleasant technique should be avoided if possible. Once anesthesia has been induced, the concentration of halothane should be decreased.

3. **Steal induction:** may be used if the child is already sleeping. Inhalational induction is accomplished by holding the mask away from the child's face and gradually increasing the concentration of halothane. The goal is to induce anesthesia without awakening the child.

4. **Intravenous induction:** used in a child who already has an intravenous line in place and in older children (> 10 years). The same drugs and techniques used in adults are used in children. EMLA cream (eutectic mixture of local anesthesia) applied at least 90 minutes before starting the intravenous infusion makes this an atraumatic procedure.

7. How does the presence of a left-to-right shunt affect inhalational induction? intravenous induction?
A left-to-right intracardiac shunt leads to volume overload of the right side of the heart and the pulmonary circulation. Patients develop congestive heart failure and decreased lung compliance. Uptake and distribution of inhaled agents are minimally affected; onset time for intravenous agents is slightly prolonged.

8. How about a right-to-left shunt?
Right-to-left shunting causes hypoxemia and left ventricular overload. Patients compensate by increasing blood volume and hematocrit. It is important to maintain a high systemic vascular resistance to prevent increased shunting from right to left. Such shunts may slightly delay inhalation induction and shorten the onset time of intravenous induction agents.

9. What other special precautions need to be taken in a child with heart disease?
1. The **anatomy** of the lesion(s) and **direction of blood flow** should be determined. Pulmonary vascular resistance (PVR) needs to be maintained. If the PVR increases, right-to-left shunting may increase and worsen oxygenation, whereas a patient with a left-to-right shunt may develop a reversal in the direction of blood flow (Eisenmenger's syndrome). If a patient has a left-to-right shunt, decreasing the PVR may increase blood flow to the lungs and lead to pulmonary edema. Decreasing the PVR in patients with a right-to-left shunt may improve hemodynamics.

Conditions that Can Increase Shunting

LEFT-TO-RIGHT SHUNT	RIGHT-TO-LEFT SHUNT
Low hematocrit	Decreased SVR
Increased SVR	Increased PVR
Decreased PVR	Hypoxia
Hyperventilation	Hypercarbia
Hypothermia	Acidosis
Anesthetic agent:	Anesthetic agents:
Isoflurane	? Nitrous oxide
	? Ketamine

SVR = systemic vascular resistance; PVR = pulmonary vascular resistance.

2. **Air bubbles** should be meticulously avoided. If there is a communication between the right and left sides of the heart (ventricular septal defect, atrial septal defect), air injected intravenously may travel across the communication and enter the arterial system. This may lead to central nervous system symptoms if the air obstructs the blood supply to the brain or spinal cord (paradoxical air embolus).
3. **Prophylactic antibiotics** should be given to prevent infective endocarditis. Specific recommendations for medications and doses can be found in the American Heart Association guidelines.
4. **Avoid bradycardia**.
5. **Recognize and be able to treat a "tet spell."** Children with tetralogy of Fallot have right outflow tract (RVOT) obstruction, an overriding aorta, ventricular septal defect, and pulmonary stenosis/atresia. They may or may not have cyanosis at rest. However, many are prone to hypercyanotic spells ("tet spells") with stimulation as they get older. Such episodes are characterized by worsening RVOT obstruction, possibly as a result of hypovolemia, increased contractility, or

tachycardia during times of stimulation or stress. Patients are frequently treated with beta block-ers, which should be continued perioperatively. Hypovolemia, acidosis, excessive crying or anxi-ety, and increased airway pressures should be avoided. The systemic vascular resistance (SVR) should be maintained. If a hypercyanotic spell occurs in the perioperative period, treatment in-cludes maintaining the airway, volume infusion, increasing the depth of anesthesia, or decreasing the surgical stimulation. Phenylephrine is extremely useful in increasing SVR. Additional doses of beta blockers also may be tried. Metabolic acidosis should be corrected.

10. How does one choose an endotracheal tube of appropriate size?

Guidelines for Endotracheal Tube (ETT) Size

AGE	SIZE (MM INTERNAL DIAMETER)
Newborns	3.0–3.5
Newborn–12 months	3.5–4.0
12–18 months	4.0
2 years	4.5
> 2 years	ETT size = $\dfrac{16 + \text{age}}{4}$

1. An ETT ½ size above and ½ size below the estimated size should be available.
2. The leak around the tube should be < 30 cm H_2O.
3. The ETT should be placed to a depth of approximately 3 times its internal diameter.

11. How does the pharmacology of commonly used anesthetic drugs differ in children?
    1. The minimal alveolar concentration (MAC) of the volatile agents is higher in children than adults. The highest MAC is in infants aged 1–6 months. Premature babies and neonates have a lower MAC for isoflurane and halothane.
    2. Children have a higher tolerance to the dysrhythmic effects of epinephrine during general anesthesia with volatile agents.
    3. In general children have higher drug requirements (mg/kg) because they have a greater volume of distribution (more fat, more body water).
    4. *Opioids* should be used carefully in children less than 1 year old, who are more sensitive to the respiratory depressant effects.

12. How is perioperative fluid managed in children?
    1. Maintenance is calculated as follows:
        Infant < 10 kg   4 ml/kg/hr
        10–20 kg   40 + 2 ml/kg/hr for every kg < 10
        Child > 20 kg   60 + 1 ml/kg/hr for every kg > 20
    2. Estimated fluid deficit (EFD) should be calculated and replaced as follows:
        EFD = maintenance × hours since last oral intake
        ½ EFD + maintenance given over the 1st hour
        ¼ EFD + maintenance given over the 2nd hour
        ¼ EFD + maintenance given over the 3rd hour
    3. All EFD should be replaced for major cases. For minor cases, 10–20 ml/kg of a balanced salt solution with or without glucose is usually adequate.
    4. Estimated blood volume (EBV) and acceptable blood loss (ABL) should be calculated for every case.

13. What is the most common replacement fluid used in children? Why?
A balanced salt solution (BSS) such as lactated Ringer's with glucose (D5LR) or without glucose (LR) is recommended. Welborn showed that hypoglycemia may occur in healthy children under-going minimally invasive procedures if glucose-containing fluids are not used. However, she also

found that administration of 5% glucose-containing solutions resulted in hyperglycemia in the majority of children. Some authors recommend using fluid containing 1% or 2.5% glucose. Others still use 5% glucose solutions for maintenance but recommend non–glucose-containing BSS for third space or blood loss. In major operations it is prudent to check serial glucose levels and to avoid hyper- or hypoglycemia.

14. What is the estimated blood volume in children?

Guidelines for Estimated Blood Volume in Children

AGE	EBV (ML/KG)
Neonate	90
Infant up to 1 year old	80
Older than 1 year	70

15. How is acceptable blood loss calculated?

$$ABL = \frac{EBV \times (pt\ hct - lowest\ acceptable\ hct)}{average\ hct}$$

where ABL = acceptable blood, EBV = estimated blood, pt = percent, and hct = hematocrit. The lowest acceptable hematocrit varies with individual circumstances. Blood transfusion is usually considered when the hematocrit is less than 21–25%. If problems with vital signs develop, blood transfusion may need to be started earlier. For example, a 4-month-old infant is scheduled for craniofacial reconstruction. He is otherwise healthy, and his last oral intake was 6 hours before arriving in the operating room. Weight = 6 kg, preoperative hct = 33%, lowest acceptable hct = 25%.

$$
\begin{aligned}
\text{Maintenance} &= \text{weight} \times 4\ ml/hr = 24\ ml/hr \\
\text{EFD} &= \text{maintenance} \times 6\ kg = 144\ ml \\
\text{EBV} &= \text{weight} \times 80\ ml/kg = 480\ ml \\
\text{ABL} &= \frac{EBV \times (pt\ hct - lowest\ acceptable\ hct)}{average\ hct} \\
&= \frac{480 \times (33 - 25) = 132\ ml}{29}
\end{aligned}
$$

16. How do the manifestations of hypovolemia differ in children?

Healthy children compensate for acute volume loss of 30–40% before blood pressure changes. The most reliable early indicators of compensated hypovolemic shock in a child are persistent tachycardia, cutaneous vasoconstriction, and diminution of pulse pressure.

17. What are the systemic responses to blood loss?

Systemic Response to Blood Loss in Children

ORGAN SYSTEM	< 25% BLOOD LOSS	25–40% BLOOD LOSS	> 45% BLOOD LOSS
Cardiac	Weak, thready pulse; ↑ HR	↑ HR	↓ BP, ↑ HR, bradycardia indicates severe blood loss and impending circulatory collapse
Central nervous system	Lethargic, confused, irritable	Change in LOC, dulled response to pain	Comatose
Skin	Cool, clammy	Cyanotic, ↓ capillary refill, cold extremities	Pale, cold
Kidneys	↓ UOP; ↑ specific gravity	Minimal UOP	Minimal UOP

HR = heart rate, BP = blood pressure, LOC = level of consciousness, UOP = urine output.

18. What is the most common type of regional anesthesia performed in children?
Caudal epidural block is the most common regional technique performed in children. It is usually performed in an anesthetized child and provides good adjunct intraoperative and postoperative analgesia. It is used most commonly for surgery of the lower extremities, perineum, and lower abdomen.

19. Which local anesthetic is usually used?
Bupivacaine in a concentration of 0.125–0.25% is the most commonly used local anesthesia. Bupivacaine 0.25% produces good adjunct intraoperative analgesia and decreases the required MAC of volatile anesthetic. However, it may produce postoperative motor blockade that interferes with hospital discharge of outpatients. Bupivacaine 0.125% causes minimal postoperative motor block but may not provide intraoperative analgesia or decrease the MAC requirements. Gunter showed that 0.175% bupivacaine produces good intraoperative analgesia and minimal motor block and decreases the required MAC of volatile anesthetics.

20. What is the dose?

Commonly Used Doses of Local Anesthetic for Caudal Block

DOSE (CC/KG)	LEVEL OF BLOCK	TYPE OF OPERATION
0.5	Sacral/lumbar	Penile, lower extremity
1	Lumbar/thoracic	Lower abdominal
1.2	Upper thoracic	Upper abdominal

Toxic dose of bupivacaine in the child is 2.5 mg/kg; in the neonate, 1.5 mg/kg.

21. Describe the common postoperative complications.
1. **Nausea and vomiting** continue to be the most common cause of delayed discharge or unplanned admission in children. The best treatment for postoperative nausea and vomiting is prevention. Prophylactic administration of an antiemetic should be considered for patients at high risk for emesis. Avoiding opioids will decrease the incidence of postoperative nausea and vomiting as long as pain relief is adequate (e.g., patient has a functioning caudal block). Management includes administering intravenous fluid and stopping oral intake. If vomiting persists, metoclopramide, droperidol, or ondansetron can be tried. If the vomiting does not resolve, the patient should be admitted for observation.

Factors Associated with Increased Incidence of Postoperative Nausea and Vomiting

PATIENT FACTORS	SURGICAL/ANESTHETIC FACTORS
Patient age > 6 yr	Length of surgery > 20 min
Previous history of postoperative nausea and vomiting	Eye surgery
History of motion sickness	Tonsillectomy/adenoidectomy
Preoperative nausea	Use of narcotics
Extreme preoperative anxiety	? Nitrous oxide

2. **Respiratory problems,** particularly laryngospasm and stridor, are more common in children than in adults. Management for laryngospasm includes oxygen, positive pressure, the Fink maneuver (painful jaw thrust), succinylcholine, and reintubation if necessary. Stridor is usually treated with humidified oxygen, steroids, and racemic epinephrine.

CONTROVERSIES

22. What is the significance of masseter muscle rigidity?
1. Rigidity of the masseter muscles occurs in 1% of children receiving halothane and succinylcholine. Addition of sodium thiopental may decrease the incidence, although its mechanism of action is unknown.

2. Masseter muscle rigidity may be the first symptom of malignant hyperthermia (MH), but it also may occur in patients who are not susceptible to MH.

23. How is the patient who develops masseter muscle rigidity managed?

1. The incidence of MH after masseter muscle rigidity is a source of controversy. Most authors believe that the incidence is 1% or less; however, one recent study showed that it may be as high as 59% in patients referred for muscle biopsy.

2. When masseter muscle rigidity develops, the major issue is whether to substitute a nontriggering technique or to stop the procedure. The author usually switches to a nontriggering technique and continues with the operation unless other signs of possible MH develop or such severe masseter muscle spasm occurs that intubation is impossible.

3. Patients should be admitted and followed postoperatively for increased levels of creatine phosphokinase (CPK) and other signs of MH (heart rate, blood pressure, temperature, urine myoglobin). If the postoperative CPK levels are > 20,000, the patient should be managed and diagnosed with MH. If the CPK is < 20,000 but still significantly elevated, an MH work-up should be considered, including a muscle biopsy. If CPK is normal or minimally elevated, the patient is probably not at increased risk for MH.

24. Describe the management of a patient with an upper respiratory infection.

1. The risk of adverse respiratory events is 9–11 times greater up to 2 weeks after an upper respiratory infection (URI). Underlying pulmonary derangements include:
   - Decreased diffusion capacity for oxygen
   - Decreased compliance and increased resistance
   - Decreased closing volumes
   - Increased shunting (ventilation-perfusion mismatch), lung oxygen uptake
   - Increased incidence of hypoxemia
   - Increased airway reactivity
2. Endotracheal intubation increases the risks of such respiratory events.
3. General recommendations for a child with mild URI
   - Discuss increased risk with parents
   - Try to avoid intubation
   - Use anticholinergics to help to decrease secretions and airway reactivity
4. The child who has a fever, rhonchi that do not clear with coughing, an abnormal chest x-ray, elevated white count, or decreased activity levels should be rescheduled.

25. What are the advantages and disadvantages of the pediatric circle system and the Bain circuit?

Advantages and Disadvantages of the Pediatric Circle System and Bain Circuit

CIRCUIT	ADVANTAGES	DISADVANTAGES
Circle system	Relatively constant inspired concentration of gases. Conservation of moisture and heat. Minimal pollution in operating room	Complex design, with unidirectional valves. Small babies (< 10 kg) may have an increased work of breathing to overcome resistance of valves
Bain circuit	Lightweight. Good for spontaneous or controlled ventilation. Minimal resistance. Exhaled gases in outer tubing add warmth and humidity to inspired gases (in theory)	Most anesthesia machines require special attachment for this circuit. Inner tubing may kink or become disconnected

26. Should parents be allowed to accompany children for induction of anesthesia?

Young children may become extremely anxious and frightened when they are separated from their parents before surgery. Allowing parents to accompany children to the operating room may facilitate induction of anesthesia in some cases. Parents and children should be educated and prepared for what to expect. Parents should be prepared to leave when the anesthesiologists believe that it is appropriate. Highly anxious, reluctant, or hysterical parents are a hindrance. An anesthesiologist who is not comfortable with allowing parents to be present during induction probably should not allow them to be so. An uncooperative or frightened child may or may not benefit from parental presence.

BIBLIOGRAPHY

1. Berry FA (ed): Anesthetic Management of Difficult and Routine Pediatric Patients, 2nd ed. New York, Churchill Livingstone, 1990.
2. Cohen MM, Cameron CB: Should you cancel the operation when a child has an upper respiratory tract infection? Anesth Analg 72:282–286, 1991.
3. Gregory GA (ed): Pediatric Anesthesia, 3rd ed. New York, Churchill Livingstone, 1994.
4. Gunter JB, Dunn CM, Bennie JB, et al: Optimum concentration of bupivacaine for combined caudal-general anesthesia in pediatric patients. Anesth Analg 66:995–998, 1982.
5. Motoyama EK, Davis PJ (eds): Smith's Anesthesia for Infants and Children, 5th ed. St. Louis, Mosby, 1990.
6. O'Flynn RP, Shutack JG, Rosenberg H, Fletcher JE: Masseter muscle rigidity and malignant hyperthermia susceptibility in pediatric patients: An update on management and diagnosis. Anesthesiology 80:1228–1233, 1994.
7. Vetter TR: The epidemiology and selective identification of children at risk for preoperative anxiety reactions. Anesth Analg 77:96–99, 1993.
8. Welborn LG, McGill WA, Hannallah RS, et al: Perioperative blood glucose concentrations in pediatric operations. Anesthesiology 65:543–547, 1986.

64. FUNDAMENTALS OF OBSTETRIC ANESTHESIA

Ana M. Lobo, M.D., M.P.H.

1. What are the cardiovascular changes associated with pregnancy?

Cardiovascular Changes Associated with Pregnancy

Heart rate	↑ (15–20 bpm)
Cardiac output	↑ (40–50%)
Stroke volume	↑ (50% by term)
Systemic vascular resistance	↓ (21%)
Pulmonary vascular resistance	↓ (34%)
Uterine blood flow	↑ (40%)
Mean arterial blood pressure	↓ 15 mmHg (normal by 2nd trimester)
Arterial blood pressure	↓ (normal by 2nd trimester)
Vascular tone	↓
Central venous pressure	No change

In pregnancy, the heart may appear enlarged on chest x-rays, as the diaphragmatic rise shifts the heart position to the left. There is a high incidence of asymptomatic pericardial effusion during pregnancy. Because of increased blood flow and vasodilation, a low grade (I to II) systolic murmur may be heard. The ECG may show benign dysrhythmias and left axis deviation. Despite a decrease in vessel tone (both pulmonary and systemic), hemodynamic stability is more dependent on the vasomotor response in the pregnant patient. In general, pregnant women are less responsive to chronotropes and vasopressors. As vascular tone is decreased, it is important to administer fluids to the patient prior to a regional anesthetic. Sympathetic blockade may aggravate hypotension because compensatory mechanisms are diminished.

2. Discuss the respiratory changes associated with pregnancy.

Changes in the Respiratory System at Term in Pregnant Women

Diaphragm	Elevates 4 cm
Minute ventilation	↑ (50%)
Alveolar ventilation	↑ (70%)
Tidal volume	↑ (50%)
Oxygen consumption	↑ (20%)
Respiratory rate	↑ (15%)
Arterial PO_2	↓ (10 mmHg)
Serum bicarbonate (HCO_3)	↓ (4 mEq/L)
Arterial pH	No change
Arterial PCO_2	↓ (10 mmHg)
Dead space	No change
Lung compliance	No change

Continued on following page.

Changes in the Respiratory System at Term in Pregnant Women (Continued)

Total compliance	↓ (30%)
Chest wall compliance	↓ (45%)
Airway resistance	↓ (36%)
Total pulmonary resistance	↓ (50%)
Expiratory reserve volume	↓ (20%)
Residual volume	↓ (20%)
Closing volume	No change or ↓
Inspiratory lung capacity	↑ (5%)
Vital capacity	No change
Diffusing capacity	No change
Maximum breathing capacity	No change
Total lung capacity	↓ (0–5%)
Functional residual capacity	↓ (20%)

The respiratory changes that occur during pregnancy are of special concern to the anesthesiologist. Ventilation increases during pregnancy, and shortness of breath may occur toward term. Nasal congestion, voice changes, and symptoms of upper respiratory tract infection are common because of swelling in the nasal and oral pharynx and trachea (due to capillary engorgement of the mucosa). A compromised airway may result if these changes are exacerbated by an upper respiratory tract infection, fluid overload, or edema (secondary to preeclampsia). Respiratory tract mucous membranes are friable, and airway placement and laryngoscopy may result in trauma and bleeding. Airway and false vocal cord swelling may decrease the glottic area. Use of a small endotracheal tube (such as ≤ 7.0 mm) is prudent. A stubby laryngoscope handle is useful when the patient's enlarged breasts prevent laryngoscopy with a common handle. A respiratory alkalosis is normal in pregnant patients, as minute ventilation is increased (primarily due to an increased tidal volume). Arterial PCO_2 is approximately 32 mmHg. With labor pain, maternal hypocarbia may become severe, and pH may increase to > 7.55. Pregnant patients desaturate quickly as functional residual capacity is decreased and oxygen consumption is increased. Apnea quickly causes hypoxemia. A low threshold for oxygen administration is recommended. Early airway closure (smokers, obesity, kyphoscoliosis) aggravates hypoxemia, as do the Trendelenburg and supine positions. It is crucial to preoxygenate pregnant patients before general anesthesia to decrease the risk of hypoxia on induction.

3. What gastrointestinal changes occur with pregnancy?

Pregnancy alters gastrointestinal function in several ways that are of concern to the anesthesiologist. Pregnant patients are prone to silent regurgitation, active vomiting, and aspiration when they are rendered unconscious. The uterus causes a shift in stomach position, which decreases the oblique angle of the gastroesophageal junction, frequently resulting in incompetence of this mechanism. Gastric reflux may result in heartburn and/or esophagitis. A decrease in gastric motility and emptying time also increases the risk of aspiration. Gastrin produced by the placenta raises the acid content of the stomach. A gastric volume > 25 ml and a gastric pH < 2.5 are associated with an increased risk of aspiration pneumonitis. Intragastric pressure is increased during the last weeks of pregnancy. All parturients are classified as "full stomachs" (regardless of time of last oral intake) and are at risk for aspiration. Rapid-sequence inductions are a must. Prior to any anesthetic, the patient should receive aspiration prophylaxis, including an H_2 blocker, sodium citrate, and metoclopramide. Cholecystectomy is a frequent nonobstetric procedure during pregnancy, as is appendectomy.

4. List the central nervous system changes that occur during pregnancy.

Pregnancy causes a decrease in anesthetic requirements. The minimum alveolar concentration for inhalational agents is decreased by as much as 40%. The mechanism for this decrease is uncertain, but hormonal influences may be involved. Progesterone has sedative properties and increases up to 20-fold in pregnancy. The parturient requires less local anesthetic to produce the same anesthetic level via spinal or epidural routes. This decrease in local anesthetic requirement may be due to a decrease in epidural space volume (due to epidural vein engorgement) and/or an increase in nerve sensitivity to local anesthetics. The lumbar lordosis of pregnancy may increase cephalad spread of local anesthetics placed in the subarachnoid space. Also, an increase in cerebrospinal fluid pressure caused by labor may contribute to reduced local anesthetic requirements during spinal anesthesia.

5. How is the hematologic system changed by pregnancy?

Hematologic and Metabolic Changes in Pregnancy

Erythrocyte volume	↑ (20%)
Plasma volume	↑ (45%)
Blood volume	↑ (35%)
Hemoglobin	↓
Hematocrit	↓ (31.9–36.5%)
Blood urea nitrogen	↓ (33%)
Plasma cholinesterase	↓ (25%)
Total protein	↓
Albumin	↓ (14%)
AST, ALT, LDH	↑
Cholesterol	↓
Alkaline phosphatase	↑
Platelets	No change or ↓
Factors I, VII, VIII, IX, X, XII	↑
Fibrinogen	↑
Fibrinolysis	↓

AST = aspartate aminotransferase, ALT = alanine aminotransferase, LDH = lactate dehydrogenase.

Blood volume, plasma volume, and erythrocyte volume all increase during pregnancy. Plasma volume increases from 40 to 70 ml/kg and red blood cell (RBC) volume increases from 25 to 30 ml/kg. Near term, blood volume increases by 1000 ml to 1500 ml compared to the nonpregnant state; with contractions, approximately 300 to 500 ml of blood enters the vascular system from the uterus. The relative anemia of pregnancy is caused by a relatively slower rise in RBC mass compared to plasma volume. Maternal anemia, usually due to iron deficiency, occurs if the hemoglobin falls below 10 gm or the hematocrit is less than 30%. Hemodilution and decreased blood viscosity may decrease the risk of intervillous thrombosis and infarction.

6. Is coagulation affected during pregnancy?

Parturients are hypercoagulable and at risk for thrombotic events (such as deep venous thrombosis). Platelet activation and consumption are increased during pregnancy. Increased platelet consumption is compensated for by increased platelet production, and the platelet count usually remains unchanged or slightly reduced. Thrombocytopenia (platelet count < 100,000/mm^3) occurs in approximately 0.9% of normal parturients. Bleeding time is shortened during pregnancy.

The concentration of most coagulation factors increases during gestation. Fibrinolysis increases, and fibrin degradation products and plasminogen levels are increased. Prothrombin and partial thromboplastin times are shortened. These changes result in a hypercoagulable state.

7. Do plasma proteins change during pregnancy?

Plasma albumin concentrations decrease during pregnancy. Free fractions of protein-bound drugs increase with falling albumin levels. Total protein levels also decrease during pregnancy, as does maternal colloid osmotic pressure (by approximately 5 mmHg). Plasma cholinesterase concentrations decrease by about 25% before delivery and 33% by 3 days postpartum. Prolonged respiratory impairment rarely occurs after an appropriate dose of succinylcholine. Prolonged neuromuscular blockade (rarely lasting more than 20 minutes) occurs in 2–6% of patients having normal pseudocholinesterase. Conditions interfering with serum cholinesterase activity may decrease its function and prolong recovery from succinylcholine; these include dehydration, acidosis, diabetes mellitus, electrolyte abnormalities, magnesium and trimethaphan use and cholinesterase inhibitors. Monitoring muscle twitch in these patients is recommended to decrease the occurrence of prolonged muscle weakness.

8. Discuss the hepatic changes of pregnancy.

Liver size, blood flow, and liver morphology do not change during pregnancy. Lactate dehydrogenase (LDH), serum bilirubin, alanine aminotransferase (ALT, SGPT), aspartate aminotransferase (AST, SGOT), and alkaline phosphatase increase during pregnancy. Alkaline phosphatase activity increases mostly due to production of this compound by the placenta. Gallbladder emptying slows, and the bile tends to be concentrated. These changes predispose the parturient to gallstone formation.

9. How is the renal system altered in pregnancy?

Renal calices, pelvices, and ureters dilate after the third trimester due to progesterone production. Later in pregnancy, the enlarged uterus compresses the ureter at the pelvic brim, leading to urinary stasis and contributing to the frequency of urinary tract infections during pregnancy.

Renal blood flow and glomerular filtration rate increase with pregnancy. Aldosterone levels also increase, causing increased total body sodium and water. Creatinine clearance is increased as a result of increased renal blood flow and glomerular filtration rate; therefore, serum creatinine and blood urea nitrogen levels are decreased. Glucosuria (1–10 gm/day) and proteinuria (<300 mg/day) are not pathologic in the pregnant patient. Bicarbonate excretion is increased in compensation for the respiratory metabolic alkalosis.

10. How does the musculoskeletal system change during pregnancy?

Lumbar lordosis is enhanced during pregnancy to keep the woman's center of gravity over the lower extremities. This lordosis causes low back discomfort and may make regional anesthesia more challenging. Ligamentous relaxation occurs, causing increased mobility of the sacrococcygeal, sacroiliac, and pubic joints. The pubic symphysis widens. These changes also may contribute to low back pain.

11. What causes labor pain?

During the first stage of labor, pain is caused by cervical dilation and effacement and dilation of the lower uterine segment. This pain is mediated by C-fiber stimulation as afferent nociceptive impulses from the uterus enter the dorsal horn of the spinal cord at T11–T12. It is usually described as a dull, aching pain. Throughout the second stage of labor, the pain is mediated via A-delta fiber stimulation, which enters the spinal cord through the posterior roots of S2–S4 as the lower vagina, vulva, and perineum are distended. This pain is usually sharp in nature.

12. Describe the most important intrapartum physiologic changes and their significance.

The physiologic variables altered during pregnancy are magnified by active labor. Cardiac output increases to two times the prelabor value during active labor, with the maximal increase occurring immediately after delivery. This rise in cardiac output is due to pain and anxiety (increasing circulating catecholamine levels) and the autotransfusion cycle (increasing central venous blood volume during uterine contractions). Hyperventilation is common during active labor and may magnify the preexistent respiratory alkalosis, producing uterine vasoconstriction and compromised placental perfusion, hypoxemia, and fetal distress. Markers for physiologic stress increase during active labor (epinephrine, norepinephrine, cortisol). Metabolic acidosis during active labor may be caused by elevated lactate and pyruvate levels (due to prolonged labor with inadequate hydration) and a compensatory response to maternal alkalemia. Circumstances which aggravate the pH balance (dehydration, hypothermia, hemorrhage, vomiting) may be poorly tolerated during the intrapartum period. Regional anesthesia during the intrapartum period may attenuate the hemodynamic changes, hyperventilation, and stress response associated with active labor.

13. How quickly do the organ systems recover after delivery?

Cardiac output rises immediately after birth because of autotransfusion of 500–750 ml of blood from the sustained contraction of the empty uterus (patients with pulmonary hypertension and stenotic valvular lesions are at risk during this time). Cardiac output returns to normal about 4 weeks postpartum. Functional residual capacity and residual volume rapidly return to normal. Many of the pulmonary changes due to mechanical compression by the gravid uterus resolve quickly. Alveolar ventilation returns to normal by 4 weeks postpartum, and there is a rise in maternal arterial pCO_2 as the progesterone level decreases. The "dilutional" anemia of pregnancy resolves and the hematocrit returns to normal within 4 weeks, due to a postpartum diuresis without a significant change in red cell mass. Serum creatinine, glomerular filtration rate, and blood urea nitrogen return to normal levels in less than 3 weeks. Mechanical effects of the gravid uterus on the gastrointestinal system resolve within 2–3 days postpartum, although gastric emptying may be delayed for several weeks as serum progesterone levels are maintained. Therefore, precautions against pulmonary aspiration of gastric contents should be continued for several weeks postpartum.

14. How is the aortocaval compression syndrome treated?

Aortocaval compression becomes a significant concern by the second trimester and occurs when a pregnant woman assumes the supine position. Signs and symptoms of aortocaval compression are similar to those of shock—hypotension, tachycardia, pallor, sweating, nausea, vomiting, and changes in cerebration. These are caused by lack of venous return to the heart. The gravid uterus compresses the inferior vena cava, decreasing venous return and resulting in these symptoms. If the gravid uterus compresses the aorta, compromising aortic blood flow, there may be a decrease in uterine and placental blood flow resulting in fetal distress. Aortocaval compression is prevented by keeping the patient in a tilted or lateral position. It is treated with uterine displacement (lateral position) to increase venous return, fluids and a pressor (ephedrine) to increase blood pressure quickly, and oxygen to improve fetal oxygenation.

15. What are the three stages of labor?

The first stage begins with the onset of regular contractions and ends with full cervical dilation (10 cm at term). The second stage of labor begins with full cervical dilation and is complete with delivery of the infant. The period of time from delivery of the infant to delivery of the placenta is referred to as the third stage of labor.

16. Describe the phases of cervical dilation in first-stage labor.

Cervical dilation in the first stage of labor occurs over time in an S-shaped curve. This stage is separated into latent and active phases. During the latent phase, many hours of painful uterine contractions may occur with little change in cervical dilation. The cervix effaces and becomes softer during this preparatory phase. The transition between the latent and active phases of the first stage of labor does not occur at a specific cervical dilation but is distinguished by a change in the slope of the cervical dilation curve over time. The active phase is often entered abruptly, and consistent changes in cervical dilation should occur. Peisner and Rosen, evaluating the progress of labor in nulliparous women and parous women, found that 60% of women reached the transition phase to active labor by 4 cm of cervical dilation and 89% reached it by 5 cm.

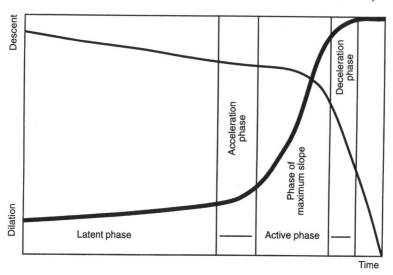

The first stage of labor—The Friedman curve. (From Friedman EA. Patterns of labor as indicators of risk. Clin Obstet Gynecol 16:172–183, 1973, with permission.)

17. Does pregnancy affect a patient's recommended drug dose?

In general, drug dosages are decreased in pregnancy. In pregnant ewes, the minimal alveolar concentration of isoflurane is decreased up to 40%, possibly due to effects of progesterone. Similarly, lower doses of local anesthetics are required for regional anesthesia as early as the first trimester, because there is greater sensitivity to these agents.

18. Describe the anatomy of the maternal-placental-fetal unit.

Maternal component: Uterine blood flow increases from a nonpregnancy rate of 50 ml/min to 500–700 ml/min during pregnancy. The uteroplacental circulation uses up to 20% of maternal cardiac output at term. Eighty percent of uterine blood flow goes to the placenta, whereas the myometrium receives only 20%. Uterine weight increases from 70 gm to 1100 gm at term (not including placental and fetal tissues). The arterial blood supply to the gravid uterus is chiefly provided by the uterine arteries (originating from the hypogastric and ovarian arteries), and these branch to form the arcuate, radial, and spiral arteries, which extend into the placental tissue ending in the intervillous space. The gravid uterus is drained by the decidual veins, which eventually form the uterine and ovarian veins and empty into the inferior vena cava.

Placental component: Both maternal and fetal tissues form the placenta, where the maternal and fetal circulations join. The placenta, which weighs approximately 500 gm at term, is composed of a basal plate (maternal tissue) and a chorionic plate (fetal tissue) separated by an intervillous space. The chorionic plate consists of three layers and includes the fetal chorionic villi (the unit of fetal exchange), which protrude into the intervillous space. Maternal blood enters the intervillous space via the spiral arteries and spreads over the fetal chorionic villi, as fetal blood moves across the umbilical capillaries in the chorionic villi (villous stream pattern). Maternal-to-fetal placental transfer occurs across the chorionic membrane.

Fetal component: Fetal blood, containing the byproducts of fetal metabolism, leaves the fetus via the internal iliac arteries, which give rise to *two umbilical arteries*. These umbilical arteries carry blood away from the fetus via the umbilical cord into the placenta, where they become smaller and give rise to the umbilical capillaries. These capillaries travel through the chorionic villi, where fetal blood is cleansed and oxygenated. Oxygenated blood returns to the fetus via a *single umbilical vein*, with 50% entering the fetal portal circulation (which varies with reactivity of the ductus venosus) and the rest entering the fetal inferior vena cava. At the level of the right atrium, oxygenated blood from the inferior vena cava mixes with poorly oxygenated blood from the superior vena cava (from the head and upper extremities) and is shunted to the left atrium via the open foramen ovale. From here, blood enters the left ventricle and is distributed throughout the fetal body. Fetal lungs do not have a respiratory function in utero and receive only a small amount of perfusion via the right ventricle and pulmonary outflow tract. The *ductus arteriosus* permits this pulmonary blood flow to empty into the fetal aorta.

19. What is the uterine perfusion equation?

$$UBF = (MMAP - UVP)/UVR$$

The vascular bed of the uterus is maximally dilated and therefore is not autoregulated. Uterine blood flow (UBF) is directly related to the mean maternal arterial blood pressure (MMAP). The MMAP is the driving pressure at the level of the spiral artery (average, 80 mmHg) during uterine rest. Resting uterine venous pressure (UVP) is approximately 10 mmHg. Therefore, resting uteroplacental pressure is 70 mmHg. Uterine vascular resistance (UVR) is affected by tension in the myometrium and by vasoconstriction of the uterine, ovarian, arcuate, and radial arteries. Uterine vasculature actively responds to alpha-adrenergic stimulation. During catecholamine release, UBF will decrease and fetal compromise may result.

20. Which five factors influence uteropalcental perfusion?

1. **Aortocaval compression:** When lying supine, gravid patients compress their abdominal aorta, decreasing uteroplacental perfusion.

2. **Hypotension:** A fall in MMAP of 25% is associated with a decrease in uterine blood flow. Uteroplacental perfusion is compromised at MMAP of 100 mmHg systolic.

3. **Increases in uterine vascular resistance:** Increases in uterine vascular resistance occur during contractions and parturition, with use of intravenous ketamine (> 1.5 mg/kg) and oxytocin, and with abruptio placentae.

4. **Maternal hypoxia, hypercarbia, and hypocarbia:** These changes are associated with decreased uteroplacental perfusion.

5. **Catecholamines** (increased uterine vascular resistance): Exogenous or endogenous catecholamines decrease uteroplacental perfusion. Ephedrine and phenylephrine maintain uteroplacental perfusion. Ephedrine acts indirectly and increases MMAP by stimulating a release of catecholamines, not by adrenergic receptor agonism. Phenylephrine is a direct-acting alpha-adrenergic agonist but may be contraindicated because it decreases uterine blood flow in pregnant sheep and decreases placental and myometrial blood flow. Ephedrine affects uterine blood flow less than the other vasopressor agents, and for this reason it is usually used to increase blood pressure in pregnant patients.

21. Describe the fetal umbilical-placental circulation and its influences.

The umbilical-placental circulation uses approximately one-half of the fetal cardiac output (approximately 250 ml/min at term). It is less variable and reactive to stimuli than the maternal uteroplacental circulation. It is a low-pressure system and changes throughout gestation. Early in gestation, asphyxia causes an increase in heart rate without a change in fetal blood pressure. As the fetus matures, bradycardia, with an increase in blood pressure, occurs in response to asphyxia. Continuous fetal heart rate monitoring can detect changes in this circulation. The umbilical-placental circulation is influenced by direct effects on umbilical vessels (mechanical compression with cord prolapse, vasospasm secondary to placental transfer of local anesthetics, vasopressors, maternal hypocarbia and norepinephrine release) and by alterations in the fetal neuroendocrine axis caused by drugs (morphine and diazepam given to the mother decrease fetal heart rate variability).

22. How is placental transfer of substances, including anesthetic compounds and inhaled gases, accomplished?

Placental transfer of substances is accomplished by simple diffusion, active transport, bulk flow, facilitated diffusion, and "breaks" in the chorionic membrane. Anesthetic compounds cross the placenta mostly by simple diffusion, as described by the Fick equation:

$$Q/t = [k \times A \times C_m - C_f)]/D$$

This equation states that the quantity of free drug (nonionized and nonprotein bound, Q) that crosses the placenta per unit of time (t) is directly proportional to the diffusion coefficient of the drug (k), the total area of the chorionic membrane available for transfer (A), and the difference between the maternal (C_m) and fetal concentrations (C_f) of free drug (both in µg/ml) and is indirectly proportional to the distance across the membrane $(D$, in µm).

23. How do the factors contained in the Fick equation affect placental drug transfer?

A drug's molecular weight, spatial configuration, degree of ionization, and lipid solubility determine its diffusion coefficient (k). The greater the diffusion coefficient, the greater the quantity of drug transferred. Compounds that are low in molecular weight, small in spatial configuration, poorly ionized, and lipid soluble have high rates of placental transfer. Most anesthetic drugs are highly lipid soluble and have molecular weights < 600, and for this reason their rates of placental transfer are high. The rate of drug transfer also increases with increasing placental area, with decreasing distance for diffusion, and with increasing maternal free drug concentration. Maternal drug concentrations are dependent on the site of drug administration and the degree of protein binding, tissue redistribution, clearance, metabolism, and blood pH. Drug administration into a densely vascular area increases peak blood levels (intravenous > caudal epidural > paracervical block > lumbar epidural > intramuscular > subarachnoid block). Adding a vasoconstrictor to a local anesthetic may decrease the peak blood level of the drug.

24. Describe the management of the pregnant patient undergoing nonobstetric surgery.

In the pregnant patient, nonemergent surgery should be avoided to protect the developing fetus. If a procedure must be done, the second trimester is the safest time, because the use of drugs during organogenesis and hypoxia during the first trimester can cause congenital anomalies. Surgery during pregnancy increases perinatal mortality, and manipulation of the uterus should be minimal to decrease the risk of premature labor. The most common surgical condition in this population is appendicitis, followed by torsion, rupture, or hemorrhage of ovarian cysts. Cholecystectomies and trauma-related surgery are not uncommon.

When performing regional anesthesia, the following should be accomplished: avoid hypotension, hydrate the patient prior to the block, decrease local anesthetic dose by 30%, keep the patient in the left uterine displacement position, and treat hypotension with ephedrine. If general anesthesia is needed, the patient should be well preoxygenated and undergo rapid-sequence induction and intubation with cricoid pressure. The patient must be extubated awake when protective airway reflexes are intact. If the surgical procedure takes place during the first trimester, drugs with an established safe history should be used. Maternal PaO_2 should be kept between 100 and 200 mmHg. The fetal heart rate should be monitored perioperatively after the 16th week of gestation.

25. What are the anesthetic concerns in pregnant women undergoing nonobstetric surgery?

Anesthetic considerations include the pregnant patient's altered physiology, response to anesthetic drugs, and effects of the anesthetic on the developing fetus. Most anesthesiologists prefer to use local or regional anesthesia when possible, which allows the administration of drugs with no evidence of teratogenicity and is associated with fewer maternal respiratory complications than general anesthesia. If general anesthesia is necessary, drugs with a long history of safe use are preferred, such as thiopental, morphine, meperidine, fentanyl, succinylcholine, curare, pancuronium, and low concentrations of nitrous oxide and isoflurane. A common technique employs a high concentration of oxygen, an opioid, and/or a moderate concentration of an inhalational agent and a muscle relaxant. The use of nitrous oxide is generally not contraindicated after the sixth week of pregnancy, but its use should be limited to a concentration of 50% or less in short operations and avoided during long operations. Nitrous oxide use during early pregnancy (the first 6 weeks) should be avoided, because it may inhibit DNA synthesis with significant exposures.

Although a definitive correlation has not been established between anesthetic drugs and fetal anomalies, minor tranquilizers, such as diazepam, used during the first trimester of pregnancy have been associated with fetal abnormalities (cleft lip and palate). No anesthetic in itself currently appears to be a potent teratogen. If depth of anesthesia is not adequate, catecholamine production resulting from painful surgical stimulation may cause uterine artery vasoconstriction, compromising uterine perfusion. High oxygen concentrations should be maintained and hypotension avoided by aggressive use of fluid administration and divided doses of ephedrine as needed. Epinephrine and norepinephrine may decrease uteroplacental perfusion.

26. How is fetal monitoring used to evaluate fetal well-being?

Fetal heart rate (FHR) monitoring provides important information regarding intrauterine fetal health. The most important index is the relationship of FHR patterns to maternal uterine contractions. The *baseline FHR* is evaluated between contractions and is normally 120–160 bpm. Fetal tachycardia (> 160 bpm) may be caused by fever, hypoxia, beta-sympathomimetic agents, maternal hyperthyroidism, or fetal hypovolemia. Fetal bradycardia (< 120 bpm) may result from hypoxia, complete heart block, beta blockers, local anesthetics, or hypothermia. The moment-to-moment change in FHR is the *beat-to-beat variability*. Fetal well-being is associated with a normal fetal pH and normal FHR variability. Increased variability is seen with uterine contractions and maternal activity. Decreased variability may be due to central nervous system depression, hypoxia, acidosis, sleep, narcotic use, vagal blockade, and magnesium therapy for preeclampsia.

27. Name the different types of fetal heart rate decelerations.

Early decelerations in FHR are caused by head compressions (vagal stimulation), are uniform in shape, begin near the onset of a uterine contraction, and are benign.

Variable decelerations are caused by umbilical cord compression, are nonuniform in shape, abrupt in onset and cessation, and severe if the FHR is < 70 bpm and of duration > 60 seconds. They usually do not reflect fetal acidosis.

Late decelerations are caused by uteroplacental insufficiency, are uniform in shape and are severe when the FHR decreases by > 45 beats below baseline. When severe, they are associated with fetal acidosis. These decelerations are associated with maternal hypotension, hypertension, diabetes, preeclampsia, or intrauterine growth retardation. These are ominous patterns and indicate that the fetus has inadequate reserves (it is not able to maintain normal oxygenation and pH in the face of decreased blood flow). If fetal distress is present, the anesthesiologist should administer oxygen to the mother, maintain maternal blood pressure, and place the parturient in the left uterine displacement position.

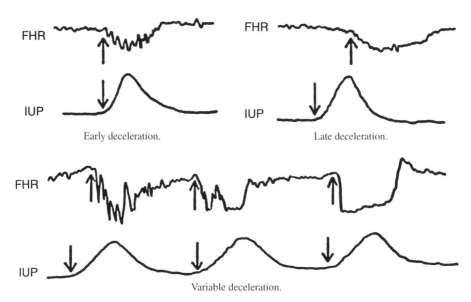

FHR

IUP

Early deceleration.

FHR

IUP

Late deceleration.

FHR

IUP

Variable deceleration.

Early, late, and variable FHR decelerations during labor. (IUP = intrauterine pressure). (From Ackerman WE, Juneja MM: Obstetric Anesthesia Pearls. East Norwalk, CT, Appleton & Lange, 1992, pp 98–100, with permission.)

28. What are normal fetal capillary pH and arterial blood gas values at birth and at 30 minutes of life?

Normal fetal capillary pH is ≥ 7.25. Fetal acidosis is diagnosed when the pH is < 7.20. At birth, normal values for arterial blood gases are pH 7.25, PCO_2 of 40 mmHg, and PO_2 of 60 mmHg. At 30 minutes of life, the normal values are 7.33, 35, and 68, respectively.

29. How does one evaluate the neonate?

The Apgar score, originally introduced in 1952, is the most frequently used index for evaluating neonatal well-being and the fetal effects of medications administered to the mother before birth. This score can also be used as a guide to the success of neonatal resuscitation. The Apgar score is measured at 1 and 5 minutes of life and gives a value to five physiologic variables, with a possible total score of 10. Heart rate and respiratory effort are the most important evaluations. In premature infants, the Apgar score often is low at 1 minute, even when fetal pH is ≥ 7.25, and some Apgar responses may not be elicited. Thus, the 1-minute score in this group may not reflect acid-base status. Infants exposed to general anesthesia in utero also have lower 1-minute Apgar scores, but after effective resuscitation, the 5-minute Apgar score is not significantly different. The 5-minute score is believed to be a predictor of neurologic abnormalities and survival. An Apgar score of 0–3 indicates a severely depressed neonate, whereas a score of 7–10 is considered normal.

The Apgar Score

	0	1	2
Heart rate	Absent	< 100 bpm	> 100 bpm
Respirations	Absent	Irregular, shallow	Good, crying
Reflex irritability	No response	Grimace	Cough, sneeze
Muscle tone	Flaccid	Good tone	Spontaneous flexed arms/legs
Color	Blue, pale	Body pink, extremities blue	Entirely pink

From Chantigan RC: Neonatal evaluation. In Ostheimer GW (ed): Manual of Obstetric Anesthesia. New York, Churchill Livingstone, 1992, p 49, with permission.

30. What drugs are useful in neonatal resuscitation?

Drugs Used in Neonatal Resuscitation

DRUG	DOSE	ROUTE	INDICATION
Atropine	0.02 mg/kg (max 1 mg)	IV/ETT/IM	Bradycardia
Epinephrine	0.01 mg/kg	IV/ETT	Asystole
CaCl$_2$	5–20 mg/kg	IV	Low cardiac output, hypermagnesemia
Isoproterenol	Titrate to 16 µg/kg/min	IV	Persistent bradycardia
Lidocaine	1 mg/kg	IV/ETT	Ventricular arrhythmia
NaHCO$_3$	1–2 mg/kg	IV	Acidosis (pH < 7.1)
Naloxone	0.1 mg/kg	IV	Reverse narcotic-related depression
	0.2 mg/kg	IM	

IV = intravenous, IM = intramuscular, ETT = endotracheal tube.

A mnemonic for remembering which drugs may be administered via endotracheal tube is **LANE** (**l**idocaine, **a**tropine, **n**aloxone, **e**pinephrine).

31. What are the major concerns of anesthesiologists during neonatal resuscitation?

1. **Airway/breathing:** Laryngoscope blade size 0; endotracheal tube 2.5–3.5 mm; suction trachea to prevent aspiration; administer 100% oxygen.

2. **Circulation:** Cardiac compressions 100/min; defibrillation dose 2 J/kg once, then 4 J/kg.

3. **Hypovolemia:** Poor capillary refill; usually blood pressure 50–70 mmHG systolic, 35–50 mmHG diastolic; treat with volume expansion (10 ml/kg).

4. **Hypothermia:** Neonates lose heat quickly because of their large body surface area to mass ratio; blankets, humidified oxygen, and heating lamp should be available.

5. **Hypoglycemia:** Dextrose, 2 mg/kg intravenously, then 5–8 mg/kg/min; may be due to asphyxiation or maternal hyperglycemia; document hypoglycemia prior to dextrose use.

6. **Hypocalcemia:** Calcium chloride given to patients suspected of having low ionized calcium levels contributing to poor cardiac function, for prolonged persistent asystole, and for the urgent treatment of hyperkalemia.

BIBLIOGRAPHY

1. Ackerman WE, Juneja MM: Obstetric Anesthesia Pearls. Norwalk, CT, Appleton & Lange, 1992.
2. Burger GA: Anatomy of the maternal-placental-fetal unit. In Ostheimer GW (ed): Manual of Obstetric Anesthesia. New York, Churchill Livingstone, 1992, pp 32–35.
3. Burger GA: Physiology of the maternal-placental-fetal unit. In Ostheimer GW (ed): Manual of Obstetric Anesthesia. New York, Churchill Livingstone, 1992, pp 35–37.
4. Burger GA: A model of placental transfer of anesthetics. In Ostheimer GW (ed): Manual of Obstetric Anesthesia. New York, Churchill Livingstone, 1992, pp 37–40.
5. Cammann WR, Ostheimer GW: Physiologic adaptions during pregnancy. In Ostheimer GW (ed): Manual of Obstetric Anesthesia. New York, Churchill Livingstone, 1992, pp 1–12.
6. Chantigian RC: Neonatal evaluation. In Ostheimer GW (ed): Manual of Obstetric Anesthesia. New York, Churchill Livingstone, 1992, pp 49–54.
7. Cheek TG, Gutsche BB: Maternal physiologic adaptations during pregnancy. In Shnider SM, Levinson G (eds): Anesthesia for Obstetrics, 3rd ed. Baltimore, Williams & Wilkins, 1993, pp 3–17.
8. Chetham PM: Obstetric anesthesia and uteroplacental blood flow. In Ostheimer GW (ed): Manual of Obstetric Anesthesia. New York, Churchill Livingstone, 1992, pp 41–47.
9. Conklin KA: Physiologic changes of pregnancy. In Chestnut DH (ed): Obstetric Anesthesia Principles and Practice. St. Louis, Mosby-YearBook, 1994, pp 24–28.
10. Friedman EA: Patterns of labor as indicators of risk. Clin Obstet Gynecol 16:172–183, 1973.
11. Palahniuk RJ, Shnider SM, Eger EI: Pregnancy decreases requirements for inhaled anesthetic agents. Anesthesiology 41:82–83, 1974.
12. Peisner DB, Rosen MG: Transition from latent to active labor. Obstet Gynecol 68:448–451, 1986.
13. Rosenfeld CR: Circulatory response to systemic infusion of norepinephrine in the pregnant ewe. Am J Obstet Gynecol 127:376–383, 1977.
14. Santos AC, Mieczyslaw F, Pedersen H: Obstetric anesthesia. In Barash PG, Cullen BF, Stoelting RK (eds): Clinical Anesthesia, 2nd ed. Philadelphia, J.B. Lippincott, 1992, pp 1267–1306.

65. OBSTETRIC ANALGESIA AND ANESTHESIA

Ana M. Lobo, M.D., M.P.H.

1. What are the most commonly used parenteral opioids for labor analgesia? Which side effects are of special concern to the parturient?

Intravenous and Intramuscular Analgesics for Labor

DRUG	USUAL DOSE	ONSET	DURATION	COMMENTS
Meperidine	25 mg IV 50 mg IM	5–10 MIN IV 40–45 min IM	2–3 hr	Active metabolite is normeperidine; neonatal effects most likely if delivery occurs between 1 and 4 hr after administration.
Morphine	2–5 mg IV 10 mg IM	5 min IV 20–40 min IM	3–4 hr	Infrequent use during labor; greater respiratory depression in neonate than with meperidine
Fentanyl	25–50 µg IV 100 µg IM	2–3 min IV 10 min IM	30–60 min	Short-acting, potent respiratory depressant, used as continuous infusion and/or PCA; cumulative effect with large doses over time.
Nalbuphine	10–20 mg IV/IM	2–3 min IV 15 min IM/SQ	3–6 hr	Agonist/antagonist, less nausea and vomiting than with meperidine.
Butorphanol	1–2 mg IV/IM	5–10 min IV/IM	3–4 hr	Agonist/antagonist; maternal sedation similar to meperidine plus phenothiazine.
Pentazocine	20–40 mg IV/IM	2–3 min IV 15–20 min IM/SQ	2–3 hr	Agonist/antagonist; psychomimetic effects possible with usual doses but more frequent after large doses; infrequent use.

IV = intravenous; IM = intramuscular, PCA = patient-controlled analgesia, SQ = subcutaneous.
(From Wakefield ML: Systemic analgesia. Opioids, ketamine and inhalational agents. In Chestnut DH (ed): Obstetric Anesthesia: Principles and Practice. St. Louis, Mosby, 1994, p 341, with permission.)

In general, the above intravenous (IV) drugs help the parturient to tolerate labor pain but rarely provide complete analgesia. The incidence of side effects and efficacy of analgesia are dose-dependent, not drug-dependent. Opioids easily cross the placenta and may cause a decrease in fetal heart rate with beat-to-beat variability. In addition, IV opioids may cause neonatal respiratory depression and neurobehavioral changes.

2. What advantages does patient-controlled analgesia (PCA) offer over conventional intermittent bolus dosing?
PCA has been associated with greater patient satisfaction, less risk of maternal respiratory depression, less placental drug transfer, less need for antiemetic use, and better pain relief with lower drug doses. PCA is especially useful if epidural anesthesia is contraindicated or not available or has not been successful.

3. Discuss the benefits of epidural anesthesia for labor and delivery.
In most laboring women, epidural analgesia is effective, reduces maternal catecholamine levels, and improves uteroplacental perfusion. Induction of catecholamine secretion as a result of

painful contractions may prolong labor by adversely affecting uterine contractility. In addition, painful contractions may lead to maternal hyperventilation and respiratory alkalosis, which in turn shifts the oxyhemoglobin dissociation curve to the left, increasing maternal oxygen affinity and decreasing delivery of oxygen to the fetus. Between contractions, hypocarbia leads to maternal hypoventilation, which may result in decreased maternal oxygenation. Epidural analgesia may stop this cycle.

4. What are the indications and contraindications for epidural anesthesia in labor and delivery?

The treatment of labor pain is an indication for epidural anesthesia. Traumatic vaginal breech delivery and vaginal delivery of twins are made easier by epidural anesthesia. In addition, epidural anesthesia facilitates instrumental delivery and helps to control hypertension in preeclamptic patients. Epidural analgesia is also useful in patients with certain medical problems (e.g. mitral stenosis and other cardiac disease), because it blunts the hemodynamic effects that accompany uterine contractions (increased preload, tachycardia, increased systemic vascular resistance [SVR], hypertension, and hyperventilation). The contraindications to epidural anesthesia include patient refusal, coagulopathy, uncontrolled hemorrhage, increased intracranial pressure due to a mass lesion or cerebral edema, skin or soft-tissue infection at the site of needle introduction, and inexperience of the anesthesiologist with this technique. Relative contraindications include systemic maternal infection and neurologic disease.

5. Discuss the importance of a test dose and suggest an epidural test-dose regimen. When and why is this regimen used?

The idea behind administering a test dose of local anesthetic is to recognize subarachnoid or intravenous placement of the epidural catheter, thereby preventing total spinal anesthesia or systemic toxicity, respectively. A test dose may be 3 ml of 1.5% lidocaine with 1:200,000 epinephrine. If the dose of local anesthetic is given in the subarachnoid space, a spinal block will appear within 3–5 minutes. Sacral, lumbar, or thoracic sensory blockade may result. If the local anesthetic is injected intravenously, tachycardia may result within 45 seconds (increase in heart rate of 30 bpm) because of the epinephrine additive. This test may not be specific, however; other causes of tachycardia during labor (e.g., pain) may elicit the same response. A test dose should be given before each subsequent bolus of local anesthetic, because the epidural catheter may migrate intrathecally or intravascularly. Aspiration of the catheter is not adequate to identify all cases of intrathecal or intravascular catheter placement. If there is any doubt in the anesthesiologist's mind about the exact site at which the epidural catheter is placed, the catheter should be removed and replaced. Subjective symptoms may also indicate an intravascular injection of local anesthetic (e.g., dizziness, tinnitus, somnolence).

6. What are the characteristics of the ideal local anesthetic for use in labor? Discuss the three most common local anesthetics used in obstetric analgesia. How does epinephrine affect the action of local anesthetics?

The ideal local anesthetic in labor would have rapid onset of action, minimal risk of toxicity to mother and fetus, minimal motor blockade with effective sensory blockade, and a minor effect on uterine activity and placental perfusion. Bupivacaine, lidocaine and chloroprocaine are most commonly used in obstetric analgesia.

Bupivacaine is an amide type of local anesthetic and is the most commonly used local anesthetic for obstetric analgesia. Pain relief is first noted by the patient after 10 minutes; twenty minutes are required to achieve peak effect. Analgesia usually lasts approximately 2 hours. Dilute solutions provide excellent sensory analgesia with minimal motor blockade. During early labor a 0.125% solution is often adequate, whereas a 0.25% solution is usually required during the active phase. Because bupivacaine is highly protein-bound, its transplacental transfer is limited.

Lidocaine is also an amide local anesthetic used in concentrations of 0.75–1.5% for sensory analgesia. It crosses the placenta more readily than bupivacaine and may not provide analgesia comparable to that of bupivacaine. Analgesia lasts approximately 1½ hours and is usually apparent within 10 minutes.

2-Chloroprocaine is an ester local anesthetic. Onset of analgesia is rapid. Effective analgesia is provided for approximately 40 minutes; this short duration limits its usefulness in labor. The efficacy of bupivacaine or opioids is diminished by prior use of chloroprocaine. Chloroprocaine 3% is frequently used to increase the anesthetic level quickly for cesarean section or instrumental vaginal delivery. Chloroprocaine has a very short half-life in maternal and fetal blood. Back pain may occur with epidural injection of large volumes of nesacaine R (a new formulation of 2-chloroprocaine) and is thought to be caused by disodium ethylenediaminetetraacetic acid (EDTA) which is added as an antioxidant to stabilize the nesacaine R formulation. The pain is usually severe and may last several hours. It is relieved by a further dose of epidural local anesthetic or by 100–200 µg epidural fentanyl.

Addition of epinephrine (1:200,000) to bupivacaine speeds its onset and lengthens its duration of action. Epinephrine also increases the intensity of motor blockade (which is not desirable in laboring patients).

7. Name three methods of maintaining an epidural block. State the concerns and appropriate doses associated with each.
The three methods of maintaining an epidural block include intermittent bolus injection, continuous infusion, and patient-controlled epidural anesthesia (PCEA).

Intermittent injection requires that the catheter be checked for migration into the subarachnoid space or a blood vessel via aspiration and a repeat test dose. After multiple injections, the patient may develop intense motor block and blockade of sacral segments.

Maintenance of epidural anesthesia also may be accomplished by a continuous infusion of dilute local anesthetic (with or without added opioid). The possible benefits of this method include (1) less need to give bolus injections of local anesthetic (with inherent risk of systemic toxicity), (2) maintenance of a stable level of analgesia, (3) maintenance of stable maternal hemodynamics with decreased risk of hypotension, and (4) improved patient satisfaction. The patient should be assessed hourly for signs of catheter migration and adequacy of analgesia, as well as progress of labor. The infusion tubing used should be labeled and have no side injection ports. The infusion pump should be different from that of intravenous infusion lines to minimize the chance of accidental injection of other substances into the epidural space.

With PCEA, each patient may adjust the dose that she receives to control her level of analgesia. PCEA may result in greater patient satisfaction and less total dose of drug than other techniques. Errors may occur in pump programming, however. As with a continuous infusion, the above precautions apply to PCEA, and the patient should be checked frequently for catheter migration and degree of analgesia.

Maintaining an Epidural Block: Intermittent Injection and Continuous Infusion Techniques

DRUGS	INTERMITTENT INJECTION	CONTINUOUS INFUSION
Bupivacaine	5–10 ml of a 0.125–0.375% solution every 90–120 minutes	0.0625–0.25% solution at 8–15 ml/hr
Lidocaine	5–10 ml of a 0.75–1.5% solution every 60–90 minutes	0.5–1.0% solution at 8–15 ml/hr
2-Chloroprocaine	5–10 ml of a 1–2% solution every 45–60 minutes	0.75% solution at 27 ml/hr

From Glosten B: Epidural and spinal anesthesia/analgesia—local anesthetic techniques. In Chestnut DH:Obstetric Anesthesia Principles and Practice. St. Louis, Mosby, 1994, p 363, with permission.

8. Describe three different techniques used to provide analgesia for vaginal delivery.
During vaginal delivery, pain is due to distention of the perineum and vagina, mediated via the pudendal nerve (S2–S4). The nerve fibers are somatic and large. Larger doses of local anesthetic

are frequently required for blockade at a time when a motor block is not desirable because the patient needs to push. Perineal analgesia may be augmented by a bolus dose of local anesthetic via a lumbar epidural catheter (e.g., 10-15 ml of 1–2% lidocaine). This is especially useful if instrumentation is used during delivery. If no lumbar epidural catheter is in place, a caudal epidural catheter may be placed. Currently this type of analgesia is not frequently used because it is technically difficult (85% failure rate) and involves an increased risk of injecting local anesthetic directly into the fetus. Spinal anesthesia (saddle block) also may be used via a subarachnoid catheter or as a single injection (intrathecal injection of 25–50 mg hyperbaric lidocaine, 4–6 mg of hyperbaric tetracaine, or 6–8 mg of hyperbaric bupivacaine). This technique blocks the sacral spinal segments and facilitates atraumatic delivery, especially if instrumentation or forceps are required.

9. Discuss the complications of epidural anesthesia and their treatments.

Complications of epidural anesthesia include hypotension, inadequate analgesia, intravenous injection of local anesthetic, unintentional dural puncture, unexpected high block, unexpected prolonged block, extensive motor block, urinary retention, and back pain.

Hypotension (systolic blood pressure [SBP] < 100 mg or SBP decrease of 20–30%) may accompany dosing of the epidural catheter with local anesthetic. Epidurally administered local anesthetics cause sympathetic blockade, peripheral venodilation, and decreased venous return to the heart, which results in a drop in maternal cardiac output and blood pressure. Uncorrected hypotension results in decreased uteroplacental perfusion, which leads to fetal distress. Treatment involves volume expansion, supplemental oxygen, and placement of the mother in the full lateral and Trendelenburg positions. Ephedrine (5–10 mg) IV should be administered if blood pressure does not promptly return to normal.

Inadequate analgesia may result. The epidural catheter may be misplaced initially or the catheter may migrate out of the epidural space. The failure rate during placement is up to 5% and depends on the skill of the anesthesiologist. Analgesia may also be incomplete (unilateral, asymmetric, or missed segments) because of the position of the catheter in relation to other epidural structures that affect the spread and quality of analgesia. Opioids may be given (in addition to local anesthetic) to augment a marginal block.

Intravenous injection of large amounts of local anesthetic causes central nervous system and cardiovascular (CV) symptoms. Dizziness, restlessness, tinnitus, seizures, and loss of consciousness may occur. CV effects begin with an increase in blood pressure (due to sympathetic stimulation) and eventually result in bradycardia, decreased ventricular function, ventricular tachycardia, and ventricular fibrillation. Bupivacaine toxicity is especially severe and may be fatal. Treatment includes the following:

1. Stop convulsions with a barbiturate or a benzodiazepine.
2. Give the patient 100% O_2 and intubate if necessary (to oxygenate, ventilate, and protect the airway).
3. Support blood pressure (IV fluids and pressors).
4. Treat bradycardia with atropine.
5. Treat ventricular tachycardia with bretylium.
6. Treat ventricular fibrillation with bretylium, epinephrine and defibrillation.
7. Use cardiopulmonary resuscitation if necessary.
8. Delivery of the fetus may help resuscitation of the mother.
9. Prolonged resuscitative efforts should ensue if bupivacaine is involved.

Unintentional dural puncture may occur during attempts to identify the epidural space. The incidence of this complication is about 1–8% in obstetric patients. If cerebrospinal fluid (CSF) is noted with the epidural needle, the needle should be removed and the epidural catheter placed at an alternate interspace. Whether a postdural puncture headache may be prevented by injecting saline or blood via the epidural catheter is controversial. Local anesthetic subsequently injected epidurally may pass into the subarachnoid space and result in a block that is unexpectedly high. After a dural puncture, the catheter may be threaded into the subarachnoid space and produce spinal anesthesia, which may be used for analgesia. The continuous spinal technique is usually reserved for patients who have poor anatomy or are at risk for another wet tap.

An **unexpected high block** also may occur during epidural anesthesia. The epidural catheter may be placed unintentionally into the subdural or subarachnoid space, or the catheter may migrate into the subarachnoid space during the course of labor and delivery. Injection of an epidural dose of local anesthetic in the above cases may lead to an unexpected high block. The incidence of a high or total spinal block is approximately 1 in 4,500 lumbar epidurals during labor. Risk is minimized by aspirating the catheter and giving a test dose each time the catheter is bolused. The signs and symptoms of a total spinal include hypotension, dyspnea, inability to speak, and loss of consciousness. Treatment includes oxygen administration, intubation, ventilation and support of maternal circulation with IV fluids and ephedrine or epinephrine if needed until the block recedes. Subdural (potential space between the dura and arachnoid mater) injection of local anesthetic may also result in a high block which has a slow onset and an unexplained high, patchy block. This block may rise cephalad to involve the brainstem (causing apnea and loss of consciousness) and frequently spares the sacral nerves. These catheters are not useful for labor and delivery and should be replaced.

An **unexpected prolonged block** may occur in patients who are particularly sensitive to the anesthetic used. Unless a peripheral nerve injury has occurred or an epidural hematoma or abscess is present, an unexpected prolonged block is usually the result of the use of a high concentration of local anesthetic with epinephrine. Epidural hematoma or abscess should be suspected if the patient has back pain or bilateral block and symptoms worsen (as the mass expands). Peripheral nerve injuries are common during difficult deliveries or improper positioning. The result is a neurologic deficit contained only within the distribution of the nerve.

Extensive motor block may occur after several hours of epidural bupivacaine (especially with epinephrine) or after repeated bolus doses. If motor block occurs, stop the infusion for 30 minutes and resume with a more dilute concentration of local anesthetic or at a reduced rate.

Urinary retention sometimes occurs after vaginal delivery. Difficulty in voiding often occurs after perineal edema, hematoma, and trauma. Currently, it has not been established whether epidural analgesia is associated with postpartum urinary retention, although dense analgesia decreases the patient's urge to void. Treatment of prolonged urinary retention is catheterization.

The association between epidural anesthesia for labor and delivery and **postpartum back pain** is controversial.

10. How does epidural analgesia affect placental and fetal blood flow, neonatal outcome, and maternal body temperature?

Uteroplacental blood flow and umbilical artery vascular resistance are not adversely affected by epidural analgesia for labor (in the absence of maternal hypotension). The association between epidural analgesia and neonatal outcome is controversial. No conclusive evidence indicates that epidural analgesia negatively affects neonatal outcome; in fact, it may be beneficial. Epidural anesthesia may decrease core maternal body temperature (causing a shivering response) by heat redistribution to the periphery. Epidural opioids suppress shivering.

11. Explain the mechanism of action of intrathecal and epidural opioids. What effect do they have on pain perception, sympathetic tone, sensation, and movement?

Opioids administered intrathecally or epidurally provide excellent analgesia under certain circumstances without appreciably affecting sympathetic tone, sensation, and voluntary motor function. Opioids given via these routes bind to presynaptic and postsynaptic receptor sites in the dorsal horn of the spinal cord (Rexed laminae I, II, V) and in the brainstem nuclei, periventricular gray matter, and medial thalamus. Within the spinal cord, opioids bind to different types of opioid receptors (i.e. mu, kappa, epsilon, gamma, sigma), resulting in varied physiologic responses. In this manner, opioids block transmission of pain-related information. Opioids given epidurally first penetrate the dura, then pass through CSF, and eventually bind to the above receptor sites.

12. What opioids are used to provide spinal and epidural analgesia during labor? Name their most common side effects. Do they provide adequate analgesia for labor and delivery when used alone?

The most commonly used epidural opioids include fentanyl, sufentanil, morphine, and meperidine. Pruritus, nausea, and vomiting are the most common side effects; delayed respiratory depression is the most serious complication. Intrathecal or epidural opioids alone may provide adequate relief for the early stages of labor, but they are unreliable in producing adequate analgesia for the late first stage and second stage of labor. Concurrent administration of local anesthetic is recommended for late cervical dilation and delivery of the infant. However, opioids alone are useful in patients who cannot tolerate sympathetic blockade. The coaxial technique (see question 24) frequently involves the use of intrathecal opioid for analgesia during the first stage of labor.

Opioids Used to Provide Intrathecal Analgesia During Labor

DRUG	DOSE
Morphine	0.25–0.3 mg
Fentanyl	10–20 µg
Suftentanil	5–10 µg
Meperidine	10 mg

From Ross BK: Epidural and spinal anesthesia/analgesia—opioid techniques. In Chestnut DH (ed): Obstetric Anesthesia Principles and Practice. St. Louis, Mosby, 1994, p 382, with permission.

Opioids Used to Provide Epidural Analgesia During Labor

OPIOID	LIPID SOLUBILITY*	DOSE	ONSET (min)	DURATION (hr)
Morphine	1.4	3–5 mg	30–60	4–12
Meperidine	39	25–50 mg	5–10	2–4
Methadone	116	5 mg	15–20	6–8
Butorphanol	140	2-4 mg	10–15	6–12
Diamorphine	280	5 mg	9–15	6–12
Fetanyl	816	50–100 µg	5–10	1–2
Sufentanil	1727	5–10 µg	5–10	1–3

From Ross BK: Epidural and spinal anesthesia/analgesia—opioid techniques. In Chestnut DH (ed): Obstetric Anesthesia Principles and Practice. St. Louis, Mosby, 1994, p 382, with permission.

13. What are the major advantages of using a dilute local anesthetic-opioid solution for epidural administration during labor?

A solution of 0.0625% bupivacaine plus 2 µg/ml of fentanyl administered at 10–14 ml/hr provides excellent analgesia. It minimizes the amount of local anesthetic that the patient receives and the development of motor block. Side effects of both agents are also lessened.

14. Is there a cause-and-effect relationship between epidural anesthesia and prolonged labor or operative delivery?

This issue is highly controversial. Research attempting to answer this question is fraught with inadequacies. For ethical reasons, controlled trials of patients randomized to receive epidural anesthesia or another form of pain relief are scarce. Multiple reports in the obstetric literature state that epidural anesthesia is associated with prolonged labor or operative delivery. Recently, Hawkins et al. retrospectively reviewed the charts of 14,804 women and found that after a 10-fold increase in its use, the association between epidural anesthesia and instrumental delivery remained the same. In addition, they found that gestational age > 41 weeks, a second stage of labor

> 2 hours, an occiput posterior or transverse fetal position, previous cesarean section, and epidural anesthesia are independently and individually associated with an increase in the incidence of instrumental delivery. Maintenance of dense anesthesia may prolong the second stage of labor. However, a prolonged second stage per se does not appear to harm the mother or the infant. Few controlled studies have addressed the relationship of epidural analgesia to the incidence of cesarean section, and the results of uncontrolled studies are contradictory. In a recent study, Chestnut et al. randomized healthy nulliparous women with vertex presentation of a single fetus of at least 36 weeks' gestation, whose labor required oxytocin augmentation, to receive early (3–5 cm) or late (> 5 cm cervical dilation) epidural analgesia. They concluded that early epidural administration did not prolong labor or increase the incidence of malposition at delivery or the cesarean rate. The current belief of most anesthesiologists is that it is not humane to withhold anesthesia during the first stage of labor until a patient is dilated to an arbitrary amount or to stop analgesia during the second stage.

15. What alternative regional anesthetic techniques can be used in patients who have a contraindication to epidural and spinal anesthesia?

Alternative techniques include paracervical block, lumbar sympathetic block, pudendal nerve block, and perineal infiltration.

Paracervical blocks are used to control pain resulting from the first stage of labor (T10–L1). The goal is to block transmission of pain fibers through the paracervical ganglion. Fear of fetal injury has limited the application of paracervical blocks. Fetal bradycardia is an adverse effect. Fetal scalp injection of local anesthetic results in toxicity and possibly death.

Lumbar sympathetic block interrupts the transmission of pain impulses from the cervix and lower uterine segment to the spinal cord (stage 1). There is less risk of fetal bradycardia with lumbar sympathetic block. Afferent sensory fibers from the lower uterus and cervix join the sympathetic chain at L2–L3. This block is technically difficult and has mostly been abandoned in the United States.

The **pudendal nerve** (S2–S4) carries the primary sensory nerve fibers from the lower vagina, vulva, and perineum and provides motor innervation to the perineal muscles and external anal sphincter. Pudendal nerve block is useful for analgesia during delivery. Maternal and fetal complications are rare.

The most common local anesthetic technique used today is **perineal infiltration**, which provides anesthesia only for episiotomy and repair.

16. What factors are of special importance in the preanesthetic evaluation of the obstetric patient?

A thorough history and physical examination should be done before the administration of *any* anesthetic to *any* patient. It is important to ask the patient about her medical history and to review any previous anesthetic records available (see table, top of next page). The patient also should be asked if she has had any allergies to medications, previous operations or problems with anesthesia (including an anesthetic history of her family), obstetric difficulties and modes of delivery (including anesthetic type), and above average weight gain with pregnancy (>25 lbs). A review of the patient's previous anesthetic records may indicate a potential problem with intubation, placement of a regional anesthetic, and/or particular sensitivity or reaction to a previously administered drug.

During the physical examination of the pregnant patient, it is particularly important to evaluate the vital signs, head, neck, heart, lungs, back, and extremities. Blood pressure measurement may reveal hypertension. The airway must be thoroughly evaluated by noting mouth opening, jaw range of motion, thyromental distance, neck extension, condition of teeth, size of tongue, and visualization of the uvula, tonsils and hard and soft palates. Pregnant patients may be difficult to intubate, because their airways are frequently edematous and enlarged breasts may interfere with proper exposure of the airway on laryngoscopy. Auscultation of the heart may reveal a moderate systolic murmur frequently present in pregnant patients. The lung exam should note the presence

Important Historical Information for the Preanesthetic Evaluation to the Obstetrical Patient.

SYSTEM	SPECIFIC ELEMENTS
Head and neck	Limitations in mouth opening and jaw range of motion, neck extension, loose teeth, dental prostheses, mental status changes, headaches, seizures, psychiatric disorders
Respiratory	Smoking, asthma, cough, dyspnea, recent respiratory infection
Cardiovascular	Rheumatic fever, murmur, angina, palpitations, orthopnea
Endocrine	Thyroid disorder, diabetes mellitus
Hepatic	Jaundice, hepatitis
Renal	Kidney or bladder disorders
Hematologic	Thromboses, bleeding disorders
Gastrointestinal	Last food or beverage intake, nausea, vomiting, hiatal hernia, heartburn
Musculoskeletal	Lumbar lordosis, back pain, radicular pain, rheumatic disorders
Genitourinary	Herpes simplex virus labialis (epidural morphine may cause a postpartum recurrence)

of rhonchi, rales, or wheezes. The back should be palpated to evaluate the degree of difficulty that can be expected in performing regional anesthesia and inspected for signs of infection or evidence of previous surgery. Deformities or restriction of movement in the extremities should be noted. A neuromuscular examination to test the patient's reflexes should be performed before delivery of a regional anesthetic. Peripheral nerves that should be evaluated include the obturator, femoral, sciatic, and deep peroneal nerves.

Based on the patient's history and physical examination, appropriate laboratory studies must be ordered. An initial hemoglobin concentration and hematocrit are useful to evaluate the need for a blood transfusion both intra- and perioperatively (based on the estimated blood loss during the procedure).

17. How should the pregnant patient be prepared for anesthesia? Which premedications should be given?

The patient and anesthesiologist should agree on the type of anesthetic that will be administered. It is necessary that all risks of anesthesia be clearly explained and understood by the patient. She also should be told what to expect from the anesthetic agreed upon. General anesthesia is indicated if the patient is hypovolemic and/or significantly bleeding, has a significant bleeding disorder or elevated intracranial pressure, or refuses a regional block or if an emergency situation may necessitate a general anesthetic. General anesthesia in the obstetric patient requires rapid-sequence induction with cricoid pressure to minimize the risk of pulmonary aspiration (pregnant patients are "full stomachs"). Regional anesthesia is preferred whenever possible. When the procedure is performed correctly, the patient's airway reflexes are preserved and pulmonary aspiration is minimized compared with general anesthesia.

Before any anesthetic is administered, the patient must have a large-bore intravenous line (18 gauge or greater) for hydration and drug and blood administration. Dextrose-containing solutions should be avoided, because they may result in maternal hyperglycemia and hyperinsulinemia with subsequent neonatal hypoglycemia (especially in patients with gestational diabetes). Hypovolemia before a general or regional anesthetic should be avoided to prevent hypotension associated with anesthetic administration.

All patients should be premedicated with an antacid before receiving any type of anesthetic. Antacid administration decreases morbidity if the patient aspirates. **Sodium citrate** is a nonparticulate antacid frequently used to elevate the gastric pH without increasing gastric volume. Gastric pH should be higher than 2.5 to decrease the morbidity of pulmonary aspiration. **Metoclopramide** should be given (10 mg IV) before emergency cesarean sections to accelerate gastric emptying and to increase lower esophageal sphincter tone. Its onset of action with IV administration is 1–3 minutes. **Cimetidine** and **ranitidine** are H2 receptor antagonists that decrease gastric acidity and gastric volume. Both also may be given for aspiration prophylaxis, although their time of onset is 60 to 90 minutes. **Alka-Seltzer** (2 tablets) dissolved in a small amount of water may be given to patients before a regional anesthetic for labor to buffer the acidity of the contents of the patient's stomach.

18. What preoperative preparations should be made before cesarean section?

In addition to the preoperative preparations discussed above, the following steps should be taken before cesarean section.

1. If the patient will have regional anesthesia, approximately 15–20 ml/kg of a balanced salt solution should be administered within 30 minutes of surgery. For general anesthesia, less volume is required.

2. A blood type and screen should be readily available, because blood loss may be significant (usually 500–1000 ml).

3. Avoid aortocaval compression by providing left uterine displacement continuously during patient transport and throughout the procedure.

4. Intraoperative monitoring should include blood pressure, ECG, pulse oximetry, arterial oxygen saturation (SaO_2), temperature, and fetal heart rate (FHR) for all anesthetics. Cesarean sections under general anesthesia also should include an end-tidal carbon dioxide monitor, a precordial stethoscope, and nerve stimulator.

19. Name several preventative measures that help to avoid the most common maternal complications during cesarean section.

Acid aspiration prophylaxis should be given to every patient (regardless of anesthetic technique) to decrease gastric volume and acidity (sodium citrate, H2 receptor antagonist, and metoclopramide). Other measures used to prevent aspiration include rapid-sequence induction with cricoid pressure, avoidance of general anesthesia (if possible), and awake intubations in patients with difficult airway. Orogastric tubes may be used to empty the stomach before emergence.

A difficult and complicated intubation may be avoided by thorough examination of a patient's airway and neck mobility. A plan should be in mind to deal with the recognized and unrecognized difficult airway. To prevent hypotension, give IV fluids and a vasopressor, when necessary, in addition to keeping the patient positioned with uterine displacement in mind. To prevent a high spinal or systemically toxic reaction, use a test dose when planning an epidural anesthetic. The most common causes of a failed spinal anesthetic include inadequate dose of local anesthetic, forgetting to put the local anesthetic into the drug mixture, incorrect placement of the local anesthetic (anywhere other than the subarachnoid space), and, rarely, a large volume of a low-potency drug. Spinal anesthesia may be repeated if it does not work. General anesthesia may be used if the patient refuses a second attempt. Epidural anesthesia fails in 2–6% of cases. Epidural anesthesia can be repeated or another technique chosen. If spinal anesthesia is performed after inadequate epidural anesthesia, a high spinal block may result. A large volume of local anesthetic in the epidural space from the previous attempt may decrease the volume in the lumbar subarachnoid space, causing a high spinal block. In this instance, it is prudent to assess the level of block (from the epidural local anesthetic) and reduce accordingly the amount of local anesthetic injected intrathecally (usually about 20–30% less).

20. What types of anesthetic techniques are appropriate for routine cesarean and emergent section?

In choosing an anesthetic technique, one must consider the health of the mother and fetus, the indication for abdominal delivery, the degree of urgency of the procedure, and the mother's wishes.

Spinal anesthesia is usually a good choice for most urgent and elective procedures if an epidural catheter is not in place or is not functioning properly. Epidural anesthesia is a good choice if one is concerned about sympathetic blockade that is too rapid and hypotension or if the patient cannot handle a dense motor blockade of the thoracoabdominal musculature because of preexistent respiratory compromise.

General anesthesia is indicated for truly emergent cesarean sections. In cases of fetal distress or stress, the choice of anesthesia depends on the severity of fetal compromise vs. the risks of general anesthesia to the mother. Regional spinal anesthesia has not been found to place the fetus at increased risk.

For patients with medical problems, the choice of anesthesia depends on the degree and type of illness. Maternal hemorrhage usually requires general anesthesia. In patients who are extremely debilitated, local anesthesia may be indicated. It may also be used to supplement an incomplete epidural or spinal block.

21. Relate the advantages and disadvantages of spinal anesthesia for cesarean section. Which drugs are frequently used in the technique?

Spinal anesthesia produces a dense neural blockade, is relatively easy to perform, has a rapid onset, and results in a negligible risk of infant local anesthetic depression and maternal systemic local anesthetic toxicity. The development of small-gauge, noncutting needles has significantly reduced the incidence of postdural-puncture headache (PDPH). Spinal anesthesia is frequently used in elective cesarean sections. Disadvantages include rapid onset of sympathectomy and hypotension and the possibility that if the surgical procedure is prolonged, supplemental analgesia or general anesthesia may become necessary.

Drugs Used for Spinal Anesthesia for Cesarean Section

DRUG	DOSAGE RANGE (mg)	DURATION (min)
Lidocaine	60–75	45–75
Bupivacaine	7.5–15.0	60–120
Tetracaine	7.0–10.0	60–120
Procaine	100–150	30–60
Adjuvant drugs		
Epinephrine	0.2	–
Morphine	0.25–0.4	360–1080
Fentanyl	0.015–0.025	180–240

From Reisner LS: Anesthesia for cesarean section. In Chestnut DH (ed): Obstetric Anesthesia: Principles and Practice, St. Louis, Mosby, 1994, p 468, with permission.

22. What drugs can be added to the local anesthetic to enhance the quality of the spinal block and/or provide postoperative analgesia?

Preservative-free morphine and epinephrine enhance the quality of spinal anesthesia. Epinephrine prolongs the duration of a tetracaine spinal by up to 50%. Morphine and fentanyl provide postoperative analgesia.

23. What are the advantages and disadvantages of cesarean section with epidural anesthesia? What are the most commonly used local anesthetics?

Epidural anesthesia is frequently used for labor and delivery, and the same catheter can be used for operative delivery. Epidural catheters allow the local anesthetic to be given in increments so that the dose can be titrated to the desired sensory level. Titration of local anesthetic dose and a slow onset of block result in more controlled sympathetic blockade. Thus, the risk of hypotension is decreased, as is the risk of reduced uteroplacental blood flow. This technique is useful in patients who have cardiovascular disease or preeclampsia. Epidural anesthesia may be maintained via repeated dosing if surgical time is prolonged. Typically, epidural blocks produce a less intense motor blockade than spinal anesthesia. This may be advantageous in patients with respiratory compromise.

Disadvantages include slower onset of analgesia, large local anesthetic dose requirement, and risk of total spinal anesthesia or systemic toxicity if the epidural catheter migrates. Unintentional dural puncture usually occurs in < 1% of patients, but 50–85% of such patients experience headache.

Drugs commonly used for cesarean section via epidural include 0.5% bupivacaine, 2% lidocaine, and 3% chloroprocaine. Epinephrine (1:200,000) may be added to prolong the duration of the block, to decrease vascular absorption of the local anesthetic and to improve the quality of the block. The addition of epinephrine to a local anesthetic (with subsequent systemic absorption) does not appear to affect uterine blood flow adversely. Fentanyl, morphine, and meperidine enhance intraoperative analgesia and provide postoperative pain relief (see question 12). The addition of 1 mEq of sodium bicarbonate per 10 ml of lidocaine hastens the onset of anesthesia. It is frequently necessary to add epinephrine to lidocaine for cesarean section, because lidocaine alone is unreliable in providing consistently satisfactory anesthesia.

24. How is combined spinal and epidural anesthesia performed? What are its advantages?
The anesthesiologist first finds the epidural space by loss-of-resistance technique with a Touhy needle. Subsequently, a long (4¹/₂ in), small-gauge (24 G), noncutting (Sprotte) spinal needle is advanced through the epidural needle and clear CSF is noted. A spinal dose of local anesthetic (plus narcotic, if desired) is injected into the subarachnoid space, and the spinal needle is removed. The epidural catheter is subsequently threaded into the epidural space. The major advantage of this coaxial technique is that rapid onset and dense analgesia (spinal anesthesia) are combined with the ability to dose the epidural sequentially to the desired level. This technique also results in a low incidence of PDPH.

25. List the indications for general anesthesia for cesarean section.
Extreme fetal distress (in the absence of a functioning epidural catheter)
Significant coagulopathy
Inadequate regional anesthesia
Acute maternal hypovolemia/hemorrhage
Patient refusal of regional anesthesia

26. What concerns the anesthesiologist when he or she administers general anesthesia for cesarean section? How is it performed?
General anesthesia is best avoided in patients with difficult airways, severe asthma, or a history of malignant hyperthermia. The goal is to minimize maternal risk of aspiration and neonatal depression. This goal is accomplished by following certain guidelines. After monitors are placed, while the patient is being preoxygenated for a full 4 minutes, the abdomen is prepared and draped, and the obstetricians are ready to begin. Rapid-sequence induction is always used, and incision occurs when correct endotracheal tube placement is verified. Frequently used induction agents include thiopental, propofol, ketamine, and etomidate. Succinylcholine is the muscle relaxant of choice for most patients (1–1.5 mg/kg), and only small amounts cross the placenta. To prevent maternal awareness until the neonate is delivered, frequently a combination of 30–50% nitrous oxide in oxygen is used with a low concentration of a halogenated agent (0.5 MAC). Larger concentrations of a volatile agent may cause vasodilation of the uterus and excessive uterine bleeding.

After delivery of the child, the concentration of nitrous oxide is increased, opioids and nondepolarizing muscle relaxant (lower doses, remember!) are administered, and concentrations of volatile agents are decreased to avoid uterine atony. Pitocin is also administered. At the conclusion of the procedure, the neuromuscular blockade is reversed, and the awake patient is extubated after thorough orogastric and airway suctioning.

BIBLIOGRAPHY

1. Bromage PR: Choice of local anesthetics in obstetrics. In Shnider SM, Levinson G (eds): Anesthesia for Obstetrics, 3rd ed. Baltimore, Williams & Wilkins, 1993, p 84.
2. Chestnut DH, Vincent RD, McGrath JM, et al: Does early administration of epidural analgesia affect obstetric outcome in nulliparous women who are receiving intravenous oxytocin? Anesthesiology 80:1193–1200, 1994.
3. Chestnut DH: Epidural and spinal anesthesia/analgesia—effect on the progress of labor and method of delivery. In Chestnut DH (ed): Obstetric Anesthesia: Principles and Practice. St. Louis, Mosby, 1994, pp 403–419.
4. Chestnut DH: Alternative regional anesthetic techniques. In Chestnut DH (ed): Obstetric Anesthesia: Principles and Practice. St. Louis, Mosby, 1994, pp 420–431.
5. Chestnut DH: Vaginal birth after cesarean section. In Chestnut DH (ed): Obstetric Anesthesia: Principles and Practice. St. Louis, Mosby, 1994, pp 432–442.
6. Glosten B: Epidural and spinal anesthesia/analgesia—local anesthetic techniques. In Chestnut DH (ed): Obstetric Anesthesia: Principles and Practice. St. Louis, Mosby, 1994, pp 354–378.
7. Hawkins JL, Hess KR, Kubicek MA, et al: A re-evaluation of the association between instrumental delivery and epidural analgesia. Reg Anesth 20:50–56, 1995.
8. Horowitz IR, Gomella LG (eds): Obstetrics and Gynecology on Call. Norwalk, CT, Appleton & Lange, 1993, pp 83–87.
9. Ostheimer GW, Leavitt KA: Lumbar epidural anesthesia. In Ostheimer GW (ed): Manual of Obstetric Anesthesia. New York, Churchill Livingstone, 1992, pp 168–179.
10. Ostheimer GW, Leavitt KA: Subarachnoid anesthesia. In Ostheimer GW (ed): Manual of Obstetric Anesthesia. New York, Churchill Livingstone, 1992, pp 168–179.
11. Reisner LS, Lin D: Anesthesia for cesarean section. In Chestnut DH (ed): Obstetric Anesthesia: Principles and Practice. St. Louis, Mosby, 1994, pp 459–486.
12. Ross BK: epidural and spinal anesthesia/analgesia—opioid techniques. In Chestnut DH (ed): Obstetric Anesthesia: Principles and Practice. St. Louis, Mosby, 1994, pp 379–403.
13. Santos AC, Mieczyslaw F, Pedersen H: Obstetric Anesthesia. In Barash PG, Cullen BF, Stoelting RK (eds): Clinical Anesthesia, 2nd ed. Philadelphia, J.B. Lippincott, 1992, pp 1267–1306.
14. Wakefield ML: Systemic analgesia: Opioids, ketamine and inhalational agents. In Chestnut DH (ed): Obstetric Anesthesia: Principles and Practice. St. Louis, Mosby, 1994, p 341.

66. HIGH-RISK OBSTETRICS AND COEXISTING DISEASE

Ana M. Lobo, M.D., M.P.H.

1. Define high-risk pregnancy.

A pregnant patient is placed into the high-risk category when she has a condition(s) that significantly increases the likelihood of maternal or fetal morbidity and/or mortality.

High-risk Conditions in Pregnancy

Hypertension 7% of all pregnancies
Preeclampsia 5–7% of all pregnancies
Preterm birth 7–10% of all births
Abruptio placentae 0.2–2.4% of all pregnancies
Placenta previa 0.5% of term deliveries
Uterine atony 2–5% of all vaginal deliveries
Gestational diabetes mellitus 1–5% of all pregnancies
Hyperthyroidism 0.2% of all pregnancies
Obesity 6% of all pregnancies
Morbid obesity 1–2% of all pregnancies
Renal disease 1–2% of all pregnancies
Cardiac disease 1–2% of all pregnancies

2. Describe the four categories of hypertension associated with pregnancy.

Hypertension occurs in 7% of pregnancies and may result in perinatal death and prematurity. **Gestational hypertension** is characterized by an increase in mean arterial pressure after 20 weeks' gestation, without proteinuria. **Preeclampsia**, also known as pregnancy-induced hypertension, is characterized by hypertension and proteinuria with or without edema. **Chronic hypertension** may also be present during pregnancy, as can **chronic hypertension with superimposed preeclampsia.**

3. What is the etiology of preeclampsia?

Preeclampsia is characterized by vasoconstriction, hypovolemia, coagulation abnormalities, and poor organ perfusion. Although the etiology is unknown, many theories have been proposed. Circulating vasoconstrictive toxins have been isolated from the blood, placenta, and amniotic fluid of women with preeclampsia. The immunologic theory states that circulating immune complexes, which result in vascular damage, are formed in response to an inadequate maternal antibody response to the fetal allograft. Others propose that primary endothelial damage causes an increase in thromboxane A_2 (vasoconstrictor) and a decrease in prostacyclin production (vasodilator). Some theorize that primary disseminated intravascular coagulation, causing the formation and deposition of microvascular thrombin, is responsible. Endogenous vasoconstrictors have also been implicated, as these patients are particularly sensitive to norepinephrine, epinephrine, and vasopressin and have an increased hypertensive response to angiotensin II. Uteroplacental insufficiency is thought to occur in these patients, although the precise etiology is unclear.

4. What clinical findings are present in preeclampsia?

Preeclampsia consists of the triad of hypertension, proteinuria, and edema developing after 20 weeks' gestation. It usually occurs after the 24th week of gestation. It is seen more frequently in nulliparous black women and in women at the extremes of child-bearing age, of lower socioeconomic status, and with underlying chronic hypertension, multiple gestations, diabetes mellitus, and hydatidiform moles. Clotting factors may be decreased in up to 20% of patients. Pulmonary edema and left ventricular failure are common if the patient is fluid-overloaded.

Symptoms and Signs of Preeclampsia

SYMPTOM/SIGN	MILD	SEVERE
Headache	—	+
Visual disturbances	—	+
Cerebral disturbances	—	+
Seizures (eclampsia)	—	+
Serum creatinine	N	↑
Thrombocytopenia	—	+
Hyperbilirubinemia	—	+
AST (SGOT) elevation	N	—
Fetal growth retardation	—	+
Epigastric pain	—	+

Adapted from Horowitz IR, Gomella LG: Obstetrics and Gynecology on Call. Norwalk, CT, Appleton & Lange, 1993, p78.

5. List the criteria for diagnosing preeclampsia.

Criteria for Diagnosing Preeclampsia

	MILD	SEVERE
Systolic blood pressure*	> 140 mmHg or increase of 30 mmHg	> 160 mmHg
Diastoic blood pressure*	> 90 mmHg or increase of 15 mmHg	> 110 mmHg
Proteinuria*	> 300 mg in 24-hr urine Trace, 1+, or 2+ semiquantitative	> 5 gm in 24-hr urine 3+ or 4+ semiquantitative
Oliguria	—	>400 ml/ 24 hr
Pitting edema	1+	> 2+

* Values must be duplicated at least 6 hr after the initial reading.
Adapted from Horowitz IR, Gomella LG: Obstetrics and Gynecology on Call. Norwalk, CT, Appleton & Lange, 1993, p 77.

6. What conditions contribute to maternal and perinatal mortality in preeclampsia?

Preeclampsia is the leading cause of maternal mortality in pregnancy and results in death in 0.4–11.9% of patients who develop it. Maternal mortality may be the result of cerebral hemorrhage, hepatic rupture, myocardial infarction with cardiac arrest, or pulmonary edema. Perinatal mortality occurs in 20–30% of affected mothers and may be due to placental infarction or placental growth retardation.

7. What is the HELLP syndrome?

The HELLP syndrome is characterized by **H**emolytic anemia, **E**levated **L**iver enzymes, and **L**ow **P**latelets occurring in the setting of preeclampsia and is associated with high maternal and fetal mortality. The HELLP syndrome usually occurs before 36 weeks' gestation and is considered a severe form of preeclampsia. The most common complaints of patients with this disorder are epigastric pain (90%), malaise (90%), and nausea and vomiting (50%). Both epigastric pain and nausea/vomiting are caused by liver capsule distention (hepatic rupture may occur). Some patients present with a nonspecific viral flu-like syndrome. Hypertension and proteinuria may be very mild at first, but a rapidly accelerating downhill course is usually noted, leading to disseminated intravascular coagulation and renal and liver failure.

To prevent maternal and fetal mortality, immediate delivery is indicated upon diagnosis, regardless of the gestational age of the fetus. Platelet counts usually reach their lowest level 24–48 hours after delivery (frequently < 50,000/ml). Platelet counts recover within 11 days postpartum, depending on the severity of the thrombocytopenia.

8. How is preeclampsia managed?

Aspirin may be used in small doses prior to delivery to alter the prostacyclin/thromboxane ratio. Initial results have been positive in women who are at risk for this disorder.

Magnesium sulfate is used as prophylaxis against the development of seizures by increasing the patient's seizure threshold. Magnesium therapy is started with an IV loading dose of 4–6 gm over 15 minutes, followed by an intravenous infusion of 1–3 gm/hr. Magnesium blood levels must be monitored to prevent toxicity.

A rapid-acting **antihypertensive agent** is initiated when diastolic blood pressures are consistently high (> 110 mmHg). Hydralazine is the most commonly used drug of this class. Its vasodilating properties can increase uterine blood flow and maternal renal blood flow. The diastolic blood pressure should be maintained around 90 mmHg, as uterine perfusion may be compromised with rapid lowering of blood pressure.

Diuretics are usually avoided because patients are vasoconstricted and volume-depleted.

Invasive monitoring should be considered in patients who require vigorous hydration or remain oliguric after a fluid challenge. An arterial line should be placed in patients with severe preeclampsia and with symptoms of pulmonary edema.

Definitive treatment of preeclampsia involves **delivery** of the placenta and neonate.

9. What potential problems may occur in the patient receiving magnesium sulfate?

The therapeutic range of magnesium sulfate is 4–8mEq/L. As plasma Mg levels increase, the patient develops ECG changes with widening of the QRS complex and a prolonged P-Q interval. Deep tendon reflexes are lost at 10 mEq/L; sinoatrial and atrioventricular block as well as respiratory paralysis occur at 15 mEq/L; and cardiac arrest occurs at 25 mEq/L. In therapeutic doses, magnesium sulfate increases the sensitivity of the mother and fetus to muscle relaxants. Magnesium rapidly crosses the placenta, and as maternal magnesium serum levels increase, the newborn will be more likely to have decreased muscle tone, respiratory depression, and apnea. Intravenous calcium slowly administered to the newborn may decrease the neuromuscular-blocking properties of magnesium. Magnesium also decreases catecholamine release and systemic vascular resistance.

10. What are the anesthetic considerations in the patient with preeclampsia?

The patient should undergo a thorough preoperative evaluation. Airway evaluation is crucial, as the airway is usually edematous in these patients. As with all pregnant patients, a large-bore intravenous line should be placed (for access and resuscitation with crystalloid or blood products if necessary) and aspiration prophylaxis should be given before any anesthetic. Oxygen therapy increases oxygen delivery to the fetus. The patient's position should maximize uterine displacement. The patient's coagulation profile should be evaluated in addition to a platelet count.

Labor epidurals are usually placed when the patient enters the active phase of labor. In the preeclamptic patient, the coagulation profile must be assessed, including platelet count, prothrombin time, and partial thromboplastin time. Some clinicians also advocate obtaining a bleeding time to assess the risk of hemorrhage with regional anesthesia and will avoid regional anesthesia if the bleeding time is prolonged. In patients who have clinical signs of a coagulopathy or a platelet count < 100,000/ml, most anesthesiologists avoid inserting an epidural.

Once the epidural is in place, the epidural should be dosed slowly to avoid the rapid development of hypotension with subsequent uteroplacental insufficiency. Injudicious fluid bolusing is more likely to lead to pulmonary edema in this population. Epidural anesthesia is the preferred regional technique for cesarean section, as spinal anesthesia may quickly result in hypotension and further compromise uteroplacental blood flow.

General anesthesia is indicated in the setting of fetal distress, especially when there is no functioning epidural in place. The usual precautions for general anesthesia in the obstetrical patient should be taken. In this population, one should expect a small glottic opening on intubation (use a small endotracheal tube, such as 6.0 mm) and an edematous, friable airway. Ketamine should not be used for induction because it may aggravate hypertension. Rapid-sequence induction with cricoid pressure is indicated when using pentothal (or etomidate) as the induction agent and succinylcholine for paralysis. All doses of muscle relaxants should be decreased, as magnesium sulfate therapy potentiates their effects. The patient's degree of paralysis should be closely monitored throughout the surgery, and extubation should be accomplished only after the patient is awake and full muscle strength has returned.

If the patient's hypertension is not well controlled (preoperatively or intraoperatively), intravenous nitroglycerin or nitroprusside may be used to normalize blood pressure. Sodium nitroprusside may be used for only a short time (< 6 hours) because of concern of fetal cyanide toxicity and maternal tachyphylaxis.

11. How is eclampsia diagnosed? How does it affect different organ systems?
Eclampsia is diagnosed in the preeclamptic patient when seizures or coma develop. Cerebral edema and focal hemorrhages may occur. Liver necrosis, hemorrhage, and thrombosis may develop. Disseminated intravascular coagulation and hyaline degeneration of the kidneys may also occur.

12. How are eclamptic seizures treated?
The control of grand mal seizures in eclampsia is a priority. Maternal mortality increases (in part) with the number of convulsions the patient has experienced. Oxygen should be given during a seizure to diminish the degree of hypoxia. A rapid-acting anticonvulsant, such as thiopental (50–100 mg), diazepam (2.5–5 mg), midazolam (1–2 mg), or magnesium (2–4 gm), should be administered intravenously to stop the seizure. The patient should then receive seizure prophylaxis with magnesium sulfate. If the seizure is not stopped quickly or if there is difficulty in maintaining the airway, the patient should be intubated to prevent pulmonary aspiration and to maintain adequate ventilation.

13. Discuss preterm labor.
Preterm delivery is that occurring before 37 weeks' gestation or when the newborn weighs < 2500 gm. Frequent uterine contractions associated with progressive cervical dilatation or effacement occurring after the second trimester is known as **preterm labor**. Preterm labor is associated with placental abruption, uterine abnormalities, breech presentation, and multiple gestations. It is common following premature rupture of the membranes. This condition is seen in 5–10% of all pregnancies and is more common in women who are < 20 years of age, of low socioeconomic status, and smokers. Urinary tract infection, systemic infections, dehydration, vaginitis, or cervicitis may contribute to the development of preterm labor. Patients usually present with pelvic pressure, abdominal cramping, dull and constant back pain, and regular uterine contractions occurring every 15 minutes or less for more than 1 hour. The major consequence of preterm labor is neonatal prematurity, leading to an increased risk of neonatal mortality (due mostly to pulmonary immaturity) and morbidity.

14. How is preterm labor treated?
The treatment of preterm labor involves bedrest and parenteral or oral tocolytics. These uterine relaxants are used routinely to abolish labor prior to 34 weeks' gestation. The most widely used drugs are beta-2 adrenergic agonists and magnesium sulfate. Beta-2 adrenergic agonists, such as ritodrine and terbutaline, may be administered intravenously or orally. They cause bronchodilation, vasodilation, and uterine relaxation and are preferentially used in emergent situations. Common side effects include hypotension, tachycardia, arrhythmias, hypokalemia and pulmonary edema. Magnesium sulfate is also used for tocolysis, but serum levels must be monitored to prevent toxicity (pulmonary edema, chest tightness, nausea and vomiting). Infusions of both agents are continued for 24 hours after tocolysis is accomplished. Prostaglandin synthetase

inhibitors (indomethacin and ibuprofen) and calcium channel blockers (verapamil and nifedipine) are used as second-line tocolytics because of their respective fetal and neonatal side effects. In addition to these medications, pregnant women in preterm labor (gestational age < 34 wk) may receive steroids to improve fetal lung maturity and decrease the risk of neonatal hyaline membrane disease. If tocolysis fails, delivery of a premature neonate is certain.

15. Describe the anesthetic management of the patient with preterm labor who is proceeding to delivery.
When tocolysis fails to abolish premature labor, the patient should receive a thorough preoperative evaluation with emphasis on the airway, gestational age, anticipated neonatal weight, and prior medications used to treat this condition. As always, the patient should be positioned to maximize left uterine displacement and should receive oxygen therapy to augment fetal oxygen delivery. Prior to any anesthetic, she should receive aspiration prophylaxis and have a large-bore intravenous line placed.

An increased risk of cesarean section is seen in this population due to fetal distress, maternal hemorrhage, and breech presentation. A continuous lumbar epidural is useful to minimize maternal pushing, which may traumatize the fetal head. Care must be taken in dosing the epidural because these patients become hypotensive more easily due to a beta-2 agonist effect. Blood glucose levels should be monitored because patients who concurrently take beta-2 agonists and steroids have a higher incidence of maternal hyperglycemia and pulmonary edema. If general anesthesia is indicated, the usual precautions for all pregnant women should be taken. Care must be taken to avoid hyperventilation, which will result in hypotension and hypokalemia in the setting of beta-2 agonist therapy.

16. What is the survival rate for infants delivered prematurely?
Several factors influence the survival of a premature neonate. Birth weight is an important predictor of neonatal survival. Neonates weighing > 1000 gm have greater than 90% survival. Infants weighing < 500 gm rarely survive. Up to 50% of neonates with a gestational age < 25 weeks survive, whereas 90% of neonates with a gestational age ≥ 28 weeks survive. Better outcomes in preterm neonates are associated with an absence of congenital malformations and the availability of a neonatal specialist at delivery. Admission to a neonatal intensive care unit is not uncommon for neonates born prematurely.

17. Characterize the different grades of placental abruption.
The most common causes of third-trimester vaginal bleeding are abruptio placentae and placenta previa. Abruptio placentae is the separation of the placenta after 20 weeks' gestation and before birth of the neonate. The cause of this disorder is not completely understood, but factors associated with it include pregnancy-related and chronic hypertension, previous placental abruption, uterine abnormalities, advanced parity, smoking, and cocaine use. Perinatal mortality occurs in up to 50% of placental abruptions. Placental abruption may be internal (painful hemorrhage without external bleeding) or external (painless hemorrhage through the cervix). Abruptions are classified in terms of severity:

Grade 0	No signs or symptoms (recognized after delivery)
Grade 1 (mild)	Vaginal bleeding, abdominal pain, contractions, uterine tenderness
Grade 2 (moderate)	Same symptoms as grade 1 plus uterine tetany and fetal distress
Grade 3 (severe)	Maternal shock, uterine tetany, coagulopathy, fetal demise, distal organ necrosis, and disseminated intravascular coagulation

18. What is the anesthetic management of patients with abruptio placentae?
The usual preoperative evaluation of the pregnant patient should be done. Abruptio placentae may cause fetal distress, and cesarean section is frequently indicated. In grade 0 or 1 abruptions, regional anesthesia is appropriate. In grade 2 or 3 abruptions, general anesthesia is indicated, as

regional anesthesia is contraindicated in patients with hypovolemic shock and/or severe coagulopathies. Prior to induction of anesthesia, hemoglobin, hematocrit, platelet count, prothrombin time, partial thromboplastin time, fibrinogen level, and fibrin degradation products should be measured, although the emergent nature of this situation precludes delaying surgery for lab results. Rapid-sequence induction of anesthesia may be accomplished safely with ketamine (0.5–1 mg/kg) as it stimulates the sympathetic nervous system and increases blood pressure. Thiopental in a small dose (< 100 mg intravenously) may be used. It is crucial to have two large-bore intravenous lines for access and resuscitation, and blood products for transfusion should be readily available. After delivery, the uterus may not contract and bleeding will continue. Oxytocin should be administered (20–40 U intravenously in 500 ml of crystalloid) following delivery (see question 20).

19. What is placenta previa? How is it managed?

In placenta previa, the placenta obstructs the descent of the neonatal presenting part. Its etiology is not known, but this condition is more common in multiparous patients and those with a previous cesarean section. A partial placenta previa occurs when only part of the internal os is covered, whereas the internal os is completely covered in complete placenta previa. A marginal placenta previa occurs when the placental edge is at the os but does not cover it. The main symptom is painless vaginal bleeding. At any time, the patient may have a severe hemorrhage.

The diagnosis of placenta previa may be made with ultrasonography or by direct examination of the cervical os (usually done in an operating room with all preparations for hemorrhage and emergency cesarean section, a "double set-up"). The anesthesiologist evaluates the patient to receive an anesthetic as usual, ensuring that the patient has two large-bore intravenous lines, has blood available for transfusion, and has received aspiration prophylaxis. If the patient is actively bleeding, emergent cesarean section is performed. Regional anesthesia is contraindicated due to maternal hemorrhage and hypovolemia, and the patient is managed as for placental abruption. Rapid-sequence induction with cricoid pressure is performed using thiopental (if normotensive) or ketamine and succinylcholine. Maintenance of anesthesia is accomplished with 100% oxygen, a nondepolarizing muscle relaxant, and a low dose of a halogenated agent as tolerated. The neonate may require resuscitation at birth and intensive care. If the patient is not bleeding despite being diagnosed with placenta previa, cesarean section is still performed. Anesthesiologists disagree as to whether a regional anesthetic (spinal or epidural) should be performed if the patient requests it and she is not hypovolemic. The potential for blood loss in this setting is increased, and some argue that general anesthesia is still preferable.

20. What is postpartum uterine atony? How is it treated?

Uterine atony occurs when the uterus will not contract after delivery. This condition may result in a severe hemorrhage, with a blood loss of 2–5 L occurring in < 5 minutes from a completely atonic uterus. Overdistention of the uterus is thought to cause uterine atony in some cases. Other conditions associated with it include multiple gestation, macrosomia, polyhydramnios, high parity, prolonged labor, chorioamnionitis, precipitous labor, augmented labor, tocolytic agents, and a high concentration of a halogenated volatile anesthetic. Uterine atony may be diagnosed by observing vaginal bleeding and palpating a soft uterus postpartum.

Obstetric management of this condition includes bimanual compression, uterine massage, and administration of drugs that stimulate uterine contractions. **Oxytocin** (Pitocin), the first-line drug for treating this condition, is a synthetic hormone that is administered intravenously in a solution of 20 U/1000 ml of crystalloid, and its onset of action is immediate. If atony is severe, 1 to 2 U of oxytocin may be given as an intravenous bolus. Oxytocin may not be rapidly administered intravenously, because it causes hypotension, coronary artery spasm, and intracranial hemorrhage. **Methergine** is given in a dose of 0.2 mg intramuscularly, and its onset of effect is rapid. It may also be administered in doses of 0.02 mg intravenously with careful observation of maternal blood pressure. The combination of this drug followed by a vasopressor may lead to severe hypertension, requiring treatment with a vasodilator. **Prostaglandin F_2 alpha** (Hemabate) is used to treat refractory uterine atony. The dose is 250 µg intramuscularly or intramyometrially and may be repeated every 15–30 minutes (total dose < 2 mg). This drug may cause nausea, vomiting, and fever. If these agents are not successful, either internal iliac artery ligation or hysterectomy is indicated.

Anesthetic management for uterine atony involves evaluation of the patient, administration of oxygen and a nonparticulate antacid, and placement of a large-bore intravenous catheter. If not previously done, blood should be sent for typing and cross-matching. Aggressive volume resuscitation may be necessary. Urine output should be monitored. Medications to stop uterine atony should be given. Preparation for emergent laparotomy should be accomplished. If the hemorrhage is not controlled, the anesthesiologist should use the same precautions used in any pregnant woman undergoing general anesthesia in an emergent situation. Rapid-sequence induction with cricoid pressure is indicated.

21. Discuss the morbidity associated with gestational diabetes mellitus.

Gestational diabetes mellitus, the most common medical problem of pregnancy, occurs when a state of carbohydrate intolerance develops with pregnancy or is first recognized during pregnancy. Diagnosis is made on the basis of two abnormal venous plasma glucose values on a 3-hour glucose tolerance test. Frequently, patients are overweight. The incidence of abortion, polyhydramnios, preeclampsia, dystocia, operative delivery, and an excessively large fetus is increased in this population. Fetal effects include macrosomia, death in utero, hydramnios, malpresentation, malformation and fetal hypoglycemia. The perinatal mortality rate is 10–30%. Diabetes is classified with the modified White's classification. Treatment involves control of blood glucose levels with diet and/or pharmacologic therapy. Insulin is not always required to maintain normoglycemia. Subcutaneous human insulin is indicated if the patient has not attained euglycemia after 1–2 weeks of diet therapy.

Modified White's Classification of Diabetes Mellitus

Class A	Chemical diabetes diagnosed before pregnancy; managed by diet alone; any age of onset or duration.
Class B	Insulin treatment necessary before pregnancy; onset after age 20; duration < 10 yrs.
Class C	Onset at age 10–19; or duration of 10–19 yrs.
Class D	Onset before age 10; or duration of ≥ 20 yrs; or chronic hypertension; or background retinopathy.
Class F	Renal disease.
Class H	Coronary artery disease.
Class R	Proliferative retinopathy.
Class T	Renal transport.

From Pernoll ML, Benson RC (eds): Current Obstetrics and Gynecologic Diagnosis and Treatment, 6th ed. Norwalk, CT, Appleton & Lange, 1987.

22. What are the anesthetic concerns in managing gestational diabetes?

Patients with gestational diabetes are frequently overweight and have larger gastric volumes and delayed gastric emptying. If hydramnios is present, there is increased susceptibility to aortocaval compression and hypotension. Placental insufficiency is present in this condition, and it is aggravated by hyperglycemia.

Anesthetic management during labor and delivery may be accomplished with epidural anesthesia. Insertion of an epidural may be a challenge in this population due to poor landmarks. These patients are very sensitive to local anesthetics, so they should be dosed in a conservative manner. Epidural anesthesia may decrease maternal catecholamine release (caused by pain and anxiety) and improve placental perfusion. This regional technique is useful if a forcep delivery is indicated or emergent cesarean delivery becomes necessary for fetal distress.

For cesarean delivery, regional or general anesthesia may be used. It is important to avoid hypotension, as this may cause fetal hypoxia which in the presence of hyperglycemia may worsen fetal acidosis. Epidural anesthesia may be preferable as precipitous hypotension is less likely. These patients may be difficult to intubate (due to obesity). Delayed gastric emptying and larger gastric volumes put them at high risk for pulmonary aspiration, making aspiration prophylaxis crucial. Hyperglycemia in the prepartum period should be avoided. Blood glucose levels should be monitored prior to and during the procedure to ensure normoglycemia.

23. What is the significance of hyperthyroidism in pregnancy?

Thyroid function should remain normal during pregnancy. Hyperthyroidism complicating pregnancy is most likely caused by Graves' disease, trophoblastic disease, or excessive thyroid supplementation. Maternal hyperthyroidism secondary to Graves' disease is due to stimulation of thyroxine synthesis by autoantibodies. Maternal symptoms include heat intolerance, poor weight gain, diarrhea, nervousness, and tachycardia. These autoantibodies cross the placenta, resulting in fetal thyroid stimulation with possible fetal prematurity, in utero death, intrauterine growth retardation, goiter, and exophthalmos. A low thyroid-stimulating hormone and increased thyroxine, triiodothyronine, and free thyroid index are noted on maternal thyroid function studies. Propylthiouracil (PTU) is administered to treat this condition, and symptoms usually decrease after 4 weeks of therapy. This treatment is maintained during pregnancy, although PTU may cross the placenta and cause fetal hypothyroidism. A subtotal thyroidectomy is indicated if PTU therapy fails.

Thyroid storm, or thyrotoxicosis, is a life-threatening disorder that is precipitated by stress, such as that experienced during infection, labor, or cesarean section. Clinically it is manifested by tachycardia, atrial fibrillation, hyperpyrexia, dehydration, altered consciousness, and hemodynamic instability.

Preoperative preparation of these patients involves reducing the risk of thyroid storm. An antithyroid medication, beta-adrenergic blocking agent, glucocorticoid, and iodine should be given.

24. Describe the anesthetic management of the patient with hyperthyroidism.

Anesthetic management of these patients is affected by several features of hyperthyroidism, including the partial airway obstruction resulting from an enlarged thyroid gland, respiratory muscle weakness, electrolyte abnormalities, and hyperdynamic cardiovascular system. The safety of various anesthetic techniques in this patient population has not been thoroughly evaluated. Regional anesthesia is beneficial in that it avoids the difficult intubation, and sympathetic blockade may decrease epinephrine secretion and lower blood pressure. It is now considered safe to include epinephrine in local anesthetic solutions in hyperthyroid patients. Glucocorticoid supplementation should be given. Medications that may cause tachycardia should be avoided (ketamine, atropine, pancuronium). Thiopental is the induction agent of choice because it has an antithyroid effect. Nonemergent surgery should be postponed until the patient is clinically euthyroid. Propranolol, intravenous glucocorticoids, oral PTU, and aspiration prophylaxis should be given preoperatively to the hyperthyroid patient who needs emergent surgery.

The anesthesiologist should be prepared to treat thyroid storm, should this occur. Treatment includes oxygen supplementation, intravenous hydration with chilled crystalloid solution containing glucose, cooling blankets as needed, electrolyte replacement, glucocorticoid administration (dexamethasone, 2–4 mg intravenously), antithyroid medication (PTU, 600–1000 mg/day), sodium iodide (1 gm intravenously), and beta-adrenergic blocking agents (propranolol, esmolol). Invasive monitoring may be needed, as these patients may develop high-output cardiac failure.

25. Are there complications associated with obesity in pregnancy?

Obesity (body weight 20% above ideal) and morbid obesity (body weight twice normal) complicate both pregnancy and anesthetic management for labor, delivery, and cesarean section. These patients are at increased risk for large babies, breech presentation, oxytocin induction, and cesarean delivery. Obese parturients are frequently older and of higher parity, and they have an increased antepartum risk of diabetes mellitus, hypertension, and twin gestations. Their perioperative mortality is also increased.

Several features of obesity complicate anesthetic management. Obese pregnant patients are at increased risk for aspiration of gastric contents, perioperative respiratory failure and arrest, cardiovascular failure, pulmonary embolism, infections, hepatic and renal dysfunction, and metabolic disturbances.

Regional anesthesia is frequently challenging in this population. As with all parturients, aspiration prophylaxis must be administered prior to any anesthetic. Obese patients have delayed gastric emptying. Technical difficulties may arise in performing regional anesthesia because of poor landmarks. The patient should be placed in the sitting position to maximize respiratory function and spinal flexion. A continuous spinal anesthetic should be considered for labor and delivery if the epidural technique is not successful or results in a wet tap. The amount of local anesthetic needed to achieve a block is decreased, as these patients are more sensitive to local anesthetics and have a smaller epidural space. Oxygen should be administered during labor as these patients have increased oxygen consumption. The anesthetic level should be kept below T6 to ensure that the patient can use her intercostal muscles for respiration, including during cesarean section. Uterine displacement is more difficult to accomplish in the obese patient but should be maintained at all times. The Trendelenburg position (used to treat hypotension) should be avoided if possible, as it will promote regurgitation. Despite these problems associated with regional anesthesia, it is the technique of choice for both labor and operative delivery. These patients frequently have narrowed airways, and maintaining a patent airway is crucial to their management. Epidural anesthesia is also recommended because it decreases respiratory work and oxygen consumption.

26. Why is general anesthesia usually avoided in the obese patient?

There are many reasons why general anesthesia is not the preferred anesthetic technique in this population. Obese parturients have much soft tissue in the airway, making it narrower, and edema further complicates their airway management. A small endotracheal tube (≤ 6.5 mm) is frequently needed. A large panniculus and large breasts also may make intubation difficult (use a stubby-handle laryngoscope). Before induction, the patient's head and shoulders should be propped up by pillows to improve glottic exposure upon laryngoscopy. Obesity, as well as pregnancy, causes a decreased functional residual capacity, resulting in rapid oxygen desaturation during rapid-sequence induction. The patient should be extubated when she is fully awake and full muscle strength has returned.

Awake, fiberoptic intubations are useful in obese parturients. This intubation method may be chosen when airway evaluation suggests a very difficult (or seemingly impossible) intubation. With this method, there is less risk of pulmonary aspiration, as the patient is awake and capable of protecting her own airway because reflexes are intact.

27. How does sickle cell disease complicate pregnancy?

In sickle cell disease, the hemoglobin molecule polymerizes when exposed to low oxygen saturation and acidosis, leading to red blood cell (RBC) distortion, decreased RBC survival time, hemolysis, hyperbilirubinemia, anemia, and blood vessel occlusion causing tissue anoxia. During sickle cell crises, vessel occlusion by sickled RBC may lead to splenic infarctions, avascular necrosis, sepsis, and chest symptoms (chest pain, pulmonary infiltrates). These crises are painful. Patients may have repeated crises throughout pregnancy and have increased risk of fetal miscarriage, stillbirth, preterm labor, abruptio placentae, placenta previa, and preeclampsia.

Treatment remains supportive in nature. During pregnancy, the goal is to prevent exposure to factors that precipitate sickle cell crises. Unfortunately, pregnancy itself may increase the possibility of crises. Decreased oxygen saturation, acidosis, and dehydration should be avoided. Prophylactic and partial exchange transfusions as therapy for symptomatic crises are controversial. The goal is to lower the amount of hemoglobin S cells and increase the level of hemoglobin A to 40%.

28. What precautions should the anesthetist take in managing patients with sickle cell disease?

During labor and delivery, the patient should be kept well oxygenated and hydrated with intravenous crystalloid. A pulse oximeter should be used to guide oxygen therapy. The parturient should be kept warm (use warm intravenous fluids), and shivering should be prevented. Left uterine displacement should be maintained. Regional anesthesia is safe in the patient with sickle cell disease. It is important to ensure that the patient is well hydrated prior to regional or general anesthesia. A labor epidural is useful in that it alleviates pain, thereby increasing oxygen supply and decreasing oxygen demand. Epidural or spinal anesthesia may be used for cesarean section. Care must be taken to avoid hypotension, and if it occurs it should be immediately treated with intravascular volume expansion. Vasopressors, causing peripheral vasoconstriction, may aggravate blood stasis. General anesthesia is indicated for emergent abdominal delivery, and precautions and problems with this technique are similar to those in other parturients. Blood transfusion may be necessary to maximize oxygen-carrying capacity, so blood typing and cross-matching should be done prior to the procedure.

29. What causes disseminated intravascular coagulation in the obstetric patient?

Disseminated intravascular coagulation (DIC) is the result of abnormal activation of the coagulation system. This causes the formation of large amounts of thrombin, decreasing coagulation factors, activation of the fibrinolytic system, and hemorrhage. In pregnant women the most frequent causes of DIC include shock, infection, abruptio placentae, amniotic fluid embolism, intrauterine fetal death, and preeclampsia or eclampsia.Increased prothrombin (PT), partial thromboplastin (PTT), and thrombin (TT) times and a decreased platelet count and fibrinogen level are seen on laboratory examination. Treatment involves removing the precipitating cause, providing multisystem organ support, and replacing depleted coagulation factors. The medical management of these patients is controversial, as is the use of heparin.

Before performing any procedure in a patient, the anesthesiologist must weigh the potential risks and benefits. Epidural or spinal anesthesia is contraindicated in the patient with a frank coagulopathy. If the patient has received anticoagulation therapy, the anesthesiologist may assess the degree of anticoagulation currently present with a measurement of PT and PTT. The question of whether to perform a regional anesthetic (spinal or epidural) in a patient with laboratory evidence of a coagulopathy is a difficult one, because the benefits of regional anesthesia must be weighed against the risk of hemorrhage and/or spinal or epidural hematoma formation. Isolated laboratory evidence of thrombocytopenia (without clinical manifestations) may occur in women with preeclampsia or in healthy obstetric patients, and there is always a small risk of causing an epidural hematoma in thrombocytopenic patients. Clinical judgment is the most important way of assessing the risk of epidural hematoma formation in a patient.

Should a coagulopathy occur after the placement of an epidural catheter, the catheter should be left in place until one of two events occurs. Some recommend removing the catheter immediately after delivery (but an epidural vein may be injured in removing the catheter at this time). Others recommend keeping the catheter in place until the coagulation profile has normalized.

30. What types of renal disease are most frequently seen in the obstetric patient?

Glomerular disease and acute renal failure are the most common renal disorders observed during pregnancy. **Glomerular disease** may be secondary to infection, inflammatory processes, or systemic diseases such as diabetes mellitus or systemic lupus erythematosus. Hypertension and proteinuria may also accompany this disorder. Preeclampsia occurs in up to 50% of patients with glomerular disease, hypertension, and proteinuria. Deterioration of renal function with pregnancy may occur in patients with glomerular disease. Nephrotic syndrome is frequently caused by glomerular disease. Hypoproteinemia may result in altered drug binding.

Acute renal failure may occur in patients with preexisting renal disease who experience the superimposed stress of pregnancy. It is usually due to complications that occur late in pregnancy (such as abruption, hemorrhage, amniotic fluid embolism, or preeclampsia/eclampsia). Renal failure is treated in a supportive fashion.

31. How is anesthetic management affected in patients with renal disorders?

Regional anesthesia in patients with renal impairment is generally considered safe. If hemodynamic stability is maintained, there are minimal effects on renal blood flow and glomerular filtration rate (GFR). The method of choice for labor and delivery is **epidural analgesia**. In providing analgesia, this technique decreases catecholamine secretion, which reduces renovascular resistance and increases renal blood flow. It is preferred over spinal anesthesia because the level of sympathetic blockade can be increased slowly, avoiding hypotension. In patients with impaired renal function, fluid overload must be avoided prior to epidural insertion. In general, intravenous fluid should not contain potassium, as these patients tend to be hyperkalemic. Clotting abnormalities frequently accompany renal disease, and decreased platelet adhesiveness (uremia) and coagulopathies may preclude the use of a regional technique. A coagulation profile should be done. Both amino and ester local anesthetics are safe in these patients. In patients with uremic neuropathy, sodium bisulfite-containing chloroprocaine anesthetics should not be used (they can produce chronic neurologic damage).

In the parturient with renal disease, **general anesthesia** should be avoided, unless it is an emergent situation or regional anesthesia is contraindicated. Inhalational agents may cause vasodilation and myocardial depression, resulting in increased renovascular resistance and decreased renal blood flow and GFR. Anemia (which occurs in both pregnancy and renal disease) in the setting of intrapulmonary shunting may result in an increase in hypoxemia. Ethrane should be avoided because it is partially metabolized to nephrotoxic fluoride ions. Renal patients frequently have electrolyte and acid-base abnormalities. In these patients, halothane may produce arrhythmias resulting from myocardial irritability. The hypoalbuminemia found in these patients requires that the barbiturate dose for induction be reduced (fewer molecules are protein bound). In patients who are normokalemic, succinylcholine may be used for rapid-sequence induction. If the patient is hyperkalemic, vecuronium (0.28 mg/kg) or rocuronium should be used. These drugs may cross the placenta and cause neonatal weakness at birth, however. Blood pressure control during induction and general anesthesia is important and may be accomplished with small doses of hydralazine or labetolol. Nitroglycerin and nitroprusside may be used for short-term reduction in blood pressure.

32. Which cardiac disease most commonly complicates pregnancy?

Valvular heart disease is the most common cardiac disease in obstetric patients. Most valvular lesions are due to rheumatic heart disease, with mitral stenosis being the predominant lesion (in up to 90% of cases) and also the most clinically important one. Half of all deaths in patients with valvular heart disease occur within 24 hours after delivery, and 30% occur within the following 4 days, usually from pulmonary edema and congestive heart failure (75%). Mortality approaches 1–3%.

33. How is mitral stenosis managed?

Mitral stenosis (MS) prevents filling of the left ventricle, resulting in decreased stroke volume and cardiac output, and prevents emptying of the left atrium, resulting in increased left atrial and pulmonary artery pressures (PAP). Signs and symptoms include a diastolic murmur, dyspnea, hemoptysis, chest pain, right heart failure, and thromboembolism. Normal pregnant patients have increased cardiac output, heart rate, and blood volume. Pregnancy aggravates MS because an increased heart rate limits ventricular filling, further increases left atrial pressure, and increases PAP. MS limits the patient's ability to increase her cardiac output despite an increase in blood volume. Atrial fibrillation may occur, increasing the risk of maternal morbidity, mortality, and systemic emboli. The sudden increase in preload following delivery may cause pulmonary edema.

Medical management of MS includes beta-adrenergic receptor blockade (propranolol, atenolol) to prevent tachycardia and digoxin to treat atrial fibrillation. During labor, delivery, or cesarean section, symptomatic patients may require hemodynamic monitoring. During the second stage of labor, the patient should not be encouraged to push (which increases venous return), and delivery should be accomplished by the force of uterine contractions alone. Oxygen supplementation should be given throughout labor and delivery.

Anesthetic goals include the following: maintain a slow heart rate (to increase ventricular filling time), maintain sinus rhythm (to improve cardiac output), avoid aortocaval compression, maintain normal PAP, maintain an adequate systemic vascular resistance (SVR) (a decreased SVR will lower perfusion and a high SVR will decrease cardiac output), and prevent increases in pulmonary vascular resistance (PVR) (due to pain, hypoxemia, hypercarbia, or acidosis). **Epidural analgesia** reduces preload and prevents postpartum pulmonary edema. A combined **spinal-epidural technique** is useful in providing good pain relief during the first stage of labor with a combination of epidural opioids and a low concentration of local anesthetic (to prevent a dramatic decrease in SVR). Intravenous administration of crystalloid should be judiciously given (hemodynamic monitoring helps here). If **general anesthesia** is indicated, drugs that produce tachycardia (atropine, ketamine, pancuronium) should be avoided. A beta blocker, such as esmolol, is useful in slowing the heart rate. These patients should be monitored closely during the postpartum period.

34. Do any other cardiac diseases complicate pregnancy?

Congenital heart disease may also complicate pregnancy. Parturients with corrected congenital heart lesions require no special treatment other than a pediatrician present at delivery (there is a high incidence of congenital cardiac lesions in their offspring). They may also require antibiotic prophylaxis. Some women may present with uncorrected congenital lesions. Both atrial and ventricular septal defects in pregnant patients are not uncommon. With either epidural or general anesthesia, the goal of anesthetic management is to avoid changes in SVR and PVR. Such changes alter and/or reverse shunts present. PVR increases with hypoxia, hypercarbia, acidosis, and high airway pressures.

BIBLIOGRAPHY

1. Ackerman WE, Juneja MM: Obstetric Anesthesia Pearls. Norwalk, CT, Appleton & Lange, 1992, pp 111–207.
2. Biehl DR: Antepartum and postpartum hemorrhage. In Shnider SM, Levinson G (eds): Anesthesia for Obstetrics, 3rd ed. Baltimore, Williams & Wilkins, 1993, pp 389–391.
3. Busch, RL: Valvular disease. In Ostheimer GW (ed): Manual of Obstetric Anesthesia. New York, Churchill Livingstone, 1992, pp 276–280.
4. Cox K: Preterm labor. In Frederickson HL, Wilkins-Haug L (eds): Ob/Gyn Secrets. Philadelphia, Hanley & Belfus, 1991, pp 239–244.
5. Datta S: Diabetes mellitus. In Ostheimer GW (ed): Manual of Obstetric Anesthesia. New York, Churchill Livingstone, 1992, pp 298–299.
6. Gutsche BB, Cheek TG: Anesthetic considerations in preeclampsia-eclampsia. In Shnider SM, Levinson G (eds): Anesthesia for Obstetrics, 3rd ed. Baltimore, Williams & Wilkins, 1993, pp 305–329.
7. Gutsche BB, Samuels P: Anesthetic considerations in premature birth. Int Anesthesiol Clin 28:33, 1990.
8. Hartigan P: Prematurity. In Ostheimer GW (ed): Manual of Obstetric Anesthesia. New York, Churchill Livingstone, 1992, pp 240–250.
9. Horowitz IR, Gomella LG (eds): Obstetrics and Gynecology On Call. Norwalk, CT, Appleton & Lange, 1993, pp 40–43, 76–80.
10. LaPorta RF, Johnson MD: Hematologic disease. In Ostheimer GW (ed): Manual of Obstetric Anesthesia. New York, Churchill Livingstone, 1992, pp 302–305.
11. Lechner RB: Hematologic and coagulation disorders. In Chestnut DH (ed): Obstetric Anesthesia: Principles and Practice. St. Louis, Mosby-Yearbook, 1994, pp 826–828.
12. Mayer DC, Spielman FJ: Antepartum and postpartum hemorrhage. In Chestnut DH (ed): Obstetric Anesthesia: Principles and Practice. St. Louis, Mosby-Yearbook, 1994, pp 708–709.
13. Santos AC, Mieczyslaw F, Pedersen H: Obstetric anesthesia. In Barash PG, Cullen BF, Stoelting RK (eds): Clinical Anesthesia. Philadelphia, J.B. Lippincott, 1992, pp 1267–1306.
14. Thornhill ML, Camann WR: Cardiovascular disease. In Chestnut DH (ed): Obstetric Anesthesia: Principles and Practice. St. Louis, Mosby-Yearbook, 1994, pp 747–760.

67. THE GERIATRIC PATIENT

David E. Strick, M.D.

1. How do we define the geriatric patient?

Historically the definition of the geriatric patient has been determined arbitrarily and has undergone repeated modification over the years. Currently age 65 is considered the beginning of the geriatric period. The process of aging results in a progressive deterioration in organ system function. The physiologic age of a patient, however, is more significant than the chronologic age in terms of the effects of aging because there is great variation in the progression of loss of organ system function among aging individuals.

2. In what ways does body composition change with aging?

- Increase in the proportion of body fat
- Diminished skeletal muscle mass (approximately 10%)
- Reduction in intracellular water

Although intracellular volume contracts with age, in otherwise healthy individuals, intravascular volume is preserved. In chronically ill, hypertensive, or otherwise debilitated patients, in addition to those on diuretics, the plasma volume may be contracted.

3. What are the anesthetic implications of the changes in body composition?

Changes in body composition can affect the distribution and elimination of anesthetic drugs. The **increase in the percentage of body fat** leads to a larger proportion of total body mass that can serve as a reservoir for lipid-soluble drugs. Thus, elderly patients may have an extended elimination time for these drugs, which results in prolongation of effect. The effect of the **loss of skeletal muscle** is a decrease in maximal and resting oxygen consumption, a slightly lowered resting cardiac output, and diminished production of body heat. Despite a smaller muscle mass, elderly patients are not more sensitive to muscle relaxants, probably because of fewer receptors at the neuromuscular junction. Patients who do have a **diminished plasma volume** may develop higher than expected plasma concentrations of drugs if dosing is based on body weight alone. Therefore, these patients may have a greater than anticipated response to drugs and thus appear to be more sensitive.

4. What changes in pulmonary function are seen with advancing age?

Total lung capacity	Decreased	Residual volume	Increased
Vital capacity	Decreased	Functional residual capacity	Increased
FEV_1	Decreased	Dead space	Increased
		Closing capacity	Increased

Aging affects chest wall mechanics, lung function, gas exchange, and ventilatory regulation that in general result in decreased lung volumes and reduced efficiency of gas exchange. The bellows function of the lung is reduced by fibrosis and calcification of the thoracic cage, loss of height of intervertebral disks, and declining mass and strength of the respiratory muscles. The lung itself undergoes a loss of elastic recoil secondary to diminishing amounts of elastin and increasing fibrous connective tissue. The breakup of alveolar septa leads to enlarged alveoli with diminished surface area. The lungs become more compliant but lose their ability to keep small airways open. Airway collapse leads to air trapping and uneven inhaled gas distribution, whereas parenchymal changes cause abnormal blood flow patterns. This produces ventilation/perfusion ($\dot{V}/\dot{Q}$) mismatching and less efficient alveolar gas exchange, resulting in a decrease in resting arterial partial pressure of oxygen (Pao_2). Older patients also have a reduced ventilatory response to hypercarbia and hypoxia in the awake state.

5. List dominant changes that occur in the cardiovascular system with aging.
- Myocardial infarction
- Ventricular hypertrophy
- Valvular calcification
- Loss of vascular elasticity
- Decreased baroreceptor responsiveness

6. Describe the effects of a reduced vascular elasticity.
Inelastic vasculature creates increased afterload for the heart and leads to elevated systolic blood pressures. As a result of the increased work against noncompliant vessels, the left ventricle becomes hypertrophied and the aorta dilates. Inadequate control of chronic hypertension can lead to a contracted intravascular volume, which contributes to intraoperative blood pressure lability.

7. What changes occur in the autonomic function of the elderly?
The changes in autonomic function seen in geriatric patients have been referred to as a **physiologic beta blockade.** Elderly patients, despite having higher levels of endogenous catecholamines, develop lower maximal heart rates in response to stress. Elderly patients also have a reduced chronotropic and inotropic response to exogenous beta-adrenergic agonists. Possible explanations include a reduced number of receptors, abnormal receptor affinity, or reduced cAMP production after receptor activation. A reduced affinity of beta-adrenergic receptors to both agonists and antagonists has definitely been documented. In addition, the elderly have fewer responsive vascular adrenergic receptors, as demonstrated by requiring higher doses of phenylephrine to attain a given blood pressure rise when compared with younger patients.

8. What are the consequences of physiologic beta blockade?
The decline in autonomic function impairs the cardiovascular reflexes that normally maintain hemodynamic stability. Inadequate autonomic responses during periods of stress can lead to cardiovascular decompensation. Elderly patients have a diminished heart rate response to hypotension produced by postural changes or alpha-antagonists as well as to acute hemodilution. Drugs or anesthetic techniques (e.g., spinal or epidural anesthesia) that reduce or block autonomic function tend to cause more hypotension in older patients.

9. Is there a change in cardiac output with aging?
Studies on active, otherwise healthy older subjects have shown that cardiac output at rest and during moderate exercise does not significantly decline with age. Maximal cardiac output does decline with age owing to the progressive decrease in maximum heart rate.

10. Is coronary artery disease easy to detect in the aging population?
The incidence of coronary artery disease increases with age secondary to a progressive worsening of coronary artery stenosis. Because coronary artery disease does not become clinically apparent until a critical stenosis develops, many older, inactive patients may have occult disease and be asymptomatic. Consequently the incidence of coronary artery disease in the elderly is underestimated if it is based only on history and resting ECG criteria. The incidence of silent myocardial infarction also increases with age. Thus ECG findings during the preoperative evaluation of an asymptomatic elderly patient may reveal a prior unrecognized myocardial infarction. In addition, peripheral vascular disease is an important prognostic factor for the presence of coronary artery disease.

11. Discuss the disturbances in cardiac rhythm associated with aging.

Signs of aging:	Common disturbances in rhythm:
• Fibrosis of the sinoatrial node	• Sick sinus syndrome
• Atrophy of conduction pathways	• Hemiblocks
• Loss of normal pacemaker cells	• Bundle-branch blocks
	• Supraventricular and ventricular ectopic beats

The findings of left anterior hemiblock, atrioventricular conduction delays, and atrial flutter or fibrillation suggest underlying cardiac disease and should prompt additional evaluation. Right bundle-branch block does not appear to be associated with an increased incidence of cardiac disease. Premature ventricular and supraventricular beats are common in the elderly and are not necessarily pathologic in healthy elderly individuals. These ectopic beats, however, may indicate underlying coronary artery disease or left ventricular hypertrophy in some individuals.

12. Why is the hepatic clearance of drugs diminished in the elderly?
Decreased clearance is most likely due to the marked reduction in the size of the liver that accompanies aging. By age 80, liver mass may be reduced by as much as 40%. Hepatic blood flow declines proportionately to the loss of liver mass. This decline in hepatic blood flow results in elevated blood levels of drugs that undergo extensive first-pass metabolism. Qualitatively the microsomal and nonmicrosomal enzymatic function of elderly patients is preserved.

13. What changes occur in the kidneys of geriatric patients?
The kidneys become smaller with age. As much as 30% of an adult's renal mass can be lost by the age of 70. By age 80, the number of functioning glomeruli may be one half that of a young adult. Renal blood flow also decreases with age and is associated with a glomerular filtration rate (GFR) that declines by 1% to 1.5% per year. Creatinine clearance decreases by approximately 1% per year after age 40 and can be estimated by the following formula:

$$\text{creatinine clearance} = \frac{(140 - \text{age}) \times \text{wt (kg)}}{72 \times \text{serum creatinine}}$$

Serum creatinine levels usually remain within normal limits despite the lower GFR because of reduced creatinine production from a declining muscle mass. Thus, unless the serum creatinine is elevated, it is not a sensitive test of renal function in the elderly. The kidneys of geriatric patients are also less responsive to antidiuretic hormone and have an impaired ability to concentrate urine.

14. How do the changes in renal function affect anesthetic management?
Deterioration of renal function leaves geriatric patients with minimal renal reserve and places them at risk for intraoperative fluid and electrolyte disturbances. In addition, renal blood flow, which diminishes with age, may be further compromised by dehydration or congestive heart failure. These factors contribute to an increased risk for acute renal failure, which is responsible for 20% or more of perioperative deaths in geriatric surgical patients. Thus, the anesthetic plan must include careful management of fluids and electrolytes as well as maintenance of urine output of at least 0.5 ml/kg/hour. One must also take into account the pharmacokinetic effects of impaired renal clearance. Anesthetic drugs and their metabolites that depend on renal clearance have prolonged elimination half-lives and longer durations of action.

15. Why is intraoperative body temperature difficult to control in older patients?
During general anesthesia, older patients have a greater decrease in body temperature when compared with younger patients and are less likely to reestablish normal body temperature in the recovery phase. Elderly patients have a reduced basal metabolic rate and thus produce less body heat, in addition to a diminished ability to retain their body heat. Elderly patients tend to have smaller amounts of subcutaneous tissue, which provides insulation, as well as diminished reflex cutaneous vasoconstriction to prevent heat loss.

16. What is so bad about postoperative shivering?
Shivering, which has been shown to increase oxygen consumption up to 400%, places enormous requirements on both the pulmonary and the cardiac systems. In the elderly, who may not be able to compensate adequately for this increased oxygen demand, arterial hypoxemia can result. Patients with known or occult coronary artery disease can develop myocardial ischemia owing to the demands placed on the heart by postoperative shivering.

17. Do anesthetic requirements increase or decrease with advancing age?
Anesthetic requirements progressively decrease. This decrease occurs for both inhalational agents as measured by minimum alveolar concentration (MAC) and intravenous agents as measured by ED_{50}. The MAC for volatile anesthetics decreases 4% to 5% per decade after age 40. The basis for this change is unclear, but the fact that this decrease in anesthetic requirement occurs with a wide variety of agents suggests a physiologic as opposed to a pharmacologic cause.

18. Are geriatric patients more at risk for pulmonary aspiration?
Older patients have been shown to have attenuated airway reflexes, and this places them at increased risk for pulmonary aspiration. This risk is compounded by sedatives commonly used for premedication. Routine use of antacids is warranted as well as waiting to extubate until airway reflexes are fully recovered.

19. How are the pharmacokinetics and quality of spinal anesthesia affected by age?
Elderly patients have decreased blood flow to the subarachnoid space, resulting in slower absorption of anesthetic solutions. Older patients also have a smaller volume of cerebrospinal fluid, the specific gravity of which tends to be higher than that of younger patients. This leads to a higher final concentration for a given dose and may alter the spread of the anesthetic. Elderly patients may have accentuated degrees of lumbar lordosis and thoracic kyphosis, increasing cephalad spread and pooling in the thoracic segments. Thus, one might see higher levels of spinal anesthesia, accompanied by faster onset of action and prolonged duration. Finally, older patients have a lower incidence of postdural puncture headaches when compared with younger patients.

20. Do the dynamics of epidural anesthesia change with age?
Older patients require a smaller local anesthetic dose to achieve the same level of block when compared with younger patients. This change in dose requirement is magnified when larger volumes of anesthetic solution are used and may be the result of narrowing of the intervertebral spaces.

BIBLIOGRAPHY

1. Baker AB: Physiology and pharmacology of aging. In International Anesthesia Research Society 1995 Review Course Lectures. Cleveland, International Anesthesia Research Society, 1995, pp 106–109.
2. Brommage PR: Aging and epidural dose requirements. Br J Anaesth 41:1016–1022, 1969.
3. Lakatta EG: Heart and circulation. In Schneider EL, Rowe JW (eds): Handbook of the Biology of Aging, 3rd ed. San Diego, Academic Press, 1990, pp 181–216.
4. McLeskey CH: Anesthesia for the geriatric patient. In Barash PG, Cullen BF, Stoelting RK (eds): Clinical Anesthesia, 2nd ed. Philadelphia, J.B. Lippincott, 1992, pp 1353–1387.
5. Muravchick S: Anesthesia for the elderly. In Miller RD (ed): Anesthesia, 4th ed. New York, Churchill Livingstone, 1994, pp 2143–2156.
6. Stevens WC, Dolan WM, Gibbons RT, et al: Minimum alveolar concentrations (MAC) of isoflurane with and without nitrous oxide in patients of various ages. Anesthesiology 42:197–200, 1975.
7. Stiff J: Evaluation of the geriatric patient. In Rogers MC (ed): Principles and Practice of Anesthesiology. St. Louis, Mosby-Year Book, 1993, pp 480–492.
8. Stoelting RK, Dierdorf SF: Physiologic changes and disorders unique to aging. In Stoelting RK, Dierdorf SF (eds): Anesthesia and Co-Existing Disease, 3rd ed. New York, Churchill Livingstone, 1993, pp 631–637.
9. Vaughn MS, Vaughn RW, Cork RC: Postoperative hypothermia in adults: Relationship of age, anesthesia, and shivering to rewarming. Anesth Analg 60:746–751, 1981.
10. Wahba WM: Influence of aging on lung function-clinical significance of changes from age twenty. Anesth Analg 62:764–776, 1983.

68. OUTPATIENT ANESTHESIA

Lora Manning, B.S.N., M.S.N.A.

1. What percentage of surgical cases are currently performed on an outpatient basis?

Approximately 22 million surgical procedures are performed each year, and 50% of these are conducted in outpatient facilities. From 1990–1994 outpatient surgeries increased by 80%. As many as 70% of anesthetics are administered to patients discharged later in the day or admitted on the day of surgery. This trend is expected to increase. In addition, monitored anesthesia care has increased (approximately 32% of all surgical cases at one large institution).

2. What types of operative procedures can be performed on an outpatient basis?

Many types of operations are successfully completed in ambulatory surgery, including pediatric, ophthalmic, gynecologic, orthopedic, ENT, abdominal, diagnostic, and reconstructive procedures. Both general and regional anesthetics are routinely performed in ambulatory settings.

3. What physical status, as defined by the American Society of Anesthesiologists (ASA), is appropriate in candidates for outpatient surgery?

It is common practice for relatively healthy ASA I and II patients to return home the day of surgery, provided complications from surgery or anesthesia do not arise. More controversial are geriatric and ASA III patients scheduled for outpatient surgery. Well-controlled ASA III patients are accepted on an outpatient basis, but three important points must be kept in mind: (1) the degree to which the systemic disease is under control, (2) the complexity of the surgery, and (3) the level of postoperative care and availability of assistance at home. The clinician's responsibility to the patient is to ensure that a safe and stable postoperative course extends to the home. Patients who do not have the resources to care for themselves should not be discharged home, even if they meet discharge criteria. It is imperative that provisions for home care are made well in advance.

4. List the criteria for discharge from ambulatory settings.

In addition to an Aldrete score of 8 (see page 225) and stable vital signs, before discharge from the postanesthetic care unit, patients must demonstrate:
- Ability to ambulate
- Ability to ingest fluids without nausea and vomiting
- Ability to take oral pain medication
- Ability to verbalize adequate pain relief with oral pain medication
- Recovery of sensorimotor function after conduction block with ability to void
- Lack of respiratory distress
- Regression of upper extremity blocks and adequate protection of the arm (the patient should receive specific instructions on care)

5. What types of anesthesia are appropriate for outpatients?

Approximately 50% of all anesthetics administered are regional, and many are given to outpatients. Certainly general anesthetics, using either the laryngeal mask airway, mask, or endotracheal tube, are appropriate choices. Appropriate short-acting opioids include fentanyl in low doses of 2–5 µg/kg, sufentanil in doses up to 0 .4 µg/kg, or alfentanil in doses to 10–25 µg/kg. Morphine is a less popular opioid because of its sedating properties. Propofol, either as an induction agent or in total intravenous anesthesia (TIVA), is a popular alternative. Short-acting muscle relaxants, including succinylcholine, mivacurium, vecuronium, atracurium, and rocuronium, also may be used, with appropriate reversal if necessary. There is a trend away from dopamine antagonists, including droperidol, and the phenothiazines, because of slower awakening and extrapyramidal effects. Because of its minimal side effects, ondansetron is becoming more popular as an antiemetic. Premedication with midazolam (0.025 mg/kg IV; 0.5–0.75 mg/kg orally) or diazepam (0.1 mg/kg IV/orally) is common, but the possibility of respiratory depression must be kept in mind. Although reversal with flumazenil (0.2-mg increments every 1 minute up to 1 mg) is available, it has a shorter half-life than the anxiolytics and may need to be repeated; its duration of action is 45–90 minutes compared with 1–6 hours for diazepam and midazolam.

6. What are the most common postoperative problems in surgical outpatients? How can they be managed?

Pain, nausea, and vomiting. Local infiltration of the wound either before or after surgical incision has proved effective in relieving postoperative pain. Ejlersen et al. found that preincisional infiltration with lidocaine afforded longer-lasting analgesia than postincisional infiltration. Bupivacaine (0.25% with or without epinephrine) is also an effective local anesthetic. Ketorolac (30 mg IV; 30–60 mg IM) is an NSAID and useful analgesic adjuvant. Advantages include intact ventilatory function and decreased nausea and vomiting. As with all NSAIDs, platelet function is depressed, and patients with impaired renal function are at increased risk for renal failure. Pediatric caudal blocks are also effective in providing postoperative pain relief. Bupivacaine, 0.25%, provides analgesia to the T10–L2 sensory level.

Nausea and vomiting are among the most common postoperative complaints, with an incidence of 10–30%. The many causes include pain, dehydration, opioid use, type of surgery, and gender. Women undergoing gynecologic surgery are at increased risk for developing nausea. Women menstruating at the time of surgery demonstrate an even higher incidence, peaking at the fourth and fifth day of their cycle. Although routine prophylactic treatment may not be warranted, certain types of anesthesia (general) and certain surgeries (laparoscopy) are more prone to induce nausea and vomiting and may best be managed prophylactically. Initial treatment should include ensuring adequate hydration and pain relief, followed by any of the following:

1. Ondansetron, a serotonin antagonist, has received favorable results in studies compared with placebo and more traditional antiemetics. Doses of 4–8 mg have decreased the incidence of postoperative nausea by 57–75%. It is free of many of the side effects of older drugs; however, elevated transaminase levels have been infrequently reported. Researchers have also demonstrated prolonged (up to 24-hour) relief of nausea and vomiting. The prohibiting factor is cost.

2. Droperidol, a butyrophenone, is also commonly used in doses of 0.0625–0.125 mg/kg. However, it may cause drowsiness and extrapyramidal effects.

3. Metoclopramide, in a dose of 10 mg given close to or at the end of surgery, is also effective in reducing the incidence of nausea and vomiting. It may cause extrapyramidal symptoms and is contraindicated in patients with bowel obstruction, concomitant use of tricyclic antidepressants or monoamine oxidase inhibitors, and patients with Parkinson's disease.

4. Scopolamine and scopolamine patches have been successfully used in ambulatory surgery. The patches provide long-term (3–7 days) relief of nausea and vomiting, but undesirable side effects (dry mouth, somnolence, blurred vision, fever) may necessitate discontinuation. Patches should be applied behind the ear 4 hours before they are needed.

7. What are the common causes of an unplanned admission?

The most common causes are surgically related, but anesthetic complications may occur, with nausea and vomiting topping the list. Other common causes are (1) persistent hypoxemia, (2) unresolving conduction block, (3) postdural puncture headache, (4) pain, and (5) persistent hypertension.

8. What laboratory tests are necessary preoperatively?

A thorough history and physical exam should be the guide for deciding which, if any, lab tests are necessary. The trend is to order fewer and fewer tests, basing such evaluations on strong anticipation of abnormal findings in the history and physical exam. Chronic medical conditions require a baseline evaluation; for example, diabetics require assessment of glucose level; renal patients require an electrolyte profile, blood urea nitrogen, creatinine, and hematocrit. If a consultation is necessary, the condition requiring evaluation should be clearly described and reasons for the consultation clearly conveyed. See chapter 15 for a useful guide to appropriate preoperative testing.

9. What preoperative medications are necessary?
Medications that patients must take for chronic conditions should be continued the morning of surgery and include beta-adrenergic blockers, angiotensin-converting enzyme inhibitors, central acting antihypertensives, beta agonists, anticonvulsants, H2 blockers, corticosteroids, aminophylline, and other cardiac drugs, such as antianginal or antidysrhythmic agents. Patients taking Coumadin are evaluated on a case-by-case basis but rarely are candidates for outpatient surgery.

Non–insulin-dependent diabetics should be counseled not to take oral hypoglycemic agents in the hope of preventing perioperative hypoglycemia. Diabetics can be managed several different ways: (1) Hold morning insulin dose, and check blood sugar on arrival at ambulatory anesthesia. (2) Have the patient take one-half of the usual morning insulin dose, and check blood sugar on arrival at ambulatory anesthesia.

Routine aspiration prophylaxis is recommended for high-risk patients and obstetrics and may include a nonparticulate antacid, an H2 blocker, and a benzamide, such as metoclopramide.

10. Are patients with a history of malignant hyperthermia suitable for outpatient surgery?
This issue is controversial. If patients are permitted to go home on the day of surgery, strict guidelines must be followed: (1) avoid all triggering agents perioperatively; (2) use a clean machine (inactivate or remove vaporizors; change bellows, CO_2 absorber and breathing tubes; and flush the machine with high flow oxygen for at least 10 minutes); (3) schedule the patient as the first case of the day; (4) ensure that dantrolene is readily available; and (5) observe the patient for a minimum of 6 hours postoperatively. Some centers admit susceptible patients for overnight observation.

11. What are the current fasting guidelines for pediatric patients?
Studies indicate that clear liquid intake accelerates gastric emptying. Parents are encouraged to give clear liquid feedings up to 2–3 hour before surgery. Breast milk is considered a clear liquid. Formula or solids are withheld 6–8 hours before surgery. To prevent hypovolemia and hypoglycemia, clear liquids should continue to be given up to the prescribed times.

12. Is the patient selection different for pediatric patients?
ASA I or II patients continue to be appropriate candidates for ambulatory surgery. Pediatric patients classified as ASA III or IV may be appropriate for ambulatory surgery if their medical condition is well controlled. However, children with severe asthma may develop bronchospasm after surgery and are poor candidates for ambulatory surgery. Immunocompromised pediatric patients, however, are often well suited as outpatients, because their risk of hospital-acquired illness will be minimized. Premature infants require careful consideration because of an increased risk of apnea, poor temperature control, and immature gag reflex. Generally, term infants less than 44 weeks and ex-premature infants less than 55–60 weeks postconceptual age are at risk for developing apnea. When immaturity is combined with other medical problems, risk of morbidity increases; it is best to err on the side of caution and admit such infants for apnea monitoring.

13. What types of surgery can be performed on pediatric patients on an outpatient basis?
(1) Ophthalmic procedures, (2) lower abdominal and genitourinary surgery, (3) ENT surgeries (with the exception of patients with a history of obstructive sleep apnea or cor pulmonale secondary to enlarged adenoids or tonsils), (4) extremity surgery, (5) plastic surgery, and (6) peripheral orthopedic procedures. Exceptions include upper abdominal surgery and thoracic surgeries, which are often complicated by hypoxia or prolonged surgery time. Abdominal procedures performed laparoscopically are done more frequently as an outpatient procedure.

14. What different anesthetic techniques are common in pediatrics?
Sedatives, if used preoperatively, may be given orally, nasally, or rectally. Pediatric patients < 14 months tend not to experience separation anxiety, and sedation may not be necessary. In young

children general anesthesia is accomplished with mask induction. Halothane is less irritating to the airways and is most commonly chosen as the induction agent. After induction with halothane, anesthesia can be maintained with isoflurane or desflurane. High-flow nitrous oxide and oxygen in a 6:3 ratio speed the induction. For halothane, vaporizer settings may be increased by 0.25 vol% every 2–3 breaths. In healthy patients, minimal monitoring (pulse oximeter) is acceptable until the child is sufficiently anesthetized to permit complete monitoring. Alternatively, some centers allow the parents to be in the operating room, holding the child during induction. This approach may provide a more cooperative patient and parent. Intravenous access, if necessary, is established after the child is asleep. Most older children are allowed to choose between an IV line and mask induction so that they can maintain some sense of control. Caudal blocks with 0.25% bupivacaine are also becoming more common as an adjuvant to general anesthesia for inguinal or perineal surgery in pediatric patients. They can be administered before the start of surgery or immediately before awakening and provide postoperative analgesia for many hours. Doses are as follows: inguinal region, 0.5 ml/kg; umbilical region, 0.75 ml/kg.

15. What other special considerations should be kept in mind for pediatric patients?
Patients with a current upper respiratory infection require further consideration, because infection increases the incidence of complications when intubation is required. However, many children have frequent clear nasal discharge. It is important to question the parent further about cough, fever, purulent discharge, or any other change in symptoms. If nasal discharge is due to allergic rhinitis, surgery may continue. It is common practice to delay surgery for 2–3 weeks after a significant upper respiratory infection to prevent perioperative respiratory complications (bronchospasm, laryngospasm, hypoxemia).

16. What other trends have been observed in ambulatory surgery?
The use of local anesthesia and monitored anesthesia care has increased dramatically in the last decade and will continue to do so. New drugs are constantly under investigation, including (1) sevoflurane, a low solubility inhalation agent; (2) remifentanil, an ultrashort-acting opioid; (3) dolasetron, a serotonin antagonist; (4) dezocine, a mu receptor agonist-antagonist; and (5) mirfentanil, a piperidine derivative with agonist and antagonist properties.

BIBLIOGRAPHY

1. Apfelbaum JL: Current controversies in adult outpatient anesthesia: Administrative and clinical. 45th Annual ASA Refresher Course Lecture 141:1–7, 1994.
2. Beebe JJ, Sessler DI: Preparation of anesthesia machines for patients susceptible to malignant hyperthermia. Anesthesiology 69:395–400, 1988.
3. Ejlersen E, Andersen HB, Eliasen K, Mogensen T: A comparison between preincisional and postincisional lidocaine infiltration and postoperative pain. Anesth Analg 74:495-498, 1992.
4. Henderson JA: Ambulatory surgery: Past, present, and future. In Wetchler BV (ed): Anesthesia for Ambulatory Surgery. Philadelphia, J.B. Lippincott, 1991, pp 1–27.
5. Holzman RS: Morbidity and mortality in pediatric anesthesia.Pediatr Clin North Am 41:239–256, 1994.
6. Kapur PA: Ambulatory surgery: State of the art. What are the best drugs for ambulatory surgery? 45th Annual ASA Refresher Course Lecture 422:1–7, 1994; 102:1–6, 1994.
7. Kurth CS, Spitzer AR, Broennle AM, et al: Postoperative apnea in preterm infants. Anesthesiology 66:483–486, 1987.
8. Mulroy MF: Regional anesthetic techniques. In White PF (ed): Anesthesia for Ambulatory Surgery. Boston, Little, Brown, 1994, pp 81–98.
9. Patel R, Hannallah R: Pediatric anesthetic techniques. In White PF (ed): Anesthesia for Ambulatory Surgery. Boston, Little, Brown, 1994, pp 37–53.
10. Scuderi P, Wetchler B, Sung YF, Mingus M, et al: Treatment of postoperative nausea and vomiting after outpatient surgery with the 5-HT3 antagonist ondansetron. Anesthesiology 78:15–20, 1993.
11. Splinter WM, Stewart JA, Muir JG: The effect of preoperative apple juice on gastric contents, thirst, and hunger in children. Can J Anaesth 36:55–60, 1989.
12. Stoelting RK: Pharmacology and Physiology in Anesthetic Practice. Philadelphia, J.B. Lippincott, 1991, pp 460–461.
13. Watcha MF, White PF: Postoperative nausea and vomiting. Anesthesiology 77:162–184, 1992.

69. ANESTHESIA OUTSIDE THE OPERATING ROOM

Kevin Fitzpatrick, M.D., and Michael Duey, M.D.

1. What types of anesthetics may be performed outside of the operating room (OR)?
• General inhalational
• Monitored anesthesia care (MAC)
• Regional anesthesia, including epidural and intrathecal techniques

2. For what procedures and in what locales outside the OR or obstetric suite is anesthesia conducted?
• Diagnostic radiology, which includes angiographic procedures or sedation for computerized tomography (CT) and magnetic resonance imaging (MRI)
• Cardiac catheterizations, insertion of implantable cardiac defibrillators (ICD), and coronary arteriography
• Cardioversions, which may be conducted in various locations, including the intensive care unit (ICU)
• Therapeutic radiation
• Electroconvulsive therapy, which is usually performed in the postanesthesia care unit (PACU)
• Sedation for bone marrow biopsies and other minor procedures on the pediatric ward
• Emergency airway management anywhere in the hospital
• Transport of the anesthetized or critically ill patient

3. What factors complicate administration of anesthesia outside the OR?
Complicating factors include physical constraints imposed by the environment and different paramedical personnel; for example, lack of trained OR nurses, sophisticated and familiar monitoring equipment, or other equipment normally available in surgical suites.

4. To what safety standards must one adhere when conducting an anesthetic outside the OR?
Standards developed by the Department of Anesthesia at Harvard are the same as those used in the OR.

Requirements for the Safe Conduct of Anesthesia

Piped oxygen in addition to oxygen cylinders	Adequate illumination
Suction	Immediate access to the patient
Anesthesia machine and supplies equivalent to those in the OR	Emergency resuscitation cart with defibrillator
	Attending anesthesiologist
Sufficient electrical outlets	Two-way communication to summon help

5. What situations may interfere with maintenance of the above standards?
Most facilities for nonsurgical procedures are not designed to meet the needs of anesthesiologists. Physical space is often cramped. Limited access to the patient may pose a safety risk. During certain procedures, as in radiation therapy, the anesthesiologist may not be present in the same room as the patient. Suboptimal lighting, especially in the radiology suite, may lead to unrecognized airway obstruction or cyanosis, circuit disconnections, and exhaustion of gas (oxygen) cylinders.

6. What monitoring is necessary for administration of an anesthetic outside the OR?
Required monitoring includes (1) continuous display of ECG throughout the anesthetic; (2) determination of arterial blood pressure and heart rate at least every 5 minutes; and (3) additional evaluation of circulatory function performed by a minimum of one of the following: monitoring of peripheral pulse by palpation or ultrasound, pulse plethysmography, auscultation of heart sounds, direct monitoring of (intraarterial) blood pressure, and/or pulse oximetry. When mechanical ventilation is required, a breathing system disconnect alarm must be in continuous use. In addition, an oxygen analyzer with a low oxygen concentration alarm must be used. End-tidal carbon dioxide ($ETCO_2$) and tidal volume measurements are also strongly encouraged during administration of a general anesthetic.

7. How may the equipment necessary for the conduction of an anesthetic in a remote location be different from that in the OR?
Often, as new anesthesia machines and monitors are purchased by an anesthesia department, the older equipment is relegated to remote locations. The anesthesiologist must be familiar with the operation of such equipment before using it to provide an anesthetic.

8. What other equipment is required?

1. Tools for airway management
   - Bag/mask ventilation system
   - Oral airways of various sizes
   - Laryngoscopes
   - Endotracheal tubes

2. Medications for induction of anesthesia
3. Muscle relaxants
4. Drugs for cardiac resuscitation
   These items may be easily stored and carried in an emergency airway box to any location.

9. Which patients are most likely to require anesthetic care in the radiology suite?
Most adults are able to tolerate noninvasive procedures after adequate instruction and preparation from the appropriate caregiver without the need for an anesthetic. Anesthesia consultation may be required for confused, combative, and developmentally delayed patients, or for patients suffering from neuromuscular disorders who are unable to remain still. Trauma victims, patients with increased intracranial pressure, or patients with a compromised airway are obvious candidates, as are most pediatric patients.

10. What are the dangers of dyes (contrast agents) used in radiologic imaging?
Approximately 5–8% of patients receiving an intravenous injection of contrast medium experience an allergic reaction to the dye. The method of injection (slow or bolus), type of dye used, and dose influence the risk of systemic reaction. Patients with a prior history of allergy to shellfish or seafood are more prone to reactions.

11. What are the manifestations of an allergic reaction?

Contrast Dye Allergic Reactions

MILD	MODERATE	SEVERE (ANAPHYLAXIS)
Nausea	Bronchospasm	Prolonged hypotension
Vomiting	Hypotension	Cyanosis
Facial flushing	Tissue edema	Anoxia
Fever	Seizures	Pulmonary edema
Chills		Angina
Urticaria		Dysrhythmias

12. How are allergic reactions treated?
Therapy ranges from supportive care to administration of fluids, oxygen, and full cardiopulmonary resuscitation. Available drugs should include epinephrine, atropine, diphenhydramine, corticosteroids, and benzodiazepines.

13. How can anesthesiologists protect themselves from radiation exposure?
Protective garments, including radiation-shielding aprons, thyroid shields, and protective eye-wear, are recommended. Radiation exposure badges that measure cumulative exposure also should be considered.

14. Which patients undergoing angiography may require consultation by an anesthetist?
Most adults tolerate angiographic procedures without an anesthetic. Pediatric, uncooperative, or noncommunicative patients usually require anesthetic management, often with general anesthesia. Appropriate monitoring, as always, must be in place.

15. What specific side effects are most common during cerebral angiography?
Contrast dyes may cross the blood-brain barrier, causing seizures and increased intracranial pressure. During cerebral angiography it is advantageous to keep patients awake and talking for continuous neurologic assessment.

16. Discuss specific challenges involved in the administration of an anesthetic in the CT suite.
CT scanning under general anesthesia presents difficulties in monitoring and airway management. Movement of the patient on the CT gantry may cause kinking of oxygen tubing or disconnection of the breathing circuit. Patients receiving oral contrast or undergoing emergency procedures must be considered at risk for aspiration of gastric contents. In terrified pediatric patients anesthesia is often induced outside the CT suite. Temperature monitoring of pediatric patients is essential because of the cold temperatures required for CT equipment to function properly.

17. Define the unique problems associated with providing an anesthetic in the MRI suite.
Difficulties in providing a safe anesthetic in the MRI suite arise from the necessity of using a powerful magnetic field. The MRI suite is often located in a remote, isolated area of the hospital. The cylindrical large-bore magnet surrounding the body limits access to the patient. Ferromagnetic objects may be hurled toward the scanner, creating lethal projectiles. Large metal objects may interfere with the quality of the image. Many electronic instruments may not function normally when placed in close proximity to the magnet. Implantable ferrous magnetic devices, such as older cerebrovascular clips, surgical clips, and pacemakers, are hazardous.

18. What modifications in the anesthesia machine, ventilator, and monitoring equipment must be made to provide an anesthetic in the MRI suite?
All monitoring equipment is affected by the magnetic fields generated by the MRI machine. Monitors with ferromagnetic components must be located outside the magnetic field. The distance depends on the strength of the field and shielding in the suite. If the anesthesia machine, monitoring equipment, and ventilator are located several meters from the patient, long monitoring leads and ventilation tubing, with a large compressible volume in the circuit, are required, and risk of disconnection is increased. Anesthetic and monitoring equipment with nonferromagnetic components is available and allows much closer proximity to the patient and MRI machine. Many newer institutions have anesthesia machines built into the structure of the MRI suite, which allow easier and safer conduction of anesthesia. The lack of availability of a piped oxygen source into the MRI suite in older institutions may be a significant problem, because standard gas cylinders are ferromagnetic and may become dangerous projectiles when introduced into the magnetic environment. Aluminum cylinders are a safe alternative, but they cannot be recharged because metal fatigue from repeated pressurizations predisposes these tanks to explosion. Nonferromagnetic ventilators are available.

    Electrocardiography. Many MRI manufacturers now produce ECG and respiratory monitors compatible with their equipment. Unfortunately, these monitors do not allow reliable qualitative assessment of the ECG, but they may be used to provide an index of heart rate and to serve as a gating signal for other monitoring equipment (e.g., pulse oximeters). If such equipment is not available, modification of existing equipment is necessary. When unshielded ferromagnetic wiring is used, the ECG demonstrates significant changes in the strong magnetic field produced by the MRI scanner. Changes in ECG potentials are greatest in the early T waves and late ST segments, mimicking the changes seen in conditions such as hyperkalemia and pericarditis. The rapidly changing magnetic fields may cause spikes in the ECG trace, leading to an artificially elevated heart rate on the monitor. Positioning the electrodes as close as possible to the center of the magnetic field, keeping the limb leads close together and in the same plane, and braiding or twisting the leads help to minimize the changes produced by the magnetic field.

Pulse oximetry. Problems similar to those encountered with the ECG may be experienced. The use of nonferromagnetic probes and shielded wiring minimizes distortion of the signal.

Capnography. To function properly, the capnograph should be placed outside the magnetic field. The long connecting tubing causes significant lag and alarm times. The waveform may show a prolonged upslope, even in patients with healthy lungs. Trends and respiratory rate, however, may be observed.

Blood pressure. Noninvasive blood pressure readings may be obtained if all ferrous connections are removed from the cuff and tubing. Invasive pressure readings may be obtained if the lead from the pressure transducer is passed through a radiofrequency filter. Dampening of the waveform is minimized by resting the transducer within 1.5 meters of the patient.

Auscultation. Use of precordial or esophageal stethoscopes may be difficult because of the length of tubing required and the noise produced by the MRI machine.

19. What unique problems are encountered during the administration of anesthesia for therapeutic radiation?

For patients undergoing external beam radiation, the general principles discussed above apply, including the necessity of readily available airway control equipment, emergency drugs, appropriate monitors, and anesthesia delivery machines. Special attention must be paid to the preoperative history and physical exam. The patient's physical status may be severely compromised by neoplastic disease, chemotherapy, and previous operative procedures. After careful patient and equipment positioning, all personnel must vacate the room to avoid radiation exposure. It is important to observe the patient and monitors through closed circuit television or remote displays.

20. Why is anesthesia necessary for cardioversion? How is it conducted?

Cardioversion is a painful procedure that requires brief general anesthesia (the patient must be asleep for a brief period of time) that may include ventilation of the lungs, usually with a bag-and-mask device. All standard monitors (ECG, noninvasive blood pressure, pulse oximetry) and resuscitation equipment must be present and working. The patient is preoxygenated with 100% oxygen via mask for 4 minutes, and an intravenous general anesthesia induction agent is injected. Propofol, thiopental, methohexital, or etomidate may be used as induction agents. Midazolam, 1–5 mg IV for sedation, also may be used. If the patient becomes apneic, the ability to mask-ventilate is confirmed by attempting positive pressure ventilation and observing the rise and fall of the chest cavity and by auscultating the chest and epigastrium. All personnel then confirm that they are touching nothing metallic that may be connected to the patient, and the electroshock is delivered. Often more than one shock is necessary; amnesia, hemodynamic stability, and oxygenation must be maintained throughout the procedure.

BIBLIOGRAPHY

1. Gillies BS: Anesthesia outside the operating room. In Barash PG, Cullen BF, Stoelting RK (eds): Clinical Anesthesia. Philadelphia, J.B. Lippincott,1992, pp 1465–1477.
2. Manninen PH: Anaesthesia outside the operating room. Can J Anaesth 38: R126–R129, 1991.
3. Messick JM, MacKenzie RA, Southorn P: Anesthesia at remote locations. In Miller RD (ed). New York, Churchill Livingstone, 1994, pp 2247–2276.
4. Patteson SK, Chesney JT: Anesthetic management for magnetic resonance imaging: Problems and solutions. Anesth Analg 74:121–128, 1992.
5. Peden CJ, Menon DK, Hall AS, et al: Magnetic resonance for the anaesthetist. Part II: Anesthesia and monitoring in MR units. Anaesthesia 47:508–517, 1992.
6. Rasch DK, Bready LL: Anesthesia for magnetic resonance imaging. Prog Anesthesiol 5:158–165, 1991.

70. ARTIFICIAL CARDIAC PACEMAKERS

Kevin Fitzpatrick, M.D.

GENERAL CONSIDERATIONS

1. What are some indications for the placement of a cardiac pacemaker?

1. Acquired atrioventricular (AV) block in adults
2. AV block associated with myocardial infarction
3. Chronic bifascicular or trifascicular block
4. Sinus node dysfunction
5. AV block and dysrhythmias in children
6. Tachydysrhythmias

THE LANGUAGE OF PACEMAKERS

2. What is a lead? an electrode?

The lead is the insulating wire that connects the pacemaker to the electrode. The electrode is the metal end of the lead that makes contact with the myocardium.

3. What is unipolar pacing? bipolar pacing?

In a **unipolar pacemaker**, the stimulating electrode (negative) is located in the atrium or ventricle and the ground electrode (positive) is placed in a location distant from the heart. With **bipolar pacemakers**, both the positive and the negative electrodes are placed within the paced cardiac chamber.

4. What is a triggered pacemaker? an inhibited pacemaker?

A **triggered pacemaker** senses atrial and/or ventricular depolarization and paces immediately. An **inhibited pacemaker** senses an intrinsic atrial and/or ventricular depolarization and promptly shuts off.

5. Define R-wave sensitivity.

R-wave sensitivity describes the minimum voltage of intrinsic R-wave necessary to activate the sensing circuit of the pacemaker and inhibit it from pacing. In other words, when the intrinsic R-wave is greater in magnitude than the R-wave sensitivity programmed into the pacemaker, the pacemaker will not interfere with cardiac conduction.

TYPES OF PACEMAKERS

6. What is the 5-letter coding system used to describe cardiac pacemakers?

Most pacemakers are referred to by the first three letters of the code. The first letter indicates the location of the pacing electrode. The second letter signifies the location of the pacemaker's sensor. The third letter is indicative of the mode of activity. The fourth letter describes programmability. The fifth letter describes implantable cardioverter-defibrillators (ICD). See the table below.

Coding System Describing Cardiac Pacemakers

I	II	III	IV	V
CHAMBER PACED	CHAMBER SENSED	MODE OF RESPONSE	PROGRAMMABILITY	ANTITACHYCARDIC FUNCTIONS
O = none	0 = none	0 = none	0 = none	0 = none
A = atrium	A = atrium	T = triggered	P = simple programmable	P = pacing
V = ventricle	V = ventricle	I = inhibited	M = multiprogrammable C = communicating	S = shock
D = dual (A + V)	D = dual (A + V)	D = dual (T + I)	R = rate responsive	D = dual (P + S)

Types of Pacemakers

LETTER CODE	PACEMAKER FUNCTION
AOO	Atrial fixed-rate (asynchronous) pacemaker: it paces the atrium regardless of intrinsic cardiac activity.
VOO	Ventricular fixed-rate pacemaker: it stimulates the ventricle regardless of intrinsic cardiac activity.
AAI	Atrial demand pacemaker: it senses and paces only in the atrium; it is inhibited from pacing by intrinsic P-waves.
VVI	Ventricular demand pacemaker: it senses and paces only in the ventricle; intrinsic R-waves inhibit it from pacing.
AAT	Atrial triggered pacemaker: it senses and paces in the atrium; it is triggered to pace by sensing intrinsic (nonconducted) P-waves.
VVT	Ventricular triggered pacemaker: it senses and paces in the ventricle; it is triggered to stimulate by sensing intrinsic (nonconducted) R-waves.
DVI	Sequential pacemaker; it senses only in the ventricle; it paces the atrium and then the ventricle and is inhibited by intrinsic ventricular depolarization.
VDD	This pacemaker senses in both the atrium and ventricle and paces in the ventricle; it is able to pace the ventricle after atrial contraction, even if AV conduction is impaired; likewise, it may pace only the atrium and permit intrinsic AV conduction and ventricular contraction.

7. What is a fixed-rate pacemaker? Give an example.
These are known as asynchronous pacemakers. Electrical impulses are delivered at regular, pre-set intervals, *independent* of the patient's intrinsic heart rate. These pacemakers are good for pacing during bradycardia secondary to new-onset third degree AV block. Ventricular tachycardia may result when competition with a patient's intrinsic rate leads to a pacing spike that occurs on a T-wave.

8. What is a single-chamber demand pacemaker?
Demand pacemakers are also known as noncompetitive pacemakers. They stimulate the heart "on demand" only when spontaneous impulses do not occur during a preselected time interval. This type of pacemaker is inhibited by intrinsic R-waves when the patient's own heart rate is greater than the pre-set rate. When this occurs, the ECG will not demonstrate any pacemaker "spikes" (impulses). In order to assess whether the pacemaker is functioning properly, vagal maneuvers (Valsalva or carotid massage) may slow the intrinsic rate sufficiently so that the pacemaker begins transmitting impulses to the myocardium.

9. Why is it occasionally necessary to convert a demand pacemaker to an asynchronous pacemaker? How is this accomplished?
A demand pacemaker may malfunction due to faulty circuitry, incorrect programming, or from extrinsic radio frequency interference (see #20). Under these circumstances, it may be useful to convert the pacemaker to asynchronous mode so that the myocardium is depolarized at regular intervals and cardiac output is maintained.

Mode conversion may be achieved by reprogramming the pacemaker via an external remote control radio device or by bringing a specially designed magnet in close to the pacemaker. A pacemaker magnet should always be nearby when patients with pacemakers undergo surgical procedures.

10. What is the most common type of pacemaker?
The VVI demand pacemaker is the most commonly placed pacemaker today.

11. What are sequential pacemakers?
Sequential pacemakers are designed to preserve the AV conduction sequence. They may be useful in young, exercising patients because these pacemakers are able to increase the ventricular rate in response to increases in the intrinsic rate of atrial depolarization. The ventricle, then, may be paced independently of the atrium.

12. What type of pacemaker is known as the "universal" pacemaker?
The DDD pacemaker is the universal pacemaker. It can behave as a VDD pacemaker during normal atrial rates with abnormal AV conduction. It is an AAI pacemaker during atrial bradycardia and normal AV conduction. It becomes a DVI pacemaker during sinus bradycardia with abnormal AV conduction.

13. What is an implantable cardioverter-defibrillator (ICD)?
An ICD continuously monitors the patient's cardiac rhythm. ICDs are placed into patients prone to ventricular dysrhythmias and in whom medical management has failed. When ventricular tachycardia or fibrillation is detected, this device will deliver countershocks in an attempt to convert the heart to its baseline rhythm.

PREOPERATIVE EVALUATION IN THE PATIENT WITH A PACEMAKER

14. What kinds of diagnostic information and data from the history and physical exam are particularly relevant in these patients?
Many of these patients have multiple medical problems, including cardiovascular disease. Cardiac medications should probably be continued throughout the perioperative period. It is important for the anesthetist to know the original indications for placement of the pacemaker and whether the patient is experiencing a return of pre-pacemaker symptoms, e.g., lightheadedness, dizziness, or fainting.

A chest radiograph may be helpful to verify pacemaker lead continuity and to look for signs of congestive heart failure, e.g., cardiomegaly or prominent vascularity and pulmonary edema. These patients must have a recent electrocardiogram (ECG) available. Sample ECG tracings demonstrating pacemaker activity may be found at the end of this chapter. Do not forget to palpate the patient's pulse while watching a continuous ECG monitor. In this way, one may verify that paced cardiac beats are conducted. A recent hematocrit will serve to assess oxygen-carrying capacity in patients with cardiac disease. A serum potassium is also useful in order to identify acute changes in extracellular potassium concentration which may affect myocardial sensitivity to pacing (see #23).

15. What kind of data should be gathered regarding the pacemaker itself?
The type of pacemaker (letter code) and date of placement should be determined. If the patient cannot remember, she may be able to produce the pacemaker identification card. Otherwise, a chest x-ray will reveal not only the type of pacemaker (since the letter code is radiopaque), but also the location of the pacemaker.

16. Do these patients require any type of special monitoring?
Indicated monitoring is predicated upon the patient's overall medical condition and the operation to be performed. The presence of a pacemaker is not necessarily an indication for invasive monitoring (pulmonary artery catheter, arterial line).

INTRAOPERATIVE MANAGEMENT OF THE PATIENT WITH A PACEMAKER

17. What type of anesthetic is best for procedures involving the pacemaker?
In general, no one technique is better than another. Usually, intravenous sedation (MAC- monitored anesthesia care) with local anesthetic infiltration is performed for pacemaker placemement and battery changes. General endotracheal anesthesia (GETA) is performed for ICD placement.

18. Is succinylcholine contraindicated for general anesthetics in patients with pacemakers?
Random muscular contractions, or fasciculations, often occur after the administration of depolarizing muscle relaxants and may be perceived by the pacemaker sensor as an intrinsic cardiac impulse. Depending on the type of pacemaker, it may be inhibited from firing an impulse resulting in deleterious reductions in heart rate and cardiac output, even cardiac standstill. A "defasciculating" dose of a nondepolarizing muscle relaxant should be given 5–10 minutes before succinylcholine is administered. Additionally, the pacemaker may be reprogrammed to asynchronous (VOO) mode, so that it stimulates the ventricle regardless of intrinsic cardiac activity.

19. Can etomidate be used as an induction agent?
The myoclonus typically occurring after induction doses of etomidate and, to a lesser extent, methohexital and thiopental can also fool a pacemaker's sensor and lead to cardiac standstill. This is, however, a rare occurrence.

20. How does electrocautery affect pacemaker function?
Electromagnetic interference (EMI) from electrocautery ("Bovie") is probably the most common cause of intraoperative pacemaker failure. Its use may cause the pacemaker to stop firing because EMI is interpreted as normal intrinsic cardiac activity. The sensing function of the pacemaker may be circumvented by the application of an external magnet or by reprogramming the pacemaker to asynchronous mode. Electrocautery will not affect a VOO pacemaker.

Most demand pacemakers are programmed to institute a default rhythm in the presence of continuous EMI. **Multi-programmable** pacemakers, however, could be reprogrammed to any of a number of modes during the application of electrocautery and a magnet applied to these pacemakers can actually worsen its response to electrocautery.

21. What can be done to protect the pacemaker from the untoward effects of EMI?
An attempt should be made to use bipolar cautery. The electrocautery energy level should be kept as low as possible; short bursts are safer than continuous activation. Finally, the current dispersal unit (CDU, or "Bovie pad") should be placed remote from the pacemaker.

22. Your patient with a pacemaker is found pulseless; ECG demonstrates ventricular tachycardia. The defibrillator is charged and ready to go. Do you proceed with external defibrillation?
Yes. Most pacemakers are constructed with protective circuits designed to withstand external defibrillation. The paddles, however, should not be placed directly over the pacemaker. Pulselessness or any dysrhythmia must be confirmed by palpation of a major artery. The carotid and femoral arteries are usually the easiest to identify.

CONTROVERSY

23. Your patient with a pacemaker has a serum potassium of 2.9 mEq/L. His only medication is furosemide, which he has been taking for 2 years. Should he receive supplemental potassium before receiving an anesthetic?
Probably not. The normal intracellular-to-extracellular ratio of potassium is 30:1, which is equivalent to a –90 mV resting membrane potential (RMP). Acutely increasing extracellular potassium, e.g., rapid intravenous administration of potassium, or acidosis, will create a less negative RMP. Action potential threshold is thus lowered and, consequently, the myocardium is more sensitive to electrical depolarization. This may precipitate ventricular tachycardia or fibrillation.

Acutely decreasing extracellular potassium through, for example, hyperventilation (respiratory alkalosis), creates a more negative RMP, rendering the myocardium less excitable. Clinically, hypokalemia could increase the pacing threshold and lead to loss of pacing.

Acute changes in extracellular potassium are of concern in patients with pacemakers. Chronic imbalances invoke compensatory mechanisms which restore RMP to normal levels. With regard to this patient, he is probably chronically hypokalemic and not at increased risk. If chronic hypokalemia cannot be established, i.e., there is no previous serum potassium level available or the potassium level is less than 2.9 mEg/L, anesthetic administration should be postponed.

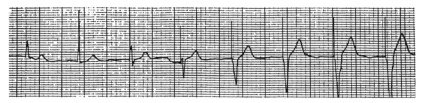

Normal VVI pacing. (From Zaidan JR: Pacemakers. In Barash PG (ed): Refresher Courses in Anesthesiology, Vol 21. Philadelphia, J.B. Lippincott, 1993, with permission.)

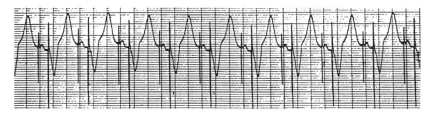

Normal atrioventricular (sequential) pacing. (From Zaidan JR: Pacemakers. In Barash PG (ed): Refresher Courses in Anesthesiology, Vol 21. Philadelphia, J.B. Lippincott, 1993, with permission.)

BIBLIOGRAPHY

1. Eckenbrecht PD: Pacemakers and implantable cardioverter defibrillators. 45th Annual Refresher Course Lectures and Clinical Update Program 234:1–7, 1994.
2. Domino KB, Smith TC: Electrocautery-induced reprogramming of a pacemaker using a precordial magnet. Anesth Analg 62:609–612, 1983.
3. Mangar D, Atlas GM, Kane PB: Electrocautery-induced pacemaker malfunction during surgery. Can J Anesth 38:616–618, 1991.
4. Stoelting RK, Dierdorf SF: Abnormalities of cardiac conduction and cardiac rhythm. In Anesthesia and Coexisting Disease, 3rd ed. New York, Churchill Livingstone, 1993, pp 63–77.
5. Zaidan JR: Pacemakers. In Barash PG (ed): Refresher Courses in Anesthesiology, Vol 21. Philadelphia, J.B. Lippincott, 1993, pp 1–12.
6. Zaidan JR: Pacemakers. Anesthesiology 60:319–334, 1984.

VIII. Regional Anesthesia

71. SPINAL ANESTHESIA

Stephanie E. May, M.S.A., CRNA., and Beth Schatzman, M.H.S., CRNA.

1. Define spinal anesthesia.

Spinal anesthesia is a type of regional anesthetic also known as a subarachnoid block (SAB); it falls under the classification of major conduction blockade, which refers to the blockade of spinal nerve roots. A local anesthetic is injected into the subarachnoid space, mixing with cerebrospinal fluid (CSF). The resultant nerve block provides surgical anesthesia as far cephalad as the upper abdomen. Uptake of the local anesthetic determines which neuronal functions—motor, sensory, or sympathetic—are affected. Distribution of the local anesthetic determines the extent of the effects, and elimination of the local anesthetic determines their duration. SAB is frequently administered as a single injection, although an indwelling catheter may be used for intermittent or continuous injections.

2. Does spinal anesthesia have advantages over general anesthesia?

Numerous studies have examined this question, and the data are conflicting. Regional anesthesia such as SAB has been shown to be of benefit in several areas:

1. The metabolic stress response to surgery and anesthesia is much more effectively reduced by SAB than general anesthesia.

2. Many studies (especially in elective hip surgery) have shown a reduction in blood loss of 20–30% in patients receiving regional anesthesia vs. general anesthesia.

3. Several studies demonstrated that regional techniques decrease the incidence of venous thromboembolic complications by as much as 50%, especially in lower extremity procedures.

4. Data regarding pulmonary complications are mixed; however, pulmonary compromise appears to be less in peripheral procedures performed under regional anesthesia. Other areas of potential benefit include avoidance of endotracheal intubation in patients with a difficult airway (although a regional anesthetic complication may necessitate emergent intubation), avoidance of airway manipulation in asthmatic patients, and decreased risk of gastric aspiration.

5. There may be a slight trend toward reduced cardiac complications in patients receiving regional vs. general anesthetics.

6. SAB is widely used in obstetric anesthesia, especially for abdominal delivery. Less medication is administered to the mother and fetus. The mother is able to remain awake and participate in the delivery.

3. What is the duration of SAB?

Duration of Spinal Anesthetic Agents

AGENT	DURATION*
Lidocaine 5%	Short-to-intermediate acting, up to 60–75 minutes; possibly 90+ minutes with a vasoconstrictor.
Tetracaine 1%	90–120 minutes; up to twice as long with a vasoconstrcitor.
Bupivacaine 0.75%	Approximately 120–150 minutes; little increase with a vasoconstrictor.

* Times are based on the more commonly used hyperbaric preparations of local anesthetics (see question 4). Isobaric solutions tend to produce a more prolonged block.

The duration depends on the particular local anesthetic and its dose. Termination of action is due to reabsorption of the agent from the CSF into the systemic circulation, where metabolism and elimination occur. Duration of neural blockade may be prolonged by addition of a vasoconstrictor, such as phenylephrine or epinephrine, to the local anesthetic solution. Vasoconstrictor efficacy varies with the type of local anesthetic.

4. Describe the factors involved in distribution (and therefore level) of spinal anesthetics.
The following factors affect distribution of local anesthetics in the CSF, which determines the level of spinal anesthesia:

1. Patient characteristics: height, position, gender (a woman in the lateral position is slightly head down because of the ratio of the width of pelvis to shoulders), intraabdominal pressure, and anatomic configuration of the spinal canal.

2. Type of needle, site of injection, and direction of needle.

3. Amount or dosage of local anesthetic (the most influential factor).

4. Physical characteristics of the local anesthetic solution. The baricity of the local anesthetic solution is defined as the ratio of the density of the local anesthetic solution to the density of CSF. A solution with a ratio > 1 is defined as hyperbaric and tends to sink with gravity in the CSF. The level of block is greatly affected by patient position (i.e., gravity). An isobaric solution has a baricity of 1 and tends to remain in the immediate area of injection. It is not significantly affected by patient position. A ratio < 1 defines a hypobaric solution, which tends to rise against gravity in the CSF. A hypobaric solution is useful when administered in unusual positions, such as the jackknife position.

5. Volume of CSF in the spinal canal. Volume may be decreased by engorgement of the epidural veins due to increased intraabdominal pressure from ascites or pregnancy.

The table below illustrates the anesthetic dermatomal levels necessary for different surgical procedures.

Dosing Guidelines for Spinal Anesthesia*

	T10	T6	T4
Dermatomal level	Umbilicus	Xiphoid	Nipple
Surgical area	Vaginal Anal/rectal Bladder Lower extremities	Small bowel Colon Appendix Pelvis	Stomach Liver Pancreas Gallbladder
Drug (mg)			
Tetracaine	6–10, 10–12, 14	12, 14, 16	12–14, 16, 18
Bupivacaine	10, 7.5–12, 14	12, 10.5–14, 16	14, 16, 20
Lidocaine	50, 50–60, 70	60, 70, 80	70, 80, 90

* Dosage given for respective patient heights of 60, 66, and 72 inches (hyperbaric solutions).

5. How and where is a spinal anesthetic administered?
A typical SAB is performed in the lumbar region below the level of the spinal cord (L3–L4 in young children, L2 in adults) to avoid direct injury to the cord. The interspace between L3–L4 is the first interspace just above an imaginary line connecting the iliac crests. The patient is positioned in the sitting or lateral decubitus position, and the lumbar spine is flexed as much as possible to open the vertebral interspaces. The spinal needle is placed midline through the skin, subcutaneous structures, interspinous ligament, ligamentum flavum, dura, and arachnoid membrane. If the patient cannot adequately flex the lumbar spine or the ligaments are heavily calcified, one may use a lateral or paramedian approach. A slight "pop" may be felt as the dura and arachnoid membranes are punctured. When flow of CSF occurs, the local anesthetic agent is injected. The patient is then properly positioned and carefully observed for adverse affects, such as a total spinal or hemodynamic instability.

6. Discuss the mechanism of action of spinal anesthesia.

After injection into the CSF, the local anesthetic solution spreads and is taken up by neural tissue. Spread may continue for up to 20 minutes. Transmission of impulses in the nerve roots or possibly the spinal cord itself is interrupted by the local anesthetic (see chapter 13 for description of mechanism of action of local anesthetics). The nerve fibers vary in function, diameter, and thickness of the myelin sheath, which affects susceptibility to local anesthetics. Preganglionic autonomic fibers (B fibers) are small and more permeable to local anesthetics than the larger sensory C fibers. As a hyperbaric anesthetic solution spreads through the CSF, a gradient of decreasing anesthetic concentration may cause sympathetic blockade 1–2 segments above the sensory block and motor blockade 1–2 segments below the sensory block.

7. List the most common complications of spinal anesthesia.

1. **Hypotension** occurs frequently with SAB. It is due to a combination of decreased vascular resistance and diminished cardiac output. Factors that increase the incidence and severity of hypotension include hypovolemia, sensory level greater than T4, increasing age, baseline systolic blood pressure below 120, performance of the block at or above L2–L3, addition of phenylephrine to the local anesthetic solution, and SAB combined with general anesthesia. Hypotension may be prevented or ameliorated with prehydration of the patient. Hypotension may be treated with volume expansion or sympathomimetics. Trendelenburg position, used to treat other forms of hypotension, may raise the level of blockade and should be used with caution. Volume loading should also be used with caution in patients with limited cardiac reserve. As the block recedes, vascular tone increases, raising the central blood volume (preload), which may precipitate heart failure.

2. **Bradycardia** also may be seen. The mechanism is usually multifactorial and may include unopposed vagal tone from a high sympathectomy, blockade of the cardioaccelerator fibers (T1–T4), and the Bezold-Jarisch reflex (slowing of the heart rate secondary to a drop in venous return). Bradycardia may be treated with anticholinergic agents, such as atropine, or beta-adrenergic agonists, such as ephedrine.

3. **Cardiac arrest** is occasionally reported during SAB. Studies have shown two major causes: oversedation and poor understanding of the physiology of sympathectomy. Oversedation is not unique to spinal anesthesia but in combination with a sympathectomy may be life-threatening. Oversedation during placement of the block (especially if one is distracted by events surrounding injection, positioning, and assessment of the level of block) may lead to respiratory compromise and hypoxemia. The patient with SAB has lost hemodynamic reserve, and this combination has led to cardiac arrest. Treatment consists of immediate assurance of adequate ventilation with reversal of hypoxia and early use of vasopressors.

4. **Nausea and vomiting** are common, perhaps because of unopposed vagal tone or hypotension that decreases cerebral blood flow. Anticholinergic medication or blood pressure elevation may be used to treat this side effect.

Total spinal, postdural puncture headache (PDPH), and other **uncommon neurologic sequelae** are discussed below.

8. What is a total spinal?

A total spinal is anesthesia to the cervical spinal cord and brainstem. It is usually caused by an overdose of local anesthetic. Signs and symptoms include dysphonia, dyspnea, upper extremity weakness, loss of consciousness, hypotension, bradycardia, and cardiopulmonary arrest. Early recognition is the key to management. Placing the patient in the reverse Trendelenburg position in an attempt to halt further rise of the block may do more harm than good. Once a high spinal occurs, the level will not immediately recede in the reverse Trendelenburg position; cardiac output will only decrease further. Treatment includes positive pressure ventilation, volume infusion, and pressor support. The patient should receive sedation once ventilation is required and hemodynamics stabilize.

9. Describe a postdural puncture headache.
A potentially severe headache may develop after dural puncture, presumably secondary to the tear in the dura and resultant CSF leak, which may cause traction on the meninges and cranial nerves. The headache typically occurs 24–48 hours after the puncture, although it may occur immediately. The headache is characteristically intense in the occipital region and neck when the patient assumes the upright position and improves when the patient is recumbent. Diplopia or blurring of vision may occur. Tinnitus and hearing loss have been reported. Cranial nerve deficits also may be seen. Patients at higher risk for PDPH include those that have been instrumented with large-bore spinal needles with sharp bevel tips. Newer pencil-point needles, ranging from 24–27 gauge, have a low incidence of PDPH. Women, younger patients, parturients, and obese patients tend to have a higher incidence of PDPH. Treatment usually begins with hydration, analgesia, and caffeine. It is important to rule out central nervous system infection as a cause of the symptoms. Refractory or severe headaches may be treated effectively with an epidural blood patch. Epidural administration of dextran, hetastarch, and even saline has been shown to be of some benefit.

10. What is the risk of neurologic injury after spinal anesthesia?
It is extraordinarily rare but has been reported. Neurologic problems after SAB may be due to nerve compression secondary to improper patient positioning, direct surgical trauma, or unrecognized preexisting neurologic disease. Direct trauma to nerve fibers may occur from the spinal needle. A paresthesia results, and the needle should be redirected before injection of the local anesthetic. Space-occupying lesions may occur after a SAB because of epidural venous bleeding (from direct trauma or coagulopathy) or abscess formation (from direct inoculation due to poor sterile technique or bacteremic seeding). Early recognition and management are imperative to avoid permanent neurologic sequelae. Adhesive arachnoiditis has been reported, presumably due to injection of an irritant into the subarachnoid space, and may be prevented by using preservative-free local anesthetics and opioids and avoiding contamination of the spinal needle with betadine and talc.

Nerve injury also has been reported from the direct effect of local anesthetics or their additives. Neurotoxicity may be due to prolonged exposure to high concentrations of local anesthetics. Evidence indicates that local anesthetics may inhibit fast axonal transport, disrupt the axonal cytoskeleton, cause axonal degeneration, and possibly contribute to ischemic nerve injury via inhibition of local vasodilating compounds. Microbore continuous spinal catheters have been associated with cauda equina syndrome, most likely due to direct high concentrations of local anesthetic at the nerve roots. Metabisulfite, a local anesthetic additive used as an antioxidant for epinephrine, has been shown to be neurotoxic in combination with the low pH of chloroprocaine. Epinephrine may increase and prolong the intraneural concentration of anesthetic, resulting in neurotoxicity. Vasoconstrictors may theoretically render ischemic injury to patients with already compromised circulation. Hyperosmolality from the addition of dextrose to local anesthetic solutions has also been suspected in the genesis of neural injury. Certain disease states such as diabetes mellitus may predispose to neural injury.

11. What are the contraindications to spinal anesthesia?
Absolute contraindications include local infection at the puncture site, bacteremia, and intracranial hypertension. **Relative contraindications** include hypovolemia, aortic stenosis, progressive degenerative neurologic disease, low back pain, and coagulopathy.

12. What risk is associated with coagulation abnormalities?
The risk of spinal hematoma and neurologic dysfunction in patients with coagulopathy is small but real. A detailed history of abnormal bleeding and medication that affects coagulation should be obtained. In patients fully anticoagulated with intravenous heparin, the infusion should be discontinued 4–6 hours before SAB. Low-dose subcutaneous heparin also should be discontinued at least 4 hours before the block. Oral warfarin therapy should be discontinued for several days, and prothrombin time should be measured before SAB. SAB followed by heparin administration is thought to be safe if heparinization occurs at least 1 hour after needle placement and excessive

anticoagulation is avoided. Patients who receive heparin after receiving NSAIDs (including aspirin) may be at higher risk for spinal hematoma. Use of NSAIDs alone probably does not pose undue risk. Bleeding times are frequently measured in such patients before the block. No data support this practice. SAB probably should be avoided in patients who have recently received thrombolytic therapy. Avoidance of SAB in patients with underlying pathologic coagulopathies, such as disseminated intravascular coagulation or thrombocytopenia, seems wise.

13. Describe the various spinal needles.

A wide range of needles of varying type and size is available for spinal anesthesia. Standard length is $3^1/_2$ inches; longer needles are available for larger patients. Needle diameter ranges from 20–27 gauge. In general, the smaller the diameter, the less the incidence of PDPH. The larger-bore needles (22 gauge and below) are useful in elderly patients, whose spinal ligaments may be calcified and who are at lower risk of PDPH or in any patient in whom placement of SAB is difficult. Tip designs may also influence the incidence of PDPH as well as CSF flow characteristics through the needle. Small (24–27 gauge) pencil-point needles, such as the Whitacre or Sprotte brands, are thought to have the lowest incidence of PDPH and the best flow characteristics.

14. Discuss briefly the use of intrathecal opioids.

Opioids may be administered into the subarachnoid space with or without local anesthetics. They cause intense visceral analgesia without affecting motor or sympathetic function. The major site of action is at the various types of opiate receptors within the second and third laminae of the substantia gelatinosa in the dorsal horn of the spinal cord. Lipophilic agents such as fentanyl and sufentanil have a much more localized effect than the hydrophilic agents such as morphine; the spread of hydrophilic agents is greater. Fentanyl and sufentanil have a rapid onset of action and a duration of 2–8 hours. Morphine lasts from 6–24 hours. The long durations of action make these drugs desirable for postoperative analgesia. Addition of these agents to local anesthetic SABs may prolong the sensory block without increasing the postoperative duration of motor blockade or time to voiding. Toxicity includes respiratory depression (which may occur late with hydrophilic agents), nausea, vomiting, pruritus, and urinary retention. Opioid antagonists or agonist/antagonists are useful in treating such complications.

BIBLIOGRAPHY

1. Abouleish E: The addition of 0.2 mg subarachnoid morphine to hyperbaric bupivacaine for cesarean delivery: A prospective study of 856 cases. Reg Anesth 16:137–140, 1991.
2. Bevacqua BK: Spinal catheter size and hyperbaric lidocaine dosing. Reg Anesth 19:136–141, 1994.
3. Brown DL: Atlas of Regional Anesthesia. Philadelphia, W.B. Saunders, 1992, pp 267–282.
4. Caldwell LE: Subarachnoid morphine and fentanyl for labor analgesia: Efficacy and adverse effects. Reg Anesth 19:2–8, 1994.
5. Caplan RA: Unexpected cardiac arrest during spinal anesthesia: A closed claims analysis of predisposing factors. Anesthesiology 68:5–11, 1988.
6. Carpenter RL: Incidence and risk factors for side effects of spinal anesthesia. Anesthesiology 76:906–916, 1992.
7. Cousins MJ, Bridenbaugh PO: Neural Blockade. Philadelphia, J.B .Lippincott, 1980.
8. de Jong RH: Local Anesthetics. St. Louis, Mosby, 1994.
9. Dripps RD: Anesthesia: The Principles of Safe Practice. Philadelphia, W.B. Saunders, 1988.
10. Grass JA: Surgical outcome: Regional anesthesia and analgesia versus general anesthesia. Anesth Rev 20:117–125, 1993.
11. Greene NM: Distribution of local anesthetic solutions within the subarachnoid space. Anesth Analg 64:713–730, 1985.
12. Horlocker TT: Effect of injection rate on sensory level and duration of hypobaric bupivacaine spinal anesthesia for total hip arthroplasty. Anesth Analg 79:773–777, 1994.
13. Jaradeh S: Cauda equina syndrome: A neurologist's perspective. Reg Anesth 18:473–480, 1993.
14. Rowlingson JC: Toxicity of local anesthetic additives. Reg Anesth 18:453–460, 1993.
15. Van Gessel EF: Influence of injection speed on the subarachnoid distribution of isobaric bupivacaine 0.5%. Anesth Analg 77:483–487, 1993.

72. EPIDURAL ANALGESIA AND ANESTHESIA

Joy L. Hawkins, M.D.

1. Where is the epidural space? Describe the relevant anatomy.

The epidural space lies just outside the dural sac containing the spinal cord and cerebrospinal fluid (CSF). As the epidural needle enters the midline of the back over the bony spinous processes, it passes through (1) skin, (2) subcutaneous fat, (3) supraspinous ligament, (4) interspinous ligament, (5) ligamentum flavum, and (6) epidural space. Beyond the epidural space lie the spinal meninges and CSF. The epidural space has its widest point (5 mm) at L2. In addition to the traversing nerve roots, it contains fat, lymphatics, and an extensive venous plexus. Superiorly the space extends to the foramen magnum, where dura is fused to the base of the skull. Caudally it ends at the sacral hiatus. The epidural space can be entered in the cervical, thoracic, or lumbar regions to provide anesthesia. In pediatric patients the caudal epidural approach is commonly used (see question 3).

2. Differentiate between a spinal and an epidural anesthetic.

For a **spinal anesthetic**, a small amount of local anesthetic drug is placed directly in the CSF, producing total neural blockade caudad to the injection site. Access of the drug to the exposed spinal nerves gives a rapid, dense, and predictable anesthetic effect. An **epidural anesthetic** requires a tenfold increase in dose of local anesthetic to fill the potential epidural space and to penetrate the nerve coverings. The onset is slower because of the required penetration. The anesthesia produced tends to be segmental; that is, a band of anesthesia is produced, extending upward and downward from the injection site. The amount of segmental spread depends largely on the volume of local anesthetic. For example, a 5-ml volume may produce only a narrow band of anesthetic covering 3–5 dermatomes, whereas a 20-ml volume may produce anesthesia from the upper thoracic to sacral dermatomes. In addition, an epidural anesthetic requires a larger needle, often uses a continuous catheter technique, and has a subtle endpoint for locating the space. The epidural space is located by the "feel" of the ligaments as they are passed through, whereas the subarachnoid space is definitively identified by CSF at the needle hub.

3. How is caudal anesthesia related to epidural anesthesia? When is it used?

Caudal anesthesia is a form of epidural anesthesia in which the injection is made at the sacral hiatus (S5). Because the dural sac normally ends at S2, accidental spinal injection is rare. Although the caudal approach to the epidural space provides dense sacral and lower lumbar levels of block, its use is limited by the major problems: (1) the highly variable anatomy in adults, (2) the risk of injection into a venous plexus, and (3) the difficulty in maintaining sterility if a catheter is used. Caudal anesthesia is primarily used in children (whose anatomy is predictable) to provide postoperative pain management after herniorrhaphy or perineal procedures. A catheter can be inserted if desired for long-term use.

4. What are the advantages of using epidural anesthesia over general anesthesia?

- Avoidance of airway manipulation; useful for asthmatics, known difficult intubations, and patients with a full stomach
- Decreased stress response; less hypertension and tachycardia
- Less thrombogenesis and subsequent pulmonary embolism; a proven benefit in orthopedic hip surgery
- Improved bowel motility with less distention; sympathetic blockade provides more parasympathetic tone

- The patient can be awake during the procedure if desired; useful for cesarean section and certain arthroscopic and laparoscopic procedures
- Less postoperative nausea and sedation
- Better postoperative pain control, especially for thoracic, upper abdominal, and orthopedic procedures
- Less pulmonary dysfunction, both from better pain control and absence of airway manipulation
- Faster turnover at the end of the case because there is no emergence time

5. What are the disadvantages of epidural compared with general anesthesia?
- Slower to initiate at the beginning of the case
- Less reliable, with higher failure rate
- Occasional contraindications, including coagulopathy, hemodynamic instability, or spinal anomalies

6. What are the advantages of epidural anesthesia over spinal anesthesia?
- Epidural anesthesia can produce a segmental block focused only on the area of surgery or pain; for example, during labor or for thoracic procedures.
- The gradual onset of sympathetic block allows time to manage hemodynamic changes such as hypotension.
- There is more flexibility to prolong the block for longer procedures with a continuous catheter technique; in other words, one can redose with more local anesthetic for longer procedures or extend postoperative pain relief as long as desired.
- There is more flexibility in the density of block; if less motor block is desired (for labor analgesia or postoperative pain management), a lower concentration of local anesthetic can be used.
- Decreased incidence of headache. Theoretically with no hole in the dura there is no spinal headache; however a wet tap occurs from 0.5–4% of the time with the large-bore epidural needle, and about 50% of such patients require treatment for headache. Because newer technology in spinal needles has decreased the incidence of headache requiring treatment to less than 1%, this advantage probably no longer holds true.

7. What are the disadvantages of epidural compared with spinal anesthesia?
- The induction of epidural anesthesia is slower because of more complex placement, the necessity of incremental dosing of the local anesthetic, and the slow onset of anesthesia in the epidural space.
- Because of the greater amounts of local anesthetic used, there is a risk of local anesthetic toxicity if a vein is accidentally entered with the needle or catheter.
- Epidural anesthesia is less reliable; it is not as dense, the block can be patchy or one-sided, and there is no definite endpoint for placement.

8. What factors should the anesthesiologist look for in the preoperative assessment before performing an epidural anesthetic? Should special laboratory tests be performed?
In addition to the general preoperative assessment of every patient before surgery, the following specific items should be assessed before performing epidural anesthesia:
History
Previous back injury or surgery
Neurologic symptoms or history of neurologic disease (e.g., diabetic neuropathy, multiple sclerosis)
Bleeding tendencies or disease associated with coagulopathy (e.g., preeclampsia)
Prior regional anesthesia and associated problems
Physical exam
Neurologic exam for strength and sensation

Back exam for landmarks and potential anatomic abnormalities (scoliosis) or pathology (infection at the site of placement)

Surgery

Expected duration and blood loss

Positioning required

Amount of muscle relaxation necessary

General

The patient should be given a detailed explanation of the procedure, risks, benefits, and options (including general anesthesia if the block fails).

Discuss the patient's desire for sedation.

Lab tests

None are specifically necessary except as based on the history and physical exam.

9. **Describe the technique for performing a lumbar epidural anesthetic.**
   - Have immediately available: oxygen, equipment for positive pressure ventilation and intubation, and pressors to treat hypotension.
   - Place a well-running intravenous (IV) line and give an appropriate preload of fluid to protect against hypotension after sympathetic blockade.
   - The patient may be sitting or in lateral position with the spinous processes aligned in the same vertical or horizontal plane and maximally flexed. Administer sedation as deemed appropriate.
   - Mark a line between the iliac crests to locate the L4 spinous process. Palpate the L2–L3, L3–L4, and L4–L5 interspaces, and choose the widest or the closest to the desired anesthetic level.
   - Make a skin wheal after sterile preparation and draping of the field. The anesthesiologist must wear a hat, mask, and sterile gloves.
   - The epidural needle is inserted in the midline through the skin wheal until increased resistance of ligaments is felt. Remove the needle stylet and attach a syringe with 3–4 ml of air or saline. When the barrel of the syringe is tapped, it should feel firm and bounce back while the tip of the needle is in ligament.
   - Advance several mm at a time, tapping the syringe intermittently. The ability to recognize the feel of various layers of ligament comes with experience. Ligamentum flavum is often described as leathery, gritty, or simply as having a marked increase in resistance. This is the last layer before the epidural space.
   - As the needle passes through ligamentum flavum and enters the epidural space, there is often a "pop" or "give," and the air or fluid in the syringe injects easily because of loss of resistance.
   - The syringe is removed, and while the nondominant hand grasps the hub of the needle to brace it, the dominant hand threads the catheter 3–5 cm into the space.
   - The epidural needle is withdrawn carefully so as not to remove the catheter. After attaching the injector port to the catheter, it is aspirated for blood or CSF; if negative, a test dose is given. The catheter is then taped in place.

10. **Are there any contraindications to epidural anesthesia?**
    Absolute contraindications
    - Patient refusal. Sometimes a more thorough explanation will allay the patient's fears and make the technique acceptable. Some common concerns include (1) having to watch surgery or remain wide awake; (2) fear of a needle in the spinal cord; and (3) pain. Reassure patients that a curtain will block their view and that the desired degree of sedation can be provided. Explain that the spinal cord ends at about L1 in adults and that the needle is placed below that level. Compare the procedure to the placement of the IV line, which also uses a 16- or 18-gauge needle, and explain that a local anesthetic will be used in the skin.

- Sepsis with hemodynamic instability. The induction of sympathetic blockade drops systemic vascular resistance (SVR) even further. There is also a remote risk of epidural abscess if bacteremic blood is introduced into the epidural space without prior antibiotic coverage.
- Uncorrected hypovolemia. With ongoing hemorrhage, the fall in SVR can produce severe refractory hypotension.
- Coagulopathy. If a vessel is injured within the epidural space, an epidural hematoma could form, causing neurologic damage.

Relative contraindications (often more medicolegal than medical)
- Elevated intracranial pressure
- Prior back injury with neurologic deficit
- Progressive neurologic disease, such as multiple sclerosis
- Chronic back pain
- Localized infection at the injection site.

11. What are the potential complications of epidural anesthesia? Can they be anticipated or prevented?
- Hypotension due to sympathetic blockade, which sometimes may be prevented by fluid preload and positioning supine.
- Intravascular injection of local anesthetic, which can be prevented by aspirating the catheter for blood, using a marker, such as epinephrine, that will cause tachycardia if injected into a vessel, and using incremental dosing (no more than 5 ml at a time). If an intravascular injection occurs, one must (1) stop convulsions with thiopental, (2) intubate the trachea, if necessary for ventilation or airway protection; and (3) treat cardiovascular collapse with pressors, inotropes, and advanced cardiac life support (ACLS) protocols if dysrhythmias are present.
- Subarachnoid injection of a large volume of local anesthetic ("total spinal"), which can be prevented by aspirating the catheter for CSF and giving a small initial dose of local anesthetic to look for rapid onset of sensory block if the drug enters the CSF (remember: the onset of an epidural anesthetic is slow). If a total spinal occurs, one must treat hypotension with pressors and support ventilation with mask ventilation or intubation.
- Postdural puncture headache due to accidental dural puncture with the large-bore epidural needle can be treated in various ways, depending on the preference of the patient and anesthesiologist. Common therapies include analgesics, caffeine, or an epidural "blood patch." Determining factors include severity of the headache and how aggressively the patient wishes to be treated. To provide a blood patch, up to 20 ml of the patient's blood is placed in the epidural space to seal the dural hole and to elevate low CSF pressure.
- Epidural hematomas, which are extremely rare and usually occur spontaneously in clinical settings outside the operating room. When they are associated with regional anesthesia, there is usually a preexisting coagulopathy. Epidural hematomas present as back pain and leg weakness and must be diagnosed by computerized tomography or magnetic resonance imaging. If the hematoma is not surgically decompressed in 6–8 hours, neurologic recovery is rare.

12. What physiologic changes should be expected after successful initiation of an epidural anesthetic?
- Decrease in blood pressure. Afterload reduction can be useful for patients with hypertension or congestive heart failure if preload is maintained.
- Changes in heart rate. Tachycardia may occur as cardiac output increases to compensate for a drop in SVR. Bradycardia may occur if blockade above T4 disrupts the cardiac sympathetic accelerator fibers.
- Ventilatory changes. In normal patients, ventilation is maintained as long as the diaphragm is not impaired (phrenic nerve: C3–C5), but patients may become subjectively dyspneic as

they become unable to feel their intercostal muscles. Patients dependent on accessory muscles of respiration may be impaired at lower levels of anesthesia. The ability to cough and protect the airway may be lost even if ventilation is adequate.

- Bladder distention. Sympathetic blockade and loss of sensation may require catheterization for urinary retention.
- Intestinal contraction. Sympathetic blockade with parasympathetic predominance contracts the bowel.
- Change in thermoregulation. Peripheral vasodilation lowers core body temperature if the patient is not covered. Shivering is common during epidural anesthesia.
- Neuroendocrine changes. Neural blockade above T5 blocks sympathetic afferents to the adrenal medulla, inhibiting the neural component of the stress response. Sympathetic and somatic pathways for pain also are blocked. Glucose control is better maintained.

13. How does one choose which local anesthetic to use?
The choice of local anesthetics usually is based on their onset, duration, and safety profile as well as on the special clinical characteristics of the patient and surgical procedure.

Local Anesthetics Commonly Used in Epidural Techniques

ANESTHETIC	SURGICAL CONCENTRATION	ONSET	DURATION	COMMENTS; MAXIMAL DOSE (WITH EPINEPHRINE)
Chloroprocaine	3%	Rapid	45 min	Ester, rapid metabolism → least toxic, intense sensory and motor block; 15 mg/kg
Lidocaine	2%	Intermediate	60–90 min	Amide, intense sensory and motor block; 7 mg/kg
Bupivacaine	0.75% 0.5% ??	Slow	2–3 hr	Amide, most cardiotoxic; motor < sensory block; 3 mg/kg

14. Why is epinephrine used? Should it be included in all cases?
Epinephrine (and phenylephrine, another adjuvant vasoconstrictor) is often added to local anesthetic solutions in a concentration of 5 μg/ml (1:200,000) or less. There are several benefits to this practice:

- Prolongs blockade, especially of lidocaine, by reducing uptake into the bloodstream and thereby metabolism.
- Improves quality and reliability of blockade, either by increasing the available local anesthetic through decreased uptake or by an intrinsic anesthetic mechanism on central alpha-adrenergic receptors.
- Reduces peak blood levels by slowing vascular absorption.
- Helps to identify an intravascular injection as a "test dose." If the epinephrine-containing solution is unintentionally injected into a blood vessel, tachycardia usually results.

Epinephrine may be added to the local anesthetic solution for all blocks except those involving end arteries (digits, penis) or for patients in whom the tachycardia and hypertension may be detrimental (coronary artery disease, preeclampsia).

15. When should opioids be included in the epidural anesthetic?
Opioids may be mixed with the local anesthetic solution to intensify the block and/or to manage postoperative pain, either alone or with a dilute local anesthetic solution. Examples of epidural bolus doses: (1) fentanyl, 50–100 μg; sufentanil, 20–30 μg; and morphine, 2–5 mg. The narcotics work on the mu receptors in the substantia gelatinosa of the spinal cord. The more lipophilic narcotics such as fentanyl and sufentanil have fast onset (5 min), short duration (2–4 hrs), and lower

incidence of side effects. Morphine is a hydrophilic drug and does not attach to the receptor as easily. It has a long onset (1 hr), long duration (up to 24 hr), and a high incidence of side effects, such as itching and nausea. Respiratory depression, although rare, is the most serious concern and requires special monitoring for the duration of the drug.

16. Why can some patients with epidural blocks move around and even walk, whereas others have a dense motor block?
Preserving motor function is especially important in postoperative patients and laboring women. The amount of motor block can be decreased by adjusting the concentration of local anesthetic and by choosing a local anesthetic with sensory-motor dissociation. As local anesthetic concentration decreases, the intensity of the block decreases and fewer motor nerves are affected. Sensory block can be augmented by the addition of epidural narcotics if desired. Bupivacaine provides relatively more sensory block for a given amount of motor block (so-called sensory-motor dissociation). This property accounts for much of its popularity in obstetric anesthesia. For example, a common epidural infusion for postoperative pain and labor is 0.1% bupivacaine with 2–5 µg/ml fentanyl.

17. When is analgesia preferable to anesthesia?
  Anesthesia implies an intense sensory and motor blockade, which is necessary to perform a surgical procedure. It usually is obtained by using the highest available concentration of local anesthetic (for example, 2% lidocaine or 3% chloroprocaine). **Analgesia** implies sensory blockade only, usually for pain or labor, and may be achieved with dilute local anesthetic and/or epidural opioids.

18. How does one know what level of anesthesia is needed for different types of surgery? What is a segmental block? When is it used?
To provide adequate surgical blockade with an epidural anesthetic, one must know the innervation of the structures stimulated during the procedure. For example, a transurethral resection of the prostate requires a T8 level because the bladder is innervated by T8 through its embryologic origins. A laparotomy such as a cesarean section requires a T4 level to cover the innervation of the peritoneum.
  Epidural anesthesia is segmental; that is, it has an upper and lower level. The block is most intense near the site of catheter insertion and diminishes caudad and cephalad. The needle and catheter should be placed as close to the site of surgery as possible; for example, a thoracic injection is used for chest surgery, whereas a midlumbar injection is used for hip surgery. In labor, the lower limit of block can be kept above the sacral nerve roots until the second stage of labor to preserve pelvic floor tone and the perineal reflex.

19. How does one know how much local anesthetic solution to use for different procedures? What factors affect spread in the epidural space?
The extent of epidural blockade is determined primarily by the volume of local anesthetic; more dermatomes are blocked by more milliliters of local anesthetic. To achieve a T4 level from a lumbar epidural catheter, 20–30 ml of solution is required. Other factors affecting spread in the epidural space include (1) age (older patients require less local anesthetic); (2) pregnancy (requires less); (3) obesity (probably requires less); (4) height (taller patients may require more).

20. What is a combined spinal-epidural anesthetic? Why use both?
For a combined spinal-epidural anesthetic, a long spinal needle is passed through an epidural needle once it has been placed in the epidural space. When CSF is obtained from the spinal needle, a dose of local anesthetic is placed in the subarachnoid space, and the spinal needle is removed. The epidural catheter is then threaded into the epidural space and the epidural needle is removed. This technique combines the advantages of both spinal and epidural anesthesia: fast onset of an intense spinal block so that the surgery can proceed quickly and an epidural catheter

to extend the length of the block if necessary for a long surgical procedure or for postoperative pain management.

21. What is a combined epidural-general anesthetic? Why give the patient two anesthetics?
In some surgical procedures, controlled ventilation may be safer for the patient or necessary for the surgical procedure. Examples may be intrathoracic or upper abdominal operations. Because these procedures often result in moderate-to-severe postoperative pain, an epidural anesthetic can be an ideal way to provide pain relief and to aid in mobilization to prevent pulmonary and thromboembolic complications. The epidural anesthetic is usually placed prior to induction of general anesthesia. By using the epidural catheter intraoperatively, smaller amounts of the general anesthetic agents are required, which may result in fewer hemodynamic consequences and faster awakening. At the same time, the patient's airway can be protected, ventilation controlled, and hypnosis and amnesia provided.

22. What should the anesthesiologist ask the patient after use of an epidural anesthetic?
- Satisfaction with the anesthetic. Was there anything that the patient would like to have been done differently? Assess patient satisfaction and try to correct any misunderstandings.
- Regression of sensory and motor block. Is there any residual blockade? Can the patient ambulate? Does the patient have any problem with bowel or bladder function? Any of these complaints requires a thorough neurologic exam to localize the deficit. Although the complaint may be due to residual local anesthetic or nerve compression during the surgical procedure (which usually resolves with time), further evaluation may be needed. Depending on the pattern and severity of the neurologic dysfunction, further evaluation by a formal neurology consultation, electromyogram, or computerized tomography may be needed to rule out pathology in the epidural space (such as hematoma).
- Complaints of back pain. Examine the site for bruising, redness, or swelling.
- Complaints of headache. If an accidental dural puncture occurred, the patient should be followed for several days; such headaches can appear up to 1 week later.
- Adequacy of postoperative pain relief. Did any side effects of epidural narcotics (itching, nausea) require treatment?

BIBLIOGRAPHY

1. Badner NH: Epidural agents for postoperative analgesia. Anesthesiol Clin North Am 10:321–337, 1992.
2. Batra MS: Epidural and spinal analgesia and anesthesia: Contemporary issues. Anesthesiol Clin North Am 10: 1992.
3. Cousins MJ, Bromage PR: Epidural neural blockade. In Cousins MJ, Bridenbaugh PO (eds): Neural Blockade, 2nd ed. Philadelphia, J.B. Lippincott, 1988, pp 253–360.
4. Mulroy MF: Regional Anesthesia. Boston, Little, Brown, 1989, pp 89–120.

73. PERIPHERAL NERVE BLOCKS

David M. Glenn, M.D., and Jose M. Angel, M.D.

1. Define peripheral nerve block.

A peripheral nerve block (PNB) involves the injection of a local anesthetic (LA) into the nerve sheath or surrounding tissue. When the nerve absorbs the LA, neural transmission ceases. The result is the prevention of the sensation of pain and often the blockade of motor and autonomic function.

2. How are peripheral nerve fibers classified? How do they differ anatomically and functionally?

Nerve roots of the spinal cord, which become the peripheral nerves, are a mix of motor, sensory and autonomic fibers. Because these fibers have individual sensitivities to LAs, the totality of block is not always uniform. The table below describes these classifications and how their anatomic features affect ease and speed of blockade. Generally speaking, small myelinated fibers are more easily blocked than large unmyelinated fibers. Each fiber has a specific minimal concentration (Cm) of LA for blockade. The Cm is higher for motor fibers than for sensory fibers and lowest for sympathetic fibers. Hence, as the LA diffuses away from the site of injection and the concentration decreases by dilution, sympathetic nerves are more completely blocked, sensation is moderately blocked, and motor function is only partially blocked.

Anatomic and Functional Classification of Peripheral Nerve Fibers

GROUP	SUBGROUP	ACTION/FUNCTION	MYELIN	SIZE	RELATIVE EASE OF BLOCKADE
A	Alpha	Motor, proprioception	Present	Large	4
	Beta	Motor, proprioception light touch, pressure	Present	Medium	3
	Gamma	Muscle tone (spindle)	Present	Medium	3
	Delta	Pain, temprature, touch	Present	Small	2
B		Preganglionic sympathetics	Present	Small	1
C		Deep pain, temperature, pressure, postganglionic sympathetics	Absent	Extra small	2

1 = most easily blocked, 4 = least easily blocked.

3. What are the advantages of PNB over central nerve (e.g., spinal and epidural) blocks?

The severely ill cardiovascular or neurosurgical trauma patient going into surgery for a lower extremity fracture has a difficult time tolerating swings in blood pressure and heart rate. Spinal and epidural anesthesia blocks sympathetic tone of the vasculature and therefore may cause a drop in blood pressure, especially if the patient is at all dehydrated or hypovolemic. A PNB of the lower extremity provides anesthesia with much less sympathectomy.

4. What are the basic principles and techniques underlying successful PNB?

1. One must have knowledge of the anatomy and landmarks (specific bones, vessels, and muscles) involved in locating the nerve to be blocked.

2. The appropriate LA, concentration, and volume must be chosen.

3. The appropriateness of additives (e.g. epinephrine, bicarbonate) must be decided.

4. The feeling of loss of resistance as the needle passes through the nerve sheath or a paresthesia when the needle touches the nerve may be helpful in localizing the nerve.

5. A nerve stimulator connected to the advancing needle and grounded to the patient may provide additional sensitivity in locating the desired nerve (twitching of the specific muscle group supplied by the nerve).

5. What are the risks in performing PNB?

Two categories of risks are involved in a PNB: anatomic and physiologic. The anatomic structures and organs surrounding the nerve to be blocked may be damaged by the needle. Examples include pneumothorax and hemothorax in a supraclavicular block, total spinal blockade in an interscalene block, and, in any nerve block, direct nerve laceration or major vessel damage resulting in pseudoaneurysm and/or hematoma. Physiologic risks may be systemic and/or local. The most common systemic side effects usually involve first the central nervous system (CNS) and then the cardiovascular (CV) system. Systemic effects occur from overdosage and circulatory absorption or inadvertent intravascular injection. Symptoms, relative to increasing plasma concentration, usually occur in the following sequence: tongue/lip numbness, tinnitus, lightheadedness, visual disturbances, muscular spasms/twitching, seizures, coma, and CV/respiratory arrest. Fortunately, the therapeutic antiarrhythmic plasma concentration of LAs is much lower than the concentration that causes toxicity. It is important to know that the slope of the toxic effect curve is not the same for every LA. More potent LAs are usually more toxic. Bupivacaine is the most cardiotoxic, not only because of its potency but also because its slow dissociation from myocardial sodium channels results in accumulation and progressive cardiac depression.

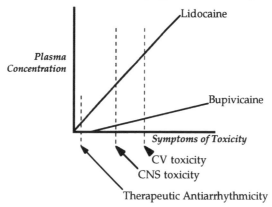

Comparison of plasma concentration to systemic toxic symptoms for licocaine vs. bupivacaine.

LAs also may cause local neurotoxic and/or myotoxic effects. In addition, the speed and completeness of absorption of LAs injected in a PNB vary greatly with the location of the block. Hence, a quantity of LA that is not toxic in one location may be toxic in another. For example, the extensive vascularity in the chest wall causes LA in an intercostal block to be absorbed rapidly; therefore, care must be taken not to use too large a dose. Last but not least are the possible allergic side effects of aminoester LAs (tetracaine, chloroprocaine, procaine, cocaine). These LAs are derivatives of para-aminobenzoic acid (PABA), a known allergen. Hypersensitivy reactions to various preservatives used in some LAs have been noted in the past.

7. How can the risks from PNB be minimized?

It is essential to ensure that the needle is placed correctly before injecting the LA. Effective methods are simple but important:

1. Continuous aspiration is mandatory while advancing the needle; a flow of blood or CSF is an obvious sign of improper needle position and indicates that the needle needs to be redirected.

2. Reports of symptoms experienced by the patient, such as paresthesia, hiccups or cough, help to determine whether the needle is touching a nerve. For this reason premedications causing oversedation are best avoided.

3. Dilute epinephrine may be added to the LA to test needle placement; it causes a momentary increase in heart rate and blood pressure if injected intravascularly. (Exception: do not use epinephrine in digital or facial blocks.)

4. Using no more than the recommended dosage (mg/kg body wt) of LA affords a good margin of safety; however, plasma levels resulting from absorption vary with the type and location (e.g. intercostal) of the block. This recognition is of vital importance to avoid toxic systemic levels from the "recommended dose."

UPPER EXTREMITIES

8. Describe the indications and landmarks for PNBs at the elbow and wrist.

PNBs at the elbow are primarily useful to supplement incomplete brachial plexus blocks. PNBs at the wrist are useful for surgery distal to the metacarpophalangeal (MCP) joints. The following table describes the useful landmarks for identifying the nerve. In practice, a large volume of LA is more likely to produce an adequate block. Blocks at the wrist and elbow are also useful for diagnosis in some chronic pain syndromes.

Landmarks for PNB Injection at the Wrist and Elbow

NERVE		LANDMARK		LANDMARK	DOSAGE OF LA
Landmark at the wrist					
Ulnar		Flexor carpi ulnaris tendon, styloid process of ulna		Ulnar artery pulsation	3–5 ml 1% lidocaine or 0.5% bupivacaine
Radial	is medial to	Anatomic snuff box	and lateral to	Radial artery pulsation	3–5 ml 1% lidocaine or 0.5% bupivacaine
Median		Flexor carpi radialis tendon		Palmaris longus tendon (identified best in the flexed wrist)	3–5 ml 1% lidocaine or 0.5% bupivacaine
Landmark at the elbow					
Ulnar		Olecranon process		Medial epicondyle of humerus	5–10 ml 1% lidocaine or 0.5% bupivacaine
Radial	is medial to	Brachioradialis muscle (antecubital space)	and lateral to	Biceps tendon (antecubital space)	5–10 ml 1% lidocaine or 0.5% bupivacaine
Median		Medial epicondyle of humerus		Brachial artery pulse	3–5 ml 1% lidocaine or 0.5% bupivacaine

9. What nerve or nerves are missed in performing brachial plexus blocks of the interscalene, supraclavicular, and axillary nerves?

A digital or terminal (radial, median, ulnar) nerve block may be all that is necessary for small, relatively simple, and quick surgeries of the fingers or hand. However, larger or more complex surgeries of the hand, forearm, or upper arm require blockade at the level of the brachial plexus by an interscalene, supraclavicular, or axillary block. The nerves of the brachial plexus originate from the spinal roots of C4–T2. They crisscross in an array of trunks, divisions, and cords; pass over the first rib and under the clavicle with the subclavian artery and vein; branch in the axilla as the ulnar, median, radial, and musculocutaneous nerves; and continue to supply the arm. Certain important anatomic factors must be considered in deciding which block is most appropriate:

- The C8–T2 roots join the plexus inferior to and distant from the site of injection of an **interscalene block**. As a result, C8–T2 roots are often missed or incompletely blocked with this approach, leaving their distribution unanesthetized, including ulnar, medial brachial, and antebrachial cutaneous nerves, certain radial and thoracodorsal nerves, and the medial aspect of the upper and lower arm, hand, and fingers. This block is therefore appropriate for surgery to the lateral aspect of the shoulder, upper arm, and hand.

- The musculocutaneous and axillary nerves exit from the plexus before entering the axilla and are therefore unaffected by an **axillary block**, leaving the shoulder and upper arm without anesthesia. The musculocutaneous nerve can be blocked by infiltration of the cora-cobrachialis muscle. If a tourniquet is expected to be used, further LA infiltration along the axillary fold is necessary for blockade of the medial brachial cutaneous and intercosto-brachial nerves. This block is best for surgery below the elbow.

- **Supraclavicular block** is most likely to anesthetize all of these nerves in a single shot and therefore is the most effective block for the entire arm (with the occasional exception of the skin overlying the shoulder, which can be blocked by a supplemental injection of the superficial cervical plexus nerves). The risk of pneumothorax, however, is greater with the supraclavicular than infraclavicular block.

10. How is a digital block performed? What is the most important thing to remember about your choice of local anesthetic?

The digital nerves of the fingers originate from the web spaces and run along both sides of each finger. They branch into dorsal and ventral arrays and are quite superficial. The best way to achieve a good block is to inject LA in a ringlike fashion around the base of the finger. Well-performed basic techniques and general principles are important:

- Continuous aspiration while advancing the needle and LA injection while withdrawing.
- Too large a volume may cause traumatic pressure injury to the nerves.
- **Do not** use vasoconstrictors, such as epinephrine, in the LA. Vasoconstriction may cause severe ischemia, necrosis, and loss of the finger. This caveat also applies to local infiltration blocks of the toes, tip of the nose, and ears.

11. Describe the Bier block. How is it performed?

Unfortunately, a Bier block does not involve consuming large quantities of foaming, fermented grain beverages until the patient is painless and stuporous. Otherwise known as intravenous regional anesthesia, the Bier block is most commonly performed on the upper extremity for forearm and hand surgery of short duration. It is reliable and safe and has a high degree of patient satisfaction. The Bier block involves the following steps:

1. A small-gauge intravenous line is placed as distally as possible, usually in a vein of the hand.

2. A double tourniquet is placed around the upper arm.

3. The arm is exsanguinated by elevating and wrapping it tightly with a wide elastic band, called an eschmark.

4. With the proximal tourniquet inflated, 40–50 ml of 0.5% lidocaine (not bupivicaine—see question 5) is injected through the intravenous catheter. Within minutes anesthesia sets in and the operation may proceed.

5. When the patient begins to experience discomfort from the proximal tourniquet, the distal cuff, under which anesthetic has been infused, is inflated; only then is the proximal cuff deflated.

6. Eventually the distal cuff becomes uncomfortable as the total allowable ischemic time limit is approached and must be deflated as well. This method enables complete anesthesia up to approximately 90 minutes.

The main side effect to watch for is LA toxicity as the tourniquet is deflated. This complication is rare unless the tourniquet time is < 30 minutes. In such cases the tourniquet may be deflated for a few seconds and then reinflated for several minutes. Repeating this procedure several times allows slower release of the LA and minimizes the risk of toxic effects. As always, constant communication with the patient is essential to detect early symptoms of toxicity. Hence oversedation is to be avoided.

A Bier block also may be performed on the lower extremities, although for surgery it is somewhat less efficacious. It is useful mostly in the diagnosis and treatment of some chronic pain syndromes in the lower extremities.

HEAD AND NECK

12. Describe the PNBs that are useful for surgery on the lateral and anterior neck.
The nerve roots arising from the plexus of cervical segments C2–C4 supply motor and sensory function to the anterior and lateral neck and some sensory function to the shoulder. Patients scheduled for surgery such as carotid endarterectomy or thyroidectomy are good candidates for cervical plexus blocks (deep and/or superficial). Bilateral blockade is necessary for midline surgery such as thyroidectomy. In nearly all cases, however, some local infiltration should be performed by the surgeons because of the innervation by cranial nerves (i.e., blockade of the glossopharyngeal innervation of the carotid bodies alleviates reflex cardiovascular changes). Interscalene or supraclavicular blocks are the preferred regional anesthesia for shoulder surgery. If the patient still experiences pain, cervical plexus blockade as a supplement usually remedies the problem.

13. Describe the PNBs that facilitate the intubation of an awake patient.
Tracheal intubation is extremely stimulating and therefore is usually performed after the induction of general anesthsia. Patients in whom a difficult tracheal intubation is anticipated (e.g., because of neck immobility or instability or obstructive airway anatomy as in morbid obesity or trauma) may necessitate intubation while the patient is awake. The oral pharynx and trachea are extremely sensitive and will not tolerate instrumentation without the help of local anesthetics. The oral and nasal cavities are easily rendered insensate with topical LAs (e.g., 4% lidocaine, tetracaine, or cocaine) that are sprayed, nebulized, or gargled and swallowed or with soaked pledgets placed in the nasal sinuses. The pterygopalantine nerves—a plexus of nerves deriving from the vagus and glossopharyngeal nerves that supply the motor and sensory function, respectively, to the pharynx—in the tonsillar arches can be blocked by direct injection. The nerves of the trachea require two separate blocks. Bilateral injection of LA between the lateral wings of the hyoid bone and the thyroid cartilage blocks the internal laryngeal branch of the superior laryngeal nerve and anesthetizes the area above the vocal cords. The external branch of the superior laryngeal nerve and the recurrent laryngeal nerve, which supplies sensation to the trachea below the vocal cords, can be blocked with a single transtracheal injection of topical LA (4% lidocaine) through the cricothyroid membrane. The aspiration of air indicates proper localization of the needle in the trachea, and with injection the patient coughs, distributing the LA. With good blockade the awake patient easily tolerates a plastic endotracheal tube in the mouth, throat, and trachea.

LOWER EXTREMITIES

14. What PNBs can be performed for surgery of the lower extremity?
As with PNBs of the upper extremity, knowledge of anatomy, especially the nerve routes and innervations, is essential. The most commonly performed and useful blocks are listedin the table below.

Lower Extremity PNBs: Examples, Innervation and Injection Sites

NERVE	EXAMPLES	INNERVATION	INJECTION SITE	LA AND DOSE
Femoral	Acute femur fracture pain for placement in traction or transport; knee surgery	Motor to quadriceps, pectineus, and sartorius muscles, sensory to medial and anterior thigh	Inferior to inguinal ligament and lateral to femoral pulse	20 ml 1% lidocaine or 0.5% bupivacaine (40 ml for 3-in-1 block)
Lateral Femoral Cutaneous	Muscle biopsy, tourniquet pain	Sensory to proximal two-thirds of lateral hip and thigh	Medial and inferior to anterior superior iliac spine through inguinal ligament	10–15 ml 1% lidocaine or 0.5% bupivacaine

Table continued on following page.

Lower Extremity PNBs: Examples, Innervation and Injection Sites (Cont.)

NERVE	EXAMPLES	INNERVATION	INJECTION SITE	LA AND DOSE
Obturator	Muscle biopsy, tourniquet pain, adductor relaxation for surgery	Sensory to medial thigh and hip, knee joint, motor to thigh adductors	"Walking" off the inferior pubic ramus into the obturator foramen	20 ml 1% lidocaine or 0.5% bupivacaine
Sciatic	All surgery of the lower extremity that does not require a tourniquet	All of the lower extremity below the knee	Anterior approach: 2 cm medial from the femoral artery at the level of and "walking" off the lesser trochanter. Posterior approach: midway between sacral hiatus and greater trochanter	20 ml 1% lidocaine or 0.5% bupivacaine
Popliteal	Surgery of ankle and foot, usually in conjunction with sural nerve block	Muscles and skin of the posterior and lateral leg and foot	Lateral to the popliteal artery and vein in the popliteal fossa	20–30 ml 1% lidocaine or 0.5% bupivacaine
Ankle block	See below			

15. Which nerves are affected by an ankle block? Where are they accessible to a needle? What region of the foot does each supply?

The table and figure below describe the three injection points for the five nerves of the ankle block.

Ankle Block Injection Site and Innervation

NERVE	LOCATION OF INJECTION	REGION OF INNERVATION
Sural	Lateral to Achilles tendon, posterior to lateral malleolus	Lateral heal ankle and foot
Posterior tibial	Medial to Achilles tendon, posterior to medial malleolus	Poterior and medial heal and plantar foot and toes
Superficial peroneal and saphenous	Subcutaneous across anterior one-third aspect of foot from lateral to medial malleolae	Top of foot and toes and medial ankle
Deep peroneal	Medial to tendon of hallucis longus	Web space of big toe

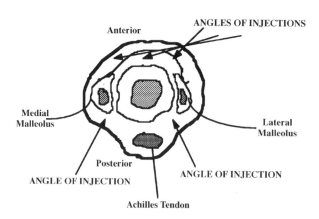

Sites of injection in an ankle block: cross-section at the level of the malleolae.

CONTROVERSIES

16. Should paresthesias be used as an indicator of nerve localizations in PNBs.

Pros: Increased certainty of nerve localization and therefore increased success rate of adequate block.

Cons: Increased risk of nerve damage/laceration, discomfort to the patient, requires greater patient cooperation than other techniques; therefore must be done with minimal sedation and reliable mental status

Note: Use of a peripheral nerve stimulator technique has not been definitively shown to be less likely to cause nerve damage than use of a paresthesia technique.

17. PNBs vs. general anesthesia: In what situations are PNBs indicated, or contraindicated, and how are they advantageous over general anesthesia?

General anesthesia (GA), although common and safely performed, is not without risks. For surgery involving a region of the body that can be anesthetically isolated from the rest of the body, a PNB avoids the potential complications of general anesthesia. The table below summarizes comparisons between GA and PNBs.

Comparison of Peripheral Nerve Blocks with General Anesthesia

	EXAMPLES
Advantages	
Patient awake, able to monitor mental status	Cerebral vascular disease
Patient with difficult airway or poor pulmonary status	Obesity, previous facial trauma or surgery, reactive airway disease, aspiration risk
Quick recovery time	Especially useful for outpatient or day surgery
More economical	Less anesthetics and use of anesthetic equipment
Increased peripheral perfusion; decreased vascular graft reocclusion	Vascular surgery of the extremities
Decreased pulmonary complications intraoperative and postoperative	Less atelectasis, avoidance of instrumentation of the airway, less risk of aspiration
Improved postoperative pain relief	Continuous infusion PNBs, less overall postoperative pain
Decreased stress response, and therefore increased intraoperative cardiovascular stability	This is true for PNB alone or combined with GA
Diagnostic/therapeutic/prognostic/ preventative	Management and possible prevention of chronic pain syndromes, i.e., reflex sympathetic dystrophy, phantom limb pain
Disadvantages	
Patient must be cooperative and willing	Mental status changes, retardation; patient refusal
Longer prep time	Efficiency-oriented, "bean counting" hospital administrators
Finite anesthetic duration in most cases	Surgeries may outlast the block, e.g., finger reattachment surgery
Patient must be able to maintain his or her own airway and tolerate surgical positioning throughout the case.	Sleep apnea, congestive heart failure, postural dyspnea, morbid obesity, musculoskeletal pain (e.g., arthritis)
Contraindications	
Abnormal anatomy	Past trauma or surgery in the site of injection, certain peripheral and central neurologic diseases
Abnormal coagulation	Coumadin, heparin, coagulopathies
Abnormal skin integrity	Infection at the site of injection

BIBLIOGRAPHY

1. Brown DL: Atlas of Regional Anesthesia. W.B. Saunders, Philadelphia, 1992.
2. Ellis H, Feldman S: Anatomy for Anesthetists. London, Saunders/Blackwell, 1977.
3. Goldberg ME, Seltzer JL, et al: A comparison of three methods of axillary approach to brachial plexus blockade for upper extremity surgery, Anesthesiology 66:814–816, 1987.
4. Miller, RD (ed): Anesthesia. New York, Churchill Livingstone, 1994.
5. Moore DC: Regional Block, 4th ed. Springfield, IL, Charles C Thomas, 1965.
6. Mulroy MF: Regional Anesthesia, An Illustrated Procedural Guide. Boston, Little, Brown, 1989.
7. Stoelting RK, Pharmacology and Physiology in Anesthesia Practice, 2nd ed. Philadelphia, J.B. Lippincott, 1991, pp 148–171, 619–626.
8. Stoelting RK, Miller RD: Peripheral nerve blocks. In Basics of Anesthesia, 2nd ed. New York, Churchill Livingstone, 1989, pp 189–200.
9. Sweitzer BJ, O'Neill C: In Davidson JK, Eckhardt WF, Perese DA (eds): Clinical Anesthesia Procedures of the Massachusetts General Hospital, 4th ed. Boston: Little, Brown, 1993, pp 197–205, pp 227–246.
10. Tetzlaff JE: Peripheral nerve blocks. In Morgan GE, Mikhail MS (eds): Clinical Anesthesia. Norwalk, Appleton & Lange, 1992, pp 230–268.
11. Tetzlaff JE, Yoon HJ, Brems J: Interscalene brachial plexus block for shoulder. Reg Anesth 19:339–343, 1994.
12. Urban MK, Urquhart B: Evaluation of brachial plexus anesthesia for upper extremity surgery. Reg Anesth 19:175–182, 1994.

IX. Anesthetic Considerations in Selected Surgical Procedures

74. CARDIOPULMONARY BYPASS

Michael Leonard, M.D.

1. What is the function of a cardiopulmonary bypass (CPB) pump?

A CPB pump functions as the temporary equivalent of an intact cardiopulmonary system. The machine perfuses the patient's vital organs, while oxygenating the blood and removing carbon dioxide (CO_2). Isolation of the cardiopulmonary system allows for surgical exposure of the heart and great vessels.

2. What are the basic components of the CPB pump?

A CPB circuit has a venous line, which siphons central venous blood from the patient into a reservoir. This blood then becomes oxygenated and has CO_2 removed before being returned to the patient's arterial circulation. Pressure to perfuse the arterial circulation is supplied by either a roller head or a centrifugal pump. The machine also has roller head pumps for cardioplegia administration, a ventricular vent to drain the heart during surgery, and a pump sucker to remove blood from the surgical field. Additionally the circuit contains filters for air and blood microemboli, because both can cause devastating central nervous system injury if delivered to the arterial circulation. A heat exchanger is present to produce hypothermia on bypass and warm the patient before separating from CPB.

3. Define the levels of hypothermia.

Mild: 32 to 35°C
Moderate: 26 to 31°C
Deep: 20 to 25°C
Profound: 14 to 19°C

4. Why is hypothermia used on CPB?

Systemic oxygen demand decreases 9% for every degree of temperature drop. The main concern on CPB is the prevention of myocardial and central nervous system injury.

5. Discuss the common cannulation sites for bypass.

Venous blood is obtained through cannulation of the superior and inferior vena cavae at the level of the right atrium. Arterial blood is returned to the ascending aorta proximal to the innominate artery. Occasionally the femoral artery and vein are used as cannulation sites. Drawbacks to femoral bypass include ischemia of the leg distal to the arterial cannula, inadequate venous drainage, possible inadequate systemic perfusion secondary to a small inflow cannula, and difficulty in cannula placement owing to atherosclerotic plaques.

6. What are the basic anesthetic techniques used in CPB cases?

Patients with poor ventricular function receive high-dose opioid anesthetics, usually with fentanyl or sufentanil. Healthier patients with reasonably good ventricular function can be given less opioid and supplemented with propofol or inhalation agents. The potential advantage of this latter approach is earlier postoperative extubation and transfer from the intensive care unit. Amnestic agents, such as midazolam, are a must to prevent intraoperative awareness. Neuromuscular blocking agents prevent shivering on bypass, which increases systemic oxygen demand, as well as contraction of the diaphragm during the surgical procedure.

7. List the two basic types of oxygenators.

1. **Bubble oxygenators** work by bubbling oxygen (O_2) through the patient's blood and then defoaming the blood to minimize air microemboli.

2. In **membrane oxygenators**, O_2 and CO_2 diffuse across a semipermeable membrane. Membrane units are generally preferable owing to a decreased risk of gas microemboli and less damage to blood elements.

8. What is meant by "pump prime," and what is the usual hemodynamic response to initiating bypass?

Priming solutions of either crystalloid or crystalloid-colloid are used to fill the CPB circuit. When bypass is initiated, the circuit must contain fluid to perfuse the arterial circulation until the patient's blood can circulate through the pump. The usual prime volume is 1.5 to 2.5 L. The acute hemodilution from the patient's circulating blood volume mixing with the prime causes an acute reduction in mean arterial pressure.

9. Why is systemic anticoagulation necessary?

Contact of the synthetic surfaces of the CPB circuit with nonheparinized blood leads to diffuse thrombosis, oxygenator failure, and frequently death. Even in a dire emergency, a minimum standard dose of 3–4 mg/kg of heparin must be given through a central line before the initiation of bypass. Postbypass, protamine is used to complex heparin and reverse the anticoagulant effect.

10. How is the adequacy of anticoagulation measured before and during bypass?

Activated clotting time (ACT) is measured about 3 to 4 minutes after heparin administration and every 30 minutes on CPB. An ACT of 400 seconds or longer is considered acceptable. Heparin levels are frequently measured, but only the ACT is a measure of anticoagulant activity. This is particularly important in patients with heparin resistance (seen with preoperative heparin infusions) and antithrombin III deficiency.

11. What must be ascertained before placing the patient on CPB?
- Adequate arterial inflow of oxygenated blood
- Sufficient venous return to the bypass pump
- ACT of at least 400 seconds
- Core temperature monitoring site
- Baseline assessment of the patient's pupils relative to size and symmetry
- Adequate depth of anesthesia

12. Why is a left ventricular vent used?

Left ventricular distention on bypass can be caused by aortic regurgitation or blood flow through the bronchial and thebesian veins. The resultant increase in myocardial wall tension can lead to serious myocardial ischemia by precluding adequate subendocardial cardioplegia distribution. A left ventricular vent, placed through the right superior pulmonary vein, decompresses the left side of the heart and returns this blood to the CPB pump.

13. Define cardioplegia.

Cardioplegia is a hypothermic, hyperkalemic solution containing some metabolic energy substrate. Perfused through the coronary arteries, cardioplegia induces diastolic electromechanical dissociation. Myocardial oxygen and energy requirements are dramatically reduced to those of cellular maintenance. Cardioplegia is perfused either anterograde via the aortic root coronary ostia or retrograde through the right atrial coronary sinus.

14. Myocardial protection refers to steps taken during bypass to minimize myocardial ischemia. What elements constitute myocardial protection?
- Cardioplegia
- Hypothermia
- Topical cooling of the heart with icy saline slush
- Left ventricular venting
- Insulating pad on the posterior cardiac surface to prevent warming from mediastinal blood flow
- Minimizing bronchial vessel collateral flow (which also rewarms the arrested heart)

15. What is the function of an aortic cross-clamp?
Clamping across the proximal aorta isolates the heart and coronary circulation. The arterial bypass perfusate enters the aorta distal to the clamp. Cardioplegia is infused between the clamp and aortic valve, thus entering the coronary circulation. This isolation of the heart from the systemic circulation allows for prolonged cardioplegia activity and profound cooling of the heart.

16. What are the pH-stat and alpha-stat methods of blood gas measurement?
In **pH-stat** measurements during hypothermic bypass, blood gases are temperature corrected to 37°C. In **alpha-stat**, blood gases are all measured as if drawn at 37°C and not temperature corrected. Some evidence suggests cerebral autoregulation of blood flow is better preserved on bypass with alpha-stat measurement of pH 7.4 and PCO_2 of 40 mmHg.

17. Develop an appropriate checklist for discontinuing bypass.
1. Check acid-base balance, hematocrit, electrolytes, platelet count.
2. Ascertain adequate systemic rewarming.
3. Recalibrate all pressure transducers.
4. Ensure adequate cardiac rate and rhythm (may require pacing).
5. Reexamine the ECG for rhythm and ischemia.
6. Remove intracardiac or intra-aortic air if aorta or cardiac chambers were opened.
7. Initiate ventilation of lungs.

18. Why is cardiac pacing frequently useful postbypass?
Between the ischemic insult of bypass and residual effect of cardioplegia, cardiac conduction may be impaired and myocardial wall motion is suboptimal. Cardiac pacing, with an atrial kick, at a rate of 80–100 beats per minute can significantly improve cardiac output.

BIBLIOGRAPHY

1. Bull BS, Korpman HA, Huse WM, Briggs BD: Heparin therapy during during extracorporeal circulation: I. Problems inherent in existing heparin protocols. J Thorac Cardiovasc Surg 69:674–684, 1975.
2. DiNardo JA: Management of cardiopulmonary bypass. In DiNardo JA, Schwartz MJ (eds):Anesthesia for Cardiac Surgery. Norwalk, CT, Appleton & Lange, 1990.
3. Hindman BJ, Lillehaug SL, Tinker JH: Cardiopulmonary bypass and the anesthesiologist. In Kaplan JA (ed): Cardiac Anesthesia, 3rd ed. Philadelphia, W. B. Saunders, 1993.
4. Murkin JM, Farrar JK, Tweed WA, et al: Cerebral autoregulation and flow/metabolism coupling during cardiopulmonary bypass: The influence of $PaCO_2$. Anesth Analg 64:576–581, 1987.
5. Robinson RJS, Boright WA, Ligier B, et al: The incidence of awareness, and amnesia for perioperative events, after cardiac surgery with lorazepam and fentanyl anesthesia. J Cardiothorac Anesth 1:524–530, 1987.

75. DOUBLE-LUMEN ENDOTRACHEAL TUBES AND ONE-LUNG VENTILATION

Matt Flaherty, M.D.

1. What is one-lung ventilation?

One lung-ventilation involves preparation of the airway so that each lung can function independently. Double-lumen endotracheal tubes have a separate lumen to each lung and thus allow ventilation of one lung while the other is collapsed or independently ventilated. Typically, one-lung ventilation is used for respiratory support when thoracic surgical procedures necessitate either partial or complete collapse, retraction, or removal of the contralateral lung. Occasionally disease states require the isolation of one lung from the other.

2 What are the absolute indications for double-lumen tubes or one-lung ventilation?

Absolute indications for isolation of one lung or one-lung ventilation include protection of a healthy lung from a contaminated lung, such as gross infection in one lung or massive hemoptysis from one side. Lavage of one lung for pulmonary alveolar proteinosis requires isolation of the affected side. Other absolute indications include bronchopleural or bronchopleural cutaneous fistulas, surgical opening of major airways, disruption of the trachea or bronchial system, and giant unilateral cyst or bulla. Such disease states generally require diversion of ventilation to avoid loss of volume at leak sites or damage to the airway or lung at fragile sites.

3. What are the relative indications for double-lumen tubes or one-lung ventilation?

Relative indications for isolation of the lungs and one-lung ventilation arise from the need to collapse one lung for surgical exposure. Procedures involving the thoracic aorta, upper lobes, or complete pneumonectomy have the highest priority among the relative indications for one-lung ventilation. Moderate need for surgical exposure arises with middle and lower lobectomies, subsegmental lung resections, esophageal surgery, thoracoscopy, and thoracic spine procedures. Lower priority still is the occasional need to separate the lungs when a chronic, unilateral, totally occluding pulmonary embolus is removed.

4. Describe common equipment used to separate the two lungs.

Separating the lungs requires either a double-lumen tube or a single-lumen tube with a blocking device (bronchial blocker) to occlude one of the mainstem bronchi. The use of a single-lumen endotracheal tube is possible if it is placed distal to the carina and the cuff isolates one side. The advantage of the double-lumen tube is the presence of a lumen to each side. The lungs can be ventilated independently and suctioned as needed, and either side may be visualized directly with a fiberoptic bronchoscope. A vent port distal to the clamp site of each lumen allows deflation of the contralateral lung.

5. What are the different types of double-lumen tubes?

There are both right- and left-sided double-lumen tubes. Robertshaw types, by far the most common, are designed with a bronchial lumen that has its own cuff and extends distal to the carina. The tracheal lumen, with its cuff, opens proximal to the carina. Carlens tubes are similar to the Robertshaw design but have a hook that catches at the carina. Carlens tubes are rarely used today, because the hook may cause airway trauma during placement. Both designs have sizes 41, 39, 37, and 35 F; the Robertshaw tubes also come in 28 F. The inflatable bronchial cuffs are a bright blue color to help visualization during positioning with the fiberoptic bronchoscope.

6. What size are the individual lumens inside the double-lumen tube?
Both lumens are the same size in double-lumen tubes. The inner diameters are 6.5, 6.0, 5.5, and 5.0 mm for the 41, 39, 37, and 35 F, respectively. Clinically, higher resistance and more frequent blockage by secretions may be noted.

7. What is the difference between a right- and left-sided double-lumen tube?
The difference between right- and left-sided double-lumen tubes is based on the difference between the length of the right and left mainstem bronchi. The right upper lobe bronchus branches from the right mainstem bronchus at about 2.1–2.3 cm. The bronchial lumen of right-sided double-lumen tubes must pass the carina far enough to let the cuff isolate the bronchial from the tracheal lumen, yet not so far that it blocks the right upper lobe take-off. The fact that the right upper lobe take-off is sometimes less than 2.1 cm or even tracheal in origin makes placement of the right-sided double-lumen tube difficult without obstructing the right upper lobe bronchus. The bronchial cuff is shaped asymmetrically, and the lumen has an additional slotted opening to help prevent this complication. The left mainstem bronchus is about 5.0–5.4 cm long and thus allows more room to place the bronchial lumen and cuff. The bronchial lumen of a left-sided double-lumen tube has a simple round opening and symmetric cuff.

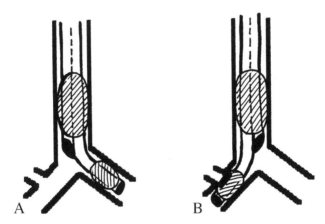

A, Left Robertshaw endotracheal tube, properly placed at the carina. *B,* Right Robertshaw endotracheal tube, properly placed at the carina.

8. When is a right-sided double-lumen tube used?
Right-sided double-lumen tubes are hard to place because of the short right mainstem bronchus. The cuff has the potential to move 1 cm or less and block the right upper lobe take-off. Because of this risk, left-sided double-lumen tubes are usually preferred. Because both right- and left-sided double-lumen tubes have a lumen to each lung, the left-sided double-lumen tube works well for procedures on either side, unless the bronchus itself is involved in the pathology or surgical procedure. When left-sided double-lumen tubes cannot be used or left bronchial surgery is planned, the right-sided double-lumen tube may be the best option.

9. What are the contraindications for use of a right- or left-sided double-lumen tube?
The left-sided double-lumen tubes cannot be used when the left mainstem bronchus is stenotic or obstructed or has an acute takeoff. For left pneumonectomy left-sided double-lumen tubes work well and can be pulled back out of the bronchus before it is stapled. The tube can be replaced with or used as a single-lumen tube. The same anatomic problems may prevent right-sided double-lumen tube placement, in addition to the technical difficulty involved in ventilation of the right upper lobe.

10. How is the double-lumen tube placed?

The double-lumen tube is supplied with a specialized stylet that, like conventional stylets, helps to stiffen the tube as it is passed through the upper airway past the vocal cords. Because it is a relatively large endotracheal tube, it should be lubricated before placement. Selecting a double-lumen tube that is too small may require excessive inflation of the cuffs to create a seal for positive pressure ventilation and increase the risk of airway injury. Tracheal cuff inflation usually requires 6–8 ml, whereas the bronchial cuff usually needs only 2–3 ml. Rupture of the mainstem bronchus due to excessive cuff inflation has been reported. The stylet also can be used to ensure the initial orientation of the longer endobronchial lumen as it is advanced toward the carina. Many anesthesiologists then remove the stylet and advance the tube blindly until it is seated in the mainstem bronchus. A possible complication is disruption of the mainstem bronchus; thus a double-lumen tube should not be forced. An alternative technique is to remove the stylet, pass a flexible fiberoptic bronchoscope through the bronchial lumen, and advance the tube with the bronchoscope as a guide. The bronchoscope also may be passed via the tracheal lumen and used to observe the endobronchial lumen as it passes into the appropriate mainstem bronchus. The placement of the right-sided double-lumen tube usually requires a fiberoptic bronchoscope; the margin for error is less because of the shorter right mainstem bronchus.

11. How does one confirm the position of a double-lumen tube?

The properly placed double-lumen tube, with both cuffs inflated, allows separation of the two lungs during ventilation; proper placement can be confirmed by auscultation and visualization of chest movement. When the bronchial lumen is clamped and the vent opened, breath sounds and chest rise should be minimal on the involved side and normal on the other. There should be no leak at the vent port. The reverse is true when the tracheal lumen is clamped and the vent opened: breath sounds and chest rise should be minimal over the tracheal side and normal over the side with the bronchial lumen. Again, there should be no leak at the vent port. Auscultation is the least sensitive method to confirm proper placement. In one study, when double-lumen tube placement was thought to be correct by auscultation, fiberoptic examination detected malpositioning in 48% of cases. Fiberoptic examination is made by passing the bronchoscope through the tracheal lumen and ensuring that the bronchial cuff (always colored bright blue) is located just distal to the carina on the desired bronchial side. The anterior trachea has complete cartilage rings, and the posterior aspect has the membranous band, which may continue down the posterior portions of the mainstem bronchi. Once the anterior tracheal wall is identified, the right and left mainstem bronchi can be positively identified. Right-sided double-lumen tubes are further examined by passing the bronchoscope through the bronchial lumen and ensuring that the slot for right upper lobe ventilation is facing and open to the right upper lobe bronchus. The final and most sensitive test of proper placement is observation of the lung when the chest is surgically opened. The double-lumen tube may move when the patient is turned to a lateral position and should be checked after the patient is in the surgical position.

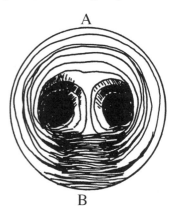

Fiberoptic bronchoscopic view of the trachea showing anterior and posterior anatomical landmarks. *A,* Cartilaginous rings, anterior. *B,* Membranous trachea, posterior.

12. Does one need a fiberoptic bronchoscope for placement and confirmation of placement?
Although double-lumen tubes can be placed blindly, if there appears to be a problem with placement, the fiberoptic bronchoscope should be used. Placement confirmation is much more sensitive with the fiberoptic bronchoscope, especially with right-sided double-lumen tubes. As mentioned above, when double-lumen tube placement was thought to be correct by auscultation, fiberoptic examination detected malpositioning in 48% of cases. Standard adult fiberoptic bronchoscopes usually have an outer diameter of 4.9 mm and barely fit through the lumens of the 37-F double-lumen tubes. If one uses a 35-F double-lumen tube or smaller, a pediatric or "slim" style bronchoscope is required.

13. How is a bronchial blocker used?
Bronchial blockers involve the placement of a Fogarty embolectomy catheter through a conventional endotracheal tube. The balloon is positioned in one of the mainstem bronchi, using the fiberoptic bronchoscope for guidance. When one-lung ventilation is desired, the balloon is inflated, blocking ventilation to that side. Venting and ventilation of the blocked lung is not possible.

14. What is a Univent tube?
The Univent tube is a endotracheal tube containing a bronchial blocker. The bronchial blocker is located in a small channel built into the wall of the endotracheal tube. The bronchial blocking balloon is connected to a venting port. Once the balloon is inflated, the blocked lung can be vented to the atmosphere and allowed to collapse. The balloon can be advanced when needed and retracted when not it use.

15. What are the common problems encountered in placing double-lumen tubes or bronchial blockers?
The most common problems involve malpositioning of the bronchial end of the double-lumen tube. If the bronchial lumen and cuff do not reach distally to either mainstem bronchus, either side may ventilate both lungs. If the bronchial lumen is in the trachea and the cuff is overinflated, it may be possible to ventilate both lungs via the bronchial lumen, whereas the tracheal lumen displays very high airway pressures and ventilates neither lung. If the bronchial lumen is placed on the wrong side, it will isolate the wrong side when one-lung ventilation is attempted. When the bronchial lumen is too far down one of the mainstem bronchi, it may block the upper lobe bronchi on the involved side, and the tracheal lumen may also ventilate the same side. Double-lumen tube cuffs may herniate like any other cuff, possibly obstructing part or all of the airway. The bronchial cuff may be overinflated and rupture the mainstem bronchus.

Bronchial blockers involve the risk of misplacement or migration into the trachea, with major airway obstruction. The balloon also can be overinflated and injure the bronchus. Univent tubes should be used only by personnel familiar with the purpose of the bronchial blocker that they contain. Usually this blocker is deflated and retracted into its channel at the end of a case. If the patient remains intubated with the Univent tube postoperatively, it may accidentally be inflated in a tracheal site and obstruct the airway.

When double-lumen tubes are placed, their shape and size lead to a higher incidence of laryngeal trauma. The incidence of trauma with Carlens tube (with the carinal hook) may be around 1.5%. An airway device in the mainstem bronchus runs a risk of being sutured into the surgical closure at that site. Endobronchial lumens of double-lumen tubes, bronchial blockers, and suction catheters have been sutured into bronchial stumps during pneumonectomy and lobectomy. When such devices are sutured into the bronchial stump, their removal may cause significant damage to the airway.

16. What are standard ventilator settings for one-lung ventilation?
Most anesthesiologists use approximately the same tidal volume for one-lung ventilation as for two-lung ventilation—typically around 10 ml/kg. Higher tidal volumes increase airway pressures and vascular resistance, which may cause more blood flow to the nonventilated lung and more

shunting. Lower tidal volumes may allow more atelectasis in the ventilated lung. The FiO_2 will usually be 0.8–1.0, giving the greatest margin of safety against hypoxia. The respiratory rate is usually adjusted to maintain a $PaCO_2$ around 40 mmHg.

17. Describe pulmonary changes that occur with one-lung ventilation.

Most thoracic surgery is performed in the lateral decubitus position with the surgical site up and nonventilated. The nonventilated lung is also referred to as the nondependent lung. When ventilation is interrupted, the remaining blood flow to the nondependent lung becomes shunted (ventilation/perfusion ratio of zero), contributing to hypoxia. Several factors help to decrease nondependent lung blood flow: gravity, which favors blood flow to the ventilated (dependent) lung; surgical compression and retraction; surgical ligation of nondependent lung blood vessels; and hypoxic pulmonary vasoconstriction. The total benefit of the above factors is a reduction of ~50% shunt to ~30%. The dependent lung physiology also changes because of loss of lung volume due to compression from the abdomen and mediastinum. Absorption atelectasis may occur in marginally ventilated areas. Hypoxic pulmonary vasoconstriction in the dependent lung may favor blood flow to the nondependent lung. Secretions in the dependent lung may be difficult to remove through the double-lumen tube.

18. Which changes more during one lung ventilation—PaO_2 or $PaCO_2$?

During one-lung ventilation change is much greater in PaO_2 than in $PaCO_2$ because of the greater diffusibility of $PaCO_2$.

19. Describe an approach to management of hypoxia during one-lung ventilation.

PaO_2 usually decreases significantly when ventilation changes to one lung. The first step is to check the FiO_2 to ensure that it is 0.8–1.0; the second is to check tidal volumes (optimal value— around 10 ml/kg). The fiberoptic bronchoscope should be used to ensure that the double-lumen tube or bronchial blocker is in proper position. The respiratory rate should be adjusted to keep the $PaCO_2$ around 40 mmHg, because hypocapnia may decrease hypoxic pulmonary vasoconstriction. The next step is to add ~5 cm H_2O pressure of continuous positive airway pressure (CPAP) to the nondependent lung. This step may expand the retracted lung and the surgeon should be informed before CPAP is initiated. CPAP supplies oxygen to some of the alveoli that are perfused in the nondependent lung by decreasing shunt. The next step is to add ~5cm H_2O pressure of positive end-expiratory pressure (PEEP) to the dependent lung; this may increase volume in the dependent lung, which is highly prone to atelectasis. The PEEP may have a negative effect, however, by increasing vascular resistance in the dependent lung and causing more blood to flow to the nondependent lung, thereby increasing shunt. For this reason CPAP should be initiated in the nondependent lung; only small increments of PEEP should be added each time. If hypoxia continues, CPAP and PEEP can be incrementally increased in the nondependent and dependent lungs, respectively. If severe hypoxia continues, the surgeon may be able to ligate or clamp the pulmonary artery to the nondependent lung (for pneumonectomy), eliminating shunt from this source. Finally, return to two-lung ventilation may be necessary.

20. Describe the extubation of patients with a double-lumen tube.

If the patient is to be ventilated postoperatively, it may be desirable to remove the double-lumen tube and replace it with a conventional endotracheal tube. Some patients are extubated in the operating room when they demonstrate usual extubation criteria. Both lumens of the double-lumen tube are suctioned. Removal of a double-lumen tube is a potent laryngeal stimulus; this stimulus may be attenuated somewhat by intravenous lidocaine, 1 mg/kg 3–5 minutes before extubation. After lobectomy and pneumonectomy, positive pressure should be limited to less than 30 cm H_2O if possible, because the bronchial stump may be damaged by high airway pressures. The stump is usually tested for a leak at 35–40 cm H_2O, under saline, before closure of the chest.

21. When should one consider leaving a double-lumen tube or bronchial blocker in place for postoperative management?

Changing to a single-lumen endotracheal tube may be undesirable for a number of reasons. Changing the double-lumen tube may entail risk of airway loss in patients with airway edema or prior difficult intubation. The lungs may benefit from continued differential ventilation modes postoperatively, as in the case of lung transplant. There may be continued risk of contamination of one lung from the other or continued bronchopleural fistula. The double-lumen tube may be used for an extended period postoperatively. Case reports describe up to 10 days' duration without tracheal or bronchial trauma. The primary difficulty is increased airway resistance and difficulty in suctioning secretions because of the relatively small lumens. Leaving a bronchial blocker in place postoperatively is not advised because of the risk of severe airway obstruction if the inflated blocker migrates into the trachea.

22. What should be done if the patient is too small for the double-lumen tube?

The smallest double-lumen tube is the 28 F. Pediatric patients requiring one-lung ventilation may be managed with a single-lumen tube and a small Fogarty embolectomy catheter, which is passed outside the lumen of th endotracheal tube. The pediatric fiberoptic laryngoscope via the endotracheal tube is used to guide placement of the bronchial blocker.

BIBLIOGRAPHY

 1. Benumof JL: Anesthesia for Thoracic Surgery. Philadelphia, W.B. Saunders, 1987, pp 223–287.
 2. Benumof JL, Partridge NL, Salvaiterra C, et al: Margin of safety in positioning modern double-lumen endotracheal tubes. Anesthesiology 67:729–738, 1987.
 3. Brodsky JB, Shulman MS, Mark JB: Malposition of left-sided double-lumen endotracheal tubes. Anesthesiology 62:667–669, 1985.
 4. Brodsky JB, Mihm FG: Split-lung ventilation. In Hall JB, Schmidt GA, Wood LDH (eds): Principles of Critical Care. New York, McGraw-Hill, 1992, pp 160–164.
 5. Eisenkraft JB, Cohen E, Kaplan JA: Anesthesia for thoracic surgery. In Barash PG, Cullen BF, Stoelting RK (eds): Clinical Anesthesia. Philadelphia, J.B. Lippincott, 1989, pp 905–946.
 6. Eisenkraft JB, Neustein SM: Anesthetic management of therapeutic procedures of the lungs and airway. In Kaplan JA (ed): Thoracic Anesthesia, 2nd ed. New York, Churchill Livingstone, 1991, pp 371–388.
 7. Lee BS, Sarnquist FH, Sarner VA: Anesthesia for bilateral single-lung transplantation. J Cardiothorac Vasc Anesth 6:201–203, 1992.
 8. Smith GB, Hirsch NP, Ehrenwerth J: Sight and sound: Can double-lumen endotracheal tubes be placed accurately without fiberoptic bronchoscopy? Br J Anaesth 58:1317–1320, 1986.
 9. Veil R: Selective bronchial blocking in a small child. Br J Anaesth 41:453–454, 1969.
10. Wilson RS: Endobronchial intubation. In Kaplan JA (ed): Thoracic Anesthesia, 2nd ed. New York, Churchill Livingstone, 1991, pp 371–388.

76. SOMATOSENSORY-EVOKED POTENTIALS AND SPINAL SURGERY

Patricia A. Gottlob, M.D.

1. What are somatosensory-evoked potentials (SSEPs)?

SSEPs are the electrophysiologic responses of the nervous system to the application of a discrete stimulus at a peripheral nerve anywhere in the body. They reflect the ability of a specific neural pathway to conduct an electrical signal from the periphery to the cerebral cortex.

2. How are SSEPs generated?

Using a skin surface disc electrode or subcutaneous fine-needle electrode placed near a major peripheral sensory nerve, a square wave electrical stimulus of 0.2–2 milliseconds is applied to the nerve at a rate of 1–2 Hz. The stimulus intensity is adjusted to produce minimal muscle contraction (usually 10–15 milliamperes). The resulting electrical potential is recorded at various points along the neural pathway from the peripheral nerve to the cerebral cortex.

3. What major peripheral nerves are most commonly stimulated?

In the upper extremity, the common sites of stimulation are the median and ulnar nerves at the wrist. In the lower extremity, the common peroneal nerve at the popliteal fossa and the posterior tibial nerve at the ankle are used. Less commonly, the tongue, trigeminal nerve, and pudendal nerve have been studied.

4. Trace the neurosensory pathway from the peripheral nerves to the cerebral cortex.

The axons of the peripheral sensory nerves enter the spinal cord via the dorsal spinal roots. These first-order neurons continue rostrally in the ipsilateral posterior column of the spinal cord until they synapse with nuclei at the cervicomedullary junction. Second-order neurons from these nuclei immediately cross to the opposite side of the brainstem, where they continue their ascent via the medial lemniscus through the midbrain, synapsing in the thalamus. Third-order neurons then travel via the internal capsule to synapse in the postcentral gyrus, the primary somatosensory cortex.

5. At what points along the neurosensory pathway are SSEPs most commonly recorded?

After upper limb stimulation, potentials are recorded at the brachial plexus (Erb's point, 2 cm superior to the clavicular head of the sternocleidomastoid muscle); the cervicomedullary junction (posterior midline of the neck at the second cervical vertebrae); and the scalp overlying the somatosensory cortex on the contralateral side.

After stimulation of the lower extremity, potentials are recorded at the popliteal fossa, lumbar spinal cord, and somatosensory cortex.

6. Describe the characteristics of the SSEP waveform.

The SSEP is plotted as a waveform of voltage versus time. It is characterized by

1. **Amplitude** (A), which is measured in microvolts from baseline to peak or peak to peak.

2. **Latency** (L), which is the time, measured in milliseconds, from onset of stimulus to occurrence of a peak or the time from one peak to another.

3. **Morphology**, which is the overall shape of the waveform, described as positive (P, below the baseline) or negative (N, above the baseline).

A waveform is identified by the letter describing its deflection above or below the baseline followed by a number indicating its latency (e.g., N20).

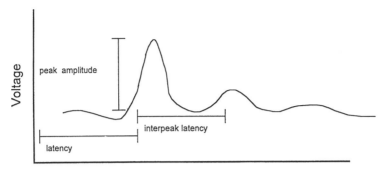

Characteristics of the SSEP waveform.

7. Name several characteristic peaks important the evaluation of SSEPs.
For median nerve stimulation:

Peak	Generator
N9	Brachial plexus (Erb's point)
N11	Dorsal root entry zone (cervical spine)
N13, 14	Posterior column (nucleus cuneatus)
P14	Medial lemniscus
N20	Somatosensory cortex

For posterior tibial nerve stimulation:

N20	Dorsal root entry zone (lumbar spine)
N40	Somatosensory cortex

8. What is the central somatosensory conduction time (CCT)?
CCT is the latency between the dorsal column nuclei (N14) and the primary sensory cortex (N20) peaks and reflects nerve conduction time through the brainstem and cortex.

9. What are the indications for intraoperative use of SSEP monitoring?
SSEP monitoring is indicated in any setting with the potential for mechanical or vascular compromise of the sensory pathways along the peripheral nerve, within the spinal canal, or within the brainstem or cerebral cortex. SSEP monitoring has been used in the following:
Orthopedic procedures
  • Correction of scoliosis with Harrington rod instrumentation
  • Spinal cord decompression and stabilization after acute spinal cord injury
  • Spinal fusion
Brachial plexus exploration
Neurosurgical procedures
  • Resection of a spinal cord tumor or vascular lesion
  • Tethered cord release
  • Resection of a sensory cortex lesion (e.g., aneurysm or thalamic tumor)
  • Repair of a thoracic or abdominal aortic aneurysm,
  • Carotid endarterectomy.

10. What constitutes a significant change in the SSEP?
Any decrease in amplitude greater than 50% or increase in latency greater than 10% may indicate a disruption of the sensory nerve pathways. The spinal cord can tolerate ischemia for about 20 minutes before SSEPs are lost.

11. Summarize the effects of anesthetic agents on the amplitude and latency of SSEPs.

Effects of Anesthetic Agents on Amplitude and Latency of SSEPs

DRUG	AMPLITUDE	LATENCY
Premedications		
Midazolam (0.3 mg/kg)	↓	0
Diazepam (0.1 mg/kg)	↓	↑
Induction agents		
Thiopental (5 mg/kg)	↑/0	↑
Etomidate (0.4 mg/kg)	↑↑↑	↑
Propofol (0.5 mg/kg)	0	↑
Ketamine (1 mg/kg)	↑	*
Opioids		
Fentanyl		↑
Sufentanil		↑
Morphine		↑
Meperidine	↑/↓	↑
Inhaled anesthetics		
Nitrous oxide	↓	↑
Isoflurane	↓	↑
Halothane	↓	↑
Enflurane	↓	↑
Desflurane	↓	↑
Others		
Droperidol	↓	↑
Muscle relaxants	0	0

↑ = increase, ↓ = decrease, 0 = no change, * = not known.

12. What is the take-home message of the effects of anesthetic agents on SSEPs?

1. All of the halogenated inhaled anesthetics probably cause roughly equivalent dose-dependent decreases in amplitude and increases in latency that are further worsened by the addition of 60% nitrous oxide.

2. If possible, bolus injections of drugs should be avoided, especially during critical stages of the surgery. Continuous infusions are preferable.

13. What other physiologic variables can alter SSEPs?

1. **Temperature:** hypothermia increases latency, whereas amplitude is either decreased or unchanged. For each decrease of 1° C, latency is increased by 1 msec. Hyperthermia (4° C) decreases amplitude to 15% of the normothermic value.

2. **Hypotension:** with a decrease of the mean arterial blood pressure (MAP < 40 mmHg), progressive decreases in amplitude are seen. The same change also is seen with a rapid decline in MAP to levels within the limits of cerebral autoregulation.

3. **Hypoxia:** decreased amplitude due to hypoxia has been reported.

4. **Hypocarbia:** increased latency has been described at an end-tidal CO_2 < 25 mmHg.

5. **Isovolemic hemodilution:** latency is not increased until the hematocrit is < 15%, and amplitude is not decreased until the hematocrit is < 7%. This effect is likely due to tissue hypoxia.

14. If SSEPs change significantly, what can the anesthesiologist and surgeon do to lessen the insult to the monitored nerves?

The **anesthesiologist** can:

1. Increase mean arterial blood pressure, especially if induced hypotension is used.

2. Correct anemia, if present.

3. Correct hypovolemia, if present.
4. Improve oxygen tension.

The **surgeon** can:
1. Reduce excessive retractor pressure.
2. Reduce surgical dissection in the affected area.
3. Decrease Harrington rod distraction, if indicated.

If changes in the SSEPs persist despite corrective measures, a wake-up test may be performed to confirm or refute the SSEP findings. The patient's anesthetic level is lightened, and a clinical assessment of neurologic function is performed.

15. Despite "normal" SSEPs, can patients awaken with neurologic deficits?

Although SSEP monitoring is a useful tool in preventing neurologic damage during spinal surgery, it is by no means fool-proof. Because motor tracts are not monitored, the patient may awaken with preserved sensation but lost motor function. The monitoring of motor-evoked potentials (MEPs) along with SSEPs provides a more complete assessment of neural pathway integrity.

BIBLIOGRAPHY

1. Black S, Cucchiara R: Neurologic monitoring. In Miller R (ed): Anesthesia, 3rd ed. New York, Churchill Livingstone, 1990, pp 1185–1207.
2. Deletic V: Evoked potentials. In Lake C (ed): Clinical Monitoring for Anesthesia and Critical Care. Philadelphia, W.B. Saunders, 1994, pp 288–314.
3. Goodrich JT: Electrophysiologic measurements: Intraoperative evoked potential monitoring. Anesthesiol Clin North Am 5:477–488, 1987.
4. Kalkman CJ: Monitoring the central nervous system. Anesthesiol Clin North Am 12:173–191, 1994.
5. McPherson R: Intraoperative neurologic monitoring. In Rogers M, Tinker J, Covino B, Longnecker D (eds): Principles and Practice of Anesthesiology. St. Louis, Mosby, 1992, pp 803–826.
6. Moller A: Evoked Potentials in Intraoperative Monitoring. Baltimore, Williams & Wilkins, 1988.
7. Schramm J, Kerthen M: Recent developments in neurosurgical spinal cord monitoring. Paraplegia 30:609–616, 1993.
8. Thiagarajah S: Anesthetic management of spinal surgery. Anesthesiol Clin North Am 5:587–600, 1987.

77. DELIBERATE HYPOTENSION

Jefferson P. Mostellar, M.D.

1. Define deliberate hypotension.
Deliberate hypotension is defined as the intentional reduction of systemic perfusion pressure.

2. Describe the indications for deliberate hypotension.
The major indication for using a deliberate hypotensive technique is to reduce intraoperative blood loss and to produce a relatively bloodless surgical site. This technique can be used in a number of different operations, including neurosurgery, orthopedic procedures, major vascular surgery, burns, plastic surgery, and craniofacial reconstruction. Deliberate hypotension also may be used to help manage patients who refuse blood transfusions (e.g., Jehovah's Witnesses).

3. What are the benefits of deliberate hypotension?
Deliberate hypotension decreases blood loss and thereby reduces the need for blood transfusion. This benefit is significant when one considers the risk of transmission of infection associated with blood transfusions, such as human immunodeficiency virus and viral hepatitis. In addition, decreasing the amount of bleeding provides the surgeon with a bloodless field that allows a clearer view of important structures and potentially decreases the duration of the procedure. However, it is important to consider the risk-benefit ratio with each individual patient.

4. What are the contraindications to deliberate hypotension?
The contraindications to deliberate hypotension include inexperience or lack of understanding of the technique; inability to monitor the patient appropriately; any systemic disease that compromises organ function (e.g., diabetes mellitus); decreased organ blood flow, either focal or generalized (coronary artery disease); decreased oxygen delivery for any reason; polycythemia; and allergy to hypotensive agents. Hypoperfusion and ischemic injury are the concerns for organ systems with compromised vascular supply. The use of deliberate hypotension in a patient with increased intracranial pressure (ICP) is controversial, because all hypotensive drugs and inhalational agents have been shown to increase ICP. These conditions listed above may cause irreversible organ damage if deliberate hypotension is inappropriately used.

5. What are the possible complications of deliberate hypotension?
Deliberate hypotension involves significant risks. The most serious risk is uncontrolled hypotension, which causes decreased cardiac output and inadequate cerebral perfusion pressure, leading to permanent brain damage. Blood pressure (BP) must be measured at the level of the brain, not heart, to ensure adequate cerebral perfusion pressure. Most complications, however, are due to inexperience of the physician with the technique or drugs or from lack of vigilance in monitoring. With a healthy patient and attention to detail, the benefits of deliberate hypotension outweigh the potential risks.

6. What is autoregulation? How is it affected by chronic hypertension?
Autoregulation is the maintenance of a constant blood flow over a wide range of pressures. Autoregulation maintains constant cerebral blood flow (CBF) in a range of cerebral perfusion pressures (CPP) from 50–150 mmHg. Outside this range, blood flow is pressure-dependent. Chronic hypertension causes a shift to the right in the autoregulation curve.

7. How is the central nervous system affected by deliberate hypotension?
The effect of deliberate hypotension on CBF is always a concern, regardless of the agents used. It is important to maintain tissue perfusion when lowering the BP. Cerebral perfusion pressure

(CPP = mean arterial pressure − ICP) should be maintained above 50 mmHg. Inhalational anesthetics and vasodilators alter the ratio of CBF to cerebral metabolic rate of oxygen consumption ($CMRO_2$). Vasodilators (e.g., sodium nitroprusside or nitroglycerin) dilate cerebral vessels directly with no effect on the $CMRO_2$. These drugs, as well as inhalational agents, attenuate the autoregulation of CBF in a dose-dependent fashion and decrease blood flow from baseline levels. The amount of decline varies with the agent and the degree of hypotension. If the decrease in CBF is greater than the decrease in $CMRO_2$, cerebral ischemia may occur. Ventilation during deliberate hypotension should be aimed at maintaining normocarbia. Hypocapnia decreases CBF by 2%/mm of mercury decline in arterial partial pressure of carbon dioxide ($PaCO_2$). Therefore, it is important to keep the $PaCO_2$ at normal levels to ensure adequate CBF and to prevent cerebral ischemia. Spinal cord blood flow (SCBF) is also affected by deliberate hypotension. Because SCBF is regulated like CBF, factors that affect CBF have similar affects on SCBF. The use of deliberate hypotension in a patient with increased ICP is controversial; if used, the technique must be done with great caution. In the presence of increased ICP, lowering the MAP may cause inadequate cerebral perfusion and resultant cerebral ischemia.

8. How is the cardiovascular system affected?

Most vasodilators improve left ventricular function by reducing afterload, which in turn decreases cardiac work. By reducing myocardial work, myocardial oxygen requirements are reduced. Coronary blood flow, which depends on diastolic filling pressure, is autoregulated, depending on metabolic demands. However, with large reductions in diastolic filling pressures, coronary blood flow is reduced; this reduction may lead to myocardial ischemia, especially in patients with coronary artery disease. Because BP depends on cardiac output and peripheral resistance, decreasing either will decrease BP. Options include decreasing myocardial contractility with beta-adrenergic blocking drugs or using higher concentrations of inhalational agents, both of which have negative inotropic effects. Vasodilation causes a relative decrease in circulating blood volume by increasing the capacitance of blood vessels. Increased capitance results in decreased venous return, which may cause baroreceptor reflex-mediated tachycardia. Drugs that cause tachycardia (atropine and pancuronium) should not be used. In addition hypercarbia causes catecholamine secretion, which increases BP and heart rate.

9. How is the pulmonary system affected?

Pulmonary blood flow is reduced by all vasodilating drugs due to redistribution of blood to the peripheral circulation. During controlled hypotension, both alveolar dead space and intrapulmonary shunting are increased. These changes are thought to be due to decreases in pulmonary artery pressures, increased blood flow through dependent areas of the lung, and inhibition of the hypoxic pulmonary vasoconstriction. Such changes, however, are usually not clinically significant, but pulse oximetry should be followed closely and arterial blood gases should be measured regularly to detect changes in oxygenation and ventilation.

10. How is the hepatic system affected?

Some oxygenated blood is received by the liver via the hepatic artery, but the majority of blood flow is derived from the portal circulation. Therefore, changes in portal blood flow (which is influenced by catecholamines, $PaCO_2$, circulating blood volume, intraabdominal procedures, and anesthetic agents) may have highly significant effects on total hepatic blood flow. Fortunately, as long as MAP is maintained within the acceptable range, hepatic oxygenation is adequate.

11. How is the renal system affected?

Autoregulation of renal blood flow occurs between a MAP of 80–180 mmHg. General anesthesia attenuates this response, depending on the anesthetic agent (inhalational, opioid). However, by simply measuring urinary output via a Foley catheter, renal perfusion and function can be monitored.

12. Describe the different techniques and agents used for deliberate hypotension.

1. **Inhalational technique.** All volatile anesthetics have been used as the sole agent in producing deliberate hypotension because of their ability to depress directly the myocardium and cardiac output and to promote vasodilation. Such effects are dose-dependent. This technique is not recommended, however, because of the inability to quickly reverse the cardiovascular depression that may accompany an inhalational overdose. The most common method of inducing deliberate hypotension uses a combination of inhalational agent and vasodilator.

2. **Vasodilator agents.** Because of their potency, vasodilators are best administered by continuous infusion, which allows easy titration through a dedicated intravenous line, which avoids inadvertent bolusing and a precipitous drop in BP. Direct, continuous arterial BP monitoring is imperative. The three commonly used vasodilators are sodium nitroprusside, nitroglycerin, and trimethaphan.

3. **Beta-adrenergic blockers.** These drugs decrease MAP by their negative inotropic properties. Labetalol and esmolol are the most commonly used beta-adrenergic blockers. Labetalol combines both alpha-1 and beta blockade and may attenuate the compensatory tachycardia associated with hypotension. Because their hypotensive potency is considerably less than that of inhalational agents and vasodilators, they usually are used as a supplement to attain the desired level of hypotension. Among their advantages are lack of rebound hypertension and absence of toxic metabolites. It must be remembered that beta blockade removes the clinical signs of hypovolemia and light anesthesia.

13. Discuss the pharmacodynamics of sodium nitroprusside.

The most commonly used drug to induce deliberate hypotension, sodium nitroprusside (SNP), is a direct vascular smooth-muscle relaxant that causes arteriolar dilation, some venodilation, and a decrease in BP. This response is due to a nitrose (-NO) group on the molecule that diffuses into the vascular smooth muscle and increases cyclic guanosine monophosphate (cGMP), thus producing relaxation. It has a rapid onset of action (seconds), brief duration of action (minutes), and minimal side effects when used appropriately. SNP tends to maintain adequate blood flow to vital organs with MAP above 50 mmHg and provides a more homogeneous distribution of cerebral blood flow by its direct cerebral vasodilating properties. It has no direct effect on $CMRO_2$ but shifts the autoregulation curve to the left in a dose-dependent fashion. Depression of myocardial contractility is minimal, and cardiac output is usually improved with decreased afterload. Coronary blood flow is maintained, and myocardial oxygen demand is reduced. Tachycardia may result from the reduced BP. SNP also decreases right ventricular afterload by directly relaxing pulmonary vasculature. Hypoxic pulmonary vasoconstriction is attenuated, causing in increase in intrapulmonary shunting. Rebound systemic and pulmonary hypertension may occur with sudden discontinuation of SNP. Tachyphylaxis is common and is usually manifested by the need for increasing doses to maintain the desired level of hypotension. It is recommended to begin infusion of SNP at 0.5–1.0 µg/kg/min and to increase the dose slowly until the desired level of hypotension is achieved. The maximal infusion rate is 10 µg/kg/min. The contraindications to SNP include liver and renal failure, anemia, unstable cardiovascular system, and Leber's optic atrophy. High doses or prolonged administration may cause toxic side effects.

14. Discuss the pharmacodynamics of nitroglycerin.

Nitroglycerin (NTG) is a direct-acting, smooth-muscle relaxant that affects primarily venous capacitance vessels, causing a decrease in preload. It also has some effect on arterial smooth-muscle, decreasing BP. NTG has a relatively rapid onset of action (minutes), brief duration of action (minutes), and lacks tachyphylaxis and toxicity. It produces a smooth reduction in BP with minimal risk of sudden hypotension. CBF is maintained in a homogeneous fashion by direct cerebral vasodilation, and $CMRO_2$ is unaffected. Coronary blood flow is increased by coronary artery vasodilation, which increases myocardial oxygen supply. Cardiac output and pulmonary artery pressure may be decreased. However, rebound hypertension due to abrupt discontinuation of NTG is usually not seen. Renal and hepatic blood flow is also well maintained. The usual starting infusion rate is 1 µg/kg/min, increasing slowly until the desired level of hypotension is reached.

15. Discuss the pharmacodynamics of trimethaphan.

Trimethaphan (TMP) is a ganglionic blocking drug with direct vasodilating properties. It decreases BP by blockade of sympathetic output, direct vasodilation, and histamine release. It has the advantages of rapid onset (minutes), brief duration (minutes), and easy titration. Because its effects are related to ganglionic blockade and sympathetic tone, the response is somewhat variable from patient to patient. CBF is reduced with a redistribution of flow away from cortical areas. Higher doses produce mydriasis, which compromises neurologic examination. Renal vascular resistance is increased with a reduction in renal blood flow. The disadvantages of TMP include impaired cerebral and spinal cord blood flow; decreases in coronary, hepatic, and renal blood flow; tachycardia; histamine release; inhibition of pseudocholinesterase enzymes; potentiation of nondepolarizing muscle relaxants; and tachyphylaxis. TMP is contraindicated in patients with asthma because of histamine release and risk of bronchospasm. Infusions are usually started at 25 µg/kg/min and titrated to effect.

16. What are the toxic side effects of agents used to induce hypotension?

Fortunately, the majority of such drugs are without toxic side effects. However, prolonged use of SNP may be associated with cyanide toxicity. Three signs should alert one to the possibility of cyanide toxicity from SNP infusion: (1) the need for doses > 10 µg/kg/min, (2) tachyphylaxis occurring within 60 minutes, or (3) immediate resistance to SNP. If any of these occurs, the infusion of SNP should be stopped. Cyanide toxicity should be suspected if unexplained metabolic acidosis occurs, if lactate levels increase, or if mixed venous oxygen content rises.

SNP is rapidly metabolized by interaction with sulfhydryl groups of red blood cells, with the resultant release of cyanide. The cyanide is converted to thiocyanate (which is nontoxic) by the rhodanase enzyme system in the liver and then excreted by the kidneys. High doses of SNP may exceed the ability of the enzyme system to metabolize cyanide to thiocyanate, thereby allowing free cyanide to bind irreversibly to the cytochrome electron transport system, resulting in cytotoxic hypoxia. This binding causes a change from aerobic to anaerobic metabolism with metabolic acidosis and death.

17. How is cyanide toxicity treated?

Treatment is directed at reversal of binding to the cytochrome system. Because cyanide binds irreversibly, treatment must be directed at introducing an alternative source of binding with greater affinity for cyanide. Administration of amyl nitrate produces methemoglobin, which has a higher affinity for cyanide than the cytochrome enzymes. Methemoglobin reacts with cyanide to form cyanmethemoglobin. Thiosulfate is then administered and reacts with cyanide to form thiocyanate, which is nontoxic and excreted by the kidneys. Therefore, the initial steps in the treatment of cyanide toxicity are to stop the infusion of SNP, to deliver 100% oxygen, and to administer amyl nitrite by inhalation for 30 seconds every 2 minutes. The next step is to give sodium nitrite in an intravenous dose of 10 mg/kg bolus, followed by an infusion of 5 mg/kg over 30 minutes. Immediately after this infusion, sodium thiosulfate, 150 mg/kg (not to exceed 12.5 gm) is given.

18. What monitoring should be used? What laboratory studies should be followed?

If the goal of deliberate hypotension is to decrease blood loss, continuous invasive monitoring of BP is indicated. Monitoring of central venous pressure (CVP) or pulmonary artery pressure (PAP) is also indicated if urine output does not accurately reflect volume status. If the goal is to improve surgical field view, only direct arterial BP monitoring is needed. Once anesthesia has been induced, baseline blood gases, oxygen saturation, hematocrit, blood glucose, and CVP or PAP should be obtained before the planned level of hypotension is reached. These values should be repeated every 30–60 minutes or sooner if necessary. Once baseline CVP or PAP has been assessed, it should be maintained throughout the procedure. Normovolemia must be maintained at all times. A change of even 1–2 mmHg in CVP or PAP may represent a significant reduction in blood volume during induced hypotension. Normocarbia and hyperoxia should be maintained to ensure adequate cerebral perfusion pressure and to prevent hypoxia due to intrapulmonary shunting. Urine output is a good monitor of renal perfusion and function. Even during deliberate hypotension, urine output should be at least 0.5–1.0 ml/kg/hr. If beta blockers are used as supplements, glucose levels need to be followed, because beta blockers inhibit glycogenolysis and hypoglycemia may develop. Temperature also must be monitored, because vasodilation results in substantial heat loss and hypothermia. Therefore, steps to ensure normothermia must be taken.

19. How does positioning affect deliberate hypotension?
Ideally, elevating the operative field to the highest point in relation to the rest of the body helps to decrease bleeding. If the head is the surgical site, the arterial transducer should be calibrated at the level of the head to ensure adequate cerebral perfusion pressure. The CVP and PAP transducers should be calibrated at the level of the heart. Posture may be a useful supplement to deliberate hypotension.

BIBLIOGRAPHY

1. Bendo AA, Hartung J, Kass IS, Cottrell JE: Neurophysiology and neuroanesthesia. In Barash PG, Cullen BF, Stoelting RK (eds): Clinical Anesthesia. Philadelphia, J.B. Lippincott, 1992, pp 871–918.
2. Brown TCK, Fisk GF: Induced hypotension. In Brown TCK, Fisk GC (eds): Anaesthesia in Children. Oxford, Blackwell, 1992, pp 324–329.
3. Collins VJ: Controlled hypotension. In Collins VJ (ed): Principles of Anesthesiology. Philadelphia, Lea & Febiger, 1993, pp 1056–1095.
4. Cote CJ: Strategies to reduce blood transfusions: Controlled hypotension and hemodilution. In Cote CJ, Ryan JF, Todres ID, Goudsouzian NG (eds): A Practice of Anesthesia for Infants and Children. Philadelphia, W.B. Saunders, 1993, pp 201–210.
5. Lerman J: Special techniques: Acute normovolemic hemodilution, controlled hypotension, and hypothermia, ECMO. In Gregory GA (ed): Pediatric Anesthesia. New York, Churchill Livingstone, 1994, pp 319–347.
6. Miller ED: Deliberate hypotension. In Miller RD (ed): Anesthesia. New York, Churchill Livingstone, 1990, pp 1347–1367.
7. Salem MR, Bikhazi GB: Hypotensive anesthesia. In Motoyama EK, Davis PJ, Cohn EL (eds): Anesthesia for Infants and Children. St. Louis, Mosby, 1990, pp 345–370.

78. ANESTHESIA FOR CRANIOTOMY

Roger A. Mattison, M.D.

1. Are there particular anesthetic problems associated with intracranial surgery?
Yes. The central nervous system disease processes that are treated operatively require specific interventions by the anesthesiologist. Space-occupying lesions of the brain are associated with disturbance in normal autoregulation in adjacent tissue, vascular malformations and aneurysms are accompanied by altered vasoreactivity (particularly if preceded by subarachnoid hemorrhage), and traumatic injuries require sometimes contradictory efforts to minimize brain swelling while maximizing systemic resuscitation. In addition, there are specific neurophysiologic concerns: control of cerebral blood flow and volume, anticipation of the effects of surgery and anesthetic management on intracranial pressure dynamics, and maintenance of adequate regional perfusion to preserve brain metabolism and function. The other requirements for general anesthesia for craniotomy are, in principle, the same as for any operative procedure: the patient should be unconscious and remain unaware of intraoperative stimuli; adrenergic responses of the patient to intraoperative events should be attenuated; and the surgeon's approach to the operative site should be facilitated.

2. How is the anesthetic requirement different in the brain and related structures?
During anesthesia for craniotomy, the level of nociceptive stimulus varies greatly. Laryngoscopy and intubation are powerful adrenergic stimuli, requiring deep levels of anesthesia to block potentially harmful increases in heart rate, blood pressure, and brain metabolic activity. These stimuli may increase cerebral perfusion and brain swelling. Except for placement of pins in the skull for head positioning, considerable time may pass during positioning and operative preparation with no noxious stimulus. Then, incision of scalp, opening of the skull, and reflection of the dura provide increased surgical stimulus, only to be followed by dissection of the brain or pathologic tissue which is almost completely free of nociceptive nerve fibers. Occasionally, vascular structures of the brain may respond with adrenergic surge during surgery, particularly if a subarachnoid hemorrhage has occurred in the region of the procedure, but this response is variable and unpredictable. Displacement or traction on the cranial nerve roots can cause specific hemodynamic alterations.

3. Should monitoring be different during a craniotomy?
The usual noninvasive monitors are used for every patient, including pulse oximetry, precordial stethoscope, noninvasive blood pressure cuff, electrocardiogram, end-tidal and inspired gas monitors, and peripheral nerve stimulator. End-tidal anesthetic agent monitoring has some theoretical value, particularly in managing emergence. Continuous arterial pressure monitoring is often used to assess hemodynamic changes, which may develop acutely with cranial nerve root stimulation or slowly because of minimal intravascular volume repletion. Some forgo the radial artery catheter for very superficial craniotomies, such as mapping of the seizure focus directly with cortical electrodes; few anesthesiologists would use a central venous catheter unless there was a high risk of air entrainment in the venous system or a likelihood of using vasoactive infusions perioperatively. Occasionally, continuous electroencephalography is used, not so much as an intraoperative monitor but rather as a means for the surgeon to localize diseased tissue. Comparison of ipsilateral and contralateral evoked potentials has been reported during aneurysm surgery. Jugular bulb venous oxygen saturation and transcranial oximetry have been described as monitors of oxygen delivery and metabolic integrity of the brain globally but are not used regularly in intraoperative settings. Some patients, especially after trauma, have subdural, intraventricular, or cerebrospinal fluid pressure monitors in use intraoperatively.

4. Discuss the considerations for fluid administration during anesthesia for a craniotomy.
During a craniotomy, intravascular volume is subject to the same changes as during the administration of other general anesthetics. Volume depletion from overnight fasting and volume redistribution from vasodilating anesthetic agents result in relative hypovolemia. Each patient should be evaluated individually to determine the hemodynamic parameters that ensure adequate myocardial, central nervous system, and renal perfusion. However, during craniotomy, special attention must be directed toward stability of intracranial volume. Prior to opening of the dura, sudden increases in intravascular volume may cause deleterious increases in intracranial pressure if the intracranial pathology is a brain contusion or malignant mass. After the brain is exposed, increases in intravascular volume may cause swelling of normal brain which the surgeon is attempting to retract. Therefore, although fluids must be given to avoid the adverse effect of hypovolemia and hypotension, sudden bolus administration is to be avoided.

The content of the fluids used during a craniotomy is also important. An isosmolar intravenous fluid should be chosen. Glucose, which increases the osmolarity, has a large volume of distribution physiologically, and glucose-containing fluids are hypotonic in vivo and very likely to cause brain edema in regions where the blood-brain barrier is impaired. Indeed, in both clinical and experimental settings where glucose is used in the resuscitation fluids after head injury, outcome is worse. Saline is the appropriate fluid for use during craniotomy. Balanced salt solutions may be used if their osmolarity approximates or exceeds that of the serum. Ringer's lactate has a slight theoretical disadvantage because lactate is metabolized and the solution becomes hypotonic. Colloid solutions or 3% NaCl are equivalent solutions for acute volume replacement prior to packed red cell administration. Often, 25% albumin is used for pressure support when blood replacement is not needed. Hetastarch solutions are generally not used during craniotomies because of concerns that they are associated with impaired coagulation in vitro.

5. When are measures for brain protection required?
"Brain protection" refers to the maneuvers by the anesthesiologist to maintain a balance between brain metabolism and substrate delivery and to prevent secondary injury to regions of the brain after an episode of ischemia. The need for brain protection should be anticipated after head trauma and brain contusion as well as during procedures for the correction of intracranial aneurysms or arteriovenous malformations.

6. How can the brain be protected?
Historically, long-acting barbiturates have been used for metabolic suppression after brain contusion and swelling. "Barbiturate coma" is easier to manage than continuous infusion of ultra-short-acting thiobarbiturates because the myocardial depression of long-acting barbiturates is less. However, the goal is the same: suppression of brain activity with resultant reduction of metabolism which is reflected by a flat electroencephalogram (EEG)

In the intraoperative setting, metabolic suppression is needed when a major artery is temporarily clipped to facilitate access to an aneurysm. The EEG correlate is "burst suppression" wherein the typical anesthetic slow-wave activity slows to random bursts of electrical activity. Burst suppression can be achieved by rapid infusion of thiopental, propofol, or etomidate. Hypothermia has long been known to reduce brain metabolism (and to slow the EEG). Recently mild to moderate hypothermia (32.5–34°C) has been found to be more useful for intraoperative brain protection. Aside from the lack of adverse hemodynamic consequences, the metabolic suppression of lowered core temperature is more global than that of pharmacologic suppression, which affects only brain structures associated with electrical activity (as opposed to membrane integrity and cellular homeostasis). Production of excitatory neurotransmitters during reperfusion after transient ischemia also may be suppressed by modest hypothermia.

Much attention has been directed to suppression of the neuroexcitation that occurs after regional or global brain ischemia. Calcium influx into glial cells and vascular smooth muscle may be suppressed by calcium channel blockade, free radicals that are generated may be "scavenged" by mannitol, and increased intracellular hyperglycemia may be prevented by treating and avoiding systemic hyperglycemia. These approaches to protection from the secondary effects of ischemia generally have been incorporated into clinical practice. Blockade of neurotransmitter receptors as a means to protect the brain from ischemia continues to be investigated.

7. How is the choice of anesthetic agent made?
Choice of anesthesia for craniotomy is based on an understanding of the pharmacologic properties of hypnotic agents, inhalation agents, opioids, and muscle relaxants and on a balancing of beneficial and potentially adverse effects.

Hypnotic agents: Thiopental effectively blocks conscious awareness and reduces the functional activity of the brain and brain metabolism. Propofol has similar effects and is eliminated more rapidly. Etomidate and midazolam are only slightly less effective in metabolic suppression. An agent is selected on the basis of associated hemodynamic effects, anticipated difficulty of regaining consciousness, and cost.

Inhalation agents: The differences between halothane, isoflurane, and desflurane concerning metabolic suppression and cerebral blood flow are slight. All cause suppression of brain activity while preserving or enhancing cerebral blood flow. Cost and speed of elimination are concerns in selection. Although a craniotomy could be completed with only an inhalation agent as the anesthetic, this is not common practice.

Opioids: All opioids have negligible effects on cerebral blood flow and small effects on cerebral metabolism. Chiefly, they block adrenergic stimulation which increases brain activity. They are useful as part of a balanced anesthesia. More fat-soluble opioids, such as morphine and hydromorphone, may be eliminated so slowly that they cause respiratory depression after the procedure is completed. Respiratory depression that causes hypercarbia results in undesirable increases in cerebral blood flow and potentially increased intracranial pressure (ICP), which is to be avoided after a craniotomy. Newer synthetic opioids that are thought of as short-acting may also cause residual respiratory depression after infusion durations of 8 hours or more. If systemic blood pressure falls during rapid infusion of a "loading" dose of synthetic opioid, especially in the face of normocapnia, ICP may be increased and cerebral perfusion pressure may be decreased transiently. Thoughtful administration of the opioid preceded by hyperventilation avoids this problem.

Muscle relaxants: Depolarizing muscle relaxants are generally not used in the setting of intracranial pathology. Although theoretical hemodynamic differences exist among the nondepolarizing muscular relaxants, these are of little importance during a craniotomy. The main criteria for choosing a nondepolarizing muscular relaxant is the duration of neuromuscular blockade and the frequency at which the clinical relaxant effect can be monitored.

Whatever combination of anesthetic agents is chosen for a craniotomy, conditions for surgery are also controlled by physiologic manipulations. Blood pressure is maintained in a narrow range (15–20% below baseline) which is well within the autoregulated limits. By use of a combination of agents, the tendency of any one agent to attenuate autoregulatory responses and CO_2 responsiveness is avoided. Respiratory rate is increased to increase minute ventilation and lower $PaCO_2$. Further increases in ventilation can be used to induce hypocarbia to reduce cerebral blood flow. If regional vascular occlusion becomes necessary, $PaCO_2$ can be increased to encourage collateral blood flow. Finally, osmotic diuresis is used to decrease the amount of interstitial fluid of intact brain tissue to improve its tolerance for retractor positioning.

8. What are the concerns for patient positioning during a craniotomy?
Because craniotomies tend to be lengthy procedures, the protection of vulnerable peripheral nerves and pressure-prone areas from injury is essential. Provisions must be made to prevent prep solutions from entering the eyes. Generally, the head is fixed in position with pins clamped against the outer table of the skull. Because the head is held in a fixed position, any movement in reaction to tracheal stimulation will stress the cervical spine. Muscle paralysis must be maintained all the time the head is secured in the holding device.

In every craniotomy, the risk of air entrainment into the venous system must be estimated. Whenever the head is positioned 10 cm above the mid-thorax (> 20° elevation), a potential negative pressure exists between the venous sinuses of the head and the central venous system. Air entrained in the central venous system may collect in the right side of the heart and interfere with preload and pulmonary flow. Air can potentially cross the intraatrial septum and, if a patent foramen ovale is present (20% of patients), become a paradoxical air embolus to the systemic circulation. This risk is very significant in sitting-position craniotomies. End-tidal CO_2, end-tidal nitrogen, and precordial Doppler are sensitive indicators of venous air. In high-risk situations, a multiorificed right atrial catheter should be placed for removal of air bubbles.

9. Why do some patients awaken slowly after a craniotomy?
Continuous infusion of opioid as part of balanced anesthesia leads to prolonged redistribution and persistent sedation. Respiratory depression from residual opioid acts synergistically with residual potent inhalation anesthetic to cause slow awakening. Residual amounts of barbiturate induction agents may further aggravate the residual sedation. However, all these residual anesthetic effects are overcome simply by waiting and providing respiratory support. Slow awakening that persists for more than 2 hours is virtually never an effect of residual anesthesia. The patient who is unresponsive for several hours after a craniotomy should be evaluated for increased ICP or brainstem ischemia. Evaluation should be a joint effort of the neurosurgeon and anesthesiologist.

10. What anesthesia problems are unique to surgery on the intracranial blood vessels?
1. **Subarachnoid hemorrhage (SAH):** Aneurysms of the intracerebral arteries may be diagnosed after SAH. Neurologic impairment after SAH ranges from headache and stiff neck (stage I) to deep coma (stage V). Initial resuscitation includes observation, control of blood pressure to avoid hypertension, and support of intravascular volume (hypervolemic, hyperosmolar, normotensive). The optimal time for surgical clipping of the aneurysm is within the first few days of hemorrhage. After 5–7 days following SAH, the risk of rebleeding remains high, but the risk of vasospasm of the vessel feeding the aneurysm markedly increases due to irritation from the breakdown of old blood. Management of craniotomy for aneurysm during the first few days after SAH requires careful hemodynamic control to avoid significant increases or decreases from resting blood pressures. Invasive monitoring of arterial pressure and central venous pressure is required. The minimal approach to brain protection is to maintain mild hypothermia. Metabolic suppression by electroencephalographic burst suppression was used previously at the time of temporary vessel clipping but has since proved to result in poorer outcome when accompanied by hypotension.
2. **Rebleeding:** Approximately 30% of intracranial aneurysms that have bled will rebleed at some time if untreated. In the initial few days, the hydrodynamic forces on the aneurysm wall are the systolic blood pressure resisted by the tension of the aneurysmal wall. Larger aneurysms have less wall tension for any part of the aneurysmal surface. When the skull is open and the dura incised, the wall tension relationship changes. For the patient, rebleeding of the aneurysm prior to the opening of the dura is catastrophic, requiring the surgeon to approach the bleeding vessel blindly, perhaps temporarily clipping major feeding vessels. Although it might seem reasonable to induce hypotension during the opening of the dura, hypotension, should a rebleed occur, adversely affects regional perfusion and may promote vasospasm.
3. **Vasospasm:** Vasospasm can occur after any SAH, regardless of clinical stage. The end result of persistent vasospasm is ischemic stroke in the region of distribution of the aneurysmal artery, resulting in permanent neurologic damage after SAH. Diagnosis is by angiography, and many times an angiogram is requested on the first postoperative day to guide therapy. Maintaining hypervolemic normotensive hemodynamic status is the first line of prevention of vasospasm and should be maintained intraoperatively. Physiologically, vasospasm is caused by mediator release in the vascular smooth muscle in response to hemoglobin in the interstitium, ending in calcium influx into the cellular walls of the artery and causing persistent vasoconstriction. Calcium channel blockade has been advocated but has shown mixed results. Thromboplastin activators have been used experimentally by irrigation in the region of the aneurysmal bleed with some success. The main line of prevention is intraoperative irrigation of the hematoma early in SAH course and maintenance of favorable hemodynamics postoperatively.

11. Are there special anesthetic problems associated with brain tumors?

Malignant mass lesions of the brain cause problems for the anesthesiologist because of their size and location. Frontal tumors grow to large size without producing neurologic symptoms or increased ICP. Supratentorial tumors of the motor and sensory cortical regions present with seizures, localizing neurologic signs, and increased ICP. Posterior fossa masses in adults cause disturbances in gait, balance, proprioception, or cranial nerve impingement. There is a "penumbra" around all intracranial tumors where the adjacent brain loses autoregulatory function. Thus, on induction, regional blood flow in these areas may increase in response to aggressive fluid replacement or increased systolic blood pressure. After the resection is completed, this penumbra may respond to reperfusion with swelling. The end result may be either preincisional or postoperative increases in ICP. Infratentorial posterior fossa tumors cause particular problems for the anesthesiologist. Tumors are generally small but may surround complex vascular channels of the basilar, posterior communicating, and cerebellar arteries. Tumors may arise from the glia surrounding the cranial nerve roots or impinge on them. Simple dissection of a brainstem tumor can cause disturbance of heart rate and rhythm or blood pressure when nerve roots are retracted. The surgical approach to the posterior fossa involves awkward positioning, from sitting to lateral to prone to "park bench." At the least, any of these positions requires careful attention to the position of the endotracheal tube to avoid migration to an endobronchial position or out of the glottis. Venous air embolism must be anticipated. The plan for anesthesia must also allow for intraoperative monitoring of auditory-evoked potentials, somatosensory-evoked potentials or motor-evoked potentials if indicated. Any of these evoked potentials can be suppressed by hypnotic and inhaled anesthetic agents.

12. Are there other anesthetic concerns during craniotomies?

Transsphenoidal surgery, although not strictly a craniotomy, involves manipulation of ventilation to raise the $PaCO_2$ and ICP, which forces the pituitary into a more easily visualized position.

Rapidly deteriorating neurologic status after closed head injury often leads to emergency intubation, neuroradiologic studies, and emergent craniotomy. The increase in ICP that causes the clinical deterioration sometimes progresses to involve brainstem compression. The physiologic response to increased ICP is systemic hypertension and, in the late stages, bradycardia known as the Cushing reflex. This reflex should be anticipated and treated by measures to reduce ICP rather than pharmacologic treatment of the hypertension per se. Typically, when the cranium is opened and brainstem pressure is reduced, the blood pressure decreases, but if aggressive treatment of elevated blood pressure has been undertaken, the drop in blood pressure may have disastrous consequences.

Craniotomies in pediatric patients are, in principle, the same as in adults but fortunately more rare. The intracranial pathology that is most common in the pediatric group is the posterior fossa tumor, particularly cerebellar astrocytoma. Positioning, cranial nerve root stimulation, and venous air embolus are concerns during posterior fossa resections in children.

BIBLIOGRAPHY

1. Drummond JC: Brain protection during anesthesia. Anesthesiology 79:877–880, 1993.
2. From RP, Warner DS, Todd MM, Sokoll MD: Anesthesia for craniotomy: A double-blind comparison of alfentanil, fentanyl and sufentanil. Anesth Analg 73:896–904, 1990.
3. Hartung J, Cottrell JE: Mild hypothermia and cerebral metabolism. J Neurosurg Anesth 6:1–3, 1994.
4. Illievich UM, Petricek W, Schramm W, et al: Electroencephalographic burst suppression by propofol in humans: Hemodynamic consequences. Anesth Analg 77:155–160, 1993.
5. Lam AM, Mayberg TS: Anesthetic management of head trauma. In Lake CL, Rice LJ, Sperry RJ (eds): Advances in Anesthesia, vol. 12, St. Louis, Mosby, 1995, pp 333–339.
6. Marx W, Shaw N, Long C, et al: Sufentanil, alfentanil and fentanyl: Impact on cerebrospinal fluid pressure in patients with brain tumors. J Neurosurg Anesth 1:3–7, 1989.
7. Prough DS, Johnson JC, Stump DA: Effects of hypertonic saline versus lactated Ringer's on cerebral oxygen transport during resuscitation from hemorrhagic shock. J Neurosurg 64:627–632, 1986.
8. Smith M-L: Cerebral ischemia and brain protection. Curr Opin Anaesth 5:626–631, 1992.
9. Todd MM, Warner DS, Sokoll MD, et al: A prospective, comparative trial of three anesthetics for elective supratentorial craniotomy. Anesthesiology 78:1005–1020, 1993.
10. Young ML: Posterior fossa: Anesthetic considerations. In Cottrell JE, Smith DS (eds): Anesthesia and Neurosurgery. St. Louis, Mosby, 1994, pp 346–356.

79. TRANSURETHRAL RESECTION OF THE PROSTATE

Lyle E. Kirson, D.D.S.

1. What is transurethral resection of the prostate?

Transurethral resection of the prostate (TURP) involves the resection of benign hypertrophic prostatic tissue by means of a movable electrocautery/cutting wire loop located at the end of a resectoscope. The resectoscope is passed through a sheath that has been positioned within the patient's
urethra. As the surgical field is visualized through the resectoscope, the cutting wire loop is
moved back and forth, carving away a small piece of prostatic tissue each time the loop is withdrawn toward the surgeon. Simultaneously, an irrigating solution flows into the surgical site via a
channel in the resectoscope to distend the bladder and to bathe the surgical site, washing away
blood and tissue debris removed by the wire loop. Thus a clear operative field is maintained for
the surgeon.

2. Describe the anatomy of the prostate gland.

The prostate gland underlies the apex of the male bladder and surrounds the prostatic portion of
the urethra. The prostate is formed by enlargement of urethral glands. A fibrous sheath surrounds
the prostate, and the body of the gland consists of a fibromuscular stroma that envelops the glandular tissue. Venous drainage is via the thin-walled veins, or sinuses, of the prostatic plexus.

Although developmentally divisible into two lobes, the prostate gland is anatomically divisible into five lobes. The median and lateral two lobes of the prostate gland most frequently undergo benign prostatic hypertrophy. The nerve supply to the prostate derives from the prostatic
plexus, which originates from the inferior hypogastric (pelvic) plexus. Afferent pain fibers of
the prostate, urethra, and mucosa of the bladder originate primarily from sacral nerves 2, 3, and
4 (S_2, S_3, and S_4). Pain impulses from an overstretched bladder travel with sympathetic fibers
that have their origin in the twelfth thoracic and first and second lumbar nerves (T_{12}, L_1, and L_2).
Proprioceptive impulses from the muscular wall of the bladder, which are activated by stretching of the muscular wall as the bladder fills, are carried by the parasympathetic fibers of S_2, S_3,
and S_4.

3. What pathologic process is treated by TURP?

Benign prostatic hypertrophy is the most common tumor of the prostate and affects a high proportion of elderly men. The hyperplasia involves growth of both smooth muscle of the prostatic
urethra and glandular tissue. Some patients appear to have a preponderance of muscle tissue
growth, whereas others may tend toward glandular development. As the hyperplasia develops,
primarily in the lateral and middle lobes, (1) the urethral orifice narrows, and (2) the normal prostatic tissue becomes compressed against the outer fibrous capsule. The compressed normal prostatic tissue and sinuses may be referred to as the surgical capsule.

The goal of TURP is to remove the hyperplastic tissue while sparing the surgical capsule.
The hyperplastic tissue does not produce a smooth junction with the compressed normal prostatic
tissue but instead involves areas of the surgical capsule. It is therefore difficult to avoid some exposure of venous sinuses of the normal prostatic tissue during transurethral resection of the hyperplastic tissue.

4. What is the primary concern and complication associated with TURP?

The primary concern associated specifically with TURP is intravascular absorption of large
volumes of irrigating fluid during the procedure. The absorption occurs predominantly through

exposed venous sinuses of the surgical capsule. A spectrum of clinical and physiologic conditions results. The clinical manifestations brought about by intravascular fluid absorption are referred to as the TURP syndrome, and the degree of symptoms depends on the type, magnitude, and extent of absorbed fluid.

Several irrigants are currently in clinical use. All irrigants are nonelectrolyte solutions, and all but one are either isoosmolar or slightly hypoosmolar in make-up. Some symptoms of TURP syndrome (discussed below) may result from the specific make-up of the irrigating solution; however, the majority of symptoms are common to all irrigants and result from the acute intravascular fluid overload and/or hyponatremia.

As the fluid is absorbed, intravascular pressure increases, and proteins, as well as electrolytes, become diluted. The cumulative effect of increased intravascular pressure, decreased protein oncotic pressure, and decreased electrolyte concentration favors the movement of fluid from the vascular compartment into the interstitial spaces. Fluid moving out of the intravascular space produces edema in various tissue beds, including the pulmonary and cerebral beds. Decline in sodium and chloride levels results in electrolyte disturbances. Myocardial contractility may diminish, and conduction disturbances may arise in the face of vascular overload, electrolyte abnormalities, and cell edema. In addition, cerebrospinal fluid (CSF) pressure increases and electrolyte disturbances occur in the CSF.

5. What are the first signs and symptoms of TURP syndrome?

The anesthesiologist must recognize signs and symptoms of developing TURP syndrome. For the patient undergoing TURP with major conduction anesthesia (subarachnoid block or epidural block), the first sign has been described classically as restlessness and mental confusion. However, presentation of symptoms is variable, and the syndrome may manifest initially in other ways, such as nausea, vomiting, dizziness, headache, unresponsiveness, or transient visual changes. Other symptoms associated with hemodynamic instability may be the first indication of a developing problem, especially in patients under general anesthesia. Signs and symptoms may include hypertension, hypotension, heart rate changes, cardiac arrhythmias, pulmonary edema, or cyanosis.

Whereas it is the responsibility of the anesthesiologist to recognize symptoms, it is the responsibility of the surgeon to notify the anesthesiologist of problems that may be evident from a surgical perspective. Excessive bleeding, deep cuts, and visualization of sinuses are signs of an increased potential for development of TURP syndrome. The anesthesiologist should take note when a surgeon states, "Let's give him a little Lasix." The surgeon has recognized that conditions may be appropriate for excessive fluid absorption.

6. Why is isoosmolar solution used for irrigation?

The irrigating solution originally used for TURP was distilled water. It was quickly recognized, however, that patients who absorbed a significant amount of distilled water developed intravascular hemolysis due to a decrease in serum osmolarity. In addition to hemolysis were signs and symptoms of (1) water intoxication and (2) renal failure, resulting from hemoglobin precipitation in the renal tubules. For these reasons, distilled water was all but abandoned as an irrigant; isoosmolar or slightly hypoosmolar irrigating solutions were developed (normal serum osmolality = 280–300 mOsml/kg).

7. Normal saline, an isoelectric solution, seems to be the safest irrigant. Why is normal saline irrigation not used for TURP?

Only nonelectrolyte solutions can be used for irrigation during TURP. Electrolyte solutions are avoided to minimize the dispersion of current throughout the bladder when electrocautery is used. Dissemination of electrocautery current would be uncomfortable for the patient and dangerous to both patient and surgeon. After completion of surgery and before the patient is moved to the postanesthesia care unit, however, bladder irrigation should be changed to normal saline. Because fluid absorption from continuous bladder irrigation may continue in the postoperative period, eliminating nonelectrolyte solutions reduces the risk of postoperative hyponatremia.

8. Is more than one type of irrigation available for TURP?

Yes. Below is a list of available irrigants for TURP.

Distilled Water. The danger of using distilled water as an irrigating solution is discussed above (see question 6). A few centers, however, still use it because it provides excellent optical qualities during resection (pH: 5.0–7.0).

Sorbitol (3% or 3.3%). Sorbitol, a nontoxic isomer of mannitol, is rapidly metabolized to 70% carbon dioxide and 30% dextrose. A small portion is excreted by the kidneys. Sorbitol at this concentration is nonhemolytic. It has a calculated osmolarity of 165 mOsml/L (pH: 5.0–7.0).

Resectisol (Mannitol 5%). Resectisol, a 5% solution of mannitol, is the only isoosmolar irrigating solution (275 mOsml/L). Mannitol is not metabolized and relies on elimination solely through renal excretion. Because resectisol is not metabolized, large intravascular volume expansion may result in cardiac decompensation if large amounts of the irrigant are absorbed (pH: 4.5–7.0).

Cytal. Cytal, a 3% solution of sorbitol and mannitol, is an attempt to combine the best qualities of both agents. The calculated osmolarity is 178 mOsml/L. Metabolism of the absorbed sorbitol portion reduces the potential for vascular overload (pH: 4.9).

Glycine. Glycine is an amino acid constituted in a 1.5% solution. The osmolarity of the solution is 200 mOsml/L. Although glycine is excreted to some extent by the kidneys, it is also metabolized to ammonia by the liver. Among the more disturbing features of glycine are the temporary visual changes (including blindness) associated with its absorption. Whether such visual changes result from the glycine itself, cortical edema, or ammonia intoxication remains unknown (pH: 4.5–6.5).

9. When is TURP syndrome likely to occur?

The time to onset of TURP syndrome depends on numerous factors, including the experience of the surgeon, the surgeon's aggressiveness with the electrocutting loop, the pathology of the gland, and the amount of tissue removed. The incidence of morbidity increases as resection time exceeds 60 minutes, and for many years it was believed that TURP syndrome was unlikely during the first hour of resection. We now recognize that TURP syndrome can develop more rapidly.

The patient is not free of risk once the resection is completed. If the integrity of the prostatic capsule or wall of the bladder is violated during surgery, irrigating fluid may be sequestered in the intraperitoneal and extraperitoneal space during resection. The fluid may be absorbed into the intravascular space during the postoperative period and result in intravascular fluid overload and symptoms of TURP syndrome.

10. What is the treatment for TURP syndrome?

Treatment of TURP syndrome should begin the moment the problem is recognized.

1. Terminate surgery as quickly as possible and switch to normal saline for continuous bladder irrigation. Be sure that the irrigation is warm, as all bladder irrigation should be, to prevent the development of hypothermia.

2. Support ventilation as needed and obtain the following baseline laboratory tests: complete blood count, platelet count, electrolytes, and clotting studies if a bleeding problem is suspected. Prothrombin time, partial thromboplastin time, and fibrinogen level should be included in the coagulopathy work-up.

3. Administration of intravenous normal saline and diuretics may be all that is needed to correct the problem. Administer furosemide, 20 mg, intravenously. If the patient is on chronic diuretics, a dose of 40 mg or more may be required, but dosing should be based on the diuresis obtained initially from 20 mg. Maintain intravascular volume with normal saline as diuresis progresses.

4. If the patient demonstrates significant effects from hyponatremia, intravenous administration of hypertonic saline may be appropriate (see question 11). Our protocol restricts the use of hypertonic saline to patients who have developed central seizures or cardiac dysfunction.

5. Consider placement of a central venous catheter to guide fluid replacement during the immediate postoperative period.

6. If hemodynamic instability develops, consider placement of an arterial catheter and pulmonary artery catheter to aid in resuscitation.

7. Monitor the serum potassium level. Patients frequently become hypokalemic as diuresis occurs.

8. Reassure patients that any symptoms, especially visual changes, are only temporary and that their symptoms will dissipate as their condition improves.

11. Why not replace sodium deficit with hypertonic saline in patients suffering from TURP syndrome?

The use of hypertonic saline for correction of hyponatremia associated with TURP syndrome should be restricted to patients demonstrating significant symptoms, namely, central seizures or cardiac dysfunction due to electrolyte imbalance. If hypertonic saline is chosen for fluid replacement, close attention must be paid to the patient's electrolyte and intravascular fluid status. The patient has not lost sodium; he has gained water. Excessive administration of hypertonic saline results in additional fluid overload and complicates an already difficult management problem. Hypertonic saline should be administered through a central line at a rate no greater than 100 ml/hr.

12. Is it possible to calculate how much irrigating fluid has been absorbed?

The amount of irrigating solution absorbed can be estimated by comparing sodium levels at any time during the procedure with levels at the start of the procedure. ECF = extracellular fluid.

Volume absorbed = (preoperative serum sodium/postoperative serum sodium × ECF) – ECF

Example: A 70-kg man undergoes transurethral resection of the prostate under subarachnoid block (spinal anesthetic). After 50 minutes of resection, he complains of headache and appears somewhat disoriented. The procedure is immediately terminated, and a blood sample is sent to the laboratory for electrolyte analysis. The patient's preoperative serum sodium concentration was 142 mEq/L compared with the immediate postoperative value of 106 mEq/L. If the patient has an extracellular fluid compartment of approximately 20% of body weight, his extracellular fluid volume at the start of the procedure was about 14 liters ($0.20 \times 70 = 14$ L). Using the above formula, $(142/106) \times 14$ L = 18.75 L. Subtracting his initial extracellular volume of 14 L from the postoperative extracellular volume of 18.75 L yields an absorption of 4.75 L. This figure represents a minimal volume of absorption, because any fluid that has shifted into the intracellular space is lost in the calculation.

A more accurate technique for calculating fluid absorption is to add a trace amount of ethanol to the irrigating solution and then to monitor and quantify the amount of ethanol that the patient expires. This technique is complex and requires special instrumentation.

13. What can be done to minimize the risk of developing TURP syndrome?

1. The patient must be prepared properly for surgery. Preparation should include adequate hydration, electrolyte analysis, and coagulation profile. Patients who are debilitated and demonstrate poor reserve benefit from the placement of hemodynamic monitors for preoperative assessment and treatment as well as for intraoperative monitoring.

2. The most important step in minimizing the risk of TURP syndrome is to limit the duration of surgery. Because fluid can be absorbed at a rate greater than 50 ml/min, it is possible to place nearly 3 L of fluid into the intravascular and interstitial spaces within 1 hour of resection time. Limit resection time to 1 hour or less.

3. The hydrostatic pressure created by the fluid irrigating the surgical site must be minimized. Because the irrigating fluid flows by gravity, the bag of irrigation should not hang higher than 60 cm above the operative field.

4. The surgeon should limit the extent of bladder distention created by the irrigant. Frequent drainage of the bladder by the surgeon reduces the amount of irrigant absorbed.

5. Careful surgical resection minimizes exposure of the venous sinuses and preserves the capsule of the prostate.

6. Blood pressure must be stable. A decrease in pressure lowers the periprostatic venous pressure and allows increased absorption of fluid.

14. How difficult is it to estimate blood loss during TURP?

It is very difficult to estimate true blood loss during TURP because of the mixing of irrigating solution with shed blood and the manner in which the irrigant/blood mixture is discarded (frequently directly into a drain). One way to calculate true blood loss is to collect all of the irrigant/blood mixture and to measure its hematocrit:

(Hematocrit of irrigant × volume of irrigant)/starting hematocrit = blood loss

Example: A 70-kg man undergoes transurethral resection of the prostate under general anesthesia. His starting hematocrit is 40%. Two liters of irrigant are used and collected during resection. A sample of the irrigant/blood mixture spun in a centrifuge reveals a hematocrit of 5%. Using the above formula: (0.05 × 2000 ml)/0.40 = 250 ml blood loss.

15. Is there a preferred anesthetic technique for TURP?

Because early recognition of the TURP syndrome is paramount in preventing significant sequelae, the anesthetic technique that lends itself to early recognition is the optimal choice. Spinal or epidural anesthesia in a patient who has received minimal sedation allows early detection of various signs and symptoms of the syndrome, especially changes in mental status (see question 5). For this reason, most clinicians agree that regional anesthesia, if not contraindicated for a particular patient, is the technique of choice for TURP.

16. What level of spinal anesthetic is required for TURP?

A spinal anesthetic with a T12 sensory level is sufficient to eliminate pain associated with resection of hypertrophied prostatic tissue as well as discomfort due to bladder distention (see question 2). It is possible, however, to perform TURP with an anesthetic level involving only the sacral nerves. In such a situation, the surgeon needs to evacuate irrigant from the bladder frequently to avoid bladder distention and the resulting discomfort.

17. What other complications are associated with TURP?

Perforation of the bladder during TURP may occur because of the proximity of the surgical site to the bladder wall (see question 9). Diagnosing bladder perforation is difficult. Symptoms may include abdominal pain, respiratory compromise, and a tense abdominal wall. If the patient has received a spinal anesthetic, abdominal pain may not become evident until the anesthetic level begins to recede. In such patients and in patients receiving a general anesthetic, difficulty in breathing or an unexplained change in airway pressure may be the first indication of bladder perforation. As fluid accumulates in the intraperitoneal cavity, abdominal compliance decreases and movement of the diaphragm becomes limited. The result is respiratory compromise. Diagnosis of bladder perforation can be confirmed by obtaining a cystogram. The sequestration of irrigating fluid into the intraperitoneal and extraperitoneal space through bladder perforation is frequently self-limiting and normally requires no treatment.

Intraoperative and postoperative hemorrhage has been associated with TURP. Bleeding may occur by several mechanisms, and it is the clinician's responsibility to identify the cause.

Thrombocytopenia may develop and produce a coagulopathy. Thrombocytopenia may be secondary to a dilutional effect from irrigant absorption or to excessive blood loss. The diagnosis of dilutional thrombocytopenia is based on platelet count, serum sodium, and hematocrit. If these indices are low in the presence of normal or elevated central venous pressure or pulmonary capillary wedge pressure, the diagnosis is dilutional thrombocytopenia secondary to irrigant absorption. Diuresis alone may correct the problem. A low platelet count and hematocrit, with a normal serum sodium level and a normal or low central venous pressure or pulmonary capillary wedge pressure, indicate thrombocytopenia secondary to blood loss. Platelet transfusion may be appropriate in this setting.

Coagulopathy may develop secondary to fibrinolysis. Tissue thromboplastin and urokinase are released from the prostate during resection and may initiate either primary or secondary fibrinolysis. The treatment for primary fibrinolysis is administration of epsilon-aminocaproic acid (EACA). EACA, however, is contraindicated in patients with secondary fibrinolysis (disseminated intravascular coagulation). Therefore, a coagulation pathologist can be very helpful in distinguishing and treating these conditions.

Late complications associated with TURP include secondary bladder neck contracture, secondary urethral stricture, and incontinence.

18. How uncomfortable are patients after TURP? What can be done to minimize their discomfort?

Postoperative pain is thought to be due primarily to the development of a surgically induced reflex arc that results in uninhibited detrusor contraction and pain, often termed bladder spasm. Current analgesic methods directed toward minimizing spasm include suppositories containing belladonna and opium.

19. What other modalities are available for postoperative pain control?

Oral and parenteral administration of narcotics is, of course, useful in controlling postoperative pain. Intrathecal narcotics also may be used. A small dose of intrathecal morphine administered concomitantly with a spinal anesthetic results in significant postoperative analgesia, even in low doses (0.1 mg) that may be inadequate for blocking pain associated with other surgical procedures. The manner in which intrathecal morphine eliminates pain associated with TURP probably involves elimination at the spinal level, via spinal opioid receptor mechanisms, of the surgically induced reflex arc and bladder spasm.

20. What alternative surgical procedures are available for the treatment of benign prostatic hypertrophy?

Open surgical procedures can be used for removal of benign hypertrophied tissue of the prostate. The choice of procedure depends on (1) surgeon preference and (2) known or presumed associated pathology. Any one of the following procedures is indicated when the amount of hypertrophied tissue is too great to remove by transurethral resection. The **transvesical or suprapubic procedure** approaches the prostate gland through the cavity of the bladder. The **retropubic approach** is through the prostatic capsule; the bladder is not opened. The **perineal prostatectomy** is used infrequently but may be indicated in obese, high-risk patients who present with a large intraurethral, hypertrophied gland.

Several transurethral procedures may have less morbidity than TURP or open surgical approaches. **Microwave-induced hyperthermic necrosis** of hypertrophic tissue and **transurethral ultrasound-guided laser-induced prostatectomy** (TULIP) are relatively new transurethral procedures currently gaining greater popularity.

An alternative to removal of hypertrophied tissue is **transurethral incision of the prostate** (TUIP). TUIP involves making one or more endoscopic-guided incisions in the bladder neck and hypertrophic tissue. This procedure is indicated only in prostate glands that have undergone minimal hyperplasia.

BIBLIOGRAPHY

1. Azar I: The transurethral prostatectomy syndrome. In Moya F (ed): Current Reviews in Clinical Anesthesia. Miami Lakes, Current Reviews, 1987, pp 167–171.
2. Defalque RJ, Miller DW: Visual disturbances during transurethral resection of the prostate. Can Anaesth Soc J 22:620–621, 1975.
3. Hahn RG, Ekengren JC: Patterns of irrigating fluid absorption during transurethral resection of the prostate as indicated by ethanol. J Urol 149:502–506, 1993.

4. Hoekstra PT, Kahnoski R, McCamish MA, et al: Transurethral prostatic resection syndrome—a new perspective: Encephalopathy with associated hyperammonemia. J Urol 130:704–707, 1983.
5. Kirson LE, Goldman JM: Low-dose intrathecal morphine for postoperative pain control in patients undergoing transurethral resection of the prostate. Anesthesiology 71:192–195, 1989.
6. Leadbetter GW Jr, Vinson RK: Urology. In Nardi GL, Zuidema GD (eds): Surgery. Boston, Little, Brown, 1982, pp 1015–1052.
7. Liu WS, Wong KC: Anesthesia for genitourinary surgery. In Barash PG, Cullen BF, Stoelting RK (eds): Clinical Anesthesia. Philadelphia, J.B. Lippincott, 1989, pp 1105–1115.
8. Maluf NSR, Boren JS, Brandes GE: Absorption of irrigating solution and associated changes upon transurethral electroresection of prostate. J Urol 75:824–836, 1956.
9. Nanninga JE, O'Conor VJ Jr: Suprapubic and retropubic prostatectomy. In Walsh PC, Gittes RF, Perlmutter AD, Stamey TA (eds): Campbell's Urology. Philadelphia, W.B. Saunders, 1986, pp 2739–2753.
10. Ovassapian A, Joshi CW, Brunner EA: Visual disturbances: An unusual symptom of transurethral prostatic resection reaction. Anesthesiology 57:332–334, 1982.
11. Takahashi S, Homma Y, Minowada S, Aso Y: Transurethral ultrasound-guided laser-induced prostatectomy (TULIP) for benign prostatic hyperplasia: Clinical utility at one-year follow-up and imaging analysis. Urology 43:802–807, 1994.
12. Yerushalmi A, Fishelovitz Y, Singer D, et al: Localized deep microwave hyperthermia in the treatment of poor operative-risk patients with benign prostatic hyperplasia. J Urol 133:873–876, 1985.

80. ANESTHETIC CONSIDERATIONS FOR LASER SURGERY

J. Todd Nilson, M.D.

1. Discuss the origins of lasers.

Einstein first conceptualized lasers in 1917; however, the first laser was not built until 1960. Lasers were not used in the operating room until about 1970.

2. What is a laser?

Laser = **l**ight **a**mplification by **s**timulated **e**mission of **r**adiation. Lasers produce coherent light, a source of light that does not occur naturally. To produce coherent light, atoms, ions, or molecules are stimulated by an energy source. The stimulated medium spontaneously radiates energy in the form of light. The radiated light is then amplified and emitted as the laser beam. Laser light has three defining characteristics:

- **Coherence**—all waves are in phase, both in time and in space.
- **Collimation**—the waves travel in parallel directions.
- **Monochromaticit**y—all waves have the same wavelength.

3. Why do surgeons use lasers?

Lasers are very precise, with minimal dissipation of damaging heat and energy to surrounding tissues. Depending on the type of laser, it is preferentially absorbed by different types of tissues. In addition, controversial issues of faster healing and fewer infections are associated with their use.

4. What makes lasers behave differently from one another?

Wavelength depends on the lasing medium (the atoms stimulated). The longer the wavelength, the more strongly it is absorbed, thus, the power of the light is converted to heat in shallower tissues. Conversely, the shorter the wavelength, the more scattered the light; therefore the light is converted to heat in deeper tissues. For example, carbon dioxide (CO_2) laser has a longer wavelength and is absorbed almost entirely at the tissue surface. As a result, precise excision of superficial lesions is possible. Conversely, Nd:YAG laser (neodymium:yttrium-aluminum-garnet) has a shorter wavelength and therefore deeper penetration. It is good for heating large tissue masses and debulking tumor.

Characteristics of Lasers Commonly Used in the Operating Room

LASER TYPE	WAVELENGTH	ABSORBER	TYPICAL APPLICATIONS
CO_2	10,600 Invisible (far infrared)	All tissues, water	General, precise surgical cutting
Nd:YAG	1,064 Invisible (near infrared)	Darkly pigmented tissues	General coagulation (via fiberoptics), tumor debulking
Nd:YAG-KTP (neodymium:yttrium-aluminum-garnet:potassium-titanate-phosphate)	532 Visible (emerald green)	Blood	General, pigmented lesions
Argon	488–514 Visible (blue-green)	Melanin, hemoglobin	Vascular, pigmented lesions
Krypton	400–700 Visible (blue-red)	Melanin	General, pigmented lesions

479

Power density (irradiance) is the energy delivered per unit area of cross-section. Power density is usually measured as watts/cm^2. Coherent light is focused into small spots of very high power density that can cut or vaporize tissue. Lower power density is used for coagulation.

Other factors that contribute to the effects of laser light at a given anatomic location include the length of time that laser contacts skin, the amount of circulating blood that cools the tissue, and the specific heat and thermal conductivity of various tissues.

5. What are the hazards of lasers?

Atmospheric contamination (particularly common in surgery for laryngeal papillomas). The vaporization of tissue and dispersion of diseased particulate matter is a hazard for all operating room personnel. The smoke produced by vaporization of tissues with lasers may be mutagenic, transmit infectious diseases, and cause acute bronchial inflammation.

Fire and explosion. Laser beam contact with flammable materials such as anesthetic gas tubing, surgical drapes, and sponges may cause fires or explosion. Endotracheal tube fires have an estimated incidence of 0.5–1.5%. Fires result in minimal or no harm to the patient if the situation is handled swiftly but may be catastrophic if not (see question 10).

Embolism. Although rare, a venous gas embolism may occur during laparoscopic surgery or hysteroscopy. Reported cases have been associated primarily with Nd-YAG lasers, in which coolant gases circulate at the probe tips. The gas from the probe tips caused embolism in the reported cases.

Inappropriate energy transfer. Laser light vaporizes whatever tissue lies in its path. Precise aim by the surgeon and a cooperative (well-anesthetized, paralyzed) patient are mandatory. In addition, laser light is easily reflected by surgical instruments and may be hazardous to all OR personnel. Laser contact with the eyes is of particular concern, because it may impair vision or cause blindness. The nature of ocular damage depends on the wavelength of the laser light. For example, CO_2 lasers cause corneal opacification, whereas Nd:YAG lasers cause damage to the retina.

Perforation. Misdirected laser energy may perforate a viscus or large blood vessel. Laser-induced pneumothorax after laryngeal surgery also has been reported. Sometimes the perforations do not occur until several days after surgery when edema and tissue necrosis are at a maximum.

6. What are the preoperative considerations for the use of lasers in airway surgery?

Airway evaluation. Assess the adequacy of the airway by evaluating the degree of obstruction, adequacy of ventilation, and feasibility of direct laryngoscopy and intubation. The quality of the patient's voice and ventilatory pattern are good indicators of the degree of obstruction. Preoperative imaging (CT, MRI) and fiberoptic examination often are helpful in assessing the degree of airway compromise.

Preparation of proper intubating instruments. Once the extent of airway obstruction is determined and the method of intubation is planned, availability and preparation of the proper intubation equipment are essential.

Premedication. Antisialogogues (glycopyrolate, atropine) help to reduce secretions and to maximize visualization of the airway during intubation and during surgery. Preoperative sedatives and opioids should **not** be administered to patients with severe obstruction, because sedation may cause total airway obstruction.

7. What is the best technique for anesthetic induction in a patient undergoing airway surgery?

In patients in whom the airway is likely to collapse after induction, an awake intubation should be strongly considered. In conscious patients with obstructive airway lesions, tracheal intubation is best performed over a fiberoptic endoscope; blind intubation may cause tissue edema or trauma and further obstruction of the airway. Sometimes awake tracheotomy is needed to secure an adequate airway before induction. When airway obstruction is mild and laryngoscopy and intubation appear feasible, preoxygenation and intravenous administration of a rapid-induction agent and succinylcholine are performed to secure intubation as quickly as possible. Regardless of whether awake or postinduction intubation is planned, a surgeon capable of emergent tracheotomy should be present during induction. Equipment for emergent cricothyrotomy also should be readily available.

8. What are the intraoperative considerations for laser surgery of the airway?

Upper airway lesions. In laser resection of upper airway lesions, tracheal intubation is optional. Techniques that do not involve an endotracheal tube allow better visualization of the operative field by the surgeon and also remove potentially flammable materials from the airway.

Lower airway lesions. Lower airway lesions are accessed via rigid bronchoscope or fiberoptically. The CO_2 laser beam is directed at the lesion via a rigid metal bronchoscope, coated with a matte finish to reduce reflected laser light. Ventilation is accomplished through the side arm of the bronchoscope, using saline-soaked gauze to form a seal around the bronchoscope. Jet ventilation (see question 9) is another option. If the lesion is to be accessed fiberoptically (e.g., lower tracheal and bronchial lesions), the Nd:YAG laser is required, because it can travel through fiberoptic cables, whereas the CO_2 laser cannot.

9. What ventilation techniques are commonly used in laser surgery of the airway?

Jet ventilation. In this technique the surgeon aims a high-velocity jet of O_2 at the airway opening. The high flow of O_2 entrains room air as a result of the Venturi effect, thus ventilating the lungs with a high volume of O_2-air mixture. Ventilation is accomplished by attaching a metal Fraser-tipped suction catheter to wall O_2 and a Sanderson-type jet injector. This apparatus is mounted to the operating laryngoscope. Sometimes the mass of the airway lesion makes this method impossible. If the jet stream is not aimed in the trachea, gastric dilatation may occur. Barotrauma to the airway and subsequent pneumothorax are also risks and may in turn lead to mediastinal or subcutaneous air.

Spontaneous ventilation. Allowing the patient to inhale volatile agents via the operating laryngoscope is also an option, although it is not feasible for some procedures. It is difficult to control the depth of anesthesia during spontaneous ventilation, and it is often necessary to paralyze the patient during many airway procedures. Of note, however, hypoventilation, hypercarbia, and aspiration (surgical debris, secretions, vomitus, and smoke) are additional complications related to both jet and spontaneous ventilation.

Endotracheal intubation. This method allows excellent ventilation and airway protection of the anesthetized patient but often obscures the operative field and puts flammable materials in the path of the laser beam.

- Flammability studies have shown that of the available pliable tubes (polyvinyl chloride [PVC], red rubber, silicone), PVC tubes are the least flammable.
- Some authors advocate wrapping the ET tube with metal tape; however, this method limits the tube's pliability and increases the risk of a reflected laser beam and loss of metal tape fragments in the trachea.
- Others advocate using a PVC endotracheal tube with an O_2/helium mixture to deliver the anesthetic agent, thus reducing flammability. Helium has a high thermal diffusivity and decreases the heat of materials in laser contact. Nitrous oxide is not used in the same fashion, because it has a much lower thermal diffusivity and supports combustion.

10. Describe the correct management of airway fires.

Two strategies minimize the potential hazard of an airway fire: (1) reduce the flammability of the airway by decreasing the O_2 concentration and covering potentially flammable tissue with wet lap sponges, and (2) remove flammable materials (such as endotracheal tubes) from the airway by using metallic Venturi jet ventilation cannulas or by ventilating with intermittent extubation.

Airway fire protocol
1. Stop ventilation.
2. Disconnect the O_2 source, remove the endotracheal tube, and flood the surgical field with saline.
3. Mask-ventilate the patient with 100% O_2, then reintubate.
4. Perform rigid laryngoscopy and bronchoscopy (using Venturi jet ventilation) to assess the damage and remove debris.
5. Monitor the patient for 24 hours.
6. Use short-term steroids.
7. Continue ventilatory support and antibiotics as needed.

BIBLIOGRAPHY

1. Geffin B, Shapshay SM, Bellack GS, et al: Flammability of endotracheal tubes during Nd-YAG laser application in the airway. Anesthesiology 65:511–515, 1986.
2. Pashayan AG: Anesthesia for laser surgery. ASA Refresher Course 215–225, 1989.
3. Pashayan AG, Gavenstein JS: Helium retards endotracheal tube fires from carbon dioxide lasers. Anesthesiology 62:274–277, 1985.
4. Rampil IJ: Anesthetic considerations for laser surgery. Anesth Analg 74:424–435, 1992.
5. Rampil IJ: Anesthesia for laser surgery. In Miller RD (ed): Anesthesia. New York, Churchill Livingstone, 1994, pp 2197–2211.
6. Van der spek AFL, Spargo PM, Norton ML: The physics of lasers and implications for their use during airway surgery. Br J Anaesth 60:709–729, 1988.
7. Wolf GL, Simpson JI: Flammability of endotracheal tubes in oxygen and nitrous oxide enriched atmosphere. Anesthesiology 67:236–239, 1987.

81. ANESTHESIA FOR ELECTROCONVULSIVE THERAPY

Steven J. Stein, M.D., and Kevin Fitzpatrick, M.D.

1. What is the historical background of electroconvulsive therapy?

Ladislas von Meduna, a Hungarian neuropsychiatrist and pathologist, erroneously believed that schizophrenia and epilepsy were mutually antagonistic and that the symptoms of schizophrenia were ameliorated by generalized seizures. In 1934 he successfully treated a catatonic man through chemically induced epileptic fits. Electrically induced seizures, first performed in 1937, are the only form of electroconvulsive therapy (ECT) used presently. Early ECTs did not involve the use of sedatives, analgesics, muscle relaxants, supplemental oxygen, or ventilation. Indeed, awareness and cyanosis were believed to be therapeutic and thus were encouraged.

2. What are the main indications for ECT?

The primary role of ECT is treatment of major depressive disorders associated with psychotic features. As many as 90% of psychotically depressed patients respond to ECT. Occasionally, ECT is used to treat nonchronic schizophrenia, mania, and catatonia unresponsive to drug therapy.

3. Describe the preanesthetic management of patients scheduled for ECT.

A preanesthetic visit with the patient and chart review are essential for administering anesthesia for ECT. Compassionate reassurance and prudent explanation of risks, benefits, and reasonable expectations of events before and after the procedure allay fears and misconceptions. The preoperative history and physical examination should concentrate on the cardiopulmonary and central nervous systems in addition to careful evaluation of the airway. In particular, the presence of hypertension, coronary artery disease, and elevated intracranial pressure must be assessed (see questions 12, 13, and 14).

4. How is anesthesia for ECT performed?

ECT is not usually performed in the operating room. However, it is often done in close proximity; for example, in the postoperative anesthesia care unit (PACU). The patient is placed on a gurney, and an intravenous infusion is started. Monitors are placed, and 100% oxygen is given by face mask. The induction agent is administered, followed by a muscle relaxant. At this point the anesthesiologist must assume control of the patient's airway via mask ventilation. The psychiatrist applies the electroshock after the muscle relaxant has taken effect, and the seizure is monitored, both centrally and peripherally (see question 6). The anesthetist continues ventilatory support until the patient is able to take control. Parameters such as vital signs and adequacy of oxygenation and ventilation must be carefully observed until the patient has safely emerged from the general anesthetic.

5. What are the requirements for monitoring the anesthetized patient during ECT?

Standard monitors include continuous electrocardiography, noninvasive blood pressure, pulse oximetry, and precordial stethoscope. Equipment and medications appropriate for full cardiopulmonary resuscitation must be readily available, including oral airways, styletted endotracheal tubes, laryngoscopes, suction, and emergency drugs (e.g., atropine, phenylephrine, ephedrine, beta blockers). The vast majority of patients do not require endotracheal intubation.

6. How is seizure activity monitored?

Centrally, an electroencephalogram (EEG) monitors the duration of the seizure. **Peripherally**, an arm or foot is isolated from the circulation with a tourniquet before injection of the muscle relaxant. Once the electroshock has been delivered, the ensuing hand or foot movement is used as an indicator of seizure duration.

7. Describe the characteristics of the seizure evoked by ECT.
The electrical stimulus is applied via electrodes that are usually fixed to the scalp by a headband. Bilateral ECT requires electrode placement over each cerebral hemisphere, whereas with unilateral ECT both electrodes are placed over a single hemisphere. The electroshock produces a grand mal seizure by acting on the cerebral cortex. A **latent period** of 2–3 seconds is followed first by a **tonic phase** of 10–12 seconds, then by a **clonic phase** lasting 30–50 seconds.

8. What are the typical electroencephalographic findings during ECT?
The EEG shows a build-up of alpha and beta rhythmic activity during the tonic phase, which is followed by repetitive polyphasic spikes and wave complexes in the clonic phase, synchronous with the clonic movements. The electrical seizure (central) always lasts longer than the clonic manifestation (peripheral).

9. Does the duration of seizure affect the therapeutic efficacy?
Most definitely. In current practice, a series of 8–12 treatments is administered at a rate of 2–3 treatments per week. It has been reported that seizures < 30 seconds in duration are not clinically effective. The cumulative seizure time over several treatments must also be noted. Cumulative seizure duration of < 210 seconds is without benefit; cumulative seizure duration of > 1000 seconds demonstrates no additional improvement in symptoms. However, many patients have had a full remission with 100 seconds of total seizure time. A 500-mg dose of intravenous caffeine is often given just before the induction of anesthesia to prolong the seizure. It is important to recognize that over the course of several treatments seizure threshold tends to increase.

10. Discuss the various induction agents used for ECT.
Methohexital (Brevital), a barbiturate, is the most commonly used induction agent. As with all barbiturates, methohexital decreases seizure duration and raises seizure threshold. Paradoxically, methohexital has been noted to induce seizures in adults and children with temporal lobe epilepsy.

Thiopental, another barbiturate, seems to offer no unique advantage over methohexital. Compared with methohexital, thiopental has a slower onset and longer duration of action. However, the incidence of hiccups, muscle twitching, and excessive salivation is lower with thiopental.

Diazepam (Valium), like thiopental, increases the seizure threshold and shortens seizure duration. Its slow onset and delayed recovery make it a poor choice.

Ketamine is the only intravenous induction agent that has been shown to increase seizure duration in both humans and animals. Unfortunately, its slow onset of action, prolonged recovery time, and association with a greater incidence of nausea and ataxia after ECT preclude its general use.

Etomidate has been used to induce general anesthesia for ECT, but it is associated with involuntary muscle movement, increased muscular tone, and longer recovery time.

Propofol has recently been shown to attenuate the hypertensive response to ECT compared with methohexital (see question 12). However, it is also associated with a shorter seizure duration. Finally, propofol in fact may behave as an anticonvulsant.

Alfentanil, a potent synthetic opioid, does not affect seizure threshold. It may substitute for a barbiturate in patients who have decreasing seizure duration over a series of ECT treatments.

11. What is the rationale for adding a muscle relaxant to the anesthetic regimen?
The violent muscular contractions accompanying the seizure may lead to skeletal injury, including vertebral fractures. Addition of succinylcholine essentially negates this risk. A bite block is placed to protect the teeth and tongue from masseter muscle contraction (which occurs even with the use of muscle relaxants) due to direct stimulation.

12. How does ECT affect the autonomic nervous system?

A **parasympathetic discharge** immediately after application of the current (coincident with the tonic phase of seizure activity) is followed seconds later by a **sympathetic surge** (coincident with the clonic phase). This parasympathetic–sympathetic sequence may cause an initial brady-cardia or even asystole, followed by tachycardia, dysrhythmias, and hypertension. Less than 1 minute after the seizure, plasma epinephrine concentrations increase about 15-fold and plasma norepinephrine 3-fold. The generalized increase in oxygen demand and pronounced sympathetic activity may result in myocardial ischemia or even infarction in patients with coronary artery disease.

13. How does ECT affect the cerebrovascular system?

An initial brief period of cerebral vasoconstriction after the electrical stimulus is followed by a sustained increase in cerebral blood flow (up to 7 times baseline) and a 400% increase in cerebral metabolism. The resulting increase in intracranial pressure (ICP) may be of concern in patients with intracranial mass lesions, vascular anomalies, or elevated ICP of any origin.

14. What can be done to treat the sympathetic response to ECT?

Labetalol (a mixed alpha and beta receptor antagonist), esmolol (a beta$_1$ selective receptor antag-onist), and fentanyl (a potent opioid) are commonly used to attenuate the sympathetic response to ECT. Clonidine (a centrally active alpha$_2$ agonist), phenoxybenzamine (an alpha receptor blocker), and trimethaphan (a ganglionic blocking agent) also have been used successfully. Nitroglycerin (a nitrate compound like nitroprusside) is an effective venodilating agent with anti-hypertensive properties.

15. How do oxygenation and ventilation affect the duration of the seizure?

Aggressive ventilation by mask after anesthetic induction and before application of the elec-troshock may increase seizure duration. This beneficial effect is associated with both oxygena-tion and hypocapnia. Conversely, hypoxemia and hypercapnia shorten seizure duration.

16. List the strong and moderate contraindications to ECT.

As with any decision-making process in medicine, the risks and benefits must be carefully con-sidered for each patient. In the case of ECT, the risks of a general anesthetic and seizure must be weighed against the benefits of potential freedom from disabling severe depression.

Strong contraindications
- Recent myocardial infarction (< 3 months)
- Recent cerebrovascular accident (< 3 months)
- Intracranial mass lesion (with or without changes in ICP)
- High risk for aspiration

Moderate contraindications
- Angina pectoris
- Congestive heart failure
- Cardiac pacemakers
- Pheochromocytoma (risk of malignant pressor crisis)
- Glaucoma (ECT elevates intraocular pressure)
- Retinal detachment
- Severe osteoporosis
- Major bone fractures
- Thrombophlebitis
- Severe acute and chronic pulmonary disease
- Pregnancy (theoretical risk of fetal hypoxemia)— fetal monitoring is essential

17. What are the anesthetic considerations for tricyclic antidepressants (TCAs), monoamine oxidase inhibitors (MAOIs), and lithium?

TCAs. Patients scheduled for ECT are frequently taking psychotropic agents. TCAs (e.g., imipramine, noripramine) are structurally related to phenothiazines and block the reuptake of norepinephrine and serotonin into presynaptic nerve terminals. The pressor response to direct-acting sympathomimetics is increased many-fold in patients taking TCAs; therefore, drugs such as phenylephrine must be administered with caution.

MAOIs. Monoamine oxidase selectively deaminates amine neurotransmitters (norepinephrine, epinephrine, dopamine, and serotonin) by oxidation. Blocking this enzyme causes accumulation of amine neurotransmitters in nerve terminals. Like TCAs, MAOIs may precipitate hypertensive crises when given in conjunction with direct or indirect sympathomimetics. Therefore, it is recommended that MAOIs be discontinued 2 weeks brefore starting ECT. Examples of MAOIs include deprenyl, isocarboxazid, phenelzine, and tranylcypromine. Both TCAs and MAOIs augment the effects of barbiturates, increasing sleep time and duration of anesthesia. Hence, lower doses of barbiturates should be used if patients are taking either of these medications.

Lithium. Lithium carbonate is occasionally used in the treatment of recurrent depression. It is associated with prolonged recovery when used in conjunction with barbiturates. In addition, it may prolong the duration of action of succinylcholine.

18. What are frequent side effects of ECT?

Muscle aches, headaches, and memory disturbances tend to be the most common side effects. Headaches may be treated with opioids. Both retrograde and anterograde amnesia may occur. The most common long-term side effect of ECT is memory disturbance, which usually improves with time and is insignificant after 6 months. In addition, many patients emerge from the anesthetic highly agitated. Agitation is treated first by reassurance and periodic reorientation of the patient. Judicious administration of midazolam or lorazepam may be indicated. Status epilepticus is a rare complication of ECT and may be treated with barbiturates, benzodiazepines, or phenytoin (Dilantin). Vertebral and long-bone fractures have not been reported since 1976. The overall mortality associated with ECT is very low—on the order of 1 in 28,000 treatments. Dysrhythmias, myocardial infarction, congestive heart failure, and cardiac arrest are the most frequent causes of death.

BIBLIOGRAPHY

1. Consensus Conference: ECT. JAMA 254:2103, 1985.
2. Gaines GY, Rees DI: Electroconvulsive therapy and anesthetic considerations. Anesth Analg 65:1345–1346, 1986.
3. Jones R, Knight P: Cardiovascular and hormonal responses to ECT. Anaesthesia 36:795, 1981.
4. Maletsky BM: Seizure duration and clinical effect in electroconvulsive therapy. Compr Psychiatry 19:541–550, 1978.
5. McPherson R, Lipsey J. Electroconvulsive therapy. In Rodgers M (ed): Current Practices in Anesthesiology. Philadelphia, B.C. Decker, 1990, pp 180–185.
6. Pitts FN, Woodruff RA, Craig AG, Rich CL: The drug modification of ECT. Part 2: Succinylcholine dosage. Arch Gen Psychiatry 19:595–598, 1968.
7. Selvin BL: Electroconvulsive therapy—1987. Anesthesiology 67:367–385, 1987.

X. Pain Management

82. ACUTE PAIN MANAGEMENT

Robin B. Slover, M.D., and Rose A. Gates, R.N., M.S.N.

1. Define acute pain.
Pain is defined as "an unpleasant sensory and emotional experience associated with actual or potential tissue damage, or described in terms of such damage." Acute pain refers to pain of short duration (< 6 weeks), usually associated with surgery, trauma, or an acute illness. Acute pain differs from chronic pain because (1) its cause is usually known; (2) it is usually temporary and located in the area of trauma or damage; and (3) it resolves spontaneously with healing.

2. Why has acute pain been undertreated?
Acute pain has been undertreated for various reasons. Training in appropriate pain assessment, and appropriate medication choices has been minimal for most health care providers. In addition, the risks associated with the use of opioids or narcotics (the most commonly used analgesics)—such as respiratory depression and addiction—are perceived as much higher than in fact they are. The fact that poorly treated pain may result in higher morbidity and mortality rates has become appreciated only recently.

3. How is pain assessed?
Pain is a subjective experience; no machine can measure pain. Changes in vital signs such as blood pressure or pulse rate correlate poorly with the degree of pain control. The only person who can determine the presence and degree of pain is the patient. However, the magnitude of pain and the response to treatment can be monitored in several ways. A scale of 10 faces, ranging from very happy to very sad, can be used in young children.

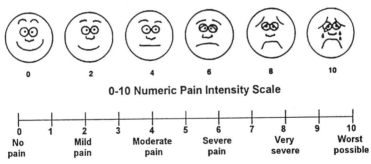

Pain scales for children and adults. (From Wong D, Whaley L: Clinical Manual of Pediatric Nursing. St. Louis, Mosby-YearBook, 1990, with permission.)

The child points to the face matching the way he or she feels. Similar scales using color (from blue for minimal pain through violet hues to bright red for maximal pain) or numbers (from zero for no pain through ten for maximal pain) have been devised for adults. A visual analog scale uses a 10-cm line on which the patient marks a point corresponding to the amount of pain. Verbal descriptive scales, such as the McGill pain questionnaire, are useful both for clinical and research purposes. Functional ability is also a useful measure of pain. In some patients, especially those who also have chronic pain, function may be more useful than pain scores. For example, in assessing a patient with chronic pancreatitis who always gives a 10/10 pain score, one can monitor the number of times the patient spontaneously leaves the room to smoke. On days with very bad pain, spontaneous activity is likely to be curtailed. In addition to documenting the current pain scale at rest, pain should also be measured during activity. The activity score may be a more sensitive measure of efficacy of pain control, because it is easier to control pain at rest. The pain scale can be used to ensure that an intervention, such as an increased dose of analgesia, is effective in decreasing the patient's pain.

4. What medications are useful in treating acute pain?

The medications useful in treating acute pain are similar to those used in treating other types of pain. The World Health Organization (WHO) analgesic ladder developed for treating patients with cancer pain also provides a useful approach to treating acute pain. At the lowest level (mild pain), nonopioid analgesics such as nonsteroidal antiinflammatory agents (NSAIDs) (e.g., ibuprofen or acetaminophen) are useful. Such drugs have an analgesic ceiling; above a certain dose, no further analgesia is expected. For moderate pain, compounds combining acetaminophen or aspirin with an opioid are useful. The inclusion of acetaminophen limits the amount of such agents that should be used within a 24-hour period, because toxic accumulations can occur. For severe levels of pain, an opioid such as morphine or hydromorphone is a better choice; such opioids have no analgesic ceiling. Most postoperative or trauma patients initially respond better to a morphine-equivalent opioid. By the time the patient is eating and ready for discharge, opioid-acetaminophen agents or NSAIDs are often adequate.

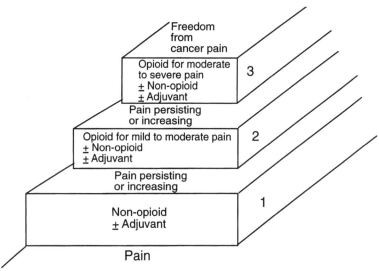

Analgesic ladder. (From Cancer pain relief and palliative care: Report of a WHO Expert Committee. Geneva, World Health Organization, 1990. Technical Report Series, No. 804, Fig. 1, with permission.)

Not all types of pain respond equally to the same medication. Opioid analgesics are helpful in controlling somatic or visceral pain. Bone pain may be helped partially by opioids. However, NSAIDs and steroids are highly effective in treating bone pain. The combination of NSAIDs and opioids is synergistic in controlling pain. Neuropathic pain, often described as pain with a burning, hyperesthetic quality, responds to a diverse group of drugs, including antidepressants (amitriptyline), anticonvulsants (carbamazepine or clonazepam), antiarrhythmics (mexiletine), baclofen, and alpha-adrenergic agonists (clonidine). Recommended regimens are listed below. Opioids may also be helpful. Frequently, pain control is improved after 1–2 days of using adjuvant drugs. Alternate medications may also help to control somatic or visceral pain. Drugs that control pain by different mechanisms may be synergistic when used together (such as NSAIDs and opioids). By using lower doses of two different agents, the patient may have good pain control with fewer side effects.

Adjuvant Drug Doses

DRUG	INITIAL DOSE	MAXIMUM DOSE
Baclofen	10 mg	40–80 mg
Clonazepam	0.5 mg	2–3 mg
Carbamazepine	100 mg twice daily	Blood level Therapeutic range
Amitriptyline	10–25 mg	100–200 mg
Clonidine patch	0.1 mg	0.1–0.3 mg
Mexiletine	150 mg twice daily	600–750 mg

5. What is the risk of addiction with opioids?
Addiction (or psychological dependence) needs to be differentiated from physical dependence. Physical dependence, a physiologic adaptation of the body to the presence of an opioid, develops in all patients maintained on opioids for a period of several weeks. If the opioid is stopped abruptly without tapering, the patient may show signs of withdrawal. The patient can stop opioids at any time and by tapering down avoids withdrawal symptoms. Tolerance is the need for a higher dose of opioid to produce the same pharmacologic effect. Neither physical dependence nor tolerance indicates addiction. The psychological dependence seen with addiction is characterized by a compulsive behavior pattern involved in acquiring opioids for nonmedical psychic effects as opposed to pain relief. The risk of iatrogenic addiction is very low; several studies have shown it to be less than 0.1%. Patients who are inadequately treated may seem to be drug-seeking, because they repeatedly request opioids and are concerned with the timing of their next dose. Such "pseudoaddiction" may mimic addictive behavior but is due to inadequate pain treatment. This iatrogenic condition can be avoided by listening to the patient and carefully assessing his or her pain. With proper doses of pain medication, pseudoaddiction disappears.

6. How should opioids be given? Are some opioids better than others?
Opioids can be given in various ways. Oral administration is usually the easiest and least expensive. Tablets should be provided on a schedule (e.g., oxycodone/acetaminophen tablets every 4 hours) rather than on an "as needed" (prn) or "as requested" basis. Many studies have shown that prn schedules usually provide only 25% of the maximal possible daily dose of opioids, despite the patient's repeated requests. If a patient cannot take medication orally, opioids can be administered intramuscularly, intravenously, (including patient-controlled analgesia [PCA] pumps), subcutaneously, rectally, transdermally, epidurally, intrathecally, and through buccal mucosa. Because PCA pumps are safe and effective, they are often used when the patient cannot take oral medication.

The opioids usually given parenterally include morphine, meperidine, and hydromorphone. Meperidine has the highest incidence of allergic reactions; in addition, its first metabolite, normeperidine, can accumulate and cause central nervous system excitation, including seizures. Normeperidine accumulation is dose-dependant and more common in patients with renal impairment. Normeperidine seizures are rare with intramuscular meperidine, because the amount of medication is small and given as needed. However, with the larger doses available through a PCA pump, more cases of normeperidine seizures have been reported. Morphine has an active metabolite—morphine-6-glucuronide—that is analgesic and has a longer half-life than morphine. This metabolite can be useful in many cases, because it allows a slow, sustained increase in analgesia. However, in patients with decreased renal function, the accumulation of an active metabolite may lead to increased side effects, including increased risk of respiratory depression. Fentanyl acts more rapidly than morphine or meperidine and has no active metabolites. It is a safer choice for patients with impaired renal or liver function. Hydromorphone also has no active metabolites. It is 5 times as potent as morphine and less dysphoric; however, its onset of action and duration are more similar to morphine than fentanyl.

7. How should a PCA pump be set?
Several decisions must be made in setting up a PCA pump. The first is what drug to use. As discussed above, the most commonly used agents are morphine and hydromorphone. The use of meperidine has decreased significantly over the last 5 years because of the risk of seizures from normeperidine. Fentanyl also can be used, particularly in patients with end-organ failure. Morphine comes prepackaged in a 1-mg/ml concentration; because hydromorphone is 5 times as potent, a 0.2-mg/ml concentration is equivalent. After choosing the drug, a decision should be made about the type of infusion: increment dosing only, basal (continuous) and incremental dosing, or incremental dosing with a basal dose only at night (between 10 p.m. and 6 a.m.) to help the patient sleep. Studies have shown no significant benefit to a basal rate, although anecdotally patients prefer a basal rate at night to help them sleep. Finally, the length of the lock-out period needs to be determined. Lock-out refers to the time between actual delivery of opioid doses; for example, if a 6-minute lock-out period is selected, the patient cannot receive opioid doses closer than 6 minutes apart, regardless of how often he or she activates the PCA pump. The lock-out period should be short enough to allow the patient to titrate the opioid level but long enough to allow the patient to feel the effect of one dose before delivering another. The usual lock-out ranges are 6–10 minutes.

PCA Opioid Guidelines for Acute Pain (Adults)

OPIOID	BASAL DOSE (AFTER LOADING)	INCREMENT DOSE	USUAL LOCK-OUT (MIN)
Morphine 1.0 mg/ml	1.0 mg	1.0–2.0 mg	6–10
Hydromorphone 0.2 mg/ml	0.2 mg	0.2–0.4 mg	6–10
Fentanyl 10–25 mcg/ml	10–25 μg	10–50 μg	6–10

8. What are common side effects of opioids? How are they treated?
The common side effects of opioids are sedation, pruritus, nausea and vomiting, urinary retention, and respiratory depression. In patients who have taken opioids previously, the risk of respiratory depression and sedation is less. Pruritus is treated by applying lotion to the affected area, by intravenous or oral delivery of diphenhydramine (25–50 mg) and, in severe cases, by using an opioid antagonist or agonist-antagonist (e.g., nalbuphine, 5 mg every 6 hours). Propofol, 10 mg every 6 hours, is also effective. Urinary retention is treated by urinary catheter drainage or nalbuphine. Nausea and vomiting respond to a decrease in opioid dose (elimination of a basal rate), nalbuphine, and antiemetics. Ondansetron, 4 mg intravenously, has proved to be a much more effective antiemetic than droperidol. Respiratory depression is treated by using an antagonist (naloxone) or agonist-antagonist (nalbuphine).

9. How do peridural opioids work?
Opioid receptors are present in levels I and II of the substantia gelatinosa of the dorsal horn. Opioids given either intrathecally or epidurally bind to these receptors. The dose of morphine can be decreased to 10% of the usual intravenous dose when given epidurally and to 1% when given intrathecally.

Approximate Equinalgesic Conversions of Morphine among Routes of Administration

PARENTERAL	EPIDURAL	SUBARACHNOID
100	10	1

The clinical behavior of the opioid can be predicted by its lipid solubility. Highly lipid-soluble opioids, such as fentanyl, pass through membranes and bind quickly. Fentanyl has a rapid onset, short duration, and limited spread. Morphine, which is highly hydrophilic, moves through membranes more slowly and has a slower onset but longer duration, because it stays suspended in solution and is released slowly to bind to the opioid receptors. Because of its poor lipid solubility, it spreads throughout the entire length of the spinal fluid and can help to control pain from several different anatomic sites. The termination of clinical activity of peridural opioids is due to vascular absorption and breakdown. Local anesthetics, such as lidocaine and bupivacaine, can be used alone or in combination with opioids (0.05–0.1% bupivacaine is used to minimize motor block).

Epidural Opioids

DRUG	ONSET (MIN)	DURATION (HR)	NUMBER OF DERMATOMES COVERED	SINGLE DOSE	INFUSION RATE
Morphine	60	12–24	All	2–5 mg	0.05–0.01 mg/ml 0.5–1.0 mg/hr
Hydromorphone	45	6–10	10–12	200–300μg	10–30 μg/ml 100–300 μg/hr
Fentanyl	5–10	3–5	5–6	50–100 μg	1–5 μg/ml 10–50 μg/hr

10. How do agonist-antagonists differ from opioids such as morphine?

Mu, delta, and kappa opioid receptors have been identified in the central nervous system. Most morphine equivalent opioids are primarily mu agonists, with some delta and kappa effect. Agonist-antagonists are mu antagonists and kappa agonists. Because kappa receptors provide weaker analgesia, agonist-antagonists are adequate for mild-to-moderate pain, whereas mu agonists are adequate for moderate-to-severe pain.

11. How should patients with epidural analgesia or PCA pumps be monitored?

Patients receiving analgesia do not need elaborate monitoring equipment. Pulse oximetry can be used if there is any question of oxygen saturation, but usually nurses are able to monitor patients safely by checking respiratory rate every hour and level of sedation every hour the patient is awake. Vital signs are taken as scheduled.

Monitoring Guidelines for Acute Pain Patients

Any additional narcotics/sedatives must be authorized by the pain service before they are administered to a patient with an epidural catheter.

Respiratory rate every 1 h × 4 h, then every 2 h × 16 after the initial dose of epidural narcotic; then every 4 h as long as epidural medications are administered:

If respiratory rate is 6–7 breaths per minute, call anesthesia pain resident.

If respiratory rate is less than 5 breaths per minute, administer naloxone, 0.2 mg (½ ampule) by intravenous push, and oxygen by mask at 6 L/min. Call anesthesia resident immediately. Arouse patient and encourage patient to breathe.

Sedation scale every 1 h × 4 h, then every 2 hr × 8 h, then every 4 h as long as epidural medications are administered.

Sedation scale: 1 = wide awake; 2 = drowsy; 3 = sleeping, arousable; 4 = difficult to arouse; 5 = not able to awaken

12. How is an oral agent chosen for a patient who preveiously received intravenous opioids?
Choice of an oral agent should be based on how much pain the patient still has and how much opioid was needed to control the pain. Opioid-acetaminophen compounds are adequate for patients whose pain required 0–2 mg/h of morphine. Hydrocodone/acetaminophen is a milder analgesic than oxycodone/acetaminophen and is useful for patients who require minimal opioids. An equal analgesic dosing chart can be used to select equivalent levels of analgesics.

Equianalgesic Doses

ANALGESIC	EQUIANALGESIC DOSES		DOSE INTERVAL (HR)
	PARENTERAL (MG)	ORAL (MG)	
Opioid agonist			
Morphine	10	30–60	3–6
Slow-release morphine	—	30–60	8–12
Hydromorphone (Dilaudid)	1.5	7.5	3–5
Fentanyl (Sublimaze, Innovar)	0.1	—	0.5–1
Transdermal fentanyl (Duragesic)	—	—	72
Levorphanol (Levo-Dromoran)	2	4	3–6
Meperidine (Demerol)	75	300	3–4
Methadone (Dolophine)	10	20	4–6
Oxycodone	—	30	3–6
Codeine	130	200	3–6
Hydrocodone	—	30	3–4
Agonist-Antagonist			
Nalbuphine (Nubain)	10	—	3–6
Butorphanol (Stadol)	2	—	3–4

Oral Drugs Approximately Equianalgesic to Aspirin (650 mg)

Codeine	50 mg	Propoxyphene	65 mg
Hydrocodone	5 mg	Acetaminophen	650 mg
Meperidine	50 mg	Ibuprofen	200 mg
Oxycodone	5 mg	Naproxen	275 mg

13. Which nonsteroidal antiinflammatory drug (NSAID) should be used?
If the patient can take oral medication, an oral agent should be used. Most oral agents have the same degree of analgesia as antiinflammatory activity. The degree of potency of analgesia parallels the risk of gastric upset with oral agents. Agents such as etodolac and nabumetone reportedly have a decreased risk of gastric upset. The number of doses needed per day also varies. Epironicam and oxaprozin are once-a-day agents. One or two specific agents may work better for a given patient, but their identification is usually a matter of trial and error. Price also may be a factor. Older NSAIDs that are off patent may be significantly cheaper and just as effective (e.g., naproxen, indomethacin, and ibuprofen).

For patients who cannot take oral medication, parenteral ketorolac is the available option. Ketorolac has a more potent analgesic than anti-inflammatory effect. It may be given intravenously (IV) or intramuscularly (IM). The dose for most patients is 30 mg IV or IM every 6 hours. For a single dose for outpatients, 30 mg IV or 60 mg IM should be used. In patients who are over 65 years old, who weigh under 100 pounds, or who are frail, 15 mg every 6 hours should be used. In patients with a creatinine ≥ 1.3 or renal failure, the use of ketorolac should be carefully considered.

The side effects of NSAIDs may be observed with either oral or parenteral use. Patients who have active gastric disease, who are anticoagulated or hypovolemic, or who have a history of triad asthma, congestive heart failure, or renal disease may have complications from NSAID use.

14. What other techniques can be used for acute pain management?

In addition to PCA pumps and epidurals, intrathecal narcotics can be used, especially if spinal anesthesia is used for the procedure. Preservative-free morphine can be used for inpatients and fentanyl for outpatients. Morphine doses of 0.1–0.3 mg are adequate for many lower extremity, urologic, and gynecologic procedures and have a minimal risk of respiratory depression. For thoracic procedures, higher doses are needed (0.3–0.75 mg) and involve a risk of respiratory depression. Fentanyl also can be used intrathecally; 10–15 µg of intrathecal fentanyl are equal to 0.1–0.3 µg of intrathecal morphine. Because fentanyl is more lipid-soluble than morphine, it does not spread as far but still may be given through lumbar spinal injection.

Other types of blocks can be useful. Intercostal blocks decrease pain and improve ventilation in patients with rib fractures or flail chests. Continuous brachial plexus blocks increase blood flow in patients with collagen vascular diseases or arterial spasm (Beuzer's disease) and patients who have digital reattachment, improving healing as well as providing good pain control.

15. How does good management of acute pain make a difference?

Pain is a form of stress and produces elevation in stress hormones and catecholamines. Good pain management has been shown to result in shorter hospital stays, improved mortality rates (especially in patients with less physiologic reserve, such as those in the intensive care unit), better immune function, less catabolism and endocrine derangements, and fewer complications. In addition, specific benefits have been shown for patients undergoing specific procedures. Patients who undergo amputation under a regional block with local anesthetic have a decreased incidence of phantom pain. Patients in whom a vascular graft is placed have a lower rate of thrombosis. A decreased mortality rate has been shown in patients with flail chests who have epidural analgesia.

Recent studies have shown the value of preemptive analgesia in some surgical situations. The blockade of the pathways involved in pain transmission before surgical stimulation may decrease the patient's postoperative pain. Local infiltration along the site of skin incision in patients having inguinal hernia repairs with general anesthesia is beneficial if the infiltration is done before the skin incision. Several studies using intravenous or epidural opiates in patients having thoracotomies and hysterectomies have also shown a preemptive effect. The use of local anesthetic with spinal and epidural anesthetics has not been shown to be preemptive. Nonsteroidal antiinflammatory drugs have not shown a preemptive effect. Further studies with larger patient groups are needed to provide definitive answers regarding preemptive analgesia.

Proper pain management not only keeps patients more comfortable; it also may decrease the risk of morbidity and mortality, thus improving utilization of health resources.

BIBLIOGRAPHY

1. Acute Pain Management: Operative or Medical Procedures and Trauma.. Clinical Practice Guideline. AHCPR Pub. No. 92-0032. Washington, DC, U.S. Department of Health and Human Services, 1992.
2. American Pain Society: Principles of Analgesic Use in the Treatment of Acute Pain and Cancer Pain, 3r ed. Skokie, IL, American Pain Society, 1992.
3. American Society of Regional Anesthesia: Comprehensive Review of Pain Management. American Society of Regional Anesthesia, 1994.
4. Batra MS (ed): Adjuvants in epidural and spinal anesthesia. Anesthesiol Clin North Am 10:13–30, 1992.
5. Goresky GV, Klassen K, Waters JH: Postoperative pain management for children. Anesthesiol Clin North Am 9:801–820, 1991.
6. Hannallah RS: Regional anesthesia. Anesthesiol Clin North Am 9:837–848, 1991.
7. Lubenow TR, McCarthy RJ, Ivankovich AD: Management of acute postoperative pain. Clin Anesth Updates 3:801–820, 1992.
8. McQuay HJ: Do preemptive treatments provide better pain control? In Gebhard GF, Hammond DC, Jensen TS (eds): Proceedings of the 7th World Congress on Pain. Seattle, IASP Press, 1993, pp 709–723.
9. Sinatra RS, Hord AH, Ginsberg B, Preble LM: Acute Pain Mechanisms and Management. St. Louis, Mosby, 1992.
10. Yaster M, Nicholas E, Maxwell LG: Opioids in pediatric anesthesai and in the management of childhood pain. Anesthesiol Clin North Am 9:745–762, 1991.

83. CHRONIC PAIN

Jose M. Angel, M.D.

1. How does normal pain perception occur?

1. A noxious stimulus causes stimulation of nociceptors (pain receptors) in the receptor organ (e.g., skin).

2. This stimulation leads to activation of cells in the dorsal horn of the spinal cord and transmission of the nerve impulse to the midbrain and cortex.

3. Transmission of sensory information is modulated (inhibited or potentiated) throughout the nervous system by neurons from the midbrain and spinal cord that release endogenous opioids, catecholamines, and other neurotransmitters.

4. Peripheral nociceptor sensitization (i.e., transmission of impulses at subnormal thresholds) occurs following release of chemical mediators (e.g., prostaglandins, leukotrienes) at the site of injury.

5. Continued stimulation by peripheral nociceptors then leads to sensitization of neurons in the spinal cord.

2. Define chronic pain.

Chronic pain is that which persists beyond the normal duration of recovery from an acute injury or disease. Chronic pain may also be due to an ongoing or intermittent disease. Although a thorough workup may reveal the presence of obvious pathology, sometimes no identifiable cause is found. Whether or not such a cause is determined, a chronic painful condition commonly also affects the patient's self-image and sense of well-being.

3. Discuss the causes of chronic pain.

Different chronic pain syndromes may involve different mechanisms. When there is clear pathophysiology, the source of pain is thought to be the constant stimulation of pain receptors, i.e., **chronic nociception**. This happens in chronic diseases such as rheumatoid arthritis or migraine headaches. The disease process may also cause a malfunction of the nervous system itself, i.e., **neuropathic pain**. A persistent pain state may follow peripheral nerve damage if there is neuroma formation (following nerve transection) or increased afferent activity (following nerve compression). Chronic neuropathic pain may also result from ongoing peripheral nociceptor input causing changes in spinal cord sensory neurons. These changes may involve increased spontaneous activity of spinal neurons or loss of inhibitory spinal neurons. When chronic pain does not have an obvious cause, other etiologies such as psychological causes must be considered.

4. How can the pain clinic help in the diagnosis of patients with chronic pain?

The pain clinic evaluation involves a multidisciplinary approach that includes anesthesiologists, neurologists, physiatrists, neurosurgeons, psychologists, and physical therapists. In addition to the history and physical examination, the diagnosis of a specific pain syndrome requires a review of available radiologic data, bone scans, and electromyographic studies. Diagnostic tests such as nerve blocks and intravenous drug infusions are also critical for an optimal evaluation.

5. Are psychological factors important in the diagnosis and therapy of chronic pain?

Because of the chronic nature of their symptoms, many aspects of patients' lives may have been profoundly affected. Often, there is associated depression, sleep disturbances, anger, and other psychological effects of chronic illness. There may also be general physical deterioration and weight gain or loss. In addition, secondary gain issues, such as a pending litigation or the need for social attention, may reinforce pain behavior and adversely affect recovery. Furthermore, some evidence suggests a higher incidence of prior physical or sexual abuse among chronic pain patients than that of the general population. All these factors must be investigated and addressed by the staff and patient to maximize the patient's chances for improvement.

6. How are nerve blocks helpful in the treatment of chronic pain?

1. **Diagnosis:** Pain relief following a series of nerve blocks can help to identify the nerve site causing the symptoms.

2. **Therapy:** Nerve blocks eliminate or reduce pain symptoms temporarily. In certain situations (e.g., sympathetically maintained pain), nerve blocks may be used in conjunction with other therapies to treat the overall pain problem.

3. **Prognosis:** Nerve blocks can help determine whether more invasive and potentially irreversible therapies, such as neurolysis or surgical neurectomy, are appropriate and amenable to the patient.

7. What is the prognosis for someone who develops back pain?

Most people experience back pain at some point in their lives; however, approximately 85% of patients recover within 2 weeks to 3 months with conservative therapy (e.g., nonsteroidal anti-inflammatory drugs, physical therapy). No known effective therapy exists for back pain that persists for more than 3 months. The prognosis is worse with increased duration of symptoms, with lower socioeconomic status, and with pending litigation.

8. Name the possible causes of chronic back pain.

Back pain (confined to the spinal and paraspinal areas) may be due to pathologic changes in the lumbar vertebrae, muscles, and nerves. These changes may result from congenital or degenerative disease, surgery, or trauma. For example, degenerative disease may lead to spinal stenosis, in which narrowing of the spinal canal or the spinal foramina causes impingement on the nerve roots. Intervertebral facet joint degeneration may also cause low back pain. Chronic pain may also result from muscle spasms owing to repetitive strain or poor posture.

9. How can pain of muscular origin be a factor in chronic pain in general and chronic back pain in particular?

Muscle fibers may become a source of localized chronic pain due to initial sprain/strain injuries or underlying bone or joint disease. It has been hypothesized that a muscle area with initial spasm may develop vasoconstriction and tissue hypoxia, which would then result in pain and tenderness. This leads to further spasm and continued vasoconstriction and hypoxia. Digital pressure over specific muscle areas, known as trigger points, causes worsening and spreading of the pain to other parts of the muscle. Therapy for this syndrome, known as myofascial pain, comprises a combination of trigger point injections and physical therapy. In chronic back pain, the lumbar paraspinal muscles and quadratus lumborum are common sites where trigger points are found.

10. Are there other causes of chronic pain of muscular origin?

Fibromyalgia presents as a diffuse bilateral muscular tenderness involving the upper and lower body and without clear trigger points. Proposed causes include intrinsic muscle cell abnormalities, changes in neurotransmitter levels, chronic sleep disruption, and changes in immune system function. Therapy with tricyclic antidepressants, muscle relaxants, physical therapy, and biofeedback, and behavioral therapy may improve symptoms significantly.

11. A patient presents with unilateral leg pain associated with a corresponding bulging or protruding herniated disc and without evidence of a neurologic deficit. Discuss treatment.

These symptoms are consistent with a radicular syndrome. The patient, however, does not present with symptoms that warrant surgical intervention. In addition to nonsteroidal anti-inflammatory drugs, the patient may benefit from a trial of lumbar epidural steroids. A series of three injections is given as close as possible to the affected root, usually 2–3 weeks apart.

12. Discuss the rationale behind the use of epidural steroids for the treatment of a radiculopathy (pain associated with a herniated disc).
Radiculopathy may be due to mechanical nerve root compression by a herniated disc; this is usually associated with a clear neurologic deficit and can be confirmed with neuroradiologic studies. Such a presentation may require surgical decompression. In some patients with radicular symptoms, however, no nerve root compression can be shown. Animal studies suggest that a ruptured disc can release substances (prostaglandin derivatives) that, in minute concentrations, cause nerve root irritation and pain. Steroids are known to be effective anti-inflammatory agents, and they have been shown in experimental animals to decrease transmission along c-fibers, which are involved in pain transmission. In addition, numerous clinical reports and some double-blind, randomized studies suggest that patients may benefit from epidural steroid therapy. Further studies are needed to determine fully the value of epidural steroids in the treatment of radicular pain. Nevertheless, this therapy remains a useful, low-risk alternative in the treatment of this syndrome.

13. Define sympathetically maintained pain (SMP).
SMP is a chronic pain associated with localized dysfunction of the sympathetic nervous system. SMP may, therefore, be considered a subset of neuropathic pain. The pain usually involves an extremity and is described as a burning sensation. In severe cases, it may be associated with other vasomotor, musculoskeletal, and neurologic changes, which may manifest as:
- A cold extremity with edema
- Muscle atrophy
- Bone resorption
- Brittle nails
- Hypersensitivity to touch or temperature

14. Does a history of severe trauma make SMP more likely to occur?
Patients with SMP usually, although not always, report a history of trauma. The severity of the injury, however, does not always correlate with the likelihood of developing symptoms. For example, SMP may develop following an ankle sprain, thrombophlebitis, or a myocardial infarction. The cause is unknown, but it may result from damage to mixed peripheral nerves (containing motor, sensory, and sympathetic fibers) that leads to aberrant function of the sympathetic nervous system.

15. What is the mechanism of SMP?
Several hypotheses, not mutually exclusive, have been proposed:
1. Damaged afferent fibers in peripheral nerves become hypersensitive to norepinephrine released from sympathetic fibers.
2. Damage to a peripheral nerve leads to abnormal healing with formation of synapses between sensory and sympathetic fibers (ephaptic transmission).
3. A hyperactive sympathetic system eventually leads to sensitization of spinal cord neurons.
The common pathway may be increased sensory fiber sensitivity to, or hyperactivity of, the sympathetic nervous system leading to pain perception in the absence of noxious stimuli. The $alpha_1$-receptor may, therefore, be important in this type of pain. Finally, it has also been proposed that over time, changes induced in the central nervous system may become irreversible, leading to a sympathetically independent pain state.

16. Why are nerve blocks useful in the treatment of SMP?
Isolated blockade of sympathetic nerves can help diagnose whether the pain symptoms are due solely or partially to a dysfunction of the sympathetic nervous system. Moreover, if the patient's pain improves after a series of diagnostic blocks, further sympathetic blockade is indicated in combination with physical therapy. This type of nerve blockade can be achieved by injection of local anesthesia in the cervical and lumbar paravertebral areas, where the sympathetic ganglia are

located. Because of the deep location of the sympathetic ganglia, performance of these blocks often requires fluoroscopic guidance to maximize success and decrease risk. The specific nerve block is chosen based on the location of the patient's pain:

Appropriate Nerve Blocks for Sympathetically Maintained Pain

PAINFUL AREA	SYMPATHETIC INNERVATION	APPROXIMATE NERVE BLOCK LOCATION
Head, neck, upper extremity	Cervicothoracic ganglia (including stellate ganglia)	Transverse process of C-6 vertebra
Chest	Thoracic ganglia	Thoracic paravertebral area
Upper abdomen	Splanchnic nerves, celiac plexus	T-12 or L-1 prevertebral area
Lower abdomen, pelvis	Hypogastric plexus	Anterolateral edge of L5–S1
Leg, lower abdomen	Lumbar plexus	Anterolateral edge of L2–L4

17. Are there other techniques available for sympathetic nerve blockade?

When pain is circumscribed to the upper or lower extremity, bretylium, which affects norepinephrine release, can be used to achieve a functional sympathetic blockade. This technique, termed **intravenous regional block**, involves the use of a tourniquet to isolate functionally the affected extremity from the rest of the body; as a result, the medication is delivered only to the affected site, which allows the concomitant use of local anesthetics and decreases the risks and incidence of side effects. When pain involves anatomically distant areas (e.g., the upper and lower body), systemic intravenous phentolamine, an alpha-adrenergic blocker, can be used as a diagnostic test. A decrease in pain with either one of these drugs suggests a sympathetically maintained cause.

18. List other medications that are helpful in the therapy of SMP.

Drugs that produce a pharmacologic blockade of the sympathetic system, such as:
- Alpha-blocking agents, including prasozin, terasozin, and phenoxybenzamine
- Clonidine (an alpha$_2$ agonist)
- Beta-blocking agents such as propranolol

19. How does damage to other parts of the nervous system result in chronic pain?

Nerve damage without significant involvement of the sympathetic nervous system may also lead to chronic pain. Such neuropathic pain may stem from a number of entities, including:

Systemic diseases (diabetes mellitus, AIDS, Friedreich's ataxia)
Trauma
Chemotherapy
Surgery
Stroke
Herpes zoster

Consequently, demyelination, axonal damage, alterations in nerve transport, and neuroma formation may all be factors in chronic pain. Neuropathy may manifest as isolated loss of sensory or motor function, but occasionally it is associated with pain described as an electric shock or pins and needles, and sometimes as burning pain as seen in patients with SMP. In contrast to SMP, however, sympathetic nerve blocks are ineffective in relieving this type of neuropathic pain. Therefore, this pain has also been termed **sympathetically independent pain**.

20. How is neuropathic pain treated?

If the pain results from a single damaged nerve, therapy includes nerve blockade with local anesthetics. Steroids are also used when neuroma formation is observed. When only short-term pain relief is obtained after several of these blocks, cryotherapy or surgical neurectomy may be used to achieve more long-lasting pain relief. Concomitant therapy with anticonvulsants such as carbamazepine and with certain antidysrrhythmics such as mexiletine may also be effective. These medications have been shown to decrease spontaneous ectopic impulse transmission while having a lesser effect on normal nerve function.

21. Are there other medications that can be used in the therapy of chronic pain?

Tricyclic antidepressants (amitriptyline, doxepin) produce analgesia at doses much lower than those required for therapy of depression. They have been shown to be superior to placebo for the treatment of several chronic pain conditions, including diabetic neuropathy, postherpetic neuralgia, migraine headaches, and possibly central pain syndrome. Anxiolytic agents (benzodiazepines) and neuroleptics (prolixin) have also been used, but their efficacy remains unproven.

22. Can spinally administered drugs be useful in the therapy of chronic nonmalignant pain?

Spinal drug administration has the potential advantage of improved analgesia with much lower dose requirements and decreased side effects. Narcotics and local anesthetics delivered into the epidural or intrathecal space have proved to be an effective therapy for patients with cancer pain who have failed to respond to more conservative therapies. In addition, epidural clonidine has also been shown to be an effective analgesic when symptoms do not improve with narcotic therapy alone and may soon be approved by the Food and Drug Administration for epidural use. Long-term use of epidural drugs, however, may be ineffective owing to the development of fibrosis. Intrathecal narcotics have been used for chronic nonmalignant pain, but their use, as is the use of narcotics in general for this type of pain, is controversial (see question 24).

23. List other common nonmalignant pain syndromes.

Neuropathic pain is also the likely cause in
    Phantom limb pain
    Trigeminal neuralgia
    Pain after spinal cord injury
    Postherpetic neuralgia
    Central pain syndrome
Syndromes in which neuropathic pain may play a role include
    Pelvic pain
    Pain from chronic pancreatitis
    Atypical facial pain

CONTROVERSY

24. Discuss the pros and cons of long-term opioids for chronic nonmalignant pain.

Traditionally, physicians have refrained from prescribing long-term opioids other than for patients with cancer. This is based on the belief that the patient is exposed to the risks of addiction, mental impairment, and decreased functioning. Moreover, physicians may have been reluctant to prescribe opioids and other "controlled substances" because of potential legal consequences. Some have proposed, however, that certain patients with chronic nonmalignant pain, who have failed to respond to other therapies, should be considered for long-term treatment with opioids. These patients would first go through a trial period that demonstrates increased comfort, increased functioning, and continued participation in other appropriate treatments, including physical therapy and psychological therapy.

BIBLIOGRAPHY

1. Abram SE: Advances in chronic pain management since gate control. Reg Anesth 18:66–81, 1993.
2. Benzon HT: Epidural steroid injections. Pain Digest 1:271–280, 1992.
3. Campbell JN, Raja SN, Selig DK, et al: Diagnosis and management of sympathetically maintained pain. In Fields HL, Liebeskind JC (eds): Pharmacological Approaches to the Treatment of Chronic Pain: New Concepts and Critical Issues. Seattle, IASP Press, 1994, pp 85–100.

4. Fishbain DA, Goldberg M, Meagher BR, et al: Male and female chronic pain patients categorized by DSM-III psychiatric diagnostic criteria. Pain 26:181–197, 1986.
5. Goldenberg DL: Management of fibromyalgia syndrome. Rheum Dis Clin North Am 15:499–512, 1989.
6. Kozin F: Reflex sympathetic dystrophy syndrome: A review. Clin Exp Rheumatol 10:401–409, 1992.
7. Lofstrom JB, Cousins JM: Sympathetic neural blockade of upper and lower extremity. In Cousins JM, Bridenbaugh PO (eds): Neural Blockade in Clinical Anesthesia and Management of Pain, 2nd ed. Philadelphia, J.B. Lippincott, 1988, pp 461–502.
8. Magni G: The use of antidepressants in the treatment of chronic pain. Drugs 42:730–748, 1991.
9. McQuay HJ: Pharmacological treatment of neuralgic and neuropathic pain. Cancer Surv 7:141–159, 1988.
10. Nachemson AL: Newest knowledge of low back pain. Clin Orthop 279:8–20, 1992.
11. Portenoy RK: Chronic opioid therapy for nonmalignant pain: From models to practice. APS Journal 1:171–186, 1992.
12. Wall PD, Melzack R (eds): Textbook of Pain, 3rd ed. New York, Churchill Livingstone, 1994.

XI. Critical Care

84. RESPIRATORY THERAPY

Mark Wilson, C.R.T.T.

1. Discuss the various oxygen (O_2) delivery devices.
There are three basic classifications for O_2 delivery devices.

1. **Low-flow systems** provide supplemental O_2 at flows ranging from 0 to 8 L/min. The nasal cannula is the most commonly employed low-flow device. The delivered O_2 concentration (FiO_2) can be estimated by adding 4% per liter of O_2 delivered. The nasopharynx acts as an anatomic reservoir that collects O_2 from the nasal cannula, enabling a maximum of 40% to 50% O_2 to be delivered.

2. **Reservoir systems** use a volume reservoir to accumulate oxygen during exhalation, thereby increasing the amount of oxygen for the next breath. The **simple mask** covers the patient's nose and mouth and provides an additional reservoir of O_2 beyond the nasal cannula. It is fed by small-bore O_2 tubing at a rate of no less than 6 L/min to ensure that exhaled CO_2 is flushed through the exhalation ports on each side of the mask and not rebreathed. An FiO_2 of 0.55 can be achieved at O_2 flow rates of about 10 L/min. The **nonrebreather mask** adds a reservoir bag and a series of one-way valves that direct gas flow from the bag on inhalation and allow egress of expired gases on exhalation. O_2 flows of 10–15 L/min are commonly needed to maintain reservoir bag inflation and should deliver FiO_2s of 0.80 to 1.00. The performance of these masks greatly depends on obtaining a tight seal between the mask and the patient's face. A poorly fitting mask allows the entrainment of room air, diluting the delivered O_2 concentration.

3. **High-flow systems** must generate a minimum of 50 to 60 L/min to be classified as such and should be sufficient to meet or exceed a patient's inspiratory flow requirement. **Air entrainment devices**, such as the large volume nebulizer, deliver high gas flows only at low to moderate FiO_2s (0.21 to 0.40). Air entrainment devices are considered high flow only at O_2 concentrations at or below 40%. The higher the FiO_2 that the device is set to deliver, the less air is entrained, and the total flow to the patient is diminished.

Approximate Air-to-Oxygen Entrainment Ratios for Common Oxygen Percentages

% FiO_2	AIR-OXYGEN ENTRAINMENT RATIO	TOTAL PARTS
1.00	0:1	1
0.80	0.3:1	1.3
0.70	0.6:1	1.6
0.60	1:1	2
0.50	1.7:1	2.7
0.45	2:1	3
0.40	3:1	4
0.35	5:1	6
0.30	8:1	9
0.28	10:1	11
0.24	25:1	26

Large-volume nebulizers produce a cool mist aerosol, which can help minimize inflammation, humidify the airway, and sooth the recently extubated pharynx. **Air-oxygen blending devices** provide complete inspiratory flow, over a full range of O_2 concentrations, and are considered the only true high-flow system.

2. Are pulmonary complications important in the postoperative patient?

Pulmonary complications are a major cause of morbidity following large surgical procedures. In elderly patients, they are the second most important cause of postoperative death. Atelectasis, aspiration, and postoperative pneumonia are the three most common pulmonary complications following surgery.

1. **Atelectasis** are areas of collapsed alveoli that usually develop within 24–48 hours after surgery and lead to approximately 90% of the febrile episodes within this time period. Atelectasis can develop in response to hypoventilation, a transient decrease in surfactant production, or obstructive factors such as copious or tenacious sputum.

2. **Aspiration** of gastric materials with a pH level below 2.5 causes an immediate chemical pneumonitis leading to inflammation, local edema, and bronchospasm. In addition to the pH of the aspirate, the extent of injury depends on the amount aspirated. Atelectasis may also develop in response to reflex bronchospasm and aspiration of large particles.

3. Gross aspiration progressing to **pneumonia** has a 30% mortality rate owing to ensuing sepsis, adult respiratory distress syndrome (ARDS), and multiorgan failure.

3. How should pulmonary complications be treated?

Prevention is the best treatment for perioperative pulmonary complications. **Atelectasis** can be minimized with good pulmonary toilet. Deep breathing and coughing, and early ambulation are probably the easiest, most effective maneuvers. Incentive spirometry, postural drainage and chest physiotherapy, proper fluid and electrolyte management, and adequate pain control are helpful. Endotracheal and nasotracheal suction may also be needed.

The risk of pulmonary **aspiration** can be minimized by avoiding general anesthesia if the patient has recently eaten. When surgery cannot be delayed, use of cricoid pressure (the Sellick maneuver) during rapid sequence induction is indicated and should be maintained until a cuffed endotracheal tube is inserted and proper position verified. Antacids, histamine$_2$ blockers, antiemetics, and gastrokinetic drugs are used to elevate stomach acid pH and reduce gastric fluid volume.

4. What is proper tracheal suctioning technique?

Always preoxygenate with 100% O_2 for 3–5 minutes before suctioning. This should reduce the risk of the most common complications, hypoxemia, and cardiac arrhythmias; however, vagal stimulation may also produce bradycardia.

Atelectasis may develop during airway suctioning and can be minimized by four methods:

1. The outer diameter of the suction catheter should not exceed ½ to ⅔ the inner diameter of the airway. A helpful formula for determining catheter size is:

$$\text{Catheter size (French)} = \frac{\text{Inner diameter (mm)} \times 3}{2}$$

2. Limit duration of suctioning to 10 to 15 seconds.

3. Avoid excessive negative pressure. The recommended negative pressure is –100 to –120 cm H_2O for adults, –80 to –100 cm H_2O for children, and –60 to –80 cm H_2O for infants.

4. Hyperinflation before and after suctioning may also help prevent atelectasis.

If elevated intracranial pressures are a concern, temporary hyperventilation before and after suctioning may be indicated. Sterile technique should always be used.

5. What role does positive end-expiratory pressure (PEEP) play in critical care ventilation?

Low to moderate levels of PEEP (5–8 cm H_2O) may help resolve atelectasis and maintain alveolar patency in conditions associated with decreased pulmonary compliance or increased capillary/alveolar wall permeability. PEEP should be used as is hemodynamically tolerated.

6. How much PEEP should be used?

This often depends on the patient's hemodynamic status. If the patient has a low intravascular volume, even low levels of PEEP can impede venous return and occlude pulmonary capillary beds, resulting in a decreased cardiac output and ventilation/perfusion mismatch. Generally the best PEEP is that level required to maintain a PaO_2 greater than 60 mmHg at an FiO_2 of less than 0.60 without compromising cardiac output. In the presence of alveolar hemorrhage or fulminant pulmonary edema, temporary PEEP levels of 20 cm H_2O are commonly employed until the alveolar capillary abnormality is corrected. Rarely, situations require levels of PEEP above 20 cm H_2O. During high PEEP therapy (> 12 cm H_2O), delivered tidal volume should be adjusted to avoid injury from overdistention of normal lung units. Data obtained from pulmonary artery catheters should also be interpreted with PEEP values taken into consideration.

7. What is a good tidal volume?

A tidal volume of 10–12 mL/kg, based on ideal body weight, is usually sufficient. Tidal volumes as low as 5 mL/kg have been used with PEEP levels of 10–15 cm H_2O in patients with ARDS. The lung with ARDS has three types of alveoli:

- **Consolidated alveoli**, which do not reexpand regardless of the amount of PEEP applied
- **Recruitable alveoli**, which respond to PEEP therapy
- **Normal functional alveoli**

Ventilating the volume-compromised lung with an otherwise acceptable tidal volume may lead to overdistention and barotrauma/volutrauma of normal alveoli.

8. Define postextubation stridor.

Stridor is a high-pitched, coarse, musical sound associated with laryngeal inflammation and edema, occurring during inspiration. Stridor is indicative of increased airway resistance and work of breathing. If the patient can move air around a deflated endotracheal tube cuff, extubation can probably be tolerated.

9. How should postextubation stridor be treated?

Aerosolized 2.25% racemic epinephrine reduces laryngeal edema via mucosal vasoconstriction. A cool mist, large-volume aerosol may also aid in reducing laryngeal inflammation. Owing to its low density, a helium and O_2 gas mixture (heliox) may enhance spontaneous ventilation but may not be tolerated if the patient has a high O_2 requirement. The most common heliox mixture is 70% helium and 30% O_2. Should a stridulous patient require intubation, reextubation becomes problematic. The risk for stridor exists for up to 24 hours postextubation. Steroid therapy for acute stridor is of questionable efficacy secondary to the delayed onset of action.

10. What is the most effective modality for delivering aerosolized bronchodilators to the mechanically ventilated patient?

The alternatives are the small volume nebulizer and the metered-dose inhaler (MDI). An MDI with an in-line spacer/reservoir has been shown to produce better particle deposition at the alveolar level, deliver a more accurate dose in half the time, and with one third the cost of the jet nebulizer system.

11. Define an in-line spacer/reservoir.

An in-line spacer is an MDI actuation device that adapts to the ventilator tubing, either between the endotracheal tube and the "Y" connector or on the inspiratory limb at the "Y" connector. The drug in an MDI is attached to a propellant that has a relatively large particle size. The larger the aerosol particle, the greater its tendency to "rain out" in the endotracheal tube or in the upper airway. Proper use of a reservoir chamber allows the initial high aerosol velocity and diameter to decrease as the propellant evaporates. The MDI should be actuated just before the inspiratory phase of ventilation, preferably a slow deep breath with an inspiratory pause.

12. How much bronchodilator therapy should be given with an MDI?

Manufacturers recommend 2–4 puffs every 3–4 hours. Clinically the dose should be titrated to effect.

Administer 5 puffs (1 puff per breath).
Wait 5 minutes.
Repeat as needed and tolerated.

It is important to shake the MDI between puffs to remix the medication and ensure proper dosing for each actuation.

13. Can principles of nebulizer therapy be useful in providing anesthesia of the airway?

Lidocaine (4%), administered via small volume nebulizer and aerosol mask, can adequately anesthetize the upper airway, facilitating awake intubation or bronchoscopy.

14. What is the oxyhemoglobin dissociation curve?

A sigmoidal curve that describes the nonlinear binding reaction or affinity of O_2 for hemoglobin. The upper, relatively flat part of the curve demonstrates that under normal conditions, minor fluctuations in PO_2 have little effect on hemoglobin saturation. When the PO_2 decreases to below 60 mmHg (as in the systemic capillary bed), the slope of the curve steepens, and hemoglobin's affinity for O_2 is decreased, allowing greater amounts of O_2 to be unloaded at the tissue level.

15. What is the P-50?

The P-50 is that O_2 tension associated with 50% hemoglobin saturation. Its utility is in describing the position of the curve and for comparing the O_2-binding characteristics of differing hemoglobin species. A normal P-50 is about 26.6 (at a pH of 7.40, $PaCO_2$ 40 mm Hg, and 37°C). The lower the P-50, the greater the affinity of hemoglobin for O_2.

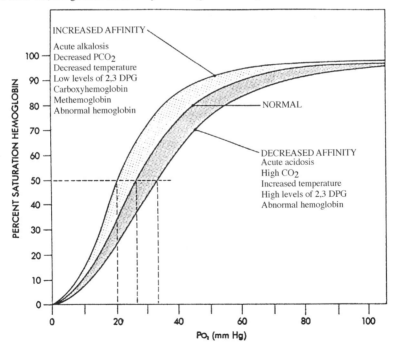

Oxyhemoglobin dissociation curve. The normal P-50 at 26.6, how its position changes with left or right shifts of the O_2 dissociation curve, and factors that affect the position of the curve. (From Egan DF: Fundamentals of Respiratory Care, 6th ed. St. Louis, C.V. Mosby, 1995, with permission.)

16. Why not induce alkalosis to shift the curve to the left, increasing hemoglobin's affinity for O_2, and increase O_2 uptake at the alveoli?
The increased affinity hinders O_2 delivery at the tissue level. At O_2 partial pressures associated with the alveoli, the dissociation curve is relatively flat, and significant changes in the degree of hemoglobin saturation do not occur.

17. Why do we give such attention to the O_2 partial pressure of blood (PaO_2) when the dissolved O_2 content of the blood is so small compared with that which is bound to hemoglobin?
A PaO_2 of 60 mm Hg correlates with hemoglobin saturation of 90% and can be found near the top of the steep portion of the oxyhemoglobin dissociation curve. As the O_2 tension decreases below 60, marked changes in the degree of saturation occur. The sigmoidal shape of the curve demonstrates that significant changes in O_2 saturation may accompany small changes in O_2 tension.

Oxyhemoglobin Dissociation Curve

pH	7.30	7.40	7.50
P_{O_2}		OXYGEN SATURATION	
10	11.7	13.3	15.4
20	31.1	35.5	40.9
30	52.4	58.0	64.1
40	68.9	73.9	78.8
44	73.9	78.4	82.7
48	78.0	82.0	85.8
52	81.4	84.9	88.2
56	84.2	87.3	90.2
60	86.5	89.3	91.8
64	88.4	90.9	93.0
68	90.0	92.3	94.0
72	91.4	93.2	94.9
76	92.5	94.1	95.6
80	93.5	94.9	96.1
90	95.3	96.3	97.2
100	96.4	97.2	97.9

Define hypoxia.
Hypoxia is a result of inadequate delivery of oxygen to maintain aerobic tissue metabolism.

19. What causes hypoxia?

Causes of Hypoxia

CAUSE	PRIMARY INDICATOR	MECHANISM	EXAMPLE
Hypoxemia			
Low P_{IO_2}	Low PaO_2 Low PaO_2	Reduced P_A	Altitude
Hypoventilation	Low PaO_2 High PCO_2	Decreased $\dot{V}_A$	Drug overdose
Diffusion defect	Low PaO_2 High $P_{(A-a)O_2}$ on air; resolves with O_2	Barrier at A-C membrane	Interstitial lung disease
Anatomic shunt	Low PaO_2 High $P_{(A-a)O_2}$ on air; does not resolve with O_2	Blood flow between right and left sides of circulation	Congenital heart disease

Table continued on following page.

Causes of Hypoxia (Continued)

CAUSE	PRIMARY INDICATOR	MECHANISM	EXAMPLE
$\dot{V}/\dot{Q}$ imbalance			
Low $\dot{V}/\dot{Q}$	Low P_{AO_2} High $P(A-a)_{O_2}$ on air; resolves with O_2	Decreased $\dot{V}a$ relative to perfusion	Chronic obstructive lung disease; aging
Physiologic shunt	Low P_{AO_2} High $P(A-a)_{O_2}$ on air; does not resolve with O_2	Perfusion without ventilation	Atelectasis
Hb deficiency			
Absolute	Low Hb content Reduced C_{aO_2}	Loss of Hb	Hemorrhage
Relative	Abnormal S_{aO_2} Reduced C_{aO_2}	Abnormal Hb	Carboxyhemoglobin
Reduced blood flow	Increased $C(a-\bar{v})_{O_2}$ Decreased $C\bar{v}_{O_2}$	Decreased perfusion	Shock; ischemia
Dysoxia	Normal C_{aO_2} Increased $C\bar{v}_{O_2}$	Disruption of cellular enzymes	Cyanide poisoning; septic shock

A-C, alveolar-capillary; Hb, hemoblogin.
From Egan DF: Fundamentals of Respiratory Care, 6th ed. St. Louis, C.V. Mosby, 1995, with permission.

20. Discuss the differences between intrapulmonary shunting and ventilation/perfusion ($\dot{V}/\dot{Q}$) mismatch.

An **intrapulmonary shunt** occurs whenever venous blood mixes with arterialized blood without participating in alveolar gas exchange. The normal anatomic shunt of 2% to 5% of cardiac output is produced by bronchial, plural, and thebesian vein drainage into the pulmonary venous system. A physiologic shunt is created under conditions of atelectasis, pulmonary edema, and pneumonia, in which venous blood perfuses nonventilated alveoli, and no gas exchange takes place. Because of the absence of gas exchange in an intrapulmonary shunt, oxygenation is not significantly improved by increasing the inspired O_2 concentration.

In contrast, a $\dot{V}/\dot{Q}$ **mismatch** responds to O_2 therapy. The most common $\dot{V}/\dot{Q}$ abnormality is a low $\dot{V}/\dot{Q}$ ratio, in which alveolar ventilation is abnormally low relative to its perfusion. A low $\dot{V}/\dot{Q}$ responds to O_2 therapy because these alveoli do participate in some gas exchange, whereas the shunted alveoli do not. Additionally, a shunt may produce hypercapnia, but a $\dot{V}/\dot{Q}$ mismatch usually does not.

CONTROVERSY

21. Discuss static (plateau) and dynamic (peak inspiratory) pressures and their significance.

Dynamic pressure is a reflection of the amount of pressure necessary to deliver a given volume and is affected by frictional resistance. The two major components of frictional resistance are tissue and airway resistance. The tissue component represents the amount of energy required to displace the muscle and organs of the thorax and abdomen, to allow for lung expansion. Tissue resistance accounts for about 20% of total frictional resistance. The remaining 80% is created by the resistance of air moving through the anatomic airways and the artificial ventilator circuit. The effect that frictional resistance has on dynamic pressure is greatly influenced by the flow characteristics of the cycling ventilator. The higher the inspiratory flow, the more turbulent the air becomes, and the more resistance it encounters.

Static pressure is a measurement taken at a point of no airflow. It is the pressure recorded during an inspiratory breath hold, or "plateau" maneuver, and represents the impedance to lung inflation caused by elastic forces. Lung compliance must be measured under static conditions to eliminate the factor of dynamic tissue and airway resistance.

Significance

Although dynamic pressure measurements are important in the detection of acute airway changes such as mucus accumulation, pneumothorax, bronchospasm, and inadvertent disconnection, they should not be the sole determinant of the patient's compliance and risk for lung injury. Situations may arise that demand high peak inspiratory flow rates, so higher dynamic pressures are to be expected from increased tubing and conducting airways resistance. Static pressures of 35–40 cm H_2O and mean airway pressures of 25–30 cm H_2O suggest a high risk for lung injury.

BIBLIOGRAPHY

1. Barash PG, Cullen BF, Stoelting RK, et al: Handbook of Clinical Anesthesia. Philadelphia, J.B. Lippincott, 1991, pp 25–27.
2. Burton GG: Respiratory Care, A Guide to Clinical Practice, 3rd ed. Philadelphia, J.B. Lippincott, 1991.
3. Corbridge TC, Wood LD, Crawford GP, et al: Adverse effects of large tidal volume and low PEEP in canine acid aspiration. Am Rev Respir Dis 142:311–315, 1990.
4. Darmon JY, Rauss A, Dreyfuss D, et al: Evaluation of risk factors for laryngeal edema after tracheal extubation in adults and its prevention by dexamethasone. Anesthesiology 77:245–251, 1992.
5. Egan DF: Fundamentals of Respiratory Care, 6th ed. St. Louis, Mosby, 1995.
6. Fuller HD, Dolovich MB, Turpie FH, et al: Efficiency of bronchodilator aerosol delivery to the lungs from the metered dose inhaler in mechanically ventilated patients. Chest 105:214–218, 1994.
7. Kiiski R, Takala J, Kari A, et al: Effect of tidal volume on gas exchange and oxygen transport in the adult respiratory distress syndrome. Am Rev Respir Dis 146:1131–1135, 1992.
8. Macdonnell SPJ, Timmins AC, Watson JD: Adrenaline administered via a nebulizer in adult patients with upper airway obstruction. Anesthesia 50:35–36, 1995.
9. Manthous CA, Chatila W, Schmidt GA, et al: Treatment of bronchospasm by metered dose inhaler albuterol in mechanically ventilatd patients. Chest 107:210–213, 1955.
10. Peterfreund RA, Niven RW, Kacmarek RM: Syringe-actuated metered dose inhalers: A quantitative laboratory evaluation of albuterol delivery through nozzle extensions. Anesth Analg 78:554–558, 1994.
11. Rau JL, Harwood RJ, Groff JL: Evaluation of a reservoir device for metered dose bronchodilator delivery to intubated adults. Chest 102:924–930, 1992.

85. PULMONARY FUNCTION TESTING AND INTERPRETATION

Theresa L. Kinnard, M.D., and William V. Kinnard, M.D.

1. What are pulmonary function tests?

The term pulmonary function test (PFT) refers to a standardized measurement of a patient's airflow (spirometry), lung volumes, and diffusing capacity for inspired carbon monoxide (DLCO). These values are always reported as a percentage of a predicted normal value , which is calculated based on the age and height of the patient. Used in combination with the history, physical exam, blood gas analysis, and chest radiograph, PFTs facilitate the classification of respiratory disease into obstructive, restrictive, or mixed disorders.

2. When are PFTs indicated as part of the preoperative evaluation?

The primary goal of preoperative pulmonary function testing is to identify a group of patients at either high or prohibitive risk of postoperative pulmonary complications in whom institution of aggressive therapy before and/or after surgery may decrease complications, or in whom surgery should be avoided entirely. Risk factors for pulmonary complications include (1) age > 70 years; (2) obesity; (3) upper abdominal or thoracic surgery; (4) history of lung disease; (5) greater than 20-pack year history of smoking; and (6) resection of an anterior mediastinal mass.

3. What factors need to be taken into consideration before interpreting PFT results?

PFTs are standardized according to predicted values based on tests of healthy individuals. The predicted values vary according to age, height, gender, and ethnicity. For example, several studies have demonstrated that vital capacity and total lung capacity is 13–15% lower in blacks than in whites. Reliable testing requires patient cooperation and understanding as well as a skilled technician.

4. What are the subdivisions of lung volumes and capacities?

The tidal volume (V_T) is the volume of air inhaled and exhaled with each breath during normal breathing. Inspiratory reserve volume (IRV) is the volume of air that can be maximally inhaled beyond a normal V_T, expiratory reserve volume (ERV) is the maximal volume of air that can be exhaled beyond a normal V_T, and residual volume (RV) is the volume of air that remains in the lung after maximal expiration. By definition, lung capacity is composed of two or more lung volumes, including total lung capacity (TLC), vital capacity (VC), inspiratory capacity (IC), and functional residual capacity (FRC).

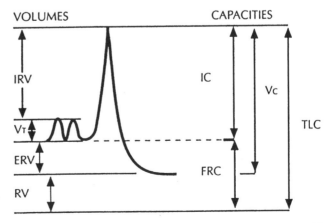

Subdivisions of lung volumes and capacities.

5. What techniques are used in the determination of lung volumes?

The determination of FRC is the cornerstone for the measurement of the remainder of the lung volumes. The FRC is the volume of air in the lung at the end of a normal expiration and is composed of RV and ERV. The FRC can be measured by three different techniques: (1) helium dilution, (2) nitrogen washout, and (3) body plethysmography. Plethysmography is more accurate for determining FRC in patients with obstructive airway disease and is considered the approach of choice. It involves a direct application of Boyle's law, which states that the volume of gas in a closed space varies inversely with the pressure to which it is subjected. All measurements of FRC, if performed correctly, are independent of patient effort.

6. What information is obtained from spirometry?

Spirometry provides timed measurements of expired volumes from the lung and forms the foundation of pulmonary function testing. With automated equipment it is possible to interpret more than 15 different measurements from spiromety alone. Forced vital capacity (FVC), forced expiratory volume in one second(FEV_1), FEV_1/FVC ratio, and flow between 25% and 75% of the FVC (MMF_{25-75}) are the most clinically helpful indices obtained from spirometry.

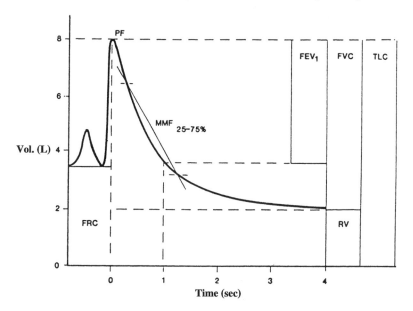

Spirogram. (Adapted from Harrison RA: Respiratory function and anesthesia. In Barash PG, Cullen BF, Stoelting RK (eds): Clinical Anesthesia. Philadelphia, J.B. Lippincott, 1989, pp 877–904.)

8. What information is not obtained from spirometry?

Spirometry may demonstrate airflow limitation but does not determine its cause (e.g., airway obstruction vs. decreased elastic recoil of the alveolus vs. decreased expiratory muscle activity). Nor does it provide information about lung volumes and capacities, which require the application of different techniques of measurement.

7. What is maximum voluntary ventilation?

Maximal voluntary ventilation (MVV) or maximal breathing capacity (MBC) is an extremely effort-dependent spirometric test that measures the maximal volume of air that a patient can expire in 1 minute by voluntary effort. This is a nonspecific test that evaluates a variety of factors important to lung function (e.g., patient motivation, strength, and endurance as well as pulmonary mechanics). A decrease in MMV has been shown to predict increased morbidity and mortality in patients undergoing thoracic surgery.

9. What is the diffusing capacity for inspired carbon monoxide (DLCO)?

The DLCO is the rate of uptake of carbon monoxide (CO) per driving pressure of alveolar CO. It is a function of both membrane diffusing capacity and pulmonary vascular components and thus is a reflection of functioning alveolar capillary units. CO is used as a nonphysiologic gas because of its affinity for hemoglobin and because it reflects the diffusing capacity of the physiologic gases (oxygen and carbon dioxide). This test has been used as an indicator of suitability for pulmonary resection and as a predictor of postoperative pulmonary morbidity.

10. What disease states cause a decrease in DLCO?

As implied above, any disease process that compromises the alveolar capillary unit may cause a decrease in DLCO. Three major types of pulmonary disorders cause a decrease in DLCO: (1) obstructive airway disease, (2) interstitial lung disease, and (3) pulmonary vascular disease. Differential diagnosis must take into account other clinical, physiologic, and radiographic findings.

11. What disease states cause an increase in DLCO?

In general, conditions that cause a relative increase in the amount of hemoglobin in the lung may result in an increased DLCO. Congestive heart failure, asthma, and diffuse pulmonary hemorrhage are the most common causes of an increased DLCO. A perforated tympanic membrane may cause an artifactually high DLCO by permitting an escape of CO by a nonpulmonary route.

12. What PFT abnormalities are present in patients with obstructive airway disease?

Obstructive airway diseases, which include asthma, chronic bronchitis, emphysema, cystic fibrosis, and bronchiolitis, exhibit diminished expiratory airflow. These conditions involve airways anatomically distal to the carina. The FEV_1, FEV_1/FVC ratio, and the FEF_{25-75} are decreased below normal predicted values. A decreased FEF_{25-75} reflects collapse of the small airways and is a sensitive indicator of early airway obstruction. The FVC may be normal or decreased due to respiratory muscle weakness, or dynamic airway collapse with subsequent air trapping. The table below grades the severity of obstruction based upon the FEV_1/FVC ratio.

Severity of Obstructive and Restrictive Airway Diseases as Measured by FEV_1/FVC and TLC

	NORMAL	MILD	MODERATE	SEVERE
FEV_1/FVC	> 73%	61–73%	51–60%	< 50%
TLC	> 81%	66–80%	51–65%	< 50%

13. What PFT abnormalities are present in patients with restrictive lung disease?

The characteristic pattern in patients with restrictive pulmonary disease is a reduction in lung volumes, particularly TLC and VC, whereas air flow rates can be normal or increased. Disorders that result in decreased lung volumes include abnormal chest cage configuration, respiratory muscle weakness, loss of alveolar air space (pulmonary fibrosis, pneumonia), and encroachment of the lung space by disorders of the pleural cavity (effusion, tumor).

14. What is a flow-volume loop and what information does it provide?

The flow-volume loop can be constructed from routine clinical spirometric data and aids in the anatomic localization of airway obstruction. Forced expiratory and inspiratory flow at 50% of FVC (FEF_{50} and FIF_{50}) are shown in the following figure. Note that expiratory flow is represented above the x-axis, whereas inspiratory flow is represented below the axis. In a normal flow-volume loop the FEF_{50}/FIF_{50} ratio is 1.0.

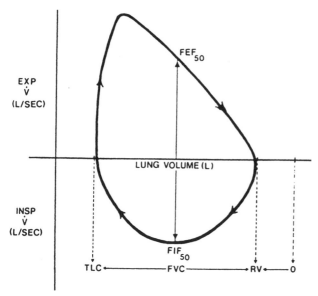

Idealized flow-volume loop. (Flow in l/sec is abbreviated v̇.) (From Harrison RA: Respiratory function and anesthesia. In Barash PG, Cullen BF, Stoelting RK (eds): Clinical Anesthesia. Philadelphia, J.B. Lippincott, 1989, pp 877–904, with permission.)

15. What are the characteristic patterns of the flow-volume loop in a fixed airway obstruction, variable extrathoracic obstruction, and intrathoracic obstruction ?

Upper airway lesions are categorized as fixed when there is a plateau during both inspiration and expiration of the flow-volume loop (tracheal stenosis). The FEF_{50}/FIF_{50} ratio remains unchanged. An extrathoracic obstruction occurs when the lesion (tumor) is located above the sternal notch and is characterized by a flattening of the flow-volume loop during inspiration. The flattening of the loop represents no further increase in airflow because the mass causes airway collapse. The FEF_{50}/FIF_{50} ratio is > 1. An intrathoracic obstruction is characterized by a flattening of the expiratory loop of a flow-volume loop, and the FEF_{50}/FIF_{50} ratio is < 1. The lesion causes airway collapse during expiration.

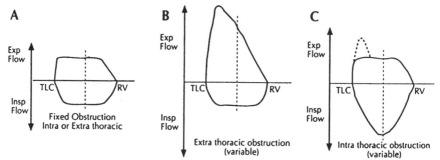

Flow-volume loops in a fixed, extrathoracic, and intrathoracic airway obstruction. (The hash marks represent flow at 50% of vital capacity.) (From Kryger M, Bode F, Antic R, et al: Diagnosis of obstruction of the upper and central airways. Am J Med 61:85–93m 1976, with permission.)

16. How can flow-volume loops be utilized in the preoperative assessment of patients with an anterior mediastinal mass scheduled for surgical resection?

General anesthesia in patients with an anterior mediastinal mass (lymphoma, thymoma, thyroid mass) may lead to a potentially catastrophic situation. After induction of anesthesia (conversion from negative-pressure to positive-pressure ventilation) the mass may compress the vena cava, pulmonary vessels, heart, or tracheobronchial tree, producing acute cardiovascular collapse. The preoperative evaluation of a flow-volume loop in different positions (sitting and supine) helps to assess potentially obstructive lesions of the airway and to identify patients in whom alternative management may be indicated.

17. What are the effects of surgery and anesthesia on pulmonary function?
All patients undergoing surgery and general anesthesia exhibit changes in pulmonary function that promote the development of postoperative pulmonary complications. Such changes, which are more significant in patients undergoing upper abdominal and thoracic procedures, include a decrease in lung volumes, particularly VC and FRC. The VC is reduced to approximately 40% of preoperative values and remains depressed for at least 10–14 days after open cholecystectomy. The FRC has been shown to decrease approximately 10–16 hours after upper abdominal surgery and gradually returns to normal by 7–10 days. The normal pattern of ventilation is also altered, with decreased sigh breaths and decreased clearance of secretions.

18. Why is the postoperative decrease in FRC important?
The decrease in FRC is important in terms of its relationship to closing volume (CV)—the volume of the lung at which small airways close. When the CV is greater than FRC, small airway collapse during normal tidal volume breathing leads to atelectasis and hypoxemia.

19. What PFT values predict increased perioperative pulmonary complications?

Pulmonary Function Criteria Suggesting Increased Risk for Abdominal and Thoracic Surgery

	ABDOMINAL	THORACIC
FVC	< 70% predicted	< 70% predicted or < 1.7 L
FEV_1	< 70% predicted	< 2 L*, < 1 L[†], < 0.6 L[‡]
FEV_1/FVC	< 65%	< 35%
MVV	<50% predicted	< 50% predicted or < 28 L/min
RV		< 47% predicted
DLCO		< 50%
VO_2		< 15 ml/kg/min

* Pneumonectomy.   [†] Lobectomy.   [‡] Segmentectomy.

Adapted from Gass GD, Olsen GN: Preoperative pulmonary function testing to predict postoperative morbidity and mortality. Chest 89:127–135, 1986, with permission.

20. What is VO_{2max}? How is it used to predict postoperative pulmonary complications?
The VO_{2max} is the maximal oxygen consumption that a patient attains during exercise. It reflects the patients pulmonary, cardiac, and peripheral vascular function as well as motivation and endurance. It has been used to predict postoperative pulmonary complications after lung resection. In a study by Bechard and Wetstein, 50 patients scheduled for lung resection who had an FEV_1 > 1.7 L underwent exercise testing. There was no morbidity or mortality in patients who could consume more than 20 ml/kg/min of oxygen. The group that could not exercise to 10 ml/kg/min had a 29% mortality rate and a 43% morbidity rate. The authors concluded that oxygen consumption should be used preoperatively in patients scheduled for lung resection.

21. Are there absolute values of specific pulmonary function tests below which the risk of surgery is prohibitive?
Multiple factors are highly predictive of postoperative pulmonary complications, but there is no preoperative pulmonary function test result that absolutely contraindicates surgery. It is ultimately the decision of the surgeon, anesthesiologist, and patient whether the risk of pulmonary complications outweighs the benefits of a surgical procedure.

BIBLIOGRAPHY

1. Bechard D, Wetstein L: Assessment of exercise oxygen consumption as preoperative criterion for lung resection. Ann Thorac Surg 44:344–349, 1987.
2. Boysen PG, Block AJ, Moulder PV: Relationship between preoperative pulmonary function tests and complications after thoracotomy. Surg Gynecol Obstet 152:813–815, 1981.
3. Craig DB: Postoperative recovery of pulmonary function. Anesth Analg 60:46–52, 1981.
4. Eisenkraft JB, Cohen E, Kaplan JA: Anesthesia for thoracic surgery. In Barash PG, Cullen BF, Stoelting RK (eds): Clinical Anesthesia. Philadelphia, JB Lippincott, 1989, pp 905–946.
5. Gass GD, Olsen GN: Preoperative pulmonary function testing to predict postoperative morbidity and mortality. Chest 89:127–135, 1986.
6. Harrison RA: Respiratory Function and Anesthesia. In Barash PG, Cullen BF, Stoelting RK (eds): Clinical Anesthesia. Philadelphia, J.B. Lippincott, 1989, pp 877–904.
7. Kryger M, Bode F, Antic R, et al.: Diagnosis of obstruction of the upper and central airways. Am J Med 61:85–93, 1976.
8. Mahler DA, Horowitz MB: Pulmonary function testing. In Bone RC (ed): Pulmonary and Critical Care Medicine. St. Louis, Mosby, 1994, pp 1–19.
9. Schoenberg JB, Beck, GJ, Bouhuys A: Growth and decay of pulmonary function in healthy blacks and whites. Respir Physiol 33:367–93, 1978.
10. Stoller JK, Holden DH, Matthay MA: Preoperative Evaluation. In Bone RC (ed): Pulmonary and Critical Care Medicine. St. Louis, Mosby, 1994, Chapter 7, pp 1–17.
11. Tisi GM: Preoperative evaluation of pulmonary function. Am Rev Respir Dis 119:293–310, 1979.

86. INTRAHOSPITAL TRANSPORT OF THE CRITICALLY ILL PATIENT

James E. Hannaford, M.A., R.R.T.

1. When should the transport of critically ill patients not be undertaken?

Perioperative transport is not associated with as many complications as transportation to and from some other areas of the hospital (e.g., radiology), but there is a risk. In any surgical procedure, when the risk of transporting the patient is greater than the risk of performing the procedure at bedside, the patient should not be moved. For example, percutaneous tracheostomy is often and readily performed at bedside in critically ill patients expected to require prolonged mechanical ventilation.

A futile or unnecessary trip to the operating rooms (OR) places the patient at risk without benefit. Transportation should not be undertaken until all individuals at the receiving end (circulating nurse and anesthesiologist) have had time to prepare the surgical suite and are briefed adequately as to the patient's condition. Likewise, when the patient is to be transported from the OR to the postanesthesia care unit or intensive care unit (ICU) after the operation, adequate time must be allowed between the notification of the receiving individuals and the transport of that patient. Total responsibility for care is not relinquished until the patient is stable in a new environment and report has been given to the new caregivers. One study has assessed the hospital's intrahospital transport cost per patient at an average of $465.

2. Describe the three levels of acuity in patient transport and their determinants.

Any patient originating from an ICU or other unit where continuous electrocardiography (ECG) has been initiated is considered critically ill. A respiratory therapist (RT) with ACLS training and instruction in transport (transport RT) and an anesthesiology resident are notified by the responsible anesthesiologist, and the patient's medical problems and management are discussed, particularly ventilator management. The transport RT's first responsibility is to assemble the monitoring equipment and supplies at the patient's bedside and assess the patient's transport situation through available nursing notes, medical record, and discussion with the bedside caregivers. The goal of this assessment is to stratify the patient transport into one of three categories:

1. **Minimal acuity patient transport**
   - ECG plus continuous pulse oximetry
   - Blood pressure stable and monitored noninvasively
   - Intravenous line or heparin lock established
   - No malignant ECG rhythms present
   - Patient cooperative and unrestrained
   - Oxygenation/ventilation are adequate
   - Patient breathing spontaneously, with minimal oxygen supplementation
2. **Moderate acuity patient transport**
   - ECG and pulse oximetry
   - Invasive blood pressure lines in use
   - May have several intravenous lines with multiple pumps
   - May be intubated and ventilated on ICU ventilator
   - Patient stable on present monitoring and therapy, but transport complicated by potential for patient decompensation or by complexity of therapy/monitoring
3. **Maximal acuity patient transport**
   - Degree of complexity of patient monitoring/therapy variable with either:
     a. Extreme degree of patient monitoring/therapy required to keep patient stable
     b. Patient unstable on present monitoring/therapy but no possibility of stabilizing condition without surgical intervention

3. What are the personnel requirements for safely transporting a critically ill patient?

MINIMAL ACUITY	MODERATE ACUITY	MAXIMAL ACUITY
Transport RT	Transport RT	Transport RT
Nonskilled help	Anesthesiology resident	Anesthesiology resident
		Attending anesthesiologist

4. What monitoring capabilities are needed during patient transport?

The Society for Critical Care Medicine states in its "Guidelines for Monitoring" that, whenever possible, the nature and extent of monitoring that has been established in an ICU (or wherever the patient is originating) should be continued while the patient is transported. Thus, the monitoring capabilities chosen for transport must have all of the modalities as the point of origin.

Most ICUs have the capability of simultaneously monitoring ECG, noninvasive blood pressure, pulse oximetry, two invasive pressure lines, and intracranial pressure. Whether the RT uses an extensive transport cart that houses every conceivable device (mini-ICU on wheels) or micro-miniaturized equipment and monitoring devices that weigh only pounds, all parameters monitored in the ICU should be continued in transport, unless the individual in charge has determined that certain monitored parameters may be safely suspended during the transport. Deviations from written policy and procedures should be well justified and documented.

5. Is a defibrillator always included as one of the pieces of equipment for transport?

Defibrillators are available in every ICU and surgical suite. If the ICU and OR are contiguous, there is usually no need to include the defibrillator during transport. However, if the ICU and OR are located apart, and a defibrillator is more than a minute away (e.g., elevator transport), inclusion of one is prudent.

For example, patients who are scheduled for placement of an automated implantable cardioverter defibrillator (AICD) are prone to malignant dysrhythmias. Clearly, they need to have an external defibrillator available during transport, and we even apply anterior and posterior defibrillator pads to a portable defibrillator before mobilizing these patients. In transporting a patient who has a significant likelihood for emergent defibrillation (frequent multifocal premature ventricular contractions [PVCs], runs of PVCs, close R on T PVCs, etc.), a defibrillator must be available.

6. A head trauma patient has an intracranial pressure (ICP) monitor in place and needs to be transported for an emergent craniotomy. How do ICP monitors work?

Two devices are commonly used to quantitate ICP. The first is a fluid-filled catheter inserted into the cranial vault, with the tip located in one of the intracerebral ventricles, the epidural or subarachnoid space. The catheter is attached to a pressure transducer of the same type used to monitor intravascular pressure. In addition, there is usually a water manometer that allows measurements of ICP without the need for electronic apparatus. Between the patient and transducer is a three-way stopcock that allows you to monitor the ICP or drain excessive cerebrospinal fluid (CSF).

The second type of device uses a pressure transducer device that transmits light along a fiberoptic tract into a distally located, miniaturized chamber in the cranial vault; the chamber is capable of changing its volume depending on the pressure around it. When the chamber changes volume, less light is reflected back along a second fiberoptic tract to the emitter/sensor. This device commonly has a catheter running along the fiberoptic tracts, through which excessive CSF can be drained.

The major advantages of the first type of ICP monitor are that it can be constructed from "spare parts" typically available in the critical care areas of a hospital, and during transport, it can be used with the water manometer to monitor ICP. The disadvantages include the risk that a fluid-filled column can introduce microorganisms into the brain due to the presence of a stopcock and the need to maintain a fluid column between the patient and transducer. The major advantages with the second type of ICP monitor are its decreased risk of introducing microorganisms and its continuous display of ICP. Disadvantages are its expense and the fragility of the fiberoptic tract.

7. Describe the problems that may develop with a patient's chest tube during transport.

The chest tube provides a route of escape for fluid or air from the pleural space so that accumulation does not impede venous return to the heart or ventilation of the lungs. The chest tube can be impaired at only a limited number of sites, so you can concentrate attention on these areas. As the tubing extends from the patient's chest wall to the chest drainage set), there usually is a low point, called the dependent loop, where some fluid accumulates. The fluid collection in the dependent loop will exhibit one of the four following behaviors. (This behavior also can be observed in the "water trap" portion of chest tube apparatus; if there is no fluid accumulation in a dependent loop.)

1. **The fluid collection moves toward the patient with each spontaneous breath and away from the patient with each ventilator- or bag-initiated positive-pressure breath.** This behavior indicates that the proximal end of the chest tube inside the patient is patent and that there is no blockage between the proximal end and dependent loop. In other words, the chest tube setup is acting as it should, with little potential for patient harm.

2. **The fluid collection moves toward the patient with each spontaneous breath, but with each positive-pressure breath, air bubbles through the standing fluid.** This behavior indicates that the proximal end of the chest tube is in proper functional order but that a bronchopleural fistula is allowing air to leak from a conducting airway into the pleural space. Without a continuous vacuum applied at the distal end of chest tube setup, air accumulates in the pleural space at a rate dependent on the size of the bronchopleural leak. A tension pneumothorax may develop if the chest tube or drainage system becomes inadvertently occluded, as when the tubing gets pinched between the bedrail and bedframe during patient mobilization or sometimes when the vacuum is disconnected from the wall source.

3. **The fluid collection does not move at all with either spontaneous or positive-pressure breaths.** This behavior indicates that the proximal end of the chest tube is blocked. If no fluid or air leaks into the pleural space, the patient is in no danger; however, if a fluid or air leak develops, the possibility of tension pneumothorax exists. Despite the presence of a chest tube, always consider the possibility of tension pneumothorax when vital signs acutely deteriorate.

4. **Air constantly bubbles through the fluid whenever active suction is applied, without regard to either spontaneous or positive-pressure ventilation.** This behavior is expected immediately after a chest tube is inserted and air from a pneumothorax is being evacuated. This behavior should revert to either condition 1 or 2 as previously outlined as the reservoir of air in the treated pneumothorax is removed. If continuous bubbling recurs, one of three possibilities is likely: a leak has developed at the connection point between the chest tube and suction tubing; the chest tube has been partially pulled out so that one of the side holes is outside the patient's chest wall; or the bronchopleural fistula has increased in size and a single chest tube system is insufficient to remove the air as fast as it is entering.

8. How is tension pneumothorax due to a bronchopleural fistula diagnosed and managed?

When the vacuum is disconnected from its wall source, collapse of a lung may produce ventilation-perfusion inequalities and hypoxemia, as well as impede pulmonary venous return to the left side of the heart. The easiest way to check for this possibility is to note the patient's arterial pressure, disconnect the vacuum, wait for a minute or so without making any other changes that might influence the patient's blood pressure, and reassess the systemic blood pressure. If the lack of an active vacuum source compromises the patient's blood pressure, make plans to obtain a portable vacuum for the transport or fluid-load the patient adequately so that left-heart filling is no longer a problem.

When a bronchopleural fistula has increased in size such that a single chest tube system is no longer sufficient to remove the air as fast as it is entering, insert another chest tube with its own vacuum source (15 L/min is maximum flow for one vacuum source) or substitute a high-flow vacuum source (maximum flow ~ 100 L/min).

9. What ventilator considerations exist in a patient with a chest tube?

　　1. **What is the set tidal volume relative to the exhaled tidal volume?** If the patient is exhaling less than the ventilator delivers, then there is a bronchopleural fistula, and the difference represents the volume lost through the chest tube. However, flow transducers are not easily calibrated ,and the accuracy of the reported flow rates may be questionable. Inequality between set and exhaled tidal volumes should simply alert you that the patient *may* have a bronchopleural fistula, but this indication must be confirmed through other means, such as inspecting the chest tube drainage system (see question 7).

　　2. **What is the peak inspiratory pressure, and what is the plateau (static) pressure?** The peak inspiratory pressure is the highest pressure during end inspiration. Static pressure is a function of the combined stiffness of the patient's lungs and chest wall and is defined as the pressure required to prevent exhalation from occurring after the delivery of a set tidal volume; this value, expressed in ml/cm H_2O, is the static lung/chest wall compliance. The greater the stiffness, the lower the compliance value will be.

　　The difference between the plateau pressure and the peak inspiratory pressure represents the work that has to be done to overcome airway resistance. Technically, airway resistance = (peak pressure − static pressure)/inspiratory flow rate, where the peak pressure is measured at a constant flow rate of 30 L/min (0.5 L/sec). The actual numbers often are not obtainable because of the necessity of measuring them at such a slow flow rate, but the wider the difference between peak and static pressures, the greater the airway resistance and the greater the danger of air trapping (auto-PEEP) unless adequate expiratory time is allowed. Expiratory time is increased by using slow respiratory rates, fast inspiratory flow rates (short I-time) and long expiratory times (long E-time).

10. What are the effects of altering a patient's rate of ventilation during transport?
Normal lung/chest wall compliance for a patient intubated and on a ventilator is 50–80 ml/cm H_2O. A stiff lung, as observed in adult respiratory distress syndrome (ARDS), tension pneumothorax, or large pleural effusion is 10–20 ml/cm H_2O. By knowing the static compliance of the patient before transport, you can better adjust your ventilating technique during transport. For instance, if you give a patient with a low compliance a large tidal volume breath, the airways will be subject to high pressures with possible **barotrauma** (new pneumothorax) or extension of an existent **bronchopleural fistula**. The safest ventilatory pattern for a patient with noncompliant, stiff lungs is rapid and shallow.

　　On the other hand, patients who have higher-than-normal lung/chest wall compliance and/or high airway resistance are placed at risk of **air-trapping** due to inadequate expiratory time if you use a rapid ventilatory pattern. If the respiratory rate is increased without increasing inspiratory flow, the result is that the expiratory time will decrease; if the patient's lungs are not allowed sufficient time to empty, then the functional residual capacity (FRC) increases and the **auto-PEEP** effect will decrease venous return to the heart. This auto-PEEP effect is commonly seen in head-injured patients, probably secondary to the relative hypovolemic state in which these patients are maintained by the neurosurgical team. Relatively small increases in the FRC in them are likely to impede venous return more readily than in normovolemic individuals.

11. How should a patient with an pulmonary artery catheter (PAC) be monitored during transport?
Displacement of the PAC tip from the pulmonary artery during transit is of major concern. The nature of the waveform displayed on the patient's monitor gives the most immediate indication of the position of the PAC tip. When the tip is in a proximal portion of a pulmonary artery, the waveform displays a systolic, diastolic, and dicrotic notch pattern. If the tip migrates more distally, the waveform becomes damped and assumes an **occluded** (wedged) **waveform** with a venous pattern characterized by a, c, and v deflections reflecting the retrograde pressure fluctuations from the left atrium. Except when obtaining a wedge reading, a spontaneous occluded waveform (without inflation of the balloon) requires the catheter be promptly withdrawn from

the occluded position. Inflation of the balloon while the PAC tip is in a small pulmonary artery can result in **pulmonary artery rupture**, and the survival of patients with this complication is less than 50%.

Conversely, the position of the PAC tip within the right ventricle is associated with **ventricular arrhythmias**, including PVCs and ventricular tachycardia. The waveform is characterized by the lack of a dicrotic notch and a lowered diastolic pressure as compared to the pulmonary artery waveform. Recognizing an unsuspected right ventricular waveform often depends on observing the change in the waveform, not the absolute appearance of the waveform. A PAC with its tip in the right ventricle should be refloated into the pulmonary artery.

Thus, pulmonary artery waveforms are usually monitored during transit. If not, close attention must be paid so that the tip of the catheter is not displaced from its normal position in the proximal pulmonary artery. One useful method that avoids the inadvertent withdrawal of the catheter is to create a loop in the PAC tube outside the insertion site and tape the loop to the patient's chest or shoulder. Unfortunately, current technology does not allow for monitoring mixed venous saturation in transit, which would be useful in detecting deterioration in the patient's condition as well as detecting inadvertent wedging of the PAC.

10. How should a patient with severe pulmonary impairment be ventilated during transport?

The adequacy of ventilation is best determined from the **$PaCO_2$**. However, most transport ventilators and monitors lack this capability, and so it is best to rely on the well-documented, inverse relationship between alveolar ventilation and $PaCO_2$; the ICU ventilator flowsheet shows arterial blood gas results and the exhaled minute volume.

The ventilatory method chosen to take the place of the ICU ventilator during transport must achieve the same **alveolar volume**. Duplicating the respiratory rate and tidal volume set on the ICU ventilator may not be an adequate substitute for the transport ventilator. Additional parameters can be set on the ICU ventilator, such as mode of inspiratory cycling, peak inspiratory flow rate, and flow pattern. Although some of these factors may not be necessary to continue in transit, some patients will have severe ventilatory impairment and be dependent on the mode of operation of the ventilator. Significant alterations in the ventilatory pattern during transit may result in hypoxemia or CO_2 retention. The physician or respiratory therapist who has been managing the patient prior to transport is the best source of information on what will work during transport.

Self-inflating resuscitation bag with an oxygen reservoir is the most common device used to transport ventilator-dependent patients. Most adult bags range from 1500–2000 ml in the total displaceable volume, but few can be collapsed sufficiently to deliver more than 1000 ml, even when a two-handed technique is used. The average tidal volume delivered with a one-handed squeeze technique is 600 ml. Patients who have a low compliance because of their disease process will benefit from small tidal volumes. Patients with high airways resistance, particularly during expiration, will benefit from larger tidal volumes, rapid inspiratory flow rates, long expiratory times, and thus a slow respiratory rate, resulting in a lower incidence of auto-PEEP and decreased venous return to the heart.

Finally, the operator should ensure the proper functioning of the bag prior to use, testing that the bag really pressurizes prior to connecting to the patient. It is also important to be familiar with the built-in pressure relief mechanism, so that these do not pop off and produce hypoventilation in patients with decreased compliance or increased airway resistance.

13. How should a patient with severe pulmonary impairment be oxygenated during transport?

A second concern to be addressed during transport is oxygenation. There are particular concerns with regard to the transport of patients with **high FiO_2 requirements**. The E-cylinders used for transport have a Bourdon gauge flowmeter that, at the highest flow, can deliver only 15 L/min (250 ml/sec). If a patient requires 100% FiO_2 and their minute ventilation exceeds 15 L/min, the resuscitation bag cannot deliver the required amount of oxygen. Unless you compensate by connecting two (or more) O_2 tanks in parallel, entrainment of room air will occur and hypoxemia will result. (This flow restriction to 15 L/min applies only to Bourdon gauge flow meters, and the Thorpe tube flowmeters found attached to central wall oxygen supplies, although calibrated to 15 L/min, can achieve flows of up to 60 L/min if opened fully.)

Many ventilator-dependent patients are on **positive end-expiratory pressure** (PEEP) to maintain oxygenation and prevent atelectasis. The removal of appropriately added PEEP may be detrimental to a patient; a patient on a given level of PEEP on an ICU ventilator should be transported with a resuscitation bag that can maintain the same level of PEEP during transport.

14. An AIDS patient with *Pneumocystis carinii* pneumonia and a positive tuberculin test is intubated and on an ICU ventilator in an isolation room. Are any special arrangements needed to transport such a patient?

Individuals at risk for infectious disease in this setting include both the patient and the health care professionals. The AIDS patient, or any other immunocompromised person, is susceptible to any number of organisms in a hospital setting. Universal precautions should be followed, with particular attention to hygenic technique as regards intravenous lines and stopcock ports. A **needleless intravenous access system** protects the patient and eliminates the possibility of a needle wound to persons transporting the patient.

The airway is another consideration. The addition to the resuscitation bag (or transport ventilator) of a bacterial/viral **airway filter**, which also acts as a heat-moisture exchanger, is invaluable for two reasons: it protects the patient from organisms that may have colonized the patient connection end of the ventilation device, and it reduces the drying of the patient's airways during transport from the cool, dry oxygen supplied by cylinder.

The possibility of spreading HIV or *P. carinii* to any health care worker is negligible in this setting, but there is a real risk of transmitting *Mycobacterium tuberculosis*. Any immunocompromised patient, particularly one with a positive tuberculin skin test, should be considered a potential carrier of this infectious agent. Because the mycobacterium is nearly always transmitted by airborne droplets, the addition of an airway filter lessens this exposure to the health care workers involved in the transport as well bystanders.

15. What are the requisite materials that should be immediately available to the physician who is responsible for the transport of any unstable (moderate or maximal acuity) patient?

Three categories of materials should be immediately available during transport: (1) airway supplies and materials; (2) vasoactive drugs; and (3) sedatives and neuromuscular blocker drugs. These materials should be carried in a "tackle box" that always accompanies patients outside the OR.

1. **Airway supplies and materials**

Laryngoscope handles (standard and stubby)	Peripheral nerve stimulator
Laryngoscope blades in both pediatric and adult sizes	Pediatric and adult McGill forceps
	Acetocaine spray
Endotracheal tubes (3.0–9.0 mm internal diameter)	Facemasks
Oro- and nasopharyngeal airways	Stylets
Transtracheal jet ventilation kit	

2. **Vasoactive drugs**

Atropine	Calcium
Epinephrine	Esmolol
Ephedrine	Labetalol
Phenylephrine	Nitroglycerin
Lidocaine	Glycopyrrolate

3. **Sedatives/neuromuscular blockers**

Vecuronium	Etomidate
Succinylcholine	Ketamine
Pancuronium	

CONTROVERSY

16. Discuss the practice of sedating or paralyzing intubated patients for transport.

Pro: ICU patients are anxious, in pain, and fighting the ventilator and endotracheal tube. Once the necessary consent forms have been signed, spare the patient any additional anxiety or agony that may endanger the hemodynamic status, airway, or intravenous lines, and sedate and paralyze the patient until after the return from the operative procedure. The transport is completed more quickly and does not require as many participants. Some believe in "total" control of the patient through sedation or paralysis while in transit.

Con: The consequences of a "lost airway" in a paralyzed, apneic patient during transport can be disastrous. There is usually no vacuum source available to suction oropharyngeal secretions, and thus the visibility to perform laryngoscopy and reinsert the tube is questionable. Paralysis and sedation also abolish the patient's airway-protective reflexes, such as cough. Some believe that although conscious, nonparalyzed patients may not be able to maintain ventilation and oxygenation for a long time, they are able to do so until reaching a more controlled environment, where the personnel and materials necessary for successful reintubation are at hand. That is, hypoventilation is better than no ventilation.

BIBLIOGRAPHY

1. Braman SS, Dunn SM, Amico CA, Millman RP: Complications of intrahospital transport of critically ill patients. Ann Intern Med 107:469–473, 1987.
2. Branson RD: Intrahospital transport of critically ill, mechanically ventilated patients. Respir Care 37:775–806,1992.
3. Crippen D: Critical care transportation medicine: New concepts in pretransport stabilization of the critically ill patient. Am J Emerg Med 8:551–554,1990.
4. Fought SG, Nemeth L: Intrahospital transport: A framework for assessment. Crit Care Nurs Q 15:87–90, 1992.
5. Guidelines Committee of the American College of Critical Care Medicine, Society of Critical Care Medicine, and American Association of Critical-Care Nurses Transfer Guidelines Task Force: Guidelines for the transfer of critically ill patients. Crit Care Med 21:931–937, 1993.
6. Indeck M, Peterson S, Smith J, Brotman S: Risk, cost, and benefit of transporting ICU patients for special studies. J Trauma 28:1020–1025, 1988.
7. Insel J, Weissman C, Kemper M, et al: Cardiovascular changes during transport of critically ill and postoperative patients. Crit Care Med 14:539–542, 1986.
8. Kissoon N, Connors R, Tiffin N, Frewen TC: An evaluation of the physical and functional characteristics of resuscitators for use in pediatrics. Crit Care Med 20:292–296, 1992.
9. Link J, Krause H, Wagner W, Papadopoulos G: Intrahospital transport of critically ill patients. Crit Care Med 18:1427–1429, 1990.
10. Nearman HK, People CG: How to transfer a postoperative patient to the intensive care unit. J Crit Illness 10:275–280, 1990.
11. Runcie CJ, Reeve WG, Reidy J, Dougall JR: Blood pressure measurement during transport. Anaesthesia 45:659–665, 1990.
12. Smith I, Flemming S, Cernaianu A: Mishaps during transport from the intensive care unit. Crit Care Med 18:278–281, 1990.
13. Venkataraman ST, Orr RA: Intrahospital transport of critically ill patients. Crit Care Clin 8:525–531, 1993.
14. Waddell G: Movement of critically ill patients within hospital. BMJ 2:417–419, 1975.
15. Youngberg BJ: Medical-legal considerations involved in the transport of critically ill patients. Crit Care Clin 8:501–514, 1993.

87. BASIC AND ADVANCED LIFE SUPPORT

Barbara Barton, R.N., B.S.N.

1. When is it acceptable to withhold basic life support (BLS)?

It is acceptable to withhold cardiopulmonary resuscitation (CPR) in patients with lividity, decapitation, and other obvious signs of death. In addition, BLS should be withheld if the rescuer's life is placed at risk. If the patient has a no-CPR order (either in-patient or prehospital) indicated by a written document, medical bracelet, or identification card, health care providers have an obligation to honor it.

2. What are the acceptable conditions for interrupting basic life support for more than 5 seconds?

1. Defibrillation
2. Placement and rhythm interpretation using an automatic external defibrillator (AED)—90-second maximum for analysis of rhythm and three-stacked shocks for ventricular fibrillation (VF)
3. Endotracheal intubation—30-second maximum
4. If the rescuer is alone, to activate emergency medical services (EMS) or call 911 for help and defibrillator
5. To move patient to a safe location as quickly as possible
6. To transport the patient up or down a flight of stairs

3. What are the current recommendations for checking a pulse? What is the best site to check a pulse during an arrest? Why?

Check for a pulse with two-rescuer CPR after the first minute and every few minutes thereafter to ensure adequate circulation during CPR; stop CPR at the same intervals to check for spontaneous return of pulse. Also check for a pulse with every change in rhythm as well as between pharmacologic or electrical interventions, except during the three-stacked defibrillations for persistent VF or pulseless VT. The recommended artery for pulse check is the carotid artery because it is easy to locate, readily accessible, and one of the largest arteries in close proximity to the heart; the pulse persists longer at the carotid artery than at peripheral sites. Another choice for health care providers is the femoral artery because most providers are trained in locating it, it is a large vessel, and it is usually easy to palpate unless the patient is obese.

4. Which cardiac arrhythmias are known as the lethal arrhythmias?

The lethal arrhythmias, which require immediate treatment for survival, include ventricular fibrillation, pulseless ventricular tachycardia, asystole, and pulseless electrical activity.

5. What are periarrest arrhythmias?

The periarrest arrhythmias are precursors to the lethal rhythms and also require prompt action to prevent deterioration of the patient's condition. Included in this category are stable and unstable tachycardias (atrial fibrillation, atrial flutter, supraventricular and ventricular tachycardias) as well as unstable bradycardias, symptomatic sinus bradycardia, second-degree atrioventricular (AV) block types I and II, and complete heart block or third-degree AV block.

6. Name the most frequent rhythm in sudden cardiac death and specify the treatment of choice.

The most frequent arrhythmia (80–90% of cases of nontraumatic sudden death in adults) is ventricular fibrillation. The treatment of choice is early defibrillation; it is the single most important intervention in determining patient survival.

7. What are the indications for use of the automatic external defibrillator?

Chances of successfully converting ventricular fibrillation to a viable rhythm decrease by 7–10% per minute. The automatic external defibrillator (AED) was designed to allow early defibrillation by first responders who are not trained in defibrillation techniques or rhythm analysis. Its use is also indicated after cardiac arrest in hospital units when there is a delay in response of personnel trained in advanced cardiac life support (ACLS).

8. Describe the correct placement of the defibrillation pads.

The placement of the AED defibrillation pads depends on the type of device. Some devices have multifunction adhesive pads for use with a transcutaneous pacemaker as well as the AED or conventional defibrillator. These pads provide immediate access for pacing or defibrillation of the high-risk patient in the operating room. The anterior electrode is placed over the apex or precordium and the posterior electrode in the left infrascapular location. Another common placement is the same as conventional paddle placement; electrodes are placed to the right of the sternum just below the clavicle and at the apex of the heart to the left of the nipple in the midaxillary line.

9. List the indications for unsynchronized cardioversion and defibrillation and the recommended energy in joules for the various rhythms.

The indications for unsynchronized cardioversion and defibrillation are pulseless ventricular tachycardia, ventricular fibrillation, or unstable tachycardia (only when there is a significant delay in synchronization and the patient's condition is critical). Unsynchronized cardioversion should be avoided except in extreme circumstances because of the possibility of R-on-T phenomenon, which creates a lethal arrhythmia. The recommended energy level for sequential defibrillation is 200, 300, and 360 joules (J). If the patient converts to a more favorable rhythm and subsequently returns to another lethal arrhythmia requiring electrical therapy, the rescuer should begin with the energy level that converted the rhythm previously. For example, if the patient is defibrillated with 300 J, converts to sinus tachycardia, and then 5 minutes later refibrillates, the rescuer should begin with delivery of 300 J.

10. List the indications for synchronized cardioversion and the recommended energy in joules for the various rhythms.

As a general rule, any tachycardia that is greater than 150 beats per minute or symptomatic is considered unstable and is treated with synchronized cardioversion. The signs and symptoms that distinguish unstable tachycardia include chest pain, shortness of breath, decreased level of consciousness, hypotension, congestive heart failure, pulmonary edema, and ischemia. If possible, sedation should be considered before cardioversion; midazolam or fentanyl is a good choice, because reversal agents are available. Paroxysmal supraventricular tachycardia and atrial flutter sometimes convert with 50 J; it is recommended to begin at this level and proceed sequentially to 100, 200, 300, and 360 J as needed. For all other unstable tachycardias, the initial cardioversion should be at 100 J and, if unsuccessful, progress upward to 200, 300, and 360 J. The only exception is polymorphic ventricular tachycardia, which rarely responds to lower energy levels; therefore, 200 J are initially recommended.

11. Describe common errors in defibrillation and synchronized cardioversion and how to troubleshoot these problems.

The most common errors occur when the operator is unfamiliar with the defibrillator and monitor and thus contributes to life-threatening delays. The American Heart Association advises that users check the equipment daily to ensure familiarity and to identify any problems. ACLS providers have the ethical responsibility to be proficient in the use of all defibrillators in their area of practice or response locale. Another potentially fatal error is failure to clear the area before delivering the shock. The arrest team should stand back, stop what they are doing, and check to ensure that the operator is not standing in water, blood, or other liquids before the electrical discharge. If the defibrillator does not charge, the battery may be weak, and the machine requires an AC power source. If it is possible to charge the defibrillator but not to deliver the shock, the team should check to see that the operator is simultaneously holding down the two buttons on the paddles until it discharges. A delay in attaching the patient to the monitor leads can be avoided by applying conductive medium to the chest, turning the lead select to paddles, placing the paddles on the chest, and obtaining a "quick look" at the patient's rhythm. If the patient's condition requires electrical therapy, a crucial delay may be avoided. Synchronized cardioversion sometimes involves a problem with synchronization on the R wave of the ECG, but this problem is usually solved easily with a few simple trials. First the team should check to see that the gain on the ECG is midrange; if this step does not help, the leads should be changed. The team must ensure that the synchronization button is on and reset after each countershock. If it still will not synchronize, possibly the rhythm has changed and is too chaotic—check the patient!

12. Explain the special considerations of defibrillator paddle placement in patients with implantable cardioverters-defibrillators and permanent pacemakers.

If the patient has either a permanent pacemaker or an implantable cardioverter-defibrillator (ICD), external defibrillator paddle placement must be altered. The paddles should be 5 inches from the site of the pulse generator to prevent pacer malfunction or increased transthoracic resistance. If the patient with an ICD has received several unsuccessful shocks at 360 J, a different paddle placement (anteroposterior or apex-sternum) should be tried. After the patient has been defibrillated, the pacemaker or the ICD should be checked for proper function and reprogrammed if necessary.

13. What are the indications for a transcutaneous pacemaker?

The two main indications for a transcutaneous pacemaker (TCP) are unstable (symptomatic) bradycardias that are atropine-refractory and early treatment of asystole. The signs and symptoms associated with an unstable bradycardic rhythm are hypotension, pulmonary edema, premature ventricular contractions (PVCs), acute myocardial infarction, chest pain, shortness of breath, dizziness, syncope, and decreased levels of consciousness. The unstable bradycardic rhythms may include sinus bradycardia with or without PVCs, first-degree AV block, second-degree AV block types I and II, and third-degree AV block. The TCP is a temporary method for increasing the heart rate until the cause can be treated, or in patients with second-degree AV block type II and complete heart block (third-degree), until a transvenous pacemaker can be placed. The asystolic heart rarely responds to pacing, but the TCP is recommended along with epinephrine and atropine early in treatment for maximal effectiveness.

14. What is the best central line placement in an arrest situation? Why?

The preferred site for central line placement in an arrest situation is controversial. Because of the lack of need to interrupt CPR and the decreased incidence of major complications on insertion, the femoral vein is often chosen. However, the femoral vein is sometimes difficult to locate with CPR in progress, because the landmark for finding the vein is the diminished femoral arterial pulsation.

15. Describe the disadvantages of central line placement with CPR in progress.

Both internal jugular and subclavian venous access involve a higher complication rate because of the close proximity of the vessels to the apices of the lung, carotid and subclavian arteries, and other important structures. Another disadvantage of attempting to place lines in the patient's upper trunk or neck is lack of sufficient space due to other participants in CPR.

16. Describe the indications for endotrachial intubation.

1. Respiratory or cardiac arrest
2. Inability to maintain or protect the airway (e.g., stroke, decreased level of consciousness, drug overdose, trauma)
3. Inability to adequately oxygenate or ventilate

17. Describe the complications of endotracheal intubation.
The complications of endotracheal intubation include trauma to the lips, teeth, tongue, trachea, or mucosa. Other problems include incorrect positioning of the tube into the mainstem bronchus (usually the right) or esophagus. Regurgitation and aspiration during intubation are concerns in patients with a full stomach. The patient also may briefly experience hypertension and/or arrhythmias in response to the stimulus of laryngoscopy or intubation. Delays in securing the airway may result in hypoxemia or hypercarbia. In addition, distortion of the airway, either from trauma, infection, obesity, or as a normal variant may pose significant difficulties.

18. What are the most common causes of airway obstruction?
The most common causes of obstructed airway in the unconscious victim are the tongue and epiglottis. Head and neck trauma are associated with hemorrhage and dental fractures that may cause obstruction of the airway, and there may be structural damage to the trachea itself. Another cause of airway obstruction is vomitus or poorly chewed food, especially in patients that cannot protect their airway. Airway obstruction frequently occurs during eating, and the offender in adults is most often meat. Loose dentures also may cause an obstructed airway.

19. Discuss the clinical assessment of the airway and explain the emergency treatment of an obstructed airway.
Obstruction of the airway by the tongue or epiglottis is often relieved by performing the head tilt and the jaw thrust or chin lift. Insertion of an oropharyngeal or nasopharyngeal airway in the unconscious person may maintain a patent airway in this setting. In partial airway obstruction, the patient most likely is wheezing audibly or has inspiratory stridor as well as an appearance of panic. A member of the team should stay with the person and encourage him or her to dislodge the foreign body by coughing forcefully. If the person is unable to clear the airway, he or she may tire and develop poor airway exchange or progress to full obstruction and cyanosis. Often the person clutches the throat (the universal distress signal) and is unable to cough, speak, or breathe. The provider should activate EMS (or call for in-hospital help) and immediately perform the Heimlich maneuver by administering subdiaphragmatic abdominal thrusts that forcefully push air out of the lungs, hopefully dislodging the foreign body and clearing the obstructed airway.

20. Describe the different ways of performing the Heimlich maneuver.
There are several different ways to perform the Heimlich maneuver, depending on the patient's level of consciousness. If the patient is still conscious and standing or sitting, put your arms around the patient's waist, place your fist midline above the patient's umbilicus but below the xiphoid process of the sternum, grasp your fist, and begin quick upward abdominal thrusts. Repeat the abdominal thrusts until the foreign body is expelled or the person becomes unconscious. If the latter occurs, carefully place the patient on the ground in the supine position, straddle the patient, place the heel of one hand on top of the other, and in the midline above the umbilicus but below the xiphoid process, press into the abdomen with 5 quick upward abdominal thrusts. The next maneuver is to perform a finger sweep to try and relieve or dislodge the obstruction; sweep the entire mouth with a hooking movement to remove the object, if possible, taking care not to push it further down. Under controlled circumstances, anesthesiologists may remove the object with a laryngoscope and Magill forceps. After the finger sweep, two rescue breaths should be attempted. If the rescuer is unable to ventilate the patient, the sequence should be repeated: 5 abdominal thrusts, a finger sweep, and 2 rescue breaths. The sequence should be continued as long as necessary. Chest thrusts (hand placement in the middle of the sternum) are recommended for markedly obese patients, women in advanced stages of pregnancy, and infants.

21. What is the first line antiarrhythmic agent used to treat wide-complex tachycardia of uncertain origin? Why?
The first line antiarrhythmic agent in wide-complex tachycardia of uncertain origin is lidocaine. Undiagnosed wide-complex tachyarrhythmia is to be treated as if ventricular in origin. If the patient

is treated as if the rhythm is paroxysmal supraventricular tachycardia (PSVT), a likely therapy is intravenous verapamil, which may be lethal to a patient with VT or Wolff-Parkinson-White (WPW) syndrome. Verapamil administered to patients with VT may cause severe hypotension and lead to VF in some cases. If verapamil is inadvertently given to patients with WPW, the ventricular rate may increase because of aberrant conduction, and the patient's condition deteriorates because of secondary hypotension or ischemia. Because lidocaine is not detrimental to the patient with PSVT, its use adheres to the principle of do no harm. If there is no response to a loading dose of lidocaine, the next drug to administer is adenosine. It is the first-line pharmacologic treatment for PSVT and is not harmful to patients with VT; it may assist with diagnosis of the rhythm as it slows.

22. What is the first drug to use for any pulseless rhythm? Why?
Epinephrine is the drug of choice in all pulseless rhythms (ventricular fibrillation, pulseless ventricular tachycardia, asystole, and pulseless electrical activity). It is probably the single most important drug in cardiac arrest because it has multiple essential actions. Epinephrine is an endogenous catecholamine with alpha- and beta-adrenergic action; it increases systemic vascular resistance, heart rate and contractility, arterial blood pressure, myocardial oxygen requirement, and automaticity (which is beneficial in converting VF to an effective rhythm). As a result, epinephrine improves cerebral and coronary perfusion pressure, which is vital to the patient's recovery.

23. Identify the causes of pulseless electrical activity (PEA) and describe the appropriate emergency treatment.

Differential Diagnosis of Pulseless Electrical Activity*

CAUSES	TREATMENT
Hypovolemia	Most common cause. Volume infusion with balanced crystalloid solutions, colloids, and blood products. Control hemorrhage if present.
Hypoxia	Oxygenation and ventilation.
Hypothermia	Passive rewarming—active external rewarming 30–36°C; if core temperature < 30°C, active internal rewarming.
Hyperkalemia	Calcium chloride, insulin, glucose, and sodium bicarbonate to force potassium into the cell.
Tension pneumothorax	14-gauge catheter over the needle inserted in the midclavicular line at the second or third intercostal space.
Cardiac tamponade	Fluid bolus, inotropes, needle pericardiocentesis.
Massive pulmonary embolus	Emergency thoracotomy for embolectomy; thrombolytics.
Drug overdoses	Immediate drug screen, gastric lavage, activated charcoal, cathartics.
Tricyclic antidepressants	Hyperventilate, sodium bicarbonate infusion.
Digoxin	Digoxin-specific antibodies.
Beta blockers	Crystalloid bolus 500–1000 cc, glucagon, epinephrine infusion, transcutaneous or transvenous pacing, calcium chloride, pressors.
Calcium channel blockers	Same as beta blockers except calcium chloride is the first-line drug.
Acidosis (preexisting)	Treat cause, hyperventilate, sodium bicarbonate.
Acute myocardial infarction	Inotropes, nitroglycerin, fluids, thrombolytics.

* A useful mnemonic is 3 Hypos, 1 Hyper, T-T, PE, D-A-M.

24. What is the drug of choice for treatment of torsades de pointes? What is the correct dose?
Torsades de pointes is a polymorphic ventricular tachycardia that appears to twist and change form and polarity. It is associated with a prolonged QT interval (> 0.40 sec) as a result of drug toxicity or electrolyte imbalances. The treatment of choice is overdrive pacing but, because of the delay this technique may involve, pharmacologic therapy is frequently indicated. The drug of choice is magnesium sulfate. The recommended dose is 1–2 gm intravenously over 1–2 minutes; the dose is repeated over 1 hour to a maximum of 4–6 gm. Additional research is needed to confirm the most efficacious dose for torsades de pointes, but this is the current recommendation.

25. Calculate the maximum dose of atropine for refractory unstable bradycardia in a 100-kg patient.

The maximum dosage is 0.04 mg/kg. Therefore a patient weighing 100 kg may receive up to 4 mg intravenously in 1-mg increments every 3–5 minutes.

26. After lidocaine and bretylium have failed, what is the next antiarrhythmic drug indicated for refractory ventricular fibrillation? How is it administered?

The third antiarrhythmic drug indicated in refractory VF is magnesium sulfate, 1–2 gm, given intravenously over 1–2 minutes.

27. Describe the treatment of a patient with a stable narrow-complex tachycardia.

The first intervention is to attempt to convert the rhythm or at least to slow it down for diagnostic purposes with vagal maneuvers. Vagal maneuvers include carotid sinus massage (after ruling out the presence of carotid bruits), Valsalva (asking the patient to bear down as if having a bowel movement), or immersion of the patient's face in ice water (contraindicated in heart disease). If vagal maneuvers are unsuccessful, pharmacologic therapy is the next choice. The initial drug in stable narrow-complex tachycardia is adenosine, 6 mg IV over 1–3 seconds. Administration may be repeated twice at increased doses of 12 mg 1–2 minutes apart. If there is still no change in rhythm and the patient continues to have an adequate blood pressure, verapamil, 2.5–5 mg by slow IV push, is the second drug of choice. Verapamil may be repeated in 15–30 minutes at a dose of 5–10 mg IV. If the patient becomes unstable, sedation and immediate synchronized cardioversion is indicated.

28. When is sodium bicarbonate *definitely* indicated in an arrest situation? Why?

If the patient is hyperkalemic, sodium bicarbonate (along with insulin and dextrose) is definitely indicated to produce an intracellular shift of potassium and hopefully to reverse the adverse cardiac effects of hyperkalemia. Blood gases should be monitored closely to prevent an iatrogenic metabolic alkalosis.

29. Explain why atropine is not the drug of choice for a heart transplant patient experiencing a symptomatic bradycardic rhythm? What treatment should be used?

Atropine is a parasympatholytic drug that increases heart rate by direct vagolytic action. The transplanted heart has been denervated and does not respond to vagolytic drugs. The treatment of choice for symptomatic bradycardia is a transcutaneous pacemaker (temporary measure). The pharmacologic intervention of choice is infusion of a catecholamine, such as epinephrine, dopamine, or isoproterenol (with extreme caution).

BIBLIOGRAPHY

1. Billi JE, Cummins RO: Instructor's Manual for Advanced Cardiac Life Support. Dallas, American Heart Association, 1994.
2. Chandra NC, Hazinski MF (eds): Basic Life Support for Healthcare Providers. Dallas, American Heart Association, 1994.
3. Cummins RO: Textbook of Advanced Cardiac Life Support. Dallas, American Heart Association, 1994.
4. Dubin DR: Update on pediatric cardiopulmonary resuscitation. Hosp Physician July:14–22, 1994.
5. Fromm RD, Varon J, Stahmer SA: Techniques in cardiopulmonary resuscitation: Past, present and future. Hosp Physician July:10–13, 1994.
6. Grauer K, Cavallaro D: ACLS Certification Preparation, vol. 1, 3rd ed.. St. Louis, Mosby, 1993.
7. Grauer K, Cavallaro D: ACLS: A Comprehensive Review, vol. 2, 3rd ed. St. Louis, Mosby. 1993.
8. Guidelines for cardiopulmonary resuscitation and emergency cardiac care. Recommendations of the 1992 national conference. JAMA 268:2171–2302, 1992.
9. Newman MN (ed): Currents in Emergency Cardiac Care, vol. 3. Dallas, American Heart Association, 1992.
10. Pollack B: Notes from an emergency room physician. Hosp Physician July:8–9, 1994.
11. Stahmer SA, Varon J, Fromm RE: Controversies in cardiopulmonary resuscitation pharmacotherapy. Hosp Physician July:23–30, 1994.

88. MODES OF MECHANICAL VENTILATION

Stuart G. Rosenberg, M.D.

1. What is mechanical ventilation?

Mechanical ventilation (MV) is a form of artificial ventilation that performs the task normally done by the respiratory muscles. It allows oxygenation and ventilation (carbon dioxide removal) of the patient. The two major types of MV are positive-pressure ventilation and negative-pressure ventilation. Positive-pressure ventilation (PPV) may be invasive (via an endotracheal tube) or noninvasive (via face mask). It also may be volume- or pressure-cycled, as discussed below. The many different modes of PPV include controlled mechanical ventilation (CMV), assist-control ventilation (ACV), intermittent mandatory ventilation (IMV), synchronized IMV (SIMV), pressure-controlled ventilation (PCV), pressure-support ventilation (PSV), inverse ratio ventilation (IRV), pressure-release ventilation (PRV), and high-frequency modes.

It is important to distinguish endotracheal intubation from MV as one does not necessarily imply the other. For example, a patient may require endotracheal intubation for airway protection and still be able to breathe spontaneously through the endotracheal tube without the need for MV.

2. Why might a patient require MV?

MV may be indicated in many disorders. In many cases, however, the indications are not clearcut. The main reasons for instituting MV are the patient's inability to oxygenate adequately and the loss of adequate alveolar ventilation, which may be secondary to primary abnormalities of the pulmonary parenchyma, such as pneumonia or pulmonary edema, or systemic disease that indirectly compromises pulmonary function, such as sepsis or central nervous system dysfunction. In addition, administration of a general anesthetic frequently requires MV, because many agents are respiratory depressants, and neuromuscular blocking drugs cause paralysis of the respiratory muscles. The principal goal of MV in the setting of respiratory failure is to support gas exchange while the underlying disease process is reversed.

3. Describe noninvasive ventilation and when it may be appropriate.

Noninvasive ventilation may be either a negative- or positive-pressure mode. Negative-pressure ventilation (usually via an iron lung or cuirass ventilator) is occasionally used in patients with neuromuscular disorders or chronic fatigue of the diaphragm due to chronic obstructive lung disease (COLD). The ventilator shell encompasses the body below the neck, and a negative pressure is generated, creating a gradient for flow of gas from the upper airway into the lungs. Exhalation is passive. This mode of ventilation avoids the need for endotracheal intubation and its attendant problems. The upper airway must be clear, and it is left unprotected from aspiration. Hypotension may occur from splanchnic pooling of blood.

Noninvasive ventilation using positive pressure (NIPPV) can be delivered in various ways, including mask continuous positive airway pressure (CPAP), mask bilevel positive airway pressure (bi-PAP), mask PSV, or combinations of these. This mode of ventilation may be used to avoid endotracheal intubation in certain subgroups of patients, such as those who are terminally ill or have certain types of respiratory failure (e.g., hypercapnic COLD exacerbation). In terminally ill patients with respiratory compromise, NIPPV has been shown to be a safe, effective, and more comfortable means of ventilatory support. It allows the patient to maintain autonomy and verbal communication and is simpler and less stressful to terminate if indicated.

4. Describe CMV, AC, and IMV, the most commonly used modes of PPV.

These three modes of conventional volume-cycled ventilation are in essence three different ways of triggering the ventilator. With CMV, the patient is entirely under the control of the preset tidal volume (V_T) and respiratory frequency (f). CMV is used in patients making no respiratory effort at all, e.g., those with respiratory depression or pharmacologically induced paralysis, as seen under general anesthesia. The ACV mode allows the patient to trigger a breath (hence, the element of assist) so that a preset tidal volume is delivered. If the patient becomes bradypneic or apneic for any reason, the ventilator provides a back-up control mode. IMV, which originally was developed as a weaning tool, allows the patient to breathe spontaneously through the ventilator circuit. The ventilator intermittently delivers positive-pressure breaths based on a preset V_T and f. SIMV prevents the ventilator from delivering a mechanical breath during a spontaneous breath.

The debate over the advantages and disadvantages of ACV and IMV continues to rage. Theoretically, IMV may allow a decreased mean airway pressure (Paw) and possibly less barotrauma, because not every breath is a positive-pressure breath. It also may be easier to synchronize the patient with the ventilator in the IMV mode. ACV probably causes respiratory alkalosis more often, because the patient receives a full V_T with every breath, even when tachypneic. Either mode requires some work of breathing on the patient's part (usually more with IMV). It may be advantageous initially to relieve as much of the work as possible in patients with acute respiratory failure (ARF) while allowing the underlying disease process to reverse itself. This usually requires sedation, occasionally muscle paralysis, and CMV.

5. What are the initial ventilator settings in ARF? What are the goals of these settings?
Most patients with ARF require full ventilatory support. The basic goals are to preserve arterial oxygen saturation and to prevent ventilator-induced complications. Complications may arise from elevated airway pressures or persistently high inspired concentrations of oxygen (FiO_2). (see below).

Most commonly one begins with the **ACV mode**, which ensures delivery of a preset volume. Pressure-cycled modes are, however, becoming more popular.

An **FiO_2** needs to be chosen. One usually starts at 1.0 and titrates downward as tolerated. Prolonged exposure to high FiO_2 values (> 60–70%) may lead to oxygen toxicity.

Tidal volume is based on body weight and the pathophysiology of lung injury. Currently, volumes in the range of 10–12 ml/kg body weight are acceptable. Conditions such as acute respiratory distress syndrome (ARDS), however, decrease the volume of the lung available for ventilation. Because large pressures or volumes may exacerbate the underlying lung injury, smaller volumes are chosen, in the range of 6–10 ml/kg body weight.

A **respiratory rate** (f) is chosen, usually in the range of 10–20 breaths per minute (bpm). Patients with high minute volume requirements may need a rate in the 20s. Carbon dioxide (CO_2) elimination does not improve significantly with rates > 25 and rates > 30 predispose to gas trapping secondary to abbreviated expiratory times.

Positive end-expiratory pressure (PEEP; see question 6) is typically chosen in small amounts initially (e.g., 5 cmH$_2$O) and may be titrated upward if necessary to improve oxygenation. A small amount of PEEP in most cases of acute lung injury helps to maintain the patency of recruitable alveoli. Recent data show that a small amount of PEEP avoids the alveolar shear forces that result from the repetitive opening and closing of alveoli. Such shear forces may aggravate lung injury.

Flow rate, pattern, and inspiratory/expiratory (I:E) ratio are frequently set by the respiratory therapist, but they should be understood also by the intensivist. The peak flow rate determines the maximal inspiratory flow rate delivered by the ventilator during the inspiratory cycle. An initial flow rate of 50–80 L/min is usually satisfactory. The I:E ratio is determined by the minute ventilation and flow rate; that is, inspiratory time is determined by flow and V_T, whereas expiratory time is determined by flow and frequency. An I:E of 1:2 to 1:3 is reasonable in most situations; however, patients with COLD may require even longer expiratory times to allow adequate exhalation of gases. This can be accomplished by increasing flow, thus decreasing the I:E ratio. High flow rates, however, may increase airway pressures and worsen gas distribution in some cases. Slower flow rates may reduce airway pressures and improve gas distribution by increasing the I:E ratio. An increased (or "reversed," as discussed below) I:E ratio increases mean

Paw but also may increase cardiovascular side effects. The shortened expiratory time is not well tolerated in obstructive airways disease. The flow pattern or waveform also has a small effect on ventilation. A constant flow pattern (square wave) provides flow at the value selected. The descending or ramp waveform may increase airway pressures yet improve gas distribution. Inspiratory hold, expiratory retard, and periodic sigh also may be chosen.

6. Explain PEEP. How is optimal PEEP determined?

PEEP is a supplement to many of the modes of ventilation whereby the airway pressure at end expiration remains above ambient pressure. PEEP tends to prevent alveolar collapse and to recruit a portion of atelectatic alveoli in acute lung injury states. Functional residual capacity (FRC) and oxygenation are increased. PEEP is applied initially at approximately 5 cmH_2O and increased in small increments to a total of 15–20 cmH_2O. High levels of PEEP may have a deleterious effect on cardiac output (see below). Optimal PEEP strives for the best arterial oxygenation, with the least decrement in cardiac output, and maintenance of acceptable airway pressures. Optimal PEEP is actually the point of maximal alveolar recruitment, which can be assessed quickly at the bedside by increasing PEEP to the point of lung inflation at which compliance (see below) begins to decrease. One simply watches the airway pressure after each incremental increase in PEEP. The airway pressure should rise only by the amount of PEEP dialed in. When the pressure begins to rise more than the amount of PEEP dialed in, the alveoli are overdistended and the point of maximal alveolar recruitment has been exceeded. Continuous positive airway pressure (CPAP) is a form of PEEP delivered throughout the respiratory cycle during spontaneous breathing.

7. What is intrinsic or auto-PEEP?

As first described by Pepe and Marini in 1982, intrinsic PEEP (PEEPi) is the development of positive pressure and continued flow within the alveoli at end expiration without application of extrinsic PEEP (PEEPe). Normally the lung volume at end expiration (FRC) is determined by the opposing forces of elastic recoil and the chest wall. These forces are normally balanced so that there is no flow or pressure gradient at end expiration. PEEPi occurs by two major mechanisms. In healthy lungs during MV, if the respiratory f is too rapid or the E time too short, there is not enough time for full exhalation before the next breath is delivered. This results in stacking of breaths and generation of positive airway pressure at end exhalation. Therefore, patients with high minute volume requirements (e.g., sepsis, trauma) or patients receiving high I:E ratios are at risk for PEEPi. Small-diameter endotracheal tubes also may limit exhalation and contribute to PEEPi. The other major mechanism for development of PEEPi is related to the underlying pulmonary pathology. Patients with increased airway resistance and pulmonary compliance (e.g., asthma, COLD) are at high risk for PEEPi. Such patients have difficulty in exhaling gas because of airway obstruction and are prone to development of PEEPi during spontaneous ventilation as well as MV. PEEPi has the same side effects as PEEPe, but it requires more vigilance. As ventilators are normally vented to ambient pressure, the only way to detect and measure PEEPi is to occlude the expiratory port at end expiration while monitoring airway pressure. This should be done routinely in all patients receiving MV, especially those at high risk. Treatment is based on etiology. Manipulating ventilator parameters (such as decreasing f or increasing inspiratory flow to decrease I:E) may allow time for full exhalation. Treatment of the underlying disease process (e.g., bronchodilators) also helps. PEEPe has been used with some benefit to relieve air trapping in patients with expiratory flow limitation from obstructive airways disease. This may work by theoretically stenting open airways to allow full exhalation. As PEEPe approaches PEEPi, however, severe hemodynamic and gas exchange compromise may occur.

8. What are the side effects of PEEPe and PEEPi?

1. Barotrauma may occur from overdistention of alveoli.

2. Cardiac output (CO) may be decreased by several mechanisms. PEEP increases intrathoracic pressure, leading to an increase in transmural right atrial pressure and a decrease in venous return. PEEP also tends to increase pulmonary artery pressure, which impedes right ventricular

output. Dilation of the right ventricle may cause bowing of the interventricular septum into the left ventricle, thus impairing filling of the left ventricle and contributing to decreased CO. Hypotension ensues, especially if the patient is hypovolemic. In a common scenario, an emergency endotracheal intubation is performed in a patient with COLD and respiratory failure. Such patients usually have been in distress for several days with decreased oral intake and increased insensible fluid losses. On intubation the patient is vigorously bagged to improve oxygenation and ventilation. Auto-PEEP rapidly worsens, and in the face of hypovolemia severe hypotension ensues. Treatment (if prevention fails) consists of rapid volume infusion, allowing a longer expiratory phase, and resolution of bronchospasm.

3. Incorrect interpretation of cardiac filling pressures (e.g., central venous pressure or pulmonary artery occlusion pressure) also may occur with PEEP. Pressure transmitted from the alveolus to the pulmonary vasculature may falsely elevate the readings. The more compliant the lung, the greater the pressure that is transmitted. A rule of thumb is to subtract one-half of the PEEP applied over five from the pulmonary artery occlusion pressure (PAOP).

4. Overdistention of alveoli from excessive PEEP decreases blood flow to these areas, increasing dead space (Vd/V_T).

5. Work of breathing may be increased with PEEP (with positive-pressure breathing that requires the patient to trigger the ventilator or with spontaneous breathing on the ventilator), because the patient is required to generate a larger negative pressure to trigger flow from the ventilator.

6. Other potential side effects of PEEP include an increase in intracranial pressure (ICP) and fluid retention.

9. Describe pressure-limited types of ventilation.

The ability to deliver pressure-limited breaths (either triggered by the patient [pressure support ventilation] or the ventilator [pressure-controlled ventilation]) has been added to most adult ventilators in recent years. Pressure-limited modes are used routinely in neonatal ventilation. With pressure support ventilation (PSV) the patient initiates the breath, causing the ventilator to deliver a preset pressure, augmenting the V_T. The positive-pressure portion of the breath is cycled off after the inspiratory flow drops to a predetermined level, typically 25% of its peak value. Note that the pressure is sustained until the flow tapers. This flow characteristic readily meets the patient's demands and results in greater comfort. This spontaneous mode of ventilation can be used to decrease work of breathing by overcoming resistance in the breathing circuit and augmenting V_T in marginal patients. It may be combined with IMV or used alone. PEEP or CPAP may be added. PSV also has been shown to expedite weaning from MV.

In pressure-controlled ventilation (PCV) the patient receives a positive-pressure breath that ceases when a preset maximal pressure is reached. Volume varies, depending on airways resistance and pulmonary compliance. PCV may be used alone or combined with other techniques such as IRV (see below). The inherent flow characteristics of PCV (high initial flow followed by a decelerating wave pattern) seem to improve compliance and gas distribution. It has been suggested that PCV may be used safely and is well tolerated as an initial mode of ventilation in patients with acute hypoxic respiratory failure. Pressure-control modes with volume-guarantee ventilators are beginning to appear on the market.

10. Does inverse ratio ventilation have a role in patient ventilation?

IRV may have some benefit in severe ARDS. It is a controversial mode of ventilation in which the I time is extended beyond the usual maximum of 50% of the respiratory cycle in a pressure- or volume-cycled mode. As the I time is prolonged, the I:E ratio inverts (e.g., 1:1, 1.5:1, 2:1, 3:1). Most intensivists do not recommend going beyond 2:1 because of the increasing risks of hemodynamic compromise and barotrauma. Oxygenation has been shown to improve by lengthening I time, although no prospective randomized trials have been done. The mechanism for improvement in oxygenation may be related to several factors: increase in mean Paw (without an increase in peak Paw), recruitment of additional alveoli with longer opening time constants due to slower inspiratory flow, and development of PEEPi. The slower inspiratory flow also may decrease the development of volutrauma or barotrauma. This technique, however, may be counterproductive in patients with airflow obstruction (e.g., COLD or asthma) by worsening PEEPi. Because IRV may be an uncomfortable mode of ventilation for patients, deep sedation or muscle paralysis may be required. In summary, although of unproven benefit, IRV may have a role in advanced ARDS.

11. Does MV cause problems in organ systems other than the cardiopulmonary system?
Yes. Increased intrathoracic pressure may cause or contribute to increased ICP. Sinusitis may result from prolonged nasotracheal intubation. Nosocomial pneumonia is always a concern in ventilated patients. Gastrointestinal bleeding is common from stress ulceration, and prophylaxis should be initiated. Water and salt retention may result from increased vasopressin secretion and decreased levels of atrial natriuretic compound. Bedridden, critically ill patients are always at risk for thromboembolic phenomena; prophylaxis is thus appropriate. Many patients receiving MV require sedation and occasionally muscle paralysis (see below).

12. What is controlled hypoventilation with permissive hypercapnia?
Controlled hypoventilation is a method used in patients requiring MV to prevent overinflation of alveoli and possible damage to the alveolar-capillary membrane. Recent data indicate that high levels of volume and pressure may induce or potentiate lung injury by alveolar overdistention. Controlled hypoventilation (or permissive hypercapnia) is a pressure-limiting, lung-protective strategy whereby less significance is given to the pCO_2 value than to the inflation pressure of the lung. Several studies in ARDS and status asthmaticus have shown a decrease in barotrauma, intensive care days, and mortality. One lowers the set V_T to a range of approximately 6–10 ml/kg in an attempt to keep the peak Paw below 35–40 cmH_2O and the static Paw below 30 cmH_2O. A small V_T is appropriate in ARDS, which is a heterogenous lung disease with small lung volumes available for ventilation. Gattinoni et al. described three zones in this disease process: a zone of consolidated diseased alveoli that cannot be recruited, a zone of collapsed yet recruitable alveoli, and a small zone (25–30% of normal) of alveoli available for ventilation. Traditional V_Ts much in excess of volume available for ventilation may cause overdistention of available alveoli, potentially exacerbating acute lung injury. Because only a small area of lung is available for ventilation, the term "baby lung" has been coined. The pCO_2 is allowed to rise slowly to a level of up to 80–100 mmHg. The pH falls and may be treated with buffer below 7.20–7.25. Alternatively one may wait for the normal kidney to retain bicarbonate in response to the hypercapnia. Permissive hypercapnia is usually well tolerated. Potential adverse effects include cerebral vasodilatation leading to increased ICP. In fact, intracranial hypertension is the only absolute contraindication to permissive hypercapnia. Increased sympathetic activity, pulmonary vasoconstriction, and cardiac arrhythmias may occur, although they are rarely of significance. Depression of cardiac contractility may be a problem in patients with underlying ventricular dysfunction.

13. Are there other methods to control pCO_2?
There are several other approaches to the control of pCO_2. Decreased production of CO_2 can be achieved by deep sedation, muscle paralysis, cooling (certainly avoiding hyperthermia), and a decrease in the amount of ingested carbohydrate. Tracheal gas insufflation (TGI) is a simple method of increasing CO_2 clearance. A small (suction-type) catheter is placed through the endotracheal tube to the level of the carina. Oxygen and blended nitrogen are insufflated at approximately 4–6 L/min. This in effect creates a wash-out of deadspace (Vd/V_T) without a change in minute ventilation or airway pressure. The average reduction in pCO_2 is 15%. This technique is helpful in head-injured patients who may benefit from controlled hypoventilation. Extracorporeal techniques for CO_2 removal are also occasionally used.

14. What is lung compliance? How is it calculated?
Compliance is a measure of distensibility and is expressed as the change in volume for a given change in pressure. Pulmonary compliance is calculated as V_T/(Paw − PEEP). Normal static

compliance is 70–100 ml/cmH$_2$O. In ARDS the compliance is less than 40–50 ml/cmH$_2$O. Compliance is a global value and does not describe what is happening regionally in the lung with ARDS, in which diseased regions are interspersed with relatively healthy regions. Trending of compliance is a useful parameter in determining the course of a patient with ARF.

15. Is ventilation in the prone position an option in patients who are difficult to oxygenate?
Studies have shown that pO$_2$ improves significantly in most patients with ARDS when they are prone, probably because of improvement in ventilation/perfusion matching in the lung. Ventilation in the prone position is not routine, however, because it makes nursing care much more difficult.

16. How does one approach the patient who is "fighting the ventilator"?
Agitation, respiratory distress, or "fighting the ventilator" must be taken seriously, because several of the causes may be life-threatening. A diagnosis must be arrived at swiftly to prevent irreversible harm to the patient. Initially, one separates the potential causes into ventilator (machine, circuit, and airway) problems and patient-related problems. The many patient-related causes include hypoxemia, secretions or mucous plugging, pneumothorax, bronchospasm, infection such as pneumonia or sepsis, pulmonary embolus, myocardial ischemia, gastrointestinal bleed, worsening PEEPi, and anxiety. The ventilator-related issues include system leak or disconnection; inadequate ventilator support or delivered FiO$_2$; airway-related problems, such as extubation, obstructed endotracheal tube, cuff herniation or rupture; or improper triggering sensitivity or flows. Until the problem is sorted out, one should ventilate the patient manually with 100% O$_2$. Breath sounds and vital signs (including pulse oximetry and end tidal CO$_2$) should be immediately checked. If time permits, an arterial blood gas analysis and portable chest radiograph should be obtained. A suction catheter may be placed rapidly through the endotracheal tube to ensure patency and to suction secretions or plugs. Suspicion of a pneumothorax with hemodynamic compromise should prompt immediate decompression before obtaining a chest radiograph. Once it is determined that the patient is well oxygenated and ventilated as well as hemodynamically stable, sedation may be administered, if required, and a more detailed assessment can be undertaken.

17. Should neuromuscular blockade be used to facilitate MV?
Neuromuscular blockade (NMB) is commonly used to facilitate MV. It modestly improves oxygenation, decreases peak Paw, and improves the patient-ventilator interface. Muscle paralysis may be of greater benefit in specific situations, such as intracranial hypertension or unconventional modes of ventilation (e.g., IRV or extracorporeal techniques). Drawbacks to the use of NMB include loss of neurologic exam; abolished cough; potential for an awake, paralyzed patient; numerous medication and electrolyte interactions; and potential for prolonged paralysis. Furthermore, improvement in patient outcome has not been scientifically proved. Use of NMB must not be taken lightly. Adequate sedation should be attempted first to avoid NMB. If deemed absolutely necessary after a careful risk-benefit analysis, NMB may be instituted. Use should be limited to 24–48 hours, if possible, to prevent prolonged paralysis.

18. Is split-lung ventilation ever useful?
Split-lung ventilation (SLV) refers to differential ventilation of each lung independently usually via a double-lumen endotracheal tube and two ventilators. Originally developed in the operating suite to facilitate thoracic surgery, its use has been extended to occasional patients in the ICU. Patients with severe unilateral lung disease may be candidates for split-lung ventilation. Split-lung ventilation has been shown to improve oxygenation in patients with unilateral pneumonia, pulmonary edema, and contusion. Isolation of the lungs can save the life of patients with massive hemoptysis or lung abscess by protecting the good lung from spillage. Patients with a bronchopleural fistula also may benefit from SLV. Different modes of ventilation may be applied to each lung individually, including V$_T$, flows, PEEP, and CPAP. The two ventilators need not be synchronized, and in fact hemodynamic stability is better maintained by using the two ventilators asynchronously.

BIBLIOGRAPHY

1. Brodsky JB, Mihm FG: Split-lung ventilation. In Hall JB, Schmid GA, Wood LDH (eds): Principles of Critical Care. New York, McGraw-Hill, 1992, pp 160–164.
2. Gattinoni L, Pesenti A, et al: Pressure-volume curve of total respiratory system in acute respiratory failure. Computed tomographic study. Am Rev Respir Dis 136:730–736, 1987.
3. Hyzy RC, Popovich J: Mechanical ventilation and weaning. In Carlson RW, Geheb MA (eds): Principles and Practice of Medical Intensive Care. Philadelphia, W.B. Saunders, 1993, pp 924–943.
4. Marini JJ: New options for the ventilatory management of acute lung injury. New Horizons 1:489–503, 1993.
5. Pappert D, Rossaint R, et al: Influence of positioning on ventilation-perfusion relationships in severe adult respiratory distress syndrome. Chest 106:1511–1516, 1994.
6. Pepe PE, Marini JJ: Occult positive end-expiratory pressure in mechanically ventilated patients with airflow obstruction. Am Rev Respir Dis 126:166–170, 1982.
7. Pilbeam SP: Mechanical Ventilation: Physiologic and Clinical Applications. St. Louis, Mosby, 1992.
8. Rappaport SH, Shpiner R, et al: Randomized, prospective trial of pressure-limited versus volume-controlled ventilation in severe respiratory failure. Crit Care Med 22:22–32, 1994.
9. Ravenscraft SA, Burke WC, et al: Tracheal gas insufflation augments CO_2 clearance during mechanical ventilation. Am Rev Respir Dis 148:345–351, 1993.
10. Shanholtz C, Brower R: Should inverse ratio ventilation be used in adult respiratory distress syndrome? Am J Respir Crit Care Med 149:1354–1358, 1994.
11. Tobin MJ: What should the clinician do when a patient "fights the ventilator"? Respir Care 36:395–406, 1991.
12. Tuxen DV: Permissive hypercapnic ventilation. Am J Respir Crit Care Med 150:870–874, 1994.
13. Williams JE, Bartolome RC: How to mechanically ventilate the critically ill patient. Intern Med 13:10–18, 1992.

89. NEUROMUSCULAR BLOCKING AGENTS IN THE INTENSIVE CARE UNIT

Stuart G. Rosenberg, M.D.

1. What are the indications for neuromuscular blocking drugs in the intensive care unit?
The main indication is facilitation of endotracheal intubation and mechanical ventilation. Ease of laryngoscopy, a flaccid patient, and prevention of laryngospasm greatly improve intubating conditions. Use of neuromuscular blocking (NMB) drugs in mechanically ventilated patients improves the patient–ventilator interface, decreases peak airway pressure, and may improve gas exchange. A flaccid, paralyzed patient is a prerequisite for newer modes such as inverse-ratio ventilation. Other indications include increased intracranial pressure (ICP), optimal oxygen transport, tetanus, hypermetabolic states, and assurance of an immobile patient for radiographic and invasive procedures. NMB drugs also control muscle activity and lactate production in status epilepticus. Electroencephalographic monitoring is required in the paralyzed patient, because the seizure activity is masked. Because of complications associated with the use of NMBs (see below), a trial of adequate sedation before instituting paralysis for any indication should be made.

2. What is the effect of NMB agents on pulmonary gas exchange?
Scant data indicate slight improvement in the partial pressure of oxygen (pO_2) and carbon dioxide (pCO_2) in some patients. This effect is thought to be due primarily to a decrease in oxygen consumption and carbon dioxide production in skeletal muscle. Lung volumes also may improve if the patient has been coughing or fighting the ventilator. On the other hand, ventilation-perfusion (V/Q) matching may worsen because of changes in diaphragmatic position secondary to paralysis. The overall net effect is variable and difficult to predict. Because some patients show improvement in gas exchange, a trial of NMBs may be worthwhile to decrease toxic oxygen concentration and other ventilatory requirements.

3. Does the use of NMB agents in mechanically ventilated patients improve morbidity or mortality?
No. Currently no evidence supports this claim.

4. What are the two major classes of NMBs?
The two classes are depolarizing and nondepolarizing agents. The only depolarizing agent currently available is succinylcholine (SCh). The nondepolarizing agents frequently used in the ICU include pancuronium, curare, atracurium, and vecuronium. Rocuronium and mivacurium are new nondepolarizers and may find an important niche in the ICU because of rapid onset of action and short half-life, respectively. The depolarizing agents act by binding to acetylcholine (ACh) receptor sites on the postjunctional neuromuscular membrane, causing depolarization and prevention of further muscle action potentials. The nondepolarizers competitively inhibit ACh at the neuromuscular junction to prevent depolarization of the postjunctional membrane.

5. What is the role of SCh in the ICU?
As in the operating room, SCh is most often used to facilitate tracheal intubation. Its onset of action is approximately 45 seconds; its duration is only 10 minutes. The quick onset of action is beneficial in patients who are at risk for pulmonary aspiration, including patients with full stomachs from recent oral intake, gastrointestinal hemorrhage, delayed gastric emptying from an ileus or autonomic dysfunction, or increased intraabdominal pressure. Its duration may be slightly prolonged in critically ill patients with decreased levels of plasma pseudocholinesterase (see question 7).

6. What are the risks of SCh?

Risks include hypoxemia and death if one is unable to secure the airway after paralysis is induced. Arrhythmias may occur, especially bradyarrhythmias, after repeated doses of SCh. Hyperkalemia may be a problem in certain pathologic states. SCh normally causes a transient rise in serum potassium of 0.5–1.0 mEq/L. Patients with large burns, spinal cord injuries, myopathies, or crush injuries may exhibit an exaggerated release of potassium after SCh administration. The ensuing hyperkalemia may lead to life-threatening arrhythmias. Calcium is the antidote. Other potential problems with SCh include increased ICP, myalgias, rhabdomyolysis, masseter muscle spasm, and malignant hyperthermia.

7. How are NMBs metabolized?

SCh is degraded rapidly by plasma pseudocholinesterase. Mivacurium is also broken down by cholinesterase. Enzyme levels may be depressed in critically ill patients. Pancuronium is mainly metabolized and excreted renally, whereas vecuronium and rocuronium are mainly cleared hepatically. Atracurium is metabolized in the plasma via two pathways, Hofmann degradation and ester hydrolysis. Atracurium and mivacurium may be the preferred agents in patients with hepatic or renal dysfunction (see question 8).

8. Do NMBs have active metabolites?

Yes. The 3-hydroxy metabolites of vecuronium and pancuronium are active at the neuromuscular junction and may accumulate in renal failure, producing a prolonged block. Laudanosine, one of the metabolites of atracurium, causes central nervous system excitation and seizures at high plasma levels in dogs. These levels have not been reached in humans, even with renal or hepatic failure. SCh, which in fact is diacetylcholine (two molecules of acetylcholine linked together), is metabolized to monoacetylcholine, which may cause bradycardia.

9. How does one determine if the patient is adequately paralyzed?

Clinical observation and direct monitoring of neuromuscular function are important to ensure that the goals of paralysis are met and to avoid overdose. Observation of a relaxed patient synchronous with the ventilator is desirable. Monitoring of depth of neuromuscular blockade is accomplished most readily with a peripheral nerve stimulator. A series of impulses (most commonly a train-of-four [TOF]) is delivered to a peripheral nerve, such as the facial, ulnar, or posterior tibial, and the muscle response in the form of contraction or twitches is measured. Typically a fading pattern develops as the block deepens, with progressive loss of twitches until complete blockade is established. The number of twitches remaining corresponds to the percentage of receptor blockade at the neuromuscular junction. In the ICU, the presence of 1–2 twitches is desirable, corresponding to an 85–90% neuromuscular junction receptor blockade. This level ensures adequate paralysis and avoids overdose and prolonged recovery.

10. What about the hemodynamic effects of nondepolarizing NMBs?

Pancuronium is vagolytic and increases circulating norepinephrine, thereby causing tachycardia and hypertension. It may be beneficial in the hypotensive, septic, or traumatized patient, because it supports blood pressure and heart rate. Bolus administration of atracurium and possibly mivacurium causes histamine release, which may lead to tachycardia, hypotension, and bronchospasm. Vecuronium has the advantage of hemodynamic stability, with little change in heart rate or blood pressure. Continuous infusion as opposed to bolus dosing decreases the hemodynamic side effects.

11. Do patients receiving NMBs require sedation?

NMBs do not provide sedation, amnesia, or analgesia. Conscious patients should not receive NMBs without the addition of a sedative, preferably one with amnestic properties, such as a benzodiazepine.

12. How does one know that the pharmacologically paralyzed patient is adequately sedated?

In patients who are unable to respond with movement or eye opening, assessment of the autonomic nervous system is necessary, just as one gauges the depth of a general anesthetic from autonomic signs. One should look for large reactive pupils, tearing, diaphoresis, piloerection, tachycardia, and hypertension as possible signs of inadequate sedation. Discontinuation of the NMB (if tolerated) allows return of skeletal muscle function and further assessment of the adequacy of sedation. Sedation may not be necessary in the unresponsive, comatose patient. Sedation also may not be tolerated if the patient is hemodynamically unstable. In this situation a cardiostable, amnestic drug such as scopolamine should be considered.

13. Do other medications used in the ICU interact with NMBs?

Yes. Many classes of drugs used in the ICU affect neuromuscular transmission and thereby interact with NMB drugs, including aminoglycosides, magnesium, class I antiarrhythmics, and calcium channel blockers. NMBs may predispose the patient receiving exogenous steroids to steroid myopathy (see question 15). Close monitoring of neuromuscular function is essential.

14. Which blood chemistry abnormalities affect NMBs?

Hypophosphatemia, hypermagnesemia, hypokalemia, respiratory acidosis, and metabolic alkalosis cause muscle weakness and potentiate NMBs. Increased creatinine or liver function tests may lead to accumulation of NMBs and their metabolites.

15. Describe the complication of prolonged muscle weakness.

Prolonged muscle weakness is a known and dreaded complication of NMBs. It may occur in patients who have received NMBs for several days to weeks. The incidence is not clear but may be as high as 10% in patients deemed at risk. More than 100 cases are documented in the literature. Prolonged muscle weakness is a proximal and distal tetraparesis that may last up to several months. It is not to be confused with the shorter-term prolonged effect of an overdose of NMBs, which usually resolves in hours to days and is due to the lingering effect of the drugs or active metabolites at the neuromuscular junction. Monitoring the TOF should prevent this shorter-term effect. Prolonged muscle weakness appears to be related to a myopathic process with normal neuromuscular transmission. The actual pathology is not well characterized but resembles a steroidlike myopathy. Patients at risk include those receiving exogenous steroids and NMBs for longer than 5 days. Asthmatics seem particularly susceptible. Concurrent aminoglycoside administration also may be a risk factor. Profound weakness may last for months, requiring ventilatory support. Many authors have recommended close monitoring of the TOF, intermittent withholding of the NMB, and physical therapy to prevent muscle atrophy with the hope of preventing prolonged muscle weakness. Unfortunately, none of these precautions has been proved to be of benefit. The use of atracurium was previously recommended to prevent prolonged muscle weakness; early reports implicated only the steroid-based NMBs, pancuronium and vecuronium, which have a steroid-ring nucleus in their structure. It was suspected that some interaction or synergistic effect between the steroidal NMBs and exogenous steroids was directly toxic to muscle tissue. More recently, however, atracurium (a nonsteroidal NMB) also has been implicated in prolonged paralysis. There is no specific treatment other than supportive measures. Prolonged ventilation may be required. Physical therapy is essential. Tapering steroids as soon as possible may be of some benefit. Survival is the rule. As the condition is so morbid, one must carefully weigh the benefits and risks of long-term neuromuscular blockade in the ICU.

16. What is the differential diagnosis of muscle weakness in the critically ill patient?

In addition to NMB-induced prolonged muscle weakness (see question 15), numerous other entities seen in the ICU lead to muscle weakness. Cervical spinal cord pathology, such as trauma, infection, or vascular accident, may lead to quadriparesis. Poliomyelitis affects the upper motor neurons and causes weakness. Peripheral neuropathies from diabetes mellitus, alcohol, human immunodeficiency virus (HIV), or porphyria cause weakness. In severely ill patients with sepsis or multiple organ failure, involvement of the peripheral nerves may lead to critical illness polyneuropathy (CIP), an axonal degeneration of motor and sensory nerves that resembles a toxic or nutritional neuropathy. Many of the above states have sensory involvement in addition to motor weakness. Prolonged muscle weakness affects motor function only. Unrecognized myasthenia gravis may cause prolonged muscle weakness after NMBs. Eaton-Lambert syndrome is a paraneoplastic syndrome that causes a decrement in neuromuscular transmission. Other myopathies, such as polymyositis, HIV-related myopathy, or alcohol-induced myopathy, should be considered. Guillain-Barré syndrome is a postinfectious ascending paralysis occasionally seen in the ICU. Of course, electrolyte abnormalities and drugs affecting neuromuscular transmission also should be considered. Prolonged muscle weakness from NMBs is a diagnosis of exclusion. Patients with weakness require a thorough neurologic exam, full chemistry panels, cranial and/or spinal cord imaging, cerebrospinal fluid examination, nerve conduction studies, electromyography, and possibly muscle or nerve biopsies. Treatment obviously depends on the specific diagnosis.

17. What other concerns are related to the patient receiving NMBs?
A major concern is the inability to perform a neurologic exam in critically ill patients. A central event such as a cerebrovascular accident may go unrecognized for some time. Patients cannot blink or protect their eyes. Drying and corneal abrasions may occur. Artificial tears and taping the eyes closed help. Inability to cough reduces the ability to mobilize pulmonary secretions. Suctioning and meticulous respiratory care are warranted. Immobile patients are prone to decubitus ulcers. An airbed may be of help in preventing ulcers. Immobile patients are also prone to thromboembolic complications. Prophylaxis of deep vein thrombosis should be instituted. Peripheral nerve injuries may occur if the patient is not positioned properly. Passive range-of-motion exercises may help to prevent muscle atrophy. Sedation may be crucial to avoid an awake, paralyzed patient. If possible, it is good practice occasionally to stop the NMB and to re-examine the patient fully.

BIBLIOGRAPHY

1. Apte-Kakade S: Rehabilitation of patients with quadriparesis after treatment of status asthmaticus with neuromuscular blocking agents and high-dose corticosteroids. Arch Phys Med Rehabil 72:1024–1028, 1991.
2. Argov Z, Mastaglia F: Disorders of neuromuscular transmission caused by drugs. N Engl J Med 301: 409–413, 1979.
3. Bishop M: Hemodynamic and gas exchange effects of pancuronium bromide in sedated patients with respiratory failure. Anesthesiology 60:369–371, 1984.
4. Durbin C: Neuromuscular blocking agents and sedative drugs, clinical uses and toxic effects in the critical care unit. Critl Care Clin 7:489–506, 1991.
5. Hansen-Flaschen J, Cowen J, Raps E: Neuromuscular blockade in the intensive care unit, more than we bargained for. Am Rev Respir Dis 147:234–136, 1993.
6. Loper K, Butler S, et al: Paralyzed with pain: The need for education. Pain 37:315–316, 1989.
7. Rosenberg S: Atracurium and prolonged muscle weakness. Anesth Analg 79:1206, 1994.
8. Segredo V, Matthay M: Prolonged neuromuscular blockade after long term administration of vecuronium in two critically ill patients. Anesthesiology 72:566–570, 1990.
9. Topulos G: Neuromuscular blockade in adult intensive care. New Horizons 1:447–462, 1993.

90. SEDATION IN THE INTENSIVE CARE UNIT

John D. Lockrem, M.D., and James Rosher, M.D.

1. Why is sedation a special problem in the intensive care unit (ICU)?

Patients in the ICU often experience pain, fear, anxiety and discomfort, all of which make sedation an important part of their medical care. The goals of sedation in the ICU are analgesia, amnesia, anxiolysis, and hypnosis. The objective is to produce a calm, comfortable, but communicative patient. Each patient presents with various medical conditions that require various levels of sedation. The needs of the patient must guide the appropriate selection of drug therapy. A patient's requirements may vary throughout the ICU stay, and the patient's condition needs to be addressed frequently. Sedation is needed for postoperative pain control; injuries received during trauma; placement and presence of endotracheal tubes, thoracotomy, and drainage catheters; endotracheal suctioning; bladder catheterization; invasive monitoring; physical therapy; and routine nursing care. Fear and anxiety are heightened by the inability to communicate during artificial ventilation, awareness of the critical situation, physical restraints, and loss of orientation to time and place. Sedation is often required for procedures such as elective cardioversion. Critically ill patients often require proper sedation for severe respiratory failure, tolerance of mechanical ventilation, neuromuscular blockade, septic shock, and combative or severely agitated states.

2. Is there an ideal sedative regimen for all ICU patients?

Unfortunately, no. Many factors play a role in selection of the sedative regimen, including age, personality, drug therapy, smoking and alcohol usage, prior experiences, surgical incision site, and current medical condition. Clinical objectives that should be considered in every ICU patient include maintenance of a relaxed state, adequate pain control, allowing sufficient cooperation for neurologic examination and therapeutic interventions, tolerance of mechanical ventilation, reduction in barotrauma, and conservation of energy. Although general recommendations can be made, the individual needs of each patient must be considered.

3. Is the best method of sedation not obvious to ICU staff?

Because a wide variety of drugs are used for ICU sedation, an adequate understanding is essential for proper usage. A recent survey in *Pain 1989* revealed that many health care workers misunderstand the sedative and analgesic properties of several commonly used medications. For example, 10% of ICU nurses and 5% of house staff physicians believed that pancuronium (a neuromuscular blocker) relieved anxiety. In the same study, 80% of physicians and 43% of ICU nurses believed that diazepam (a sedative) relieves pain. This chapter is meant to familiarize health care providers with several medications used in mechanically ventilated patients for sedation, analgesia, anxiolysis, amnesia, and hypnosis. Among the available sedatives are the **benzodiazepines, opioids, antipsychotics**, and the **nonbarbiturate anesthetic, propofol**. Various aspects of each class of drugs are discussed, including the mechanism of action, metabolism and excretion, indications, contraindications, pharmacodynamics and kinetics, cost analysis, and advantages vs. disadvantages. The use of neuromuscular blocking agents or pain management protocols is not discussed.

4. Which common characteristics of benzodiazepines affect ICU sedative choice?

Sixteen different benzodiazepines are available in the U.S.; however, the most frequently used agents in the ICU are **midazolam, lorazepam**, and **diazepam**, all of which have anxiolytic, amnestic, muscle relaxant, and hypnotic effects. They are unique in that they produce deep amnesia while the patient remains conscious. Although they do not have analgesic properties, they reduce narcotic requirements. They also possess anticonvulsant properties and are used in the prevention of alcohol withdrawal syndrome.

The administration of benzodiazepines results in minimal respiratory effects except for a decreased ventilatory response to hypoxia and hypercarbia and a decrease in minute ventilation with carbon dioxide (CO_2) retention. Cardiac effects in normovolemic patients include a mild decrease in systemic vascular resistance (SVR) secondary to venodilation, a decrease in mean arterial pressure (MAP) (10%), and an increase in heart rate (HR) (6%). In cases of hypovolemia, benzodiazepines should be used with caution, because decreases in sympathetic tone and venodilation may precipitate hypotension. A synergistic response with a further decrease in MAP is observed when opioids are used concomitantly. Central nervous system (CNS) effects include a decrease in cerebral blood flow (CBF) and cerebral metabolic rate for oxygen ($CMRO_2$). Seizure activity is promptly terminated by many benzodiazepines. Caution should be used in patients with renal and/or hepatic disease, because metabolism and excretion of most benzodiazepines occur in the kidney and liver. A dose reduction is necessary in such patients. Tolerance to benzodiazepines in general develops quickly, within 1–2 days. The most effective means of avoiding tolerance is a combination of opioids and benzodiazepines, which decreases the dosage requirement of each medication and delays the onset of tolerance. Because of withdrawal reactions after long-term therapeutic use, dosages should be tapered before discontinuation.

Potential risks include oversedation or coma, hypotension, and/or respiratory depression. Another adverse reaction, especially in the elderly, is paradoxical agitation, which is thought to result from the amnestic effects; patients may become disoriented, confused, and even combative. When reassured, they often settle down but may become restless again as they forget what they have been told. An important consideration with the use of benzodiazepines is the lack of analgesic effects; therefore, pain management remains a necessary objective in the sedated patient. By combining benzodiazepines and opioids, the dose of each can be decreased because of synergistic effects. Benzodiazepines bind to inhibitory gamma-aminobutyric acid (GABA) receptors, thereby increasing the membrane conductance of chloride ions in the CNS. The resultant change in membrane polarization inhibits normal neuronal function.

5. Describe the properties of midazolam.

Midazolam is a short-acting, water-soluble benzodiazepine with a beta elimination half-life of 1–12 hours (average: 1–4 hr). Although midazolam is water-soluble in its prepared state, its imidazole ring closes at physiologic pH, causing an increase in lipid solubility. Hepatic metabolism produces active metabolites that are excreted by the kidneys. Hepatic biotransformation results in the active metabolites alpha-1-hydroxy-midazolam and 4-hydroxy-midazolam. Midazolam and its metabolites are excreted principally by the kidneys.

With continuous infusion patients with normal liver and renal function usually awaken within 12 hours. However, in septic patients or patients with hepatic dysfunction, active metabolites may result in prolonged coma. Neither midazolam nor its metabolites are removed effectively by hemodialysis. In critically ill patients, the unpredictability and variability in duration of effect may be due to the altered volume of distribution and protein-binding. Midazolam can be administered by intermittent intravenous (IV) dosing for short-term sedation in doses of 1–2 mg every 1–4 hours. The usual sedative dose of midazolam begins by loading with 0.05–0.1 mg/kg followed by 2–3 mg/hr IV infusion with an opioid supplement. When used alone for sedation, the dose range may be as high as 10–40 mg/hr. One study reported the use of doses of 0.25–0.3 mg/kg/hr for ICU sedation of ventilated patients. The mean time to return to baseline mental status after discontinuation of the infusion was 30 hours. A drug that is usually short-acting may become long-acting under clinical conditions often encountered in the ICU.

In 1995 hospital acquisition cost of midazolam (100 mg in 100-ml bag) is approximately $120.00. A 2-mg vial costs $3.39; a 5-mg vial costs $7.50.

6. Does lorazepam have unique properties that make it useful for ICU sedation?

Yes. Lorazepam (Ativan) is an intermediate-acting, lipid-soluble benzodiazepine with a beta elimination half-life of 10–20 hr. Lorazepam is less lipid-soluble than midazolam or diazepam; hence maximal effects may not occur for 15–30 minutes after IV injection because of equilibration within the CNS. The CNS effects are attributed directly to the parent compound; no active metabolites are formed. Hepatic biotransformation by glucuronide conjugation yields lorazepam glucuronide, which is inactive. Excretion occurs primarily through the kidneys. Lorazepam is frequently administered in the ICU by intermittent injection and continuous infusions. The duration of sedation achieved by continuous infusion is much shorter than the duration of other benzodiazepines because no active metabolites are produced. Infusions of lorazepam, 1–5 mg/hr (0.01–0.1 mg/kg/hr), for ICU sedation are common. Intermittent IV boluses of 1–2 mg every 2–6 hrs also provide adequate sedation. A recent study in *Critical Care Medicine* reported doses of 0.06–0.1 mg/kg/hr for sedation of ventilated patients. The mean time to return to baseline mental status after discontinuation of lorazepam infusion was 4–5 hours. The cardiopulmonary effects of lorazepam are consistent with the features of midazolam except for the previously discussed pharmacokinetics. Care also must be taken in patients with hepatic and renal dysfunction, and dosage must be adjusted accordingly. Currently the hospital acquisition cost of lorazepam (25 mg in 100-ml bag) is approximately $60.00. A 4-mg vial of lorazepam costs $9.26.

7. Why is diazepam not used more frequently in the ICU?

Diazepam (Valium) is a long-acting, rapid-onset, highly lipid-soluble benzodiazepine with a beta elimination half-life of 20–70 hr. Diazepam is poorly dissolved in aqueous media (propylene glycol/alcohol/diazepam) and produces venous irritation and pain on IV injection. Hepatic biotransformation results in pharmacologically active metabolites, including desmethyldiazepam. These metabolites are excreted via bile into the gastrointestinal tract, where they are reabsorbed with further sedative action (half-life: 36–90 hr). Clinical activity results from a combination of the parent compound and active metabolites, which makes diazepam undesirable for repetitive IV injections. In addition, because diazepam is not soluble in aqueous solution, it cannot be given by continuous infusion. Bolus dosage of IV diazepam is 2–10 mg (average: 2.5–5 mg).

After repeated injections, diazepam may accumulate because of its long elimination half-life and active metabolites. In the ICU diazepam typically is used for treatment of muscle spasms and alcohol withdrawal syndrome, anticonvulsant therapy, and mild sedation for therapeutic interventions. Diazepam has similar characteristics to the other benzodiazepines in respect to cardiopulmonary and hepatorenal physiologic effects. The metabolism of diazepam is reduced when it is used concurrently with cimetidine; thus the amount of free diazepam is increased.

Diazepam is not used routinely for long-term sedation. However, because it is inexpensive ($0.30 for a 10-mg vial), it should be considered for intermittent sedation for specific procedures.

8. Can the effects of benzodiazepines be reversed?

Yes. Flumazenil is an imidazobenzodiazepine that acts as a specific benzodiazepine receptor antagonist. It competitively antagonizes most of the CNS effects of the benzodiazepines via a neutral receptor principle. That is, flumazenil has no direct receptor activity except to displace the active benzodiazepine from the receptor; therefore, it is not a true antagonist. The drug may be used for rapid reversal of oversedation from benzodiazepines and is helpful in differentiating the cause of coma. The dose of flumazenil is 0.2 mg IV every 1–2 minutes (maximum: 3 mg/hr). It is rapidly metabolized via the liver and has a beta elimination half-life of approximately 1–1.5 hours. Occasional side effects include anxiety, headache, dizziness, nausea and vomiting, blurred vision, pain on injection, and resedation. Hospital acquisition cost in 1995 for flumazenil (1 mg) is $35.23.

9. What role should opioids play in ICU sedation?

Because pain and discomfort are so commonly experienced by ICU patients, particularly in the postoperative period, opioids for analgesia and sedation are often primary agents in the effort to make patients more comfortable. Opioids are easy to administer and relatively inexpensive and often provide a pleasant euphoria. Most opioids have similar side effects; however, each has its own advantages and disadvantages.

10. What are the major disadvantages of opioids?
Side effects of opioids include dose-dependent respiratory depression, bradycardia, drowsiness, euphoria, dysphoria, hallucinations, cough suppression (which may be beneficial; for example, in helping a patient accommodate to a recently placed endotracheal tube), nausea and vomiting, pruritus, decreased gastrointestinal motility, constipation, urinary retention, biliary sphincter spasm, allergic reactions, and potentiation of cardiopulmonary effects of other sedatives, hypnotics, or analgesics. Opioids do not produce amnesia at commonly used doses. In large doses they significantly depress respiration and inhibit central respiratory drive. Respiratory depression may be a desirable effect in mechanically ventilated patients but may pose a problem when patients are weaned from the ventilator.

11. How are opioids administered? How do they work?
Opioids can be administered to ventilated patients by intermittent injections or continuous infusions. The mechanism of action involves opioid receptors (mu, kappa, sigma, delta) located in the brain, spinal cord, and peripheral tissues. Mu receptors mediate supraspinal analgesia, euphoria, respiratory depression, and physical dependence. Kappa receptors are involved in spinal analgesia, sedation, and miosis. Delta receptors mediate analgesia and potentiate the effects of other receptors, whereas sigma receptors play a role in hallucinations, dysphoria, and stimulation of vasomotor and respiratory centers. Opioid receptor activation inhibits the presynaptic release of and the postsynaptic response to excitatory neurotransmitters (acetylcholine and substance P). This inhibition alters the potassium and calcium ion conductance at the cellular level, resulting in central effects. Opioids also interfere with pontine and medullary respiratory control.

12. Which properties affect the use of morphine as a sedative?
Morphine is an inexpensive, reliable, commonly used opioid—the prototype to which all other opioids are compared. Its low lipid solubility results in slower onset of action and prolonged duration of effect compared with the synthetic narcotics (e.g., fentanyl). Morphine is commonly given in bolus injections of 1–5 mg every 1–2 hours.

Dosage requirements vary greatly, depending on the patient's needs. Because morphine has peak onset time of 15–20 minutes and a duration of 4–5 hours, it is easily dosed to effect. Continuous infusion is usually at rates of 2–4 mg/hr but should be titrated to effect. The pulmonary effects consist of dose-dependent respiratory depression. Minimal cardiac depression is seen in normal doses. If rapid, large doses are given intravenously, histamine release may result in hypotension and bronchospasm. The effect may be prolonged in patients with hepatic and renal disease. Metabolism occurs in the liver by conjugation with glucuronic acid to form morphine-3-glucuronide and morphine-6-glucuronide, which are minimally active metabolites. Approximately 5–10% of morphine is excreted in the urine unchanged; therefore, renal failure prolongs the effect. Less than 10% of morphine metabolites undergo biliary excretion.

Advantages of morphine are cost and duration of action. The current hospital cost of a 10-mg vial is $0.48. The continuous infusion cost of morphine (100 mg in 100-ml bag) is $4.00.

13. Does fentanyl have specific advantages and disadvantages in the ICU?
Fentanyl is a rapid-acting, potent synthetic piperidine opioid agonist that is 100 times more potent than morphine. Rapid onset and short duration of action reflect its greater lipid solubility compared with morphine and make fentanyl the preferred narcotic in the postoperative or post-traumatic period for many clinicians. Intravenous injections of fentanyl (25–50 µg every 10–20 minutes) is common for initial postoperative analgesic management. Intermittent boluses of fentanyl (50–200 µg IV every 1–4 hours) can be given once pain control is achieved. Because fentanyl has a peak onset of 5–10 minutes, it is easily titrated to effect. The beta elimination half-life is 1–3 hours; however, the analgesic duration is approximately 1 hour because of redistribution into fat and muscle. Continuous infusions are administered at rates of 0.025–0.25 µg/kg/min or 1.5–15 µg/kg/hr. Cardiovascular effects result in minimal changes in MAP, SVR, and cardiac output. Decreases in HR are caused by withdrawal of sympathetic tone and activation of vagal

efferents. Pulmonary effects include depression of ventilation by decreases in respiratory rate (RR) and increases in CO_2 retention. Maximal respiratory depression occurs in 3–5 minutes and persists for 3–4 hours. Rigidity of the abdominal and chest wall musculature may occur with large doses and may make ventilation difficult. Central nervous system (CNS) effects result in decreases in cerebral blood flow and $CMRO_2$.

Renal function is not affected by normal doses of fentanyl. Metabolism of fentanyl occurs via hepatic oxidation to norfentanyl and hydrolysis to 4-N-anilino piperidine and propionic acid (all active metabolites). Renal excretion of unchanged fentanyl accounts for 10–25% of an administered dose and of inactive metabolites for 75%. In the ICU fentanyl helps to maintain hemodynamic stability, to control tachycardia, and to suppress catecholamine release. Tachyphylaxis has been known to occur with continuous infusions of fentanyl. The hospital cost of fentanyl (1000 μg in 100-ml bag) is $2.53; 2-ml (100 μg) vial is $0.23.

14. Which drug is useful for managing the severely agitated or psychotic patient?
Haloperidol, a butyrophenone derivative, is an antipsychotic drug used in ICU patients for treatment of extreme agitation, delirium, or disorientation. Severely agitated patients require considerable nursing time to ensure that they do not pull out catheters, endotracheal tubes, or arterial or venous lines or cause physical harm to themselves or others. Haloperidol is used for elderly confused patients in whom excessive sedation or respiratory depression should be avoided. Most patients who receive haloperidol have minimal amnesia, hypnosis, or analgesia; they usually are awake and calm in appearance. The diagnosis of acute ICU psychosis is made by ruling out hypoxia, hypercarbia, electrolyte abnormalities, concurrent medication reactions, gastric or urinary distention, exacerbation of previous psychiatric conditions, septicemia, renal or hepatic dysfunction, and withdrawal symptoms. It is essential to provide adequate analgesia to patients sedated with haloperidol. It should be used with caution if at all in patients with allergic reactions to droperidol, prior history of seizures, possibility of pregnancy, or parkinsonian symptoms.

15. How is haloperidol dosed in severely agitated or psychotic patients?
Dosing regimens vary greatly among patients, and florid psychotic patients may require large amounts for adequate sedation. One rational approach is to calculate the expected dose required to achieve the effective plasma concentration of 20 ng/ml. The amount of drug is the product of weight of the patient (kg), volume of distribution (Vd), and effective plasma concentration (C_{plasma}):

$$\text{Haloperidol dose} = (kg)\,(V_d)(C_{plasma})$$

For a 70-kg person, the maximal loading dose is (70 kg) (18 L/kg) (20 ng/ml) or 25.2 mg. Haloperidol would be given at doses of 5 mg every 30 minutes, titrating to appropriate sedation up to the maximal dose calculated. The maintenance dose is one-fourth of the loading dose, given every 6 hours.

16. What complications are associated with haloperidol?
Complications of haloperidol include cardiac dysrhythmias, extrapyramidal symptoms (reversed with diphenhydramine), acute dystonic reactions, parkinsonian symptoms, tardive dyskinesias, and neuroleptic malignant syndrome. The extrapyramidal symptoms are occasionally quite troubling and hard to manage and in rare patients even permanent. Neuroleptic malignant syndrome is a rare disorder characterized by muscle tremors, catatonia, hyperthermia, autonomic dysfunction, and muscle destruction. The mortality rate is > 10%. Several incidents of cardiac dysrhythmias, including torsades de pointes, have been reported. Haloperidol has alpha-blocking properties that are associated with hypotension. Minimal respiratory effects are seen with haloperidol infusions.

17. Describe the mechanism of action, pharmacokinetics, and cost of haloperidol.
The mechanism of action of haloperidol is thought to be via central inhibition of the postsynaptic dopaminergic receptor and inhibition of catecholamine reuptake at the nerve terminals. The pharmacokinetics of haloperidol are best described by a three-compartment model. The beta elimination

half-life is 6–8 hours, and the drug may accumulate with infusions. Ninety percent is protein-bound; the large volume distribution (18 L/kg) suggests extensive tissue redistribution. Metabolism of haloperidol is via hepatic biotransformation with oxidation to inactive metabolites and reduction to hydroxyhaloperidol (minimal activity). Haloperidol and its metabolites are excreted in urine and feces. Hospital cost of haloperidol (200 mg/160 ml) is $15.00, and a 5-mg vial is $0.35.

18. What is propofol? Does it have a place in ICU sedation?

Propofol is a nonbarbiturate agent used for general anesthesia, sedation for local procedures, and ICU sedation of ventilated patients. Propofol is a milky white, lipid-soluble diisopropyl phenol. Rapid onset, rapid awakening, and minimal residual accumulation have made propofol nearly ideal for ICU sedation. Onset occurs in less than 30 seconds after IV injection, and awakening occurs in 4–8 minutes without continued infusion. Propofol can be dosed intermittently to a given effect or, more commonly, given as a continuous infusion. It is formulated in a lipid, preservative-free emulsion and must be given intravenously. The unique pharmacokinetic profile of propofol includes not only a rapid distribution phase (alpha half-life of approximately 1.8–8.3 minutes) but also a rapid metabolic elimination phase (beta half-life of approximately 34–64 minutes). Metabolism is via hepatic enzyme degradation to inactive metabolites, which are rapidly excreted by the kidney without significant accumulation, even when infused for days.

19. What are the physiologic effects of propofol? What special precautions must be observed?

Cardiovascular effects are related to dose and speed of injection. Rapid injection decreases MAP by approximately 30% in normovolemic patients. Exaggerated responses are seen with hypovolemia, depressed myocardial function, and debilitated patients; therefore, careful titration and reduced dosage are essential in these settings. Slow rates of infusion have been used in patients with poor left ventricular function and in critically ill patients; the mild negative hemodynamic effects are not statistically different from those of other sedatives.

Approximately 10–15% of patients note pain on initial injection; hence, large veins are preferred when available. No significant phlebitis occurs despite initial discomfort. Often pretreatment with opioid or lidocaine (25 mg IV) decreases the incidence of pain. Patients with renal and/or hepatic disease exhibit no adverse response or accumulation. Central nervous system effects include reduction in CBF and $CMRO_2$ corresponding to the decrease in MAP. Respiratory depression occurs acutely with intravenous doses and is directly proportional to the dose. Therefore, propofol should be used with caution in ICU patients who are not mechanically ventilated. There is no evidence of adrenal axis suppression with infusions, and propofol has no analgesic, muscle-relaxing, or amnestic properties. Propofol reduces the proliferative responses of lymphocytes and may interfere with immune function. Strict aseptic techniques must be followed in administering propofol, because no preservatives are used in the formulation. Unused propofol must be discarded every 12 hours for sterility. Caution must be exercised in patients with egg allergy; lecithin is a component of egg whites and the fat emulsion in propofol. Minimal nausea, vomiting, and pruritus have been observed with the use of propofol. Some studies demonstrate antiemetic properties.

20. What are the advantages, dosing recommendations, and cost of propofol?

Specific advantages of propofol include minimal long-term effects, rapid awakening that ensures cooperation for exams and facilitates extubation, and easy titration to the desired level of sedation. Propofol is comparable to or even less expensive than several benzodiazepine infusions. The combination of propofol and an opioid infusion allows significantly reduced doses of each. Propofol is prepared in 10% Intralipid, which provides 1 kcal/ml and may account for 10–25% of daily caloric requirements. In critically ill patients, it is best to start a slow infusion of propofol at doses of 20–40 µg/kg/min (1–2 mg/kg/hr). Most patients tolerate a maintenance infusion rate of 20–100 µg/kg/min (1.2–6.0 mg/kg/hr). The rate of infusion depends on the desired level of sedation, the patient's age and overall health, and concurrent medications. If rapid unconsciousness is desired (e.g., rapid-sequence induction), propofol should be administered at 0.5–2.0 mg/kg (mean: 1.5 mg/kg).

Hospital cost for propofol (50-ml vial) is $24.00. The average daily requirement for propofol infusion costs approximately $150–$200/day. The infusion costs of various agents are compared below.

Comparative Hospital Costs for Infusions—1994*

AGENT	ACQUISITION CHARGE	COST/MG ($)	DOSE (MG/KG/HR)	COST/HR ($)	COST/DAY ($)
Propofol	500 mg = $24	0.048	2	6.72	161.28
Midazolam	100 mg/100 ml = $120	1.2	0.15	12.6	302.40
Lorazepam	25 mg/100 ml = $60	2.4	0.08	13.44	322.56
Morphine	100 mg/100 ml = $4	0.04	0.06	0.17	4.03
Fentanyl	1 mg/100 ml = 42.53	2.53	0.0015	0.27	6.48

* Patient charges are 2–3 times the hospital cost.

21. How is the level of sedation monitored in the ICU?

Sedation scales are available to facilitate communication among the ICU staff and to standardize the assessment of sedation. The Ramsay sedation scale is easily adapted to the ICU. Most patients can be maintained at Ramsay scale level 3 (sedated, responsive to commands). At times deeper levels of sedation (levels 5 and 6) are required, such as postoperatively, after major trauma, or during use of muscle relaxants. Conversely, stable patients may benefit from level 2 (cooperative, calm) sedation. The goal of ICU sedation of mechanically ventilated patients is to achieve Ramsay scale scores of 2–3 for maximal patient comfort and cooperation.

The Ramsay Sedation Score

SCORE	CHARACTERISTICS
1	Anxious, agitated, restless
2	Cooperative, tranquil, accepting ventilator support
3	Sedated, but responsive to commands
4	Asleep, brisk response to sound or glabellar tap
5	Asleep, sluggish response to sound or glabellar tap
6	Asleep, no response to sound or glabellar tap

BIBLIOGRAPHY

1. Aitkenhead AR, et al: Comparison of propofol and midazolam for sedation in critically ill patients. Lancet 2(8665):704–708, 1989.
2. Bailie GR, et al: Pharmacokinetics of propofol during and after long term continuous infusion for maintenance of sedation in ICU patients. Br J Anaesth 68:486–491, 1992.
3. Barvais L, et al: Continuous infusion of midazolam or bolus of diazepam for postoperative sedation in cardiac surgical patients. Acta Anaesthesiol Belg 39:239–245, 1988.
4. Bell S, et al: Propofol and fentanyl anaesthesia for patients with low cardiac output state undergoing cardiac surgery: Comparison with high-dose fentanyl anaesthesia. Br J Anaesth 73:162–166, 1994.
5. Bodenham A, Park GR: Reversal of prolonged sedation using flumazenil in critically ill patients. Anaesthesia 44:603–605, 1989.
6. Carrasco G, et al: Propofol vs midazolam in short-, medium-, and long-term sedation of critically ill patients. Chest 103:557–564, 1993.
7. Degauque C, Dupuis A: A study to compare the use of propofol and midazolam for the sedation of patients with acute respiratory failure. J Drug Dev 4(Suppl 3):95–97, 1991.
8. Deppe SA, et al: Intravenous lozapam as an amnestic and anxiolytic agent in the intensive care unit: A prospective study. Crit Care Med 22:1248–1252, 1994.
9. Durbin CG Jr: Sedation in the critically ill patient. New Horizons 2:64–74, 1994.
10. Loper KA, et al: Paralyzed with pain: The need for education. Pain 37:315–316, 1989.

11. Malacrida R, Fritz ME, Suter PM: Pharmacokinetics of midazolam administered by continuous intravenous to intensive care patients. Crit Care Med 20:1123–1126, 1991.
12. McMurray TJ, et al: Propofol sedation after open heart surgery: A clinical and pharmacokinetic study. Anaesthesia 45:322–326, 1990.
13. Nimmo GR, Mackenzie SJ, Grant IS: Haemodynamic and oxygen transport effects of propofol infusion in critically ill adults. Anaesthesia 4:485–489, 1994.
14. Pirttikangas CO, Perttila J, Salo M: Propofol emulsion reduces proliferative responses of lymphocytes from intensive care patients. Intens Care Med 19:299–302, 1993.
15. Pholman AS, Simpson KP, Hall JB: Continuous intravenous infusion of lorazepam versus midazolam for sedation during mechanical ventilatory support: A prospective, randomized study. Crit Care Med 22:1241–1247, 1994.
16. Shelly MP, Mendel L, Park GR: Failure of critically ill patients to metabolize midazolam. Anaesthesia 42:619–626, 1987.
17. Simpson PJ, Eltringham RJ: Lorazepam in intensive care. Clin Ther 4:150–163, 1981.
18. Smith I, et al: Propofol: An update on its clinical use. Anesthesiology 81:1005–1043, 1994.
19. Valence JF, et al: Disadvantages of prolonged propofol sedation in the critical care unit. Crit Care Med 22:710–712, 1994.

91. SEPSIS AND THE SEPTIC INFLAMMATORY RESPONSE SYNDROME

John D. Lockrem, M.D.

1. What makes sepsis and multiple organ dysfunction an important critical care problem?
Multiple organ dysfunction has been identified as the most common cause of mortality in the surgical intensive care unit (ICU). The mortality rate for septic shock is generally reported at 50–70%. In addition to high mortality, prolonged ICU care and enormous health care costs make improvements in the treatment of sepsis a high priority.

2. Define the following terms: infection, bacteremia, systemic inflammatory response, sepsis, septic shock, and multiple organ dysfunction.
The use of varying definitions of basic terms has made the results of many studies of innovative therapies hard to interpret. The American College of Chest Physicians and the American Society for Critical Care Medicine have made a plea for consistent use of terms based on a consensus conference.

Infection: an inflammatory response to the presence of microorganisms or the invasion of normally sterile host tissue by such organisms.

Bacteremia: the presence of viable bacteria in the blood.

Systemic inflammatory response syndrome (SIRS): the systemic inflammatory response to a variety of severe clinical insults. The response is manifested by two or more of the following conditions: (1) temperature > 38°C or < 36°C; (2) heart rate > 90 beats per minute; (3) respiratory rate > 20 breaths per minute or $PaCO_2$ < 32 mmHg; and (4) white blood cell count (WBC) > 12,000/mm³, < 4,000/mm³, or > 10% immature forms.

Sepsis: the same definitions as SIRS, but limited to infection as a cause.

Septic shock: sepsis associated with hypotension, despite adequate fluid resuscitation, and perfusion abnormalities that may include, but are not limited to, lactic acidosis, oliguria, or acute alteration in mental status. Patients who are receiving inotropic or vasopressor agents may not be hypotensive at the time that perfusion abnormalities are measured.

Multiple organ dysfunction syndrome (MODS): altered organ function in an acutely ill patient such that homeostasis cannot be maintained without intervention.

3. Why is SIRS important?
The signs that for so long have been associated with infection—fever, elevated WBC count, and organ dysfunction—are actually signs of the body's inflammatory response to infection rather than a direct result of the infecting organism. Disease processes that trigger the inflammatory cascade may be clinically indistinguishable from sepsis and have the same outcome. The inflammatory cascade accounts for the clinical picture associated with trauma, pancreatitis, burns, or other noninfectious insults. Recognition that the common factor in many life-threatening illnesses is uncontrolled inflammation has led to the design of treatment strategies aimed at modulation of the inflammatory response.

4. The inflammatory response is a normal reaction to infection. Should it not be encouraged?
Yes and no. Teleologically, the classic *tumor, calor, rubor,* and *dolor* response to infection can be viewed as the organism's attempt to keep an infection localized. When, however, the response is no longer under local control (as, for example, in a swollen finger), the systemic response may be more harmful than the inciting infection. The cascading inflammatory response leads to increased capillary permeability throughout the body, and diffuse endothelial injury leads to multiple organ dysfunction.

545

5. What treatments for SIRS have proven utility?

At this point, the commonly accepted treatments are aimed mainly at the underlying condition and supporting the organism through the stressful period. Treatment of the underlying condition involves finding and treating the source of infection or inflammation, drainage of abscess, debridement of necrotic tissue, and early fixation of fractures. Essential support of vital functions includes hemodynamic support with the goal of maintaining oxygen delivery, support at stress response levels, nutritional support, and support of failing organs with appropriate therapy, including ventilation, dialysis, and replacement of platelets and clotting factors.

6. Is the exact endpoint of hemodynamic support controversial?

Yes. Several studies have shown improved survival among patients with a hyperdynamic cardiovascular performance as demonstrated by an approximately 30% increase in cardiac index (CI), oxygen delivery index (DO_2I), oxygen consumption index (VO_2I), and left ventricular stroke work index (LVSWI). Some patients with adequate cardiac reserve achieve such performance values on their own, whereas others require augmentation with inotropes or vasodilators. There is no uniform agreement that adding hemodynamic support to "supranormal" values improves outcome from sepsis, but it appears likely that the ability to respond to metabolic stress, such as sepsis, with improved hemodynamic performance is beneficial. It is possible that, in an effort to achieve a hyperdynamic state, some patients may be harmed when their cardiovascular limit is exceeded. Clearly SIRS imposes metabolic stress, but we have no way of knowing for any individual exactly what the ideal level of oxygen consumption should be; therefore, we do not know how much support is required to meet the demand.

7. What is the significance of lactic acidosis in patients with septic shock?

Experts debate how far the clinician should go to support the circulation and the specific endpoints of therapy, but in the setting of septic shock they generally agree that lactic acidosis indicates inadequate perfusion until proved otherwise. Cardiac index, DO_2I, and VO_2I should be followed and therapy directed at restoring cellular oxygen metabolism.

8. How should patients with septic shock be resuscitated?

Adequate perfusion must be restored promptly. The initial response should be fluid resuscitation, because sepsis results in increased capillary leak and increased fluid requirements. In the most severe cases or in patients at highest risk for organ damage, a pulmonary artery (PA) catheter is useful to guide therapy. The pressure recorded at the distal port of the catheter with the PA occluded (PAOP), sometimes referred to as the wedge pressure, is used as an approximation of left ventricular preload. Fluid is given until signs of shock are reversed, up to a PAOP of approximately 18–20 cm H_2O. If at that point the patient is still hypotensive or oliguric or still has altered mental status, hemodynamic parameters are measured and treatment with vasoactive infusions is begun.

9. How does one decide which vasoactive drug to use?

The choice is tempered by the situation. If the MAP is greater than 60 mmHg with a PAOP greater than 18 cm H_2O, but the CI, DO_2I, or VO_2I is low, an inotrope such as dobutamine is warranted. If the MAP is low, dopamine is useful because of its greater pressor effect. When shock is most severe, pressor and inotropic support with a norepinephrine (Levophed) infusion is indicated. When MAP and PAOP indicate adequate filling but systemic vascular resistance (SVR) is increased, the cautious use of a vasodilator may be appropriate. Most commonly, patients in septic shock have low SVR; thus the use of vasodilators is unusual.

10. Does the use of norepinephrine presage progressive deterioration?

When the rate of infusion of norepinephrine is titrated to a desired pressure, the usual result is administration of increasing amounts of drug while perfusion diminishes and vasoconstriction predominates. When, however, the goal is to maximize perfusion rather than pressure, CI and

DO_2I are monitored and maintained; with this approach, norepinephrine is a valuable aid to resuscitation.

11. What are the specific recommendations for anesthetic management in patients in septic shock?

Obviously, no elective operations are performed with a patient in septic shock, and surgery most often is related to the shock itself. Drainage of abscess, debridement of necrotic tissue, and diagnostic biopsies are often performed in hemodynamically unstable patients. In general, the anesthetic period amounts to a continuation of the resuscitation, with maintenance of perfusion a priority. The use of circulatory depressants and vasodilators should be minimized, and the use of vasoactive infusions may well be necessary intraoperatively.

12. Are steroids useful in septic shock?

Septic shock has been described as "autodigestive inflammation"; thus it is easy to understand why treatment with corticosteroids, as general antiinflammatory agents, was attempted. Although animal studies showed improved survival with steroid treatment in sepsis, several large, multicenter randomized human trials have shown no overall benefit; moreover, the mortality rate in the subset of patients with renal insufficiency was increased.

13. What is the role of monoclonal antibodies directed against proinflammatory mediators?

Many different innovative treatments have been developed in an effort to interrupt the inflammatory cycle. Monoclonal murine and human antibodies to bacterial endotoxin have been studied extensively, and although animal and early human trials generated tremendous excitement, randomized outcome trials have failed to justify clinical use. Unfortunately, the same experience has been reported for other agents, such as monoclonal antibodies to tumor necrosis factor (TNF), a soluble TNF receptor that in essence inactivates TNF, and a bioengineered receptor antagonist for interleukin-1.

14. What are the prospects for future pharmacotherapy in SIRS?

Recent research into new medical treatments for SIRS has been discouraging. Nonetheless, amazing new technologies have been developed, and much has been learned about the control of the inflammatory system. Activation of the many cytokines, the complement system, the cyclo-oxygenase pathway (which results in the generation of thromboxanes), and the many other pathways involved in the inflammatory response is a complicated and interdigitating system. Interference with one pathway is unlikely to control accelerated inflammation, and multiple treatments to block each step of the cascade, although theoretically possible, are likely to be prohibitively expensive and perhaps even harmful. Rather than trying to block each proinflammatory agent, future research may focus on attempts to stimulate the natural antiinflammatory mediators, such as interleukins 4, 8, 10 and 13, prostaglandin E_2, macrophage deactivation factor, and platelet-derived growth factor. As we learn more about the regulation and balance of the system, the likelihood of being able to modulate and control the inflammatory response should increase.

BIBLIOGRAPHY

1. Bone RC, Balk RA, Cerra FB, et al: Definitions for sepsis and organ failure and guidelines for the use of innovative therapies in sepsis. Chest 101:1644–1655,1992.
2. Eidelman LA, Sprung CL: Why have new effective therapies for sepsis not been developed? Crit Care Med 22:1330–1334, 1994.
3. Fisher CJ, Dhainau JFA, Opal SM, et al: Recombinant human interleukin 1 receptor antagonist in the treatment of patients with sepsis syndrome. JAMA 271:1836–1842, 1994.
4. Knaus WA, Sun X, Nystrum PE, et al: Evaluation of definitions for sepsis. Chest 101: 1656–1662, 1992.
5. Suffredini AF: Current prospects for the treatment of clinical sepsis. Crit Care Med 22:S12–S18, 1994.
6. Veterans Administration Systemic Sepsis Cooperative Study Group: Effect of high-dose glucocorticoid therapy on mortality in patients with clinical signs of systemic sepsis. N Engl J Med 317:653–665, 1987.
7. Ziegler, EJ, Fisher CJ, Sprung CL, et al:Treatment of Gram-negative bacteremia and septic shock with JA-1A human monoclinal antibody against endotoxin. N Engl J Med 324 :429–436, 1991.

XII. Miscellaneous Topics in Anesthesia

92. BIOETHICS AND THE CHANGING ROLE OF ANESTHESIOLOGISTS

Susan K. Palmer, M.D.

Anesthesiologists, like other physicians, may be concerned about the rapid evolution in social expectations of physicians. Changes have occurred in the perceptions of the proper role for physicians in maintaining health or preventing disability, in the value and reimbursement of their service, and in the assignment of blame for disappointing outcomes of medical care. Many physicians are concerned or angry about the rapid economic changes, the degradation in apparent respect for the medical profession, and bioethical developments that have altered medical practice in the U.S. How did bioethics develop without the understanding or approval of most members of the medical profession?

1. Define bioethics.
Ethics refers to values, to the rightness and wrongness of actions and motivations. Bioethics refers to the study of values in biologic sciences, medicine, and environmental matters. Humans of all cultures have a finely developed sense of shame when their choices are found to be bad rather than good. One feels disappointment after giving a wrong answer on a test of knowledge but shame and blameworthiness after choosing to lie or giving wrong information for personal benefit or advantage. The ability to feel and express shame and moral obligation is a universal trait among socially functioning humans and has led philosophers to believe that ethical behavior is an innate concern of all people. Ethical interactions among people require the recognition of each other's "thouness" or basic human worth. Treating each other with respect dictates that we should not force others into certain behaviors or actions. Ethics dictates that it is much better to convince or persuade (rather than coerce or force) others to adopt a certain point of view. Ethics, defined in this manner, poses special challenges to physicians.

2. Describe the special ethical dimensions of physician-patient relationships.
Relationships between physicians and patients are complicated by the fact that the two individuals are seldom equally situated. The patient is usually ill and needs advice or treatment from the physician, who is in possession of special knowledge and skills. The more knowledgeable party in a spoken, written, or understood contract is said in legal terms to have a fiduciary responsibility to the more vulnerable party. In ethical terms, physicians are obligated to put aside their own interests and to act for the benefit of their patients. This obligation forms the basis of a societal contract and perpetuates public trust in medical professionals. Physician behavior has been guided for centuries by the obligation to put patients' interests first. In addition, because physicians have had the privilege of gaining their skills at public expense (see below), they are obligated to fulfill extraordinary public responsibilities.

3. Are the ethics of physician-patient relationships the same as the ethics of business-customer relationships?
The recent and questionable assertion that medical professionals are "in business" much like the providers of commercial commodities is confusing to both doctors and patients. The ethics of

supplier-consumer relationships are quite different from the ethics of physician-patient relationships. It should be evident that *physicians have more than the usual obligation to provide a "safe product" and less than the usual freedom to charge whatever they can get.* Physicians' traditional ethics include the duty to serve and to respect others. The appearance of self-interest or economic gluttony on the part of physicians threatens to dismantle the traditional ethical dimensions of the doctor-patient relationship.

Perhaps physicians are more like public utilities than like unregulated commercial enterprises. Public utilities have a unique position: (1) they are protected from competition, (2) they provide a necessary service, and (3) their profits are closely monitored and suppressed by the people they serve. Most physicians find it difficult to view their services as analogous to public utilities. Physicians were trained to think and act independently, not to seek public approval for their services and fees.

Physicians may think that they paid for their own medical training and are therefore entitled to act like any business owner who has made a substantial investment to start a business. However, the monetary costs of training medical students and resident physicians remain largely a public expense. Programs such as Medicare and Medicaid have historically given teaching hospitals huge grants for the sole purpose of underwriting the costs of training students. In addition, there is no way to pay for the patients who allowed medical students to practice and learn medical skills on their bodies and minds because they believe that future medical care depends on such training. Graduate medical students fulfill their responsibilities in this mostly unspoken social contract by giving health care to future patients.

4. Do physicians have professional ethics that are no longer acceptable to American society at large?

Public respect for the medical profession has declined perhaps in part because of a perception that physicians have their own value system that is not in alignment with the best interests of the general public health. Has the morality of professional medicine in fact drifted so far from the morality of the general public? Have the moral understandings of the general public changed faster than those of the medical profession? To answer these questions, it is necessary to examine the ethics of professional medicine; it is necessary for physicians to reexamine the values and behaviors that they were taught during their medical training. Many of these values were taught in subtle ways and were not called "values" at the time. Nonetheless, when students are told how a "good" physician behaves, they are being instructed in the traditional ethics of the medical profession.

5. Is the Hippocratic oath still relevant?

Hippocrates' oath is often cited as a statement of professional medical ethics. It is important to reexamine this oath, which many medical school graduates recite. Hippocrates lived about 500 BC and was a member of a strict Pythagorean sect of healers who in modern times might be called ultraconservatives. The oath was not generally accepted even in its own period. Nevertheless, the oath contains descriptions of "good" physician behaviors that have profoundly influenced western medicine. Among the values expressed in the oath are selfless action for the patient's good, confidentiality about the patient's personal affairs and afflictions, refraining from criticizing other physicians, resisting temptation to engage in sexual activities with patients or members of their households, refusal to do surgery of any kind, refusal to give an abortifacient or suicidal remedy, and sharing the art of medicine only with the sons of other physicians. It should be obvious that modern physicians no longer subscribe to all of these values.

The most famous phrase of the oath is the often repeated: "First of all, do no harm." This dictate was enunciated at a time when physicians could do little good for patients. Physicians most often were called to give prognostic information or to provide pain relief. Because the therapies of the day provided little benefit, it made perfect sense to remind physicians at least not to make things worse. Modern physicians, however, "harm" patients in many ways (including surgery) in an attempt to achieve some long-term benefit requested by patients. They risk more harm because they and their patients believe that they can achieve more eventual good than the ancient Greeks could offer.

6. If physicians do not follow the Hippocratic oath, by what codes or values are they guided?

During the last 150 years professional medicine in the United States has had an interesting history and questionable ethical development. After medical education became standardized, professional codes functioned mostly to exclude practitioners who had not received the right education. Licensing battles were fought at the level of state governments, many of which at first refused to interfere with citizens' choices of medical practitioners. Eventually allopathic medicine emerged as the strongest guild and achieved recognition in the form of required state licensing of medical professionals. Special panels of allopathic physicians helped the states to decide who should receive or retain a license to practice medicine. The medical profession became responsible mostly to itself and its internal standards. Pride in the medical profession soared after World War II when penicillin was viewed as the first of the medical "magic bullets" that eventually would eliminate infectious disease. Medical professionals became increasingly more powerful and independent, and for the first time some physicians were becoming rich. In earlier times physicians seldom had more money or economic power than their patients.

Medicine has since received a series of "wake-up calls," suggesting that its actions reflected professional ethics that had wandered too far from traditional values of service and respect for patients. One such wake-up call was initiated by anesthesiologist Henry Beecher, Harvard Professor and Chair at Massachusetts General Hospital, who disparaged medical research projects that did not respect the interests or dignity of human subjects.[3] The history of medical research in the United States in the twentieth century includes many examples of research conducted on residents of mental institutions, orphanages, prisons, and poor Southern communities.[7] Beecher's courageous statement and other investigations by the press provided the impetus for the birth of modern bioethics.

The public was clearly concerned about a medical and scientific community that seemed responsible only to itself and not to the public. The President's Commission for the Study of Ethical Problems in Medicine and Biomedical and Behavioral Research[10] was purposely composed mostly of nonphysicians. Research was financed in large part by the public, which reasserted its power to direct the manner in which research would be conducted. The strict rules for subject consent and the review of research projects for ethical merit that resulted from the president's commission wounded the pride of the medical profession and for the first time limited its sense of autonomy in a meaningful way.

7. How can physicians preserve the best of traditional medical ethics and continue to develop their understanding of modern bioethics?

Rather than despair over professional medicine's past ethical failures, physicians should understand the development of bioethics and participate actively in its evolution. Philosophers, clergy, humanities specialists, and legal experts have made contributions to the development of bioethics. As in any complex area of study and research, no one has "found the answers"; the major focus is to ask the important questions. Anesthesiologists who do not understand or fail to become involved in the process of developing bioethics as they apply to anesthesiology may well become dissatisfied with changes in their professional obligations and responsibilities. Ethical problems that particularly affect anesthesiologists are discussed below.

8. What is the status of "Do Not Resuscitate" (DNR) orders for surgical patients?

Patients have the right to refuse any medical treatment. This principle of self-rule was encoded into law in 1914 by Justice Cardoza: "Every human being of adult years and sound mind has the right to determine what shall be done with their own body." Physicians find it difficult to understand why a patient would seek their advice about medical care and then refuse to follow it. However, the right to refuse any treatment, resuscitation, or food and water is a robust legal principle.

Anesthesiologists often resuscitate patients who have temporary reactions to anesthetics. It seems intrusive and illogical for patients to dictate that they cannot do a normal part of their job. However, the American Society of Anesthesiologists (ASA) has adopted "Ethical Guidelines for the Anesthesia Care of Patients with Do-Not-Resuscitate Orders or Other Directives that Limit

Treatment" (see appendix). This document, which is intended to provide ethical guidance for the reconsideration of DNR orders before the procedure is performed, emphasizes that the decision to retain or temporarily suspend DNR orders should be made by the patient in consultation with the surgeon and anesthesiologist. Other care givers, such as operating room nurses, also must be included or at least agree to honor the decision.

9. Why should patients dictate so much of their medical and surgical care?

Patients are becoming more insistent in their requests for certain types of surgical care and special techniques of anesthesia. The meaning of illness, pain, and suffering and the value assigned to their treatment or nontreatment can be determined only by the person experiencing them. Physicians are obligated to serve patients in a beneficial way, but what constitutes a benefit must be defined by the patient. This concept is difficult for physicians to understand, because medical school training emphasizes the medical response to particular disease states rather than the psychosocial response to individual patients who have a disease.

Anesthesiologists, like all other physicians, must adapt to the changing expectations and requests of their patients. However, physicians are not required to give up their own moral agency or to offer or provide types of care outside standard medical therapies. If a patient requests an anesthetic for amputation of a normal body part, physicians are not obligated to comply and in fact may be accused of unethical practice if they do. However, some physicians certainly respond to requests for alterations of normal body parts, and within current societal bounds this practice is an acceptable way to "benefit" patients. What would Hippocrates have thought of plastic surgery for normally aging faces?

10. Discuss euthanasia and the role of the physician.

Euthanasia is derived from the Greek words meaning a "good death." Greek and many other cultures valued the achievement of a good and proper end to life. Many now advocate that competent patients should be able to request their physician to provide the means and initiate the cause of their death. In Holland, under strict conditions, patients are allowed to request this service from their personal physicians. Although still illegal, the practice is tolerated when strict guidelines are followed and the physician immediately reports the act for legal review.

Rational suicide remains acceptable in many cultures. Passive physician-assisted suicide refers to physicians who assist patients with their efforts to achieve a good death. Physicians may be asked to provide the medication or the means for a patient to commit suicide, but their role is passive because they do not not initiate the suicide.

Physicians traditionally have been trained only in the preservation or prolongation of life. However, it is clear to the public that life can be prolonged in a sophisticated hospital setting far beyond the limits of the patient's ability to recover or the family's ability to suffer at the bedside. Patients seem to be calling for more control over the dying process and may be more able to accept death as a natural process than are physicians.[5]

Regardless of their current opinions about physician-assisted suicide and passive or active euthanasia, anesthesiologists need to be concerned about the public debate. They need to ask why patients ask for assisted euthanasia. Anesthesiologists already have been nominated as society's "thanatologists," because they know so much about drugs that easily induce death. If anesthesiologists do not want this role, they must enter discussions about the control of chronic or terminal suffering and recognize that the debate about assisted suicide and euthanasia is just another aspect of the debate about the role of physicians in society. Patients are demanding more control of medical decisions that affect their lives.

11. Discuss the four major principles of bioethics.

To encourage anesthesiologists to begin or continue the study of bioethics, the following glossary defines common bioethical terms as they apply to physicians. As physicians reexamine the values that direct their practice, their understanding of bioethical issues will deepen appreciation of their role as a physician. Bioethics has developed short-hand terms or principles to which one can refer during discussions of ethical dilemmas. The four principles that often are used in teaching bioethics are respect for autonomy, justice, beneficence, and nonmaleficence.[2] *A true ethical dilemma occurs when any course of action will violate at least one principle.* Because the principles have no innate priority, there is no logical way to decide which principle should prevail and which should be compromised in a given situation.

1. **Respect for autonomy.** One of the most valued characteristics of humans is their ability to develop, express, and pursue their own wishes and life plans. The personal autonomy and freedom of patients should be respected, preserved, or recovered, if possible. A physician's duty can be viewed as respecting patients and helping them to retain or recover autonomy.

2. **Justice.** This term is used by many to indicate some kind of "fairness." In general, justice means that the benefits and burdens of providing access to health care should be distributed as equally as possible. For more exhaustive exploration of the meaning of justice, the reader is referred to the following:

John Rawls, *A Theory of Justice*[8]

Rawls proposes that inequities can be justified only if they benefit the least advantaged class of society. He also proposes that if a system is truly just, anyone should be satisfied as a member of the least advantaged class.

Robert Nozick, *Anarchy, State, and Utopia*[6]

Nozick believes that inequities in the distribution of wealth can be earned. The history of how wealth was obtained is important in determining its justness.

Emmanuel Kant, *Ethical Philosophy*[4]

Kant emphasizes that if everyone acts morally, justice is always served. He proposes that in difficult situations one should apply the test of "universalizability," which involves asking, "Would I be willing for everyone to act the way I plan to act for the same reasons which guide my actions?"

3. **Beneficence.** This principle can be understood as physicians' duty to work for the good of their patients.

4. **Nonmaleficence.** This principle requires that physicians avoid doing evil directly or allowing evil to befall their patients by lack of action.

12. Discuss systems used for the ethical analysis of medical cases.

1. **Narrative or casuistic approach.** This method of discussing ethical dilemmas involves detailed case analysis and uses paradigm cases as referents. Advocates believe that "the truth is in the details." This approach builds an ethical case library by increments, much like the common law legal system. Minute differences may lead to different morally acceptable actions in cases that at first seem identical.

2. **Consequentialism.** This term applies to the philosophical position that a "good act" results in the greatest sum of positive results. The "end justifies the means" is a common description of this philosophy in its simple form.

3. **Ethics of care.** This approach to medical ethical dilemmas, which values caring human relationships as central to health and living, has been well developed in the literature of the nursing profession. It has been suggested that medicine has distanced itself unwisely from the position of "caring" for patients by becoming too concerned about prescribing technology.

4. **Virtue ethics.** This ancient Aristotelian philosophical view[1] values the development and training of the "virtuous" physician. Such physicians can then be depended on to act morally. The ancient virtues included temperance, humility, generosity, and justice.

13. What is the principle of "double effect"?

The principle of "double effect," which was developed primarily in the Roman Catholic tradition, states that if a physician's intention with a good action is to do "good," even an evil result imposes no moral responsibility. This principle is invoked to defend physicians when they "intend" to relieve suffering by administering a narcotic, a morally acceptable or good action, that has the secondary effect of depressing respiration and possibly hastening death.

APPENDIX

ETHICAL GUIDELINES FOR THE ANESTHESIA CARE OF PATIENTS WITH DO-NOT-RESUSCITATE ORDERS OR OTHER DIRECTIVES THAT LIMIT TREATMENT

(Approved by House of Delegates on October 13, 1993)

These guidelines apply to competent patients and also to incompetent patients who have previously expressed their preferences.

I. Given the diversity of published opinions and cultures within our society, an essential element of preoperative preparation and perioperative care for patients with Do-Not-Resuscitate (DNR) orders or other directives that limit treatment is communication among involved parties. It is necessary to document relevant aspects of this communication.

II. Policies automatically suspending DNR orders or other directives that limit treatment prior to procedures involving anesthetic care may not sufficiently address a patient's rights to self-determination in a responsible and ethical manner. Such policies, if they exist, should be reviewed and revised, as necessary, to reflect the content of these guidelines.

III. Prior to procedures requiring anesthetic care, any changes in existing directives that limit treatment should be documented in the medical record. These include absolute injunctions as desired by the patient (or the patient's legal representative). When appropriate, the items that should be considered are:

A. Blood product transfusion
B. Tracheal intubation or instrumentation
C. Chest compressions and direct cardiac massage
D. Defibrillation
E. Cardiac pacing, internal or external
F. Invasive monitoring
G. Postoperative ventilatory support
H. Vasoactive drug administration

IV. When relevant, the anesthesiologist should describe and discuss the appropriate use of therapeutic modalities to correct deviations of hemodynamic and respiratory variables predictably resulting from anesthetic agents and techniques.

V. Additional issues that may be relevant to discuss are perioperative placement of naso/orogastric tubes or urinary catheters, administration of antibiotics, establishment of intravenous access, maintenance of intravascular volume with non-blood products and treatment with supplemental oxygen.

VI. It is important to discuss and document whether there are to be any exceptions to the injunction(s) against intervention should there occur a specific recognized complication of the surgery or anesthesia.

VII. Concurrence on these issues by the primary physician (if not the surgeon of record), the surgeon and the anesthesiologist is desirable. If possible, these physicians should meet together with the patient (or the patient's legal representative) when these issues are discussed. This duty of the patient's physicians is deemed to be of such importance that it should not be delegated. Other members of the health care team who are (or will be) directly involved with the patient's care during the planned procedure should, if feasible, be included in this process.

VIII. Should conflicts arise, the following resolution processes are recommended:

A. When an anesthesiologist finds the patient's or surgeon's limitations of intervention decisions to be irreconcilable with one's own moral views, then the anesthesiologist should withdraw in a nonjudgmental fashion, providing an alternative for care in a timely fashion.

B. When an anesthesiologist finds the patient's or surgeon's limitation of intervention decisions to be in conflict with generally accepted standards of care, ethical practice or institutional policies, then the anesthesiologist should voice such concerns and present the situation to the appropriate institutional body.

C. If these alternatives are not feasible within the time frame necessary to prevent further morbidity or suffering, then in accordance with the American Medical Association's Principles of Medical Ethics, care should proceed with reasonable adherence to the patient's directives, being mindful of the patient's goals and values.

IX. A representative from the hospital's anesthesiology service should establish a liaison with surgical and nursing services for presentation, discussion and procedural application of these guidelines. Hospital staff should be made aware of the proceedings of these discussions and the motivations for them.

X. Modification of these guidelines may be appropriate when they conflict with local standards or policies, and in those emergency situations involving incompetent patients whose intentions have not been previously expressed.

Reprinted with permission of the American Society of Anesthesiologists. A copy of the complete text can be obtained from ASA, 520 N. Northwest Highway, Park Ridge, IL 60068-2573.

BIBLIOGRAPHY

1. Aristotle's Nichomachean Ethics, translated by Terence Irwin, Indianapolis, IN, Hackett Publishing Co, 1985.
2. Beauchamp TL, Walters L (eds): Contemporary Issues in Bioethics, 4th ed. Belmont, CA, Wadsworth Publishing, 1994.
3. Beecher H: Ethics and clinical research. N Engl J Med 274:1354–1360, 1966.
4. Kant E: Ethical Philosophy. Ellington J (ed). Indianapolis, IN, Hackett Publishing Co, 1983.
5. McCue JD: The naturalness of dying. JAMA 273:1039–1043, 1995.
6. Nozick R: Anarchy, State, and Utopia. New York, Basic Books, 1974.
7. Pence G: Classic Cases in Medical Ethics. New York, McGraw-Hill Publishing Co, 1990.
8. Rawls J A: Theory of Justice. Cambridge, MA, Harvard University Press, 1971.
9. Starr P: The Transformation of American Medicine. New York, Basic Books, 1982.
10. Summing Up: Final report on studies of the ethical and legal problems in medicine and biomedical and behavioral research. Washington D.C., U.S. Government Publishing Office, 1982.

93. STATISTICS AND CRITICAL ANALYSIS OF LITERATURE

Charles A. Tinnell, R.N., M.S.P.H.

1. Many studies report a "significant p-value." What does this mean?

The p-value is a measure of the likelihood that a given result is due to chance; p-values are usually given in regard to a statistical test between two or more groups in a study. The p-value is interpreted as the probability that one will wrongly conclude that there is a true difference between study groups when in fact no difference exists. This type of error is otherwise known as false-positive (or type I) error. The probability of false-positive error is also known as α (alpha).

For example, in a hypothetical study of blood pressure responses to an anesthetic agent, 25 previously normotensive patients were administered agent A (group A) and 25 previously normotensive patients did not receive agent A in their regimen (group B). Systolic blood pressures were measured, and an average difference between pre- and postadministration values was obtained for each group. A statistical test was performed to compare the average difference in group A with the average difference in group B; the two values were found to be different at a p-value of less than 0.001 (p < 0.001). Interpretation: the probability that the observed difference between groups A and B is due to chance is less than 0.001 (1 in a 1000).

2. Who determines what is "significant"?

By convention, p-values less than 0.05 (5% or 1 in 20) are termed "significant," although the investigator may establish the significance level wherever he or she wishes. For example, to lessen the likelihood of reporting a chance result, the significance level could be set at 0.01.

3. Does a significant p-value mean that the result is definitely due to the intervention?

Because the p-value in the example in question 1 is below 0.05, the difference is assumed to be due to the effect of the anesthetic agent. However, a word of caution is warranted: a "significant" p-value means only that the likelihood of a chance result was very low; it does not rule out the possibility. Moreover, it does not rule out the possibility that some other factor (either real or an artifact of study design) caused the result.

4. How should I interpret a "nonsignificant" p-value?

It is harder to interpret a nonsignificant p-value than it may seem. Strictly speaking, the result is nonsignificant when the p-value obtained from a statistical test fails to reach the desired level of significance (usually 0.05). However, the difficulty with interpretation comes from determining whether the nonsignificant result is due to lack of a true difference or the inability to detect a true difference, i.e., problems with study design.

This type of decision error, in which the investigator thinks that he or she has not found an effect when in fact it exists, is a false-negative (type II) error. The probability of a false-negative error is also known as ß (beta). The most common study design problem that leads to a false-negative error is insufficient sample size; other problems include bias or confounding.

5. What is statistical power?

Statistical power is the ability to detect an effect when one is present. The probability of a false-negative error is ß, and the power of a test is 1 – ß. Power of 80% is a rule of thumb for detection of a reasonable effect, but because power calculations are essentially approximate, too much emphasis should not be placed on a certain number.

6. What is a normal distribution?

A normal distribution is a statistical term for the tendency of repeated measurements to cluster in a bell-shaped curve around the mean. This property is the basis of most statistical testing, especially tests involving means and proportions. The shape of a normal curve is influenced by the variability in the measurements. High variability (large standard deviation) widens the curve, whereas low variation squeezes the curve.

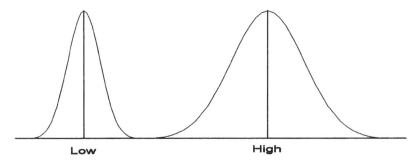

Two normal distributions: low variability and high variability.

7 What are the common "red flags" that may indicate poor study design or faulty conclusions?

Insufficient data	Many confounders	Unexplained analysis
Lone significance	Ambiguous denominators	Large samples
Unsupported conclusions	Bias	Improper generalizations
Clinical irrelevance	Uncited numbers	Lack of comparison groups
Small samples	Inappropriate tests	Lack of objectivity

The interpretation of clinical literature requires attention to study design and analysis issues as well as to biologic and clinical issues. Ideally, the article should present an objective, clear, and well-supported argument for the conclusions. In general, sufficient data should be reported to allow the reader to compute the relevant outcome measures. Often data contained in tables or graphs are sufficient for this purpose. In addition, reports of results from other studies should be properly cited.

Similarly, all conclusions should be supported with appropriate statistical tests, and the statistical tests must be appropriate for the type of outcome variable. For example, variables that are ordinal (i.e., ordered categories) should not be treated like continuous variables (variables such as temperature or blood pressure). Means can be computed on continuous variables, but it is generally invalid to compute means on ordinal variables.

A subtle problem is the lone significant result among many statistical tests. Performing many statistical tests on data is known as "fishing"—hoping to find something significant—and raises the likelihood that some tests will be significant by chance. The statistical methodology should be explained sufficiently to allow readers to replicate the process. Failure to explain the rationale or calculation of the most important outcome measure makes it difficult to determine whether the methodology was appropriate.

Very large or very small samples may affect the conclusions. Studies with very large samples may find significance in small effects. Although some small effects may be clinically relevant, other statistically significant results may be clinically insignificant or irrelevant. The problem of clinical significance vs. statistical significance may occur with any size study. However, small samples may lack the statistical power to detect an effect that is truly present.

Studies also may lack external or internal validity. Unless the study subjects have been properly sampled to be representative of the population as a whole, results cannot be generalized to the whole population (lack of external validity). Measurement imprecision, bias, confounding, improper analysis, and many other factors may render a study invalid for conclusions about the particular sample (lack of internal validity). Inferences about the relative worth of an intervention or etiology should be made in comparison with a suitable control or reference group. Similarly, in comparison of rates and proportions, the denominator should be clearly specified and valid for the comparison.

Because most disease is multifactorial, confounding variables (factors that obscure a relationship) make it hard to determine whether the effect was due to the study variable or the confounding variable. In addition, systematic factors (bias) may have distorted the results or made the study invalid.

8. What is bias?

Bias is a general term that indicates systematic factors that distort the ability to detect an effect. Bias may lead to a larger or smaller apparent effect, although bias tends to result in smaller effects. Bias is of two general types: selection and information. Selection bias refers to distortion of the study result that is due to case selection, whereas information bias refers to systematic differences in the way in which data are obtained for the study groups. Many specific subtypes of these two general types have been identified.[7]

9. What is confounding?

Confounding is the presence in a study of one or more variables that may obscure the true relationship between the study variable and the outcome. A confounding variable must be related to the study variable but also stand as an independent predictor of outcome. Confounding can be controlled in the design phase of a study and in the analysis phase.

10. What are the types of study designs?

In general, studies are experimental or observational. Observational studies may be retrospective (occurring in the past) or prospective (looking forward). An epidemiologist, statistician, or experienced researcher should be consulted to determine the appropriate design.

Experimental studies

• *Clinical trial.* Persons are assigned into study groups. Persons with the intervention are in one group, and persons without the intervention are in another group. Randomization, blinding (investigators and/or providers do not know to which group the person belongs), and complete follow-up are keys to cause-and-effect determination. Many variations in design and analysis are available for clinical trials.

Observational studies

• *Descriptive and cross-sectional studies, case reports.* The experience of a group is described. The group may be defined by personal attributes (e.g., disease, symptom, physical characteristic, cultural group), geographic attributes (from a particular community, region, or country), or temporal attributes (long-term disease or condition, short-term, epidemic). No formal comparisons are made.

• *Case-control study.* Persons with a particular outcome are found (cases) and compared with persons without the outcome (controls). Case-control studies are particularly susceptible to selection bias but are often quick and cost-effective.

• *Follow-up and cohort studies.* Persons with and without an exposure of interest are indentified and followed to ascertain outcomes. Such studies may suggest cause-and-effect but are usually expensive to perform.

• *Screening and test evaluation.* The effectiveness of diagnostic or prognostic tests is assessed. Diagnostic studies predict the presence of disease, whereas prognostic studies predict the outcome of disease. Such studies evaluate the sensitivity and specificity of tests or screening procedures.

11. What are the criteria for determining whether a cause-and-effect relationship exists?

1. Strength of association between the putative causative variable and the effect
2. Biologic plausibility

3. Consistency of association demonstrated over several studies
4. Temporal relationship: the cause precedes the effect
5. Dose-response: there is a gradient of effect as a function of cause

In general, only experimental studies can determine cause-and-effect, because observational studies do not allow manipulation of conditions. However, well-designed case-control or follow-up studies can provide strong circumstantial evidence for cause-and-effect relationships.

12. How large should the study sample be?

Sample size should be calculated during the planning of the study to determine adequate or minimal number of subjects. If the study has a fixed number of subjects, a power calculation should be done to determine the likelihood of detecting the desired effect. If adequate sample size or power is not considered, it may be too late to modify the design after the study starts, and there may be no way to compensate for low power during analysis. Power calculations should be done whenever nonsignificant results are obtained. The minimal sample size for a study is usually found by consulting the appropriate table, performing calculations by hand, or using computer software.

13. What are the major factors to consider in planning the sample size?

Planning of sample size is based on several factors. Greater variability (standard deviation or variance) in measurements leads to the need for larger numbers. In addition, the magnitude of the relative or absolute effect that the study attempts to detect inversely affects sample size. The larger the effect, the smaller the number of subjects needed to detect it. Previous studies, expertise, educated guess, or a pilot study can be used to estimate the effect size. A study with a smaller likelihood of false-positive error (i.e., a significance level of 0.01 instead of 0.05) requires larger numbers. Similarly, greater statistical power means more subjects. Sample size should account for subjects who are likely to drop out of the study. If this number is not excluded from sample size calculations, too few cases may remain at the end of the study to detect an effect. Furthermore, creating subgroups (stratifying) of subjects (e.g., by age, gender) increases sample size requirements, because each stratum must have sufficient numbers for valid comparisons. The presence of other variables that may confound (obscure) the true relationship may require a larger sample size. As a rough guide, an extra 10% should be added to sample size for each confounder that is known to be strongly related to the predictor or outcome variables. Although potentially important, this guideline is rarely done in practice.

Effects of Various Factors on Sample Size Requirements

FACTOR	EFFECT ON SAMPLE SIZE
Greater variability in measurements	↑
Larger effect size	↓
Smaller level of false-positive error	↑
Greater statistical power	↓
Losses or drop-outs	↑
Subgroups	↑
Confounding	↑

14. What can be done to improve the statistical power of a study?

1. Increase the number of subjects or amount of follow-up per subject or use multiple measurements per subject.
2. Look for a larger effect or increase the contrast between study groups.
3. Increase data precision, i.e., reduce variability (variance).
4. Make a technical adjustment to allow more false-positive (type I) error.

15. How does one decide which statistical test is appropriate?

Generally, the type of outcome measure dictates the methodology. There are three general types of measurements:

1. **Continuous (interval) measurements** involve constant interval between values. All mathematical operations are valid. Blood pressure and temperature are examples. Continuous data can be categorized (e.g., age grouping), but categorization may result in loss of statistical power. Statistical tests for continuous data include the following:

T-Test—compares means of 2 groups.

Paired T-Test—compares 2 measurements for each member of a group.

Analysis of Variance (ANOVA)—compares means of 2 or more groups.

Repeated-Measures ANOVA—compares multiple measurements from each member of a group.

Regression/Correlation—determines the association between 2 or more variables; some regression methods can be used for dichotomous (2 category) variables.

2. **Ordinal measurements**. Values are ordered without a constant interval between them. Mathematical operations (such as averaging) are generally not valid. Statistical analysis is generally the same as with categorical data. The patient classification of the American Society of Anesthesiologists is an example.

3. **Categorical (nominal) measurements**. Values are grouped in categories and named. Mathematical operations are not valid. Statistical analysis is generally the same as with ordinal data. Gender (male, female) is an example. Statistical tests for ordinal and categorical data include the following:

Chi Square—determines significance based on counts in a table.

Z Test—compares proportions.

Mantel-Haenszel—compares multiple 2 x 2 tables.

Odds Ratio/Relative Risk—determines relative strength of association between 2 proportions.

Mann-Whitney Test—compares 2 groups.

Kruskal-Wallis Test—compares 3 or more groups.

Spearman's Rank Correlation—evaluates association between 2 variables.

16. Define confidence intervals.

Confidence intervals give an indication of the precision of measurement. A large confidence interval indicates high variability. Confidence intervals are specified by giving a lower and upper bound and depend on significance level and variability of the measurement. Confidence intervals are interpreted as follows: if repeated experiments were held, there is a 95% chance that the true value of the measurement would fall within the confidence interval. Confidence intervals must not be confused with the width (usually on a graph) of the mean ± 1 standard deviation; they are not the same.

17. Define survival analysis.

Survival analysis is used to evaluate the time from entry in a study to an outcome. A graph (the survival curve) is used to show how the probability of survival changes over time. Various methodologies are available for situations in which patients are involved in the study for unequal times (e.g., not all patients enter the study at the same time, or some drop-out before the outcome occurs).

18. What is meant by "one-tailed" and "two-tailed" tests? How does one know which to use?

One- and two-tailed tests refer to the distribution of the false-positive (type I) error probabilities. In a one-tailed test, all of the false-positive error is assumed to be at one end ("tail") of the distribution. In a two-tailed test, the false-positive error is divided over both tails of the distribution. In one-tailed tests, the statistical procedure is based on the assumption that the measurement effect is either greater or less than the same effect in the baseline comparison group. In two-tailed tests, the effect measure may be greater or less than the baseline—and the analysis must account for both.

For example, in the hypothetical blood pressure study in question 1, if one knows that the effect of the agent is always to lower blood pressure, then statistical analysis of group differences can be done using a one-tailed test. If one is not sure whether the agent will raise or lower blood pressure, the analysis should be done as a two-tailed test. The direction of the effect determines whether the test is one-tailed or two-tailed.

19. Define sensitivity and specificity.

Sensitivity is the proportion of persons with the disease who test positive for the disease. Specificity is the proportion of persons without the disease who test negative for the disease The table of results used to calculate sensitivity and specificity is given below. The letters in the cells refer to counts, i.e., "a" is the number of persons who test positive and have the disease.

Sensitivity and Specificity

	DISEASE POSITIVE	DISEASE NEGATIVE
Test positive	a	b
Test negative	c	d

Calculations

Sensitivity = $a / (a + c)$
   False-negative rate = $1 -$ sensitivity = $c / (a + c)$
Specificity = $d / (b + d)$
   False-positive rate = $1 -$ specificity = $b / (b + d)$
Positive predictive value (PV+) = $a / (a + b)$
Negative predictive value (PV-) = $d / (c + d)$

The graphic relationship of false positives (1 - specificity) to true positives (sensitivity) is called a receiver–operating characteristic (ROC) curve.

BIBLIOGRAPHY

1. Freiman JA, Chalmers TC, Smith H Jr, Keubler RR: The importance of beta, the type II error and sample size in the design and interpretation of the randomized control trial: Survey of 71 'negative' trials. N Engl J Med 299:690–694, 1978.
2. Friedman GD: Primer of Epidemiology, 4th ed. New York, McGraw-Hill, 1994.
3. Glantz SA: Primer of Biostatistics. New York, McGraw-Hill, 1992.
4. Hennekens CH, Buring JE: Epidemiology in Medicine. Boston, Little, Brown, 1987.
5. Hulley SB, Cumming SR: Designing Clinical Research. Baltimore, William & Wilkins, 1988.
6. Norman GR, Streiner DL: PDQ Statistics. Toronto, B C Decker, 1986.
7. Sackett DL: Bias in analytic research. J Chron Dis [now J Clin Epidemiol] 32:51–63, 1979.

INDEX

Page numbers in **boldface type** indicate complete chapters.